D1189743

THE QUINOLONES

Third Edition

To my family
who have supported and
encouraged me always
and in everything.

To my colleague, Susan Marino,
who has assisted me in
all professional activities.

THE
QUINOLONES

Third Edition

Edited by

VINCENT T. ANDRIOLE
Yale University School of Medicine

ACADEMIC PRESS

San Diego   London   Boston   New York   Sydney   Tokyo   Toronto

Academic Press
a Harcourt Science and Technology Company
525 B Street, Suite 1900, San Diego, California 92101-4495

http://www.academicpress.com

Academic Press Limited
Harcourt Place, 32 Jamestown Road, London NW1 7BY, UK

Library of Congress Catalog Card Number: 00-106606

International Standard Book Number: 0-12-059517-6

PRINTED IN UNITED STATES OF AMERICA
01   02   03   04   05   SB   9   8   7   6   5   4   3

CONTENTS

4 Bacterial Resistance to Quinolones: Mechanisms and Clinical Implications

Thilo Köhler and Jean-Claude Pechère

5 Pharmacokinetics and Pharmacodynamics of the Fluoroquinolones

Myo-Kyoung Kim and Charles H. Nightingale

6   Use of Quinolones in Urinary Tract Infection and Prostatitis

Lindsay E. Nicolle

7   Use of the Quinolones in Sexually Transmitted Diseases

Richard P. DiCarlo and David H. Martin

8   Treatment of Respiratory Infections with Quinolones

Paul B. Iannini, Michael S. Niederman, and Vincent T. Andriole

9   Use of Quinolones in Surgery and Obstetrics and Gynecology

John Weigelt, Karen Brasel, and Sebastian Faro

13 Use of the Quinolones in Skin and Skin Structure (Osteomyelitis) and Other Infections

Adolf W. Karchmer

14 Safety Overview: Toxicity, Adverse Effects, and Drug Interactions

Ralf Stahlmann and Hartmut Lode

15 Use of the Quinolones in Pediatrics

Urs B. Schaad

16 The Quinolones: Prospects

Vincent T. Andriole

CONTRIBUTORS

Numbers in parentheses indicate the pages on which the author's contribution begin.

VINCENT T. ANDRIOLE (255, 477), Yale University School of Medicine, New Haven, Connecticut 06520-8022

PETER BALL (1), School of Biomedical Sciences, University of St. Andrews, St. Andrews, Fife KY16 9AL, Scotland, United Kingdom

KAREN BRASEL (285), Department of Surgery, Medical College of Wisconsin, Milwaukee, Wisconsin 53226

KATHERINE E. BRIGHTY (33), Department of Medicinal Chemistry, Central Research Division, Pfizer Inc., Groton, Connecticut 06340

RICHARD P. DiCARLO (227), Department of Medicine, Louisiana State University School of Medicine, New Orleans, Louisiana 70112

SEBASTIAN FARO (285), Department of Obstetrics and Gynecology, Rush Medical College, Rush Presbyterian and St. Luke's Medical Center, Rush University, Chicago, Illinois 60612

THOMAS D. GOOTZ (33), Department of Respiratory, Allergy, Immunology, Inflammation, and Infectious Diseases, Central Research Division, Pfizer Inc., Groton, Connecticut 06340

SHERWOOD L. GORBACH (303), Department of Community Health, Tufts University School of Medicine, Boston, Massachusetts 02111

DAVIDSON H. HAMER (303), Division of Geographic Medicine and Infectious Diseases, Department of Medicine, New England Medical Center, Boston, Massachusetts 02111

RODRIGO HASBUN (325), Tulane University School of Medicine, Section of Infectious Diseases, New Orleans, Louisiana 70118

PAUL B. IANNINI (255), Department of Medicine, Danbury Hospital, Danbury, Connecticut 06810, and Yale University School of Medicine, New Haven, Connecticut 06520

ADOLF W. KARCHMER (371), Division of Infectious Diseases, Beth Israel Deaconess Medical Center, and Harvard Medical School, Boston, Massachusetts 02215

MYO-KYOUNG KIM (169), Department of Pharmacy and Division of Infectious Disease, Hartford Hospital, Hartford, Connecticut 06102-5037

ANNA KING (99), Department of Microbiology, United Medical and Dental School of Guy's and St. Thomas' Hospitals, St. Thomas' Hospital, London SE1 7EH, United Kingdom

THILO KÖHLER (139), Department of Genetics and Microbiology, University of Geneva, 1211 Geneva, Switzerland

HARTMUT LODE (397), Department of Chest and Infectious Diseases, Hospital Zehlendorf, Heckeshorn Lung Clinic, 14109 Berlin, Germany

DAVID H. MARTIN (227), Department of Medicine, Louisiana State University School of Medicine, New Orleans, Louisiana 70112

LINDSAY E. NICOLLE (203), Department of Internal Medicine, University of Manitoba, Winnipeg, Manitoba, R3A 1R9, Canada

MICHAEL S. NIEDERMAN (255), Division of Pulmonary and Critical Care Medicine, Winthrop-University Hospital, Mineola, New York 11501, and Department of Medicine, State University of New York at Stony Brook, Stony Brook, New York 11794

CHARLES H. NIGHTINGALE (169), Office of Research Administration, Hartford Hospital, Hartford, Connecticut 06102-5037

JEAN-CLAUDE PECHÈRE (139), Department of Genetics and Microbiology, University of Geneva, 1211 Geneva, Switzerland

IAN PHILLIPS (99), Department of Microbiology, United Medical and Dental School of Guy's and St. Thomas' Hospitals, St. Thomas' Hospital, London SE1 7EH, United Kingdom

VINCENT J. QUAGLIARELLO (325), Section of Infectious Diseases, Department of Internal Medicine, Yale University School of Medicine, New Haven, Connecticut 06520-8022

KENNETH V. I. ROLSTON (343), Department of Medical Specialties, Section of Infectious Diseases, The University of Texas, M. D. Anderson Cancer Center, Houston, Texas 77030

URS B. SCHAAD (455), Department of Pediatrics, University of Basel, 4058 Basel, Switzerland

KEVIN SHANNON (99), Department of Microbiology, United Medical and Dental School of Guy's and St. Thomas' Hospitals, St. Thomas' Hospital, London SE1 7EH, United Kingdom

RALF STAHLMANN (397), Department of Pharmacology and Toxicology, Institute of Clinical Pharmacology and Toxicology, University Hospital Benjamin Franklin, Freie Universität Berlin, 14195 Berlin, Germany

JOHN WEIGELT (285), Department of Surgery, Medical College of Wisconsin, Milwaukee, Wisconsin 53226

PREFACE

Substantial progress has been made in the development of newer quinolones since the last edition of *The Quinolones* was published. This progress occurred because the quinolone class of antibacterial agents has captured the interest of chemists, microbiologists, pharmacologists, and clinicians. Recent progress in molecular biology has provided new information and a better understanding of structure–activity relationships of the quinolone nucleus and its radicals. This progress has resulted in the approval of a few new compounds with improved mechanism of action and the potential for delaying the development of resistance by specific bacterial pathogens. A few of the newest quinolones developed recently—moxifloxacin, gatifloxacin, and gemifloxacin—provide a more potent spectrum of activity that includes penicillin-resistant pneumococci as well as good activity against anaerobes and decreased susceptibility to the development of resistance by some bacterial species. Trovafloxacin was the first quinolone that demonstrated improved penetration into the central nervous system and cerebrospinal fluid, and early clinical studies demonstrated excellent efficacy in pediatric patients with bacterial meningitis. The newest quinolones—moxifloxacin, gatifloxacin, and gemifloxacin—broaden the clinical utility of this class of antimicrobial agents as we enter an era of increasing bacterial resistance to the previously recommended "standard therapy." During this same period, we have learned much about quinolone toxicity as it relates to quinolone chemical structure and pharmacokinetics/pharmacodynamics in treated patients. Hopefully this knowledge will provide safer molecules for use in patients.

The excellent and very recent progress that has occurred warranted an update on the quinolones. This edition is intended to provide the newest and most cogent information on the quinolones—all of it readily available in one volume.

Once again, I am much indebted to my colleagues, each of whom contributed thorough reviews on the history, chemistry, and mechanism of action, *in-vitro* properties, mechanisms of bacterial resistance, pharmacokinetics, clinical overview (described in nine separate chapters, including pediatrics), toxicity, adverse effects and drug interactions, and the future prospects of the newer quinolones.

Clearly, our hope is that this work will serve as a ready resource for new and helpful information, and, in so doing, the efforts of my colleagues most certainly will have been worthwhile.

Vincent T. Andriole
Yale University School of Medicine

CHAPTER 1

The Quinolones

History and Overview

PETER BALL

Senior Lecturer (Honorary), School of Biomedical Sciences, University of St. Andrews, St. Andrews, Fife KY16 9AL, Scotland, United Kingdom

INTRODUCTION

The development of quinolone antibacterials, since the discovery of the naph-thyridine agent nalidixic acid some 40 years ago [1], has progressed with periods of great clinical innovation, alternating with periods of apparent inactivity following unexpected recognition of rare, but severe, adverse reactions associated with specific agents. Initially, within a decade, the 4-quinolones oxolinic acid and cinoxacin, which had improved activity against a limited range of Gram-negative bacteria, had been synthesized. Parallel developments in Japan had yielded 7-piperazine-substituted compounds, such as pipemidic acid, which had limited activity against *Pseudomonas aeruginosa*. However, the breakthrough to broad-spectrum activity waited a further 10 years before fluorination, primarily at the 6-position, resulted in the fluoroquinolones. It is difficult to overestimate the clinical impact of the development of these agents.

Since the mid-1980s, the fluoroquinolones have become a major group of synthetic antibiotics with activity that ranges from the Enterobacteriaceae and opportunists such as *Pseudomonas aeruginosa*, to Gram-positive pathogens, including streptococci and staphylococci. These changes resulted in agents—for example, ciprofloxacin and ofloxacin (later the levo-isomer levofloxacin)—that are applicable across a broad range of indications, including those involving the genitourinary, respiratory, and gastrointestinal tracts, skin and soft tissues, and other structures. In most bodily tissues and fluids, the fluoroquinolones are characterized by excellent penetration and therapeutic ratios. Ciprofloxacin and ofloxacin revolutionized the management of many conditions previously amena-ble only to intravenous therapy or in which management has been compromised by bacterial resistance to standard agents, such as the β-lactams. Important examples include pyelonephritis, enteric fevers, prostatic infections, pulmonary exacerbations of cystic fibrosis, and nosocomial pneumonias.

The next significant advance occurred in the early 1990s with the synthesis of temafloxacin, which had four- to eightfold greater activity against *Streptococcus pneumoniae* and good activity against anaerobes, such as the *Bacteroides* and *Prevotella* spp. However, unexpected toxicity, in the form of hemolytic uraemic syndrome [2], resulted in its withdrawal only months after launch. In addition, the development of several other compounds with even greater anti-Gram-posi-tive potency, notably sparfloxacin, sitafloxacin, and Bay 3118, has been either delayed or discontinued due to an unacceptable incidence of phototoxicity (and other adverse effects). By the mid-1990s, clinical development appeared to have halted, although molecules with differing sidechains and laboratory activity continued to be synthesized.

However, optimism again increased with the discovery of trovafloxacin, clinafloxacin, and grepafloxacin, only to be dampened at the end of the decade by their abrupt withdrawal or suspension due to rare but severe adverse effects, including hepatotoxicity (trovafloxacin), significant QT prolongation and associated cardiac deaths (grepafloxacin), and serious phototoxicity and hypoglycemia (clinafloxacin). All of these agents had significantly greater potency against Gram-positive species, notably *S. pneumoniae*, and in the case of trovafloxacin at least proved highly clinically effective in pneumococcal infections. At a time when burgeoning global multidrug resistance among pneumococci had begun to compromise traditional therapy, this left a considerable hiatus in the range of potential alternatives to penicillin and macrolides.

Fortunately, the 8-methoxyquinolones moxifloxacin and gatifloxacin, which are highly potent against *S. pneumoniae* (10-fold greater than the earlier second-generation agents), clinically effective, and appear free from either significant or unexpected toxicity, have filled this therapeutic vacuum. Their proven activity against *S. pneumoniae*, coupled with maintained high potency against *Haemophilus influenzae* and *Moraxella catarrhalis*, and excellent penetration into respiratory tissues, including the intracellular habitat of *Chlamydia* and *Legionella* spp., suggests that, where ciprofloxacin was considered by many to be inappropriate for respiratory infections, 8-methoxyquinolone derivatives will now become agents of choice. They appear to limit emergence of resistance in Gram-positive species, which could prove a major advantage, compared with levofloxacin, which has also proven surprisingly clinically effective in respiratory infections despite a pneumococcal MIC typical of earlier second-generation agents. Further progress includes continued development of the naphthyridone subclass, notably gemifloxacin, which is characterized by a further 10-fold increase in anti-pneumococcal potency. Clinical trial results are awaited with interest.

The fluoroquinolones and their precursors have a number of predictable structure–activity and structure–adverse effect relationships relating to nuclear and sidechain configurations. Thus, design of new molecules can avoid many of the problems that have characterized previous members of the group. It may be anticipated that further modifications to the molecular structure will improve spectrum and activity while reducing the incidence of adverse effects.

STRUCTURE–ACTIVITY RELATIONSHIPS (SARs)

The 1,8 naphthyridines, 4-quinolones, cinnolines. fluoroquinolones, and fluorinated naphthyridones, together with their important sidechain substituent modifications and resultant structure–activity relationships are summarized in Table I. Modifications to the nucleus converting the naphthyridine nitrogen in the 8-position to a carbon reduced adverse reactions and increased activity against Gram-positive cocci, including both streptococci and *Staphylococcus aureus*, whereas either piperazine or other *N*-cyclic substitutions at the 7-position significantly increased potency against Gram-negative bacteria, including *P.*

TABLE I A Chemical and Functional Classification of Quinolones and Fluoroquinolones

Structure	Name	Antibacterial activity	Pharmacokinetics	Indications/comments
First-generation compounds (often all included as 4-quinolones)				
1,8 naphthyridine (carboxylic acid) 7-methyl 7-pyrrole	Nalidixic acid Piromidic acid	Enterobacteria only, no significant anti-Gram-positive activity	Orally absorbed, poor to moderate tissue penetration	UTI, shigellosis
1,2-cinnoline (carboxylic acid)	Cinoxacin			
4-quinolone (carboxylic acid)	Oxolinic acid			
7-piperazine (pyrido-pyrimidine)	Pipemidic acid	*P. aeruginosa* added		
Structure	Name	N-1 sidechain	Antibacterial activity	Pharmacokinetics	Indications/comments

Structure	Name	N-1 sidechain	Antibacterial activity	Pharmacokinetics	Indications/comments
6,7,8 sidechain substituents					
Second-generation compounds (IIA)					
A. Fluoroquinolones with enhanced but predominantly Gram-negative activity					
6-Fluoro	Flumequine	–	Gram-negative: less active than piperazinyl derivatives	Improved absorption	Limited to UTI
6-Fluoro-7-piperazinyl	Ciprofloxacin Pefloxacin Norfloxacin Ofloxacin (Levofloxacin: Rufloxacin	Cyclopropyl Ethyl Ethyl 1-8 (O) cyclic ring L-isomer) 1-8 (S) cyclic ring	Enhanced anti-Gram negative potency, including *P. aeruginosa* plus some limited anti-Gram-positive activity	High absorption, ++ tissue penetration, variable elimination (renal/metabolic) with moderate to long T/2	UTI, STD, enteric infections, RTI (not 1° pneumococcal), invasive Gram-negative infections: osteomyelitis, skin and soft tissue, etc.

Substituent	Compound	R group	Activity	Pharmacokinetics	Comments
6,8-difluoro-7-piperazinyl	Lomefloxacin Fleroxacin	Ethyl Fluoro-ethyl	Lesser anti-Gram-positive activity	Long T/2: once daily	Lomefloxacin CNS toxic significantly phototoxic

Second-generation compounds (IIB)
B. Fluoroquinolones with balanced broad spectrum activity

Substituent	Compound	R group	Activity	Pharmacokinetics	Comments
6-fluoro-7-piperazinyl 6,8-difluoro-7-dimethylpiperazinyl 6-fluoro-8-chloro-7-pyrrolodinyl 6-fluoro-7-pyrrolidinyl naphthyridone	Temafloxacin Grepafloxacin Sparfloxacin Clinafloxacin Sitafloxacin Tosufloxacin	Difluorophenyl Cyclopropyl Cyclopropyl Cyclopropyl Cyclopropyl Difluorophenyl	Enhanced anti-Gram-positive potency, broad-spectrum and anti-pneumococcal activity	Long T/2: once daily high bioavailability, excellent respiratory penetration, few interactions (except grepafloxacin)	1. All now superseded by more active third-generation agents. 2. Significantly toxic – most withdrawn from clinical use.

Third-generation compounds
Fluoroquinolones with enhanced Gram-positive activity

Substituent	Compound	R group	Activity	Pharmacokinetics	Comments
6-fluoro-7-azabicyclo naphthyridone 6-fluoro-8-methoxy-7-azabicyclo 6-fluoro-8-methoxy-7-piperazinyl and 6-fluoro-7-methoximino-naphthyridone	Trovafloxacin Moxifloxacin Gatifloxacin Gemifloxacin	Difluorophenyl Cyclopropyl Cyclopropyl Cyclopropyl	Extended activity with ++ anti-pneumococcal and potential anti-anaerobic potency	As for second-generation agents	1. Highly active respiratory quinolones CAP/AECB. 2. Potential for surgical and Ob/Gyn infections. 3. Possible pediatric use.

aeruginosa. These 7-piperazine-substituted compounds, notably pipemidic acid (a pyrido-pyrimidine), were also active against some nalidixic acid-resistant enterobacteria. Subsequent fluorination at the 6-position further improved potency and added clinically exploitable Gram-positive potency [3]. Even more potent compounds were produced by halogenation of the 8-position, notably the 8-chloro derivatives. Unfortunately, these proved highly phototoxic and have mostly been abandoned. Replacement with an 8-methoxy group has yielded the fluoroquinolones moxifloxacin and gatifloxacin, with markedly reduced phototoxic potential but similarly enhanced potency. Specific molecular configurations, now including several des-fluorinated quinolones (one with an 8-difluoromethoxy substituent), and SARs are discussed in detail in Chapter 2. It is tempting to speculate, however, on the primacy of the 1-cyclopropyl (or 1–8 cyclic) substituent in determining safety from idiosyncratic quinolone toxicity. The only compounds—that is, temafloxacin, tosufloxacin, and trovafloxacin—to depart from this configuration all had 1(2,4)-difluorophenyl substitutions and all proved to have specific, commonly immunologically mediated, severe toxicities. It seems unlikely that new molecules with either this or indeed the 8-chloro configuration will be developed.

ANTIBACTERIAL ACTIVITY

MODE OF ACTION

Quinolone antibacterials act by inhibition of bacterial topoisomerase II (DNA gyrase) and topoisomerase IV in Gram-positive species, thus inhibiting tertiary negative supercoiling of bacterial DNA [4–8]. This effect, probably associated with binding of quinolones to a DNA gyrase complex [9], is rapidly bactericidal [8]. The minimum bactericidal concentration is usually only two- to fourfold the MIC, and a prolonged post-antibiotic effect is produced at concentrations exceeding the MIC.

Fluoroquinolones only rarely demonstrate synergy or antagonism with other agents [10]. Combination therapy can be expected to enhance therapy only by the individual and additive activity of the compounds used, except possibly with imipenem in some *P. aeruginosa* infections and with rifampicin in staphylococcal disease where improved clinical outcomes may result.

SPECTRUM OF ACTIVITY

The differential activities of the original naphthyridine/quinolone derivatives, fluoroquinolones, and new naphthyridones are summarized in Table II. Individual activities are discussed in detail in Chapter 3. Significant differences are present

TABLE II Differential Activities of Representative Fluoroquinolones on Common Pathogens

Pathogen	Cipro-floxacin	Nor-floxacin	Levo-floxacin	Spar-floxacin	Grepa-floxacin	Trova-floxacin	Gati-floxacin	Moxi-floxacin	Gemi-floxacin
Staphylococcus aureus methicillin-S	0.5	2	0.5 (levo)	0.12	0.12	0.03	0.12	0.03–0.12	0.03
Staphylococcus aureus methicillin-R	16–64	>16	16	8	0.25	1–8	2→4	2–4	8
Streptococcus pneumoniae	2	16	1–2	0.5	0.25	0.12	0.5	0.25	0.016
Enterococcus faecalis	2–64	>16	1–4	0.5–1	0.25	0.25–2	4	0.5	2
Escherichia coli	0.03–0.25	0.25–1	0.06–0.25	0.25	0.25–0.5	0.05–0.5	0.05–1	0.5–1	0.016–1
Klebsiella spp.	0.03–0.25	0.25–1	0.06–1	0.5	0.25–0.5	0.5–1	0.06–0.25	0.06–0.25	0.25
Proteus mirabilis	0.06	0.12–0.5	0.12–0.25	0.5	N/A	0.25–0.5	N/A	0.25	0.25
Morganella morgani	0.06	0.12–0.5	0.12	1	N/A	1	4	0.25	0.12
Salmonella spp.	0.06	0.25	0.12	0.12	N/A	0.12	N/A	0.12	N/A
P. aeruginosa	0.5–4	2	1–8	2–8	0.5–4	1–8	4–32	8	8
Neisseria spp.	<0.01	0.03	<0.01	<0.01	0.015	<0.01	0.06	0.015	0.01
Moraxella catarrhalis	0.03	0.25	0.06	<0.01	0.015	<0.01	0.03	0.12	0.01
Haemophilus influenzae	0.015	0.06	0.03	<0.01	0.03	0.01	0.03	0.03	0.01
Bacteroides fragilis	2–16	4–32	1–8	1	8	0.25–0.5	1–2	0.25–2	2
Chlamydia pneumoniae	1	N/A	1	0.01–0.25	0.5	0.12	0.12	0.06	0.06–0.25
M. pneumoniae	1–2	N/A	0.5–1	0.12–0.25	0.06–0.5	0.25	0.06	0.12	N/A
Legionella pneumophila	0.03–0.12	N/A	0.05	0.06	0.05	0.01–0.06	0.03	0.015	0.016

Data taken from [11–15,120–128].

MICs for *E. coli* (mode) are usually <0.1 mg/liter for all agents, but resistance emergence has elevated the MIC90 to the values shown.

between the fluoroquinolones, some of which have broad-spectrum activity against both Gram-negative and Gram-positive species. Others (e.g., norfloxacin and pefloxacin) are less active against Gram-positive pathogens. Ciprofloxacin retains preeminence against Gram-negative isolates, notably against *P. aeruginosa*, for which it is the drug of choice. Levofloxacin has similar overall activity to ofloxacin (of which it is the L-isomer) but is possibly twice as active against Gram-positive isolates. Sparfloxacin is more active against the pneumococci but has been superseded by the newest agents. Trovafloxacin, moxifloxacin, and gatifloxacin have high potency and a wide spectrum including *S. pneumoniae*, against which they are 10-fold more active than ciprofloxacin and two- to fourfold more active than sparfloxacin [11–14]. Gemifloxacin continues the trend of increasing activity against respiratory pathogens [15].

The newer fluoroquinolones and naphthyridones have been specifically targeted at respiratory infections, and activity against drug- (penicillin-) resistant *S. pneumoniae* (DRSP) is of paramount importance. In this respect, all agents probably have activity against DRSP similar to their activity against sensitive strains [14,15].

Development of resistance has been a feature of fluoroquinolone therapy of staphylococcal infections [16,17]. Later agents such as clinafloxacin appear to have good activity against strains resistant to, for example, ciprofloxacin [18]. However, experience suggests that resistance would develop quickly in clinical use [15].

The new quinolones are significantly more potent than earlier class members against both *Mycoplasma pneumoniae* (MICs 0.01–0.6 mg/liter) and *Legionella pneumophila* (MICs usually <0.06 mg/liter) [14,19]. They also have improved potency against *Chlamydia pneumoniae* (14).

BACTERIAL RESISTANCE TO FLUOROQUINOLONES

Fluoroquinolone resistance may result from chromosomal mutations coding for modifications in target subunits (primarily *gyr A*, but also *gyr B*) of bacterial topoisomerase II, alterations in expression of outer membrane proteins—most importantly OmpF [8,20,21]—and, in Gram-positive species, by variations in the uptake/efflux processes [22] and mutations in topoisomerase IV [8,23]. Thus, resistance in the pneumococci requires mutations in both *par C* and *gyr A* configurations [23]. Plasmid-mediated resistance has not been confirmed to occur [24].

Resistance due to these mechanisms has now been reported in many species, not only those with initial MICs higher than average (0.5–2 mg/liter, such as *P. aeruginosa* and the staphylococci), but also in *Escherichia coli*, *Salmonella* spp.,

Neisseria gonorrhoeae, and others with MICs originally reported in the range <0.05 mg/liter [16].

Thus, by the mid-1990s various lessons had been learned regarding emergence of resistance to fluoroquinolones in a number of common pathogens [16]. Treatment of infections due to organisms with an initially high MIC (0.5–2 mg/liter or more) was likely to predispose to clinical failure, notably in infections caused by staphylococci, pneumococci, enterococci, and *P. aeruginosa* (for which spontaneous mutation leading to single-step resistance is 100 to 10,000 times— 10^6 to 10^7 vs. 10^9 to 10^{11}—more common than for other pathogens) and was often associated with a rising MIC during therapy.

Further factors predisposing to resistance development included inadequate dosage, interactions reducing bioavailability (e.g., coadministration of divalent cations), treatment of prosthetic infections, prolonged and/or repeated prescription in cystic fibrosis patients, and extensive use in veterinary practice and animal husbandry [16].

In both the United States and Europe, little significant resistance to fluoroquinolones appeared among enterobacteria up to 1990–91, despite changes appearing among *P. aeruginosa* and *S. aureus* [25–27]. However, fluoroquinolone resistance in urinary *E. coli* isolates in Spain has now risen to levels sufficient to challenge the preeminence of these agents as primary therapy [28]; it has been encountered in neutropenic patients receiving fluoroquinolone prophylaxis [29]. Much of this resistance is related to spread of resistant clones in hospitals. Indeed, the most significant factor for resistance emergence among Gram-negative pathogens in hospital patients has been prior use of fluoroquinolones [30,31]. In Spain [32] and many other countries, veterinary usage and, more importantly, use for growth promotion in animals have proved a stronger selection pressure, not only among *E. coli*, but also in *Salmonella* and *Campylobacter* spp. [15]. Furthermore, by the mid-1990s, use of drugs discarded from human use (e.g., oxolinic acid and flumequine) had already led to establishment of fluoroquinolone-resistant *E. coli* in poultry flocks [33].

CLINICAL PHARMACOLOGY

The basic pharmacokinetic parameters of fluoroquinolones are given in Table III. The newer generation, that is, sparfloxacin, trovafloxacin, grepafloxacin, clinafloxacin, moxifloxacin, and gatifloxacin, are similar in this regard to previous group members [34,37] (see Chapter 5). Levofloxacin has kinetics like those of ofloxacin.

All fluoroquinolones are well absorbed, reach peak serum concentrations within 1–2 hours (sparfloxacin 4–5 hr), and have high distribution volumes

TABLE III   Pharmacokinetic Parameters for Representative Fluoroquinolones

Fluoro-quinolone	Dose (mg)	Plasma C_{max} (mg/l)	Bioa-vaila-bility (%)	Volume of dis-tribution (l/kg)	Protein binding (%)	T½ elimin-ation (hr)	Renal elimin-ation (%)
Ciprofloxacin	500	1.5–3.0	60–80	2.5–5.0	20–40	3–5	30–50
Ofloxacin	400	3.5–5.5	85–95	1.2	25	5–7	70–85
Levofloxacin	200	2	>90	1.5	25	4–6	85–90
Norfloxacin	400	1.5–2.0	40	1.5	15	4–5	25–40
Pefloxacin	400	4.0	>90	1.5–2.0	20–30	10	30–60
Sparfloxacin	400 200	1.6 0.7	80–90	4.5	45	15–20	40
Fleroxacin	400	5.5	>90	1.0–1.5	25	9–13	60
Trovafloxacin	100–300	1.5–4.4	>90	1.5	70	10–12	23
Moxifloxacin	400	4–5	82–89	2.5–3.5	48	10–14	25
Gatifloxacin	400	3.3–4.2	96	N/A	20	7–8	85

Data taken from [8,37,38,43,78,126–131].

(1.5–4.5 liter/kg) typical of the class. Protein binding is generally 50% or less (48% for moxifloxacin and 20% for gatifloxacin), although it is higher (70%) for trovafloxacin. After oral administration, the fluoroquinolones produce levels well in excess of those required for clinical efficacy in genitourinary, gynecological, skeletal, and other important tissues and fluids [35]. They are particularly well concentrated in target tissues within the respiratory tract, matching optimal kinetics with improved potency against respiratory pathogens.

PENETRATION INTO RESPIRATORY TISSUES

Fluoroquinolones produce excellent therapeutic ratios in the respiratory tract. Bronchial mucosal concentrations are 1.5 to 2 times those in serum [36–39], although ratios between sputum/bronchial secretion concentrations and those in serum after dosage within normal clinical limits range from 0.33 to 0.5 for ciprofloxacin and sparfloxacin to almost unity for pefloxacin, ofloxacin, and lomefloxacin [36]. Concentrations in alveolar lining fluid are typically two- to threefold greater than serum [37,38] and vary between the fluoroquinolones, lung parenchymal levels ranging from 4 to 10 times that in serum [36]. The highest ratios are found in alveolar macrophages [38], where concentrations 10- to 20-fold greater than serum have been found with agents such as ciprofloxacin, levofloxacin, and temafloxacin, the recently abandoned compounds trovafloxacin, sparfloxacin, and grepafloxacin, and the newer 8-methoxyquinolones, exemplified by moxifloxacin [39].

ELIMINATION PATHWAYS

The primary route of elimination of most fluoroquinolones is via the kidney [40], the exceptions including pefloxacin, trovafloxacin, grepafloxacin, clinafloxacin, and moxifloxacin, urinary recoveries of which are 10–25% or less [34,37,38,40]. A number of agents are cleared almost exclusively by glomerular filtration and tubular secretion, notably ofloxacin (levofloxacin), lomefloxacin, and, to a lesser extent, fleroxacin. These group members require dosage modification in significant renal impairment and the elderly, leading to more complex dosage recommendations in such patients. In contrast, dose modification for agents such as ciprofloxacin, norfloxacin, and trovafloxacin is required only in patients with creatinine clearances of 20–30 ml/min or less, in whom halving the dose or extending the dosage interval is usually recommended. For pefloxacin, which is extensively metabolized, no adjustments are required. The fluoroquinolones are poorly cleared by both peritoneal dialysis and hemodialysis (<20–30%); posthemodialysis top-up dosage is not required.

The fluoroquinolones differ markedly in their degree of biotransformation, predominantly to metabolites with significantly less or absent antibacterial activity (Chapter 5). Pefloxacin is highly metabolized, principally to desmethyl (norfloxacin) and N-oxide derivatives [41], and this is its major pathway of elimination, whereas transformation of ofloxacin—and therefore levofloxacin—to similar metabolites accounts for only 6% of the dose [42]. Fleroxacin has an intermediate profile with primary renal clearance, but desmethyl (extended half-life) and N-oxide derivatives account for some 20% of the administered dose. Biotransformation of enoxacin, primarily to oxoenoxacin, accounts for some 50% of the dose. For other agents, biotransformation to drug-specific combinations of oxoquinolones (the major metabolites of ciprofloxacin and norfloxacin) and N-formyl, N-sulfonyl, N-acetyl, and desethylenyl products forms a significant but minority elimination pathway [43]. The primary metabolites of moxifloxacin are N-sulfate and acyl-glucuronide [37].

The half-lives of pefloxacin and norfloxacin are prolonged in severe liver disease, and even less highly metabolized agents, such as ciprofloxacin, may accumulate in hepatic failure [44].

Transintestinal elimination of norfloxacin and ciprofloxacin is a minor excretory pathway, which may be exploited in the management of some forms of infective diarrhoea, for example, enterotoxigenic *E. coli* (ETEC) enteritis.

PHARMACODYNAMICS OF QUINOLONES

Increasing attention has focused on prediction of outcomes by various pharmacodynamic (PD) parameters. These have been extensively reviewed by Wise and colleagues [37,38]. Quinolones exhibit concentration-dependent killing and both the serum peak concentration to inhibitory concentration (C_{max}:MIC) ratio and area under the serum inhibition curve (AUIC) can be used to model clinical and bacteriological response in community-acquired pneumonia (CAP) and acute exacerbations of chronic bronchitis (AECBs). Efficacy cutoff points of C_{max}/MIC ratios of 12 and AUIC ratios of 100–125 mg/liter·hr predict response and eradication rates of >80%, bacterial eradication within 48 hr (for fluoroquinolones), and development of resistance in <10% of cases. These indices, together with a further PD parameter—intensity of antibiotic effect (I_E)—can also be used to predict minimum dosages required to attain their cutoff points. For some of the older quinolones, PD parameters indicate unsatisfactory outcomes or the need to increase dose or dose frequency. The newest agents—moxifloxacin, gatifloxacin, and gemifloxacin—easily exceed cutoff points at current dose levels.

CLINICAL USES

URINARY TRACT INFECTIONS

The fluoroquinolones are highly effective in uncomplicated urinary tract infection and are drugs of choice where bacterial resistance compromises routine β-lactam therapy (Chapter 6). Fluoroquinolone efficacy is augmented by their ability to eliminate carriage of uropathogenic *E. coli* in the intestine [45]. Excellent results follow standard short-course and single-dose regimens [46,47].

In complicated infections and in the elderly, these agents are as or more effective than β-lactams, amoxicillin–clavulanate, nitrofurantoin, and trimethoprim–sulfamethoxazole [46,47]. Ciprofloxacin is effective in many patients with chronic infections caused by *P. aeruginosa*, including pyelonephritis, and in patients with neurologically impaired bladders. For example, oral ciprofloxacin was as effective clinically, and more so in terms of bacterial eradication, as parenteral aminoglycoside therapy in catheterized patients with multiresistant organisms causing ascending infection [48]. However, resistance in common urinary pathogens is regrettably no longer a rarity and may compromise empirical quinolone monotherapy [28].

Bacterial prostatitis is a problem to both define and treat, poor results being obtained with tetracyclines, cephalosporins, and trimethoprim–sulfamethoxazole. Oral fluoroquinolone therapy for extended periods in chronic or pseudomonal infection with adequate follow-up has given cure rates of 50–90% depending on disease and pathogen [46,47]. Failures and relapse are most likely to occur with enterococci or *P. aeruginosa* infections, but coliform prostatitis responds in 80% or more of cases.

Ciprofloxacin, pefloxacin, and ofloxacin have also been found effective in continuous ambulatory peritoneal dialysis (CAPD) infections, but their usefulness has been curtailed by the emergence of resistance in or failure to eradicate staphylococci [16,49,50].

Sexually Transmitted Diseases

All of the fluoroquinolones are effective in single-dose treatment of uncomplicated urethral, anal, and oropharyngeal gonorrhoea [51], although such regimes are ineffective for chlamydial disease. Ofloxacin for 7 days is reliably effective in chlamydial urethritis in men, although possibly less so in women, but there are little data on genital *Mycoplasma* infection. Preliminary data on trovafloxacin suggest high efficacy at low single doses in gonorrhoea [52] and, after multiple dosing, for chlamydial sexually transmitted diseases (STDs). However, fluoroquinolones are not indicated in syphilis, and results in bacterial vaginosis suggest only a secondary role.

Respiratory Infections

The use of fluoroquinolones in respiratory tract infection (RTI) has been under scrutiny since the original reports of clinical failure in, or superinfection during, ciprofloxacin therapy of pneumococcal disease [53]. Thus, despite the reality of predominantly good results in most respiratory syndromes—notably AECBs—the earlier second-generation quinolones were never accepted for use in community-acquired pneumonia (CAP). This also applied to agents such as lomefloxacin and fleroxacin that have MICs for pneumococci in the range of 4 to 16 mg/liter. In contrast, sparfloxacin, grepafloxacin, and trovafloxacin (MIC$_{90}$s of 0.12–0.5 mg/liter) were fast becoming recognized as potential agents of choice for drug-resistant infections prior to their toxicity-mediated demise [54]. Newer 8-methoxyquinolones such as gatifloxacin and moxifloxacin, which have enhanced anti-pneumococcal potency (MIC$_{90}$ = 0.12 mg/liter), will undoubtedly inherit the role of preferred drugs as penicillin and macrolide resistance continues to increase and spread. At present, levofloxacin is extensively used, giving clinical response rates of 84–96% after IV–oral switch therapy of CAP and 78–100% in AECBs [54,55]. Moxifloxacin, at present available only as an oral formulation, gives similar results (89–97%), and IV–oral switch regimes using gatifloxacin resulted in response rates of 95–97% [54,55]. New fluoroquinolones may give better results than standard therapy. For example, in CAP IV–oral levofloxacin was superior to IV ceftriaxone–oral cefuroxime [56], and oral trovafloxacin produced superior clinical response rates to amoxicillin [57]. Other measures in CAP may also reflect enhanced outcomes: mortality rates may be significantly decreased [58] and hospital admission rates, ICU admission rates, and length of stay may be reduced [59].

Fluoroquinolones are effective in legionellosis [19] and are now used, alone and in combination, as agents of choice, especially in macrolide failures. The absence of significant interaction with cyclosporin A has advantages compared with macrolide therapy.

Fluoroquinolones are now recommended for acute exacerbations of chronic bronchitis (AECBs) in patients with risk factors for poor outcome by large consensus groups [60], and both moxifloxacin and gatifloxacin give satisfactory short-term clinical outcomes of 89% in AECBs [61,62]. Preliminary data on a direct comparison over 6-month follow-up between gemifloxacin and clarithromycin appear to demonstrate a reduction in exacerbations by gemifloxacin therapy compared to clarithromycin that related to failure of pathogen eradication by the latter (data on file, SmithKline Beecham).

Comparison of ciprofloxacin with imipenem in severe pneumonia in hospitalized patients noted a significantly higher clinical response rate with the quinolone and better bacterial eradication rates for the pathogens (predominantly enterobacteria) pneumococci and *P. aeruginosa*, although eradication rates for the latter were lower (67 vs. 59% for imipenem) and resistance emerged in 33–53% of isolates [63]. Similar results were obtained with trovafloxacin, while studies of moxifloxacin and gatifloxacin are awaited.

Multidrug-resistant tuberculosis and atypical infections, for example, *Mycobacterium avium complex* (MAC), require alternatives to standard therapy, and fluoroquinolones are used widely in combination regimens despite limited efficacy data. Resistance has now been reported in *Mycobacterium tuberculosis*.

GASTROINTESTINAL INFECTIONS

The fluoroquinolones have proved a major advance in management of many forms of moderate to severe enteric infection [64]. Administered for 10 days, they are the drugs of choice for oral management of typhoid fever in both adults and children, reducing complication, relapse, and convalescent excretion rates to a greater extent than comparator antibiotics [65,66]. Ciprofloxacin has good efficacy in moderate to severe shigellosis [67], in which single-dose therapy is one of the regimens of choice [64] and is as effective as tetracyclines in cholera [68]. Fluoroquinolones are effective in both the treatment, even single-dose [69], and prophylaxis of traveler's diarrhea [70]. They are also agents of choice in the management of invasive salmonellosis in AIDS patients. However, empirical therapy of acute bacterial diarrhoea is not generally recommended, and the role of fluoroquinolones in noninvasive salmonellosis remains controversial. Early trials suggested efficacy, but failure to eradicate pathogens has proved to be a problem [64,71]. Fluoroquinolones are ineffective in campylobacteriosis.

SKIN AND SOFT TISSUE INFECTIONS

Fluoroquinolones yield similar results to standard therapy for both Gram-positive and Gram-negative infections of the skin and soft tissues [72], although emergence of resistance among both staphylococci—notably methicillin-resistant *Staphylococcus aureus* (MRSA)— and *P. aeruginosa* has been observed [25]. Treatment of diabetic infections, including polymicrobial disease, with the early fluoroquinolones gave results almost as good, but persistence and resistance acquisition proved a greater problem, most frequently in *P. aeruginosa* infections. Preliminary analyses of the therapy of diabetic foot infections with trovafloxacin and similar agents active against anaerobes, such as the *Bacteroides* spp., have indicated excellent results. The potential for early IV–oral switch therapy and discharge from hospital is a major advantage in such patients. However, the rapid emergence and spread of quinolone-resistant MRSA among patients—including those previously not exposed to fluoroquinolones—and within hospitals suggest fluoroquinolones to be inappropriate in MRSA infections [16].

Currently available fluoroquinolones have indifferent to modest activity against obligate anaerobes and microaerophilic streptococci, and are usually used in combination in infections where these organisms are involved. However, prior to its suspension, trials of trovafloxacin (MICs for anaerobes of 1 mg/liter or less) gave excellent clinical response rates in intraabdominal and pelvic anaerobic or mixed polymicrobial disease [73]. The potential future roles for other fluoroquinolones in surgery and gynecological infections are discussed in Chapter 9.

BONE INFECTIONS

The fluoroquinolones have had a major impact on the oral management of Gram-negative bacillary and polymicrobial osteomyelitis [74,75], achieving cure rates of between 65 and 95%—lower in infections caused by *P. aeruginosa*—in a disease previously requiring prolonged parenteral combination therapy. In staphylococcal osteomyelitis, notably that caused by MRSA and coagulase-negative staphylococci, fluoroquinolones should not be used routinely [16], although results with original fluoroquinolones (e.g., pefloxacin) plus rifampicin suggested potential for combination therapy [76].

NEUTROPENIC CANCER PATIENTS

Various fluoroquinolones have been used for empirical treatment of fever in neutropenic cancer patients. For ciprofloxacin, monotherapy produced less favorable results than ceftazidime alone or combination therapies [77], whereas combination therapy gave results similar to those with standard regimes [78]. Oral regimes including ciprofloxacin also proved cheaper than parenteral combinations. Resistance among *E. coli* and superinfection with Gram-positive pathogens appear likely to limit such therapy.

Since the original reports of improved efficacy of fluoroquinolones for prevention of infection in neutropenic patients compared to standard therapy [79,80], these agents—notably norfloxacin, ciprofloxacin, and ofloxacin—have become agents of choice. However, reports of fluoroquinolone-resistant *E. coli* causing bacteremia in these patients has again compromised therapy in many countries [28–31].

PROPHYLAXIS

Single-dose ciprofloxacin is a safe and effective form of prophylaxis for meningococcal infection [66,81]. It has also been used effectively for transurethral surgical procedures, in oral prophylaxis of infection complicating biliary, and, in combination with parenteral metronidazole, for colorectal surgery, in which wound infection rates are comparable to standard prophylaxis [78]. Abdominal and gynecological surgical prophylaxis using trovafloxacin were rapidly becoming established at the time of its suspension [73]. Trials of newer agents are planned.

PHARMACOECONOMIC ASPECTS OF FLUOROQUINOLONE USAGE

Fluoroquinolone antibacterial agents are expensive, especially when administered intravenously. In some indications, such as Gram-negative or polymicrobial osteomyelitis (where oral fluoroquinolone therapy can replace lengthy intravenous therapy) and enteric fevers (where the excellent clinical results and low incidence of carriage states are clearly superior to standard therapy), the benefits outweigh the additional cost. Oral fluoroquinolones are also among the agents of choice for IV–oral switch (stepdown) therapy [82–84]. Thus, Gentry and colleagues found IV-to-oral ofloxacin therapy effective for both nosocomial and community-acquired pneumonia [85].

In other indications, cost–acquisition comparison with other agents may at first sight appear unfavorable. However, when true cost–efficacy and cost–benefit studies are undertaken that effectively measure total costs—including intravenous drug preparation and administration, hospitalization and complication rates, potential for early discharge, reduced time lost from work—and subjective elements—such as quality of life, especially using IV–oral switch regimens—fluoroquinolone therapy can be a highly cost-effective proposition [84,86,87]. For example, sequential therapy using ciprofloxacin substitution after initial intravenous therapy may reduce drug costs by 45% and hospitalization costs by 20% [82]. Specific comparisons with ceftazidime and imipenem in nosocomial and severe pneumonia showed ciprofloxacin therapy to save more than US $500 per treatment [88] and to significantly reduce posttreatment days in hospital, further antibiotic costs, and repeat hospitalization [89]. In acute exacerbations of chronic bronchitis, a year-long follow-up study found oral ciprofloxacin to achieve cost savings compared to standard regimens in patients with risk factors for poor outcomes [90].

These potential savings also apply with other agents and have resulted in fluoroquinolones (e.g., ofloxacin [83]) being incorporated into IV–oral switch guidelines. Controlled use of levofloxacin in a critical pathway resulted in reduced admission rates, decreased use of resources, and shorter hospital stays compared with conventional management [91].

USE OF FLUOROQUINOLONES IN PEDIATRICS

The moratorium imposed on fluoroquinolone usage in children, relating to the potential risk of joint toxicity, has remained under review, and an expert committee has published guidelines for use in specified infections where the clinical need outweighs the theoretical risk [92]. Investigation of compounds such as nalidixic acid and flumequine in growing animals during the 1970s revealed a potential for damage to weight-bearing, di-arthrodial joints caused by effects on articular cartilage (Chapters 14, 15). Studies on juvenile beagle dogs and other species showed this effect, resulting from chronic high dosage, to be both species and compound variable, fluoroquinolones being less likely to cause the effect than the original quinolones and naphthyridines.

However, after three decades of quinolone use, including that of nalidixic acid for suppression of bacteriuria and treatment of bacillary dysentery in children, 10 years of compassionate use of fluoroquinolones (mostly ciprofloxacin) in children, and the limited licensing of norfloxacin for pediatric use in Japan, this effect has never been observed in humans [93]. Thus, retrospective database analyses of more than 1700 patients aged 17 years and under found no evidence of joint damage, nor indeed of hepatic or renal toxicity [94], and a safety analysis of compassionate use found reversible arthralgia in 1.5% (60% cystic fibrosis patients) and no evidence of arthritis [95].

Most experience has been gained in cystic fibrosis patients, where ciprofloxacin and, to a lesser extent, ofloxacin have proved valuable oral alternatives to parenteral therapy [96]. Clonal resistance emergence occurs in about 25% of *P. aeruginosa* isolates but is not invariably associated with treatment failure and may revert to previous sensitivity by the time of later exacerbations [25].

Currently, the pediatric use of fluoroquinolones is advised only for the following indications:

- Bronchopulmonary exacerbations of cystic fibrosis due to *P. aeruginosa*

- Typhoid and paratyphoid fevers in areas of high resistance prevalence

- Single-dose treatment (and prophylaxis) of cholera

- Potentially invasive shigellosis and salmonellosis

- Complicated urinary tract infection (UTI) caused by multiresistant bacteria

- Chronic suppurative otitis media caused by *P. aeruginosa*

- Osteomyelitis unresponsive to standard therapy

- Drug-resistant tuberculosis

Other indications might include invasive multiresistant infections, single-dose prophylaxis of meningococcal infection, and prophylaxis in neutropenia.

This listing may soon expand to include multiresistant pneumococcal infections in both the respiratory tract (including the middle ear) and CNS. Clinical trials of trovafloxacin in meningitis (data on file, Pfizer) reported excellent efficacy compared with ceftriaxone, but the drug was suspended prior to full evaluation. The emergence of vancomycin-tolerant pneumococci causing clinical failure or relapse in meningitis may spur investigation of some of the newer agents, notably the highly active gemifloxacin [97]. The use of combination therapy including fluoroquinolones may also increase against a background of emerging vancomycin resistance in MRSA [98]. Fluoroquinolones are already widely used for management of pediatric enteric fevers, bacillary dysentery, and cholera in developing countries [66]. It must be anticipated that extended use will follow in the Northern Hemisphere (Chapter 15).

ADVERSE DRUG REACTIONS

The main adverse drug reactions (ADRs) associated with fluoroquinolone therapy are listed with their frequencies of occurrence in Table IV [99–101]. It should be noted that different methods of assessing these effects contribute largely to the major discrepancies in incidence between agents. For example, in the 1990s, objective questioning and patient questionnaires became the norm, so that a far higher incidence of possibly related in contrast to probably related effects was noted. Equally, drugs assessed primarily in Japan tend to show lower incidences, probably related to the stoical nature of the subjects. Most quinolone ADRs are recognized class effects [99,100] that vary in frequency and degree between individual agents but are rarely sufficient to cause discontinuation. Discontinuation rates for the modern agents are usually 2–4%, although both trovafloxacin and grepafloxacin were associated with rates of 6–7% [99]. There have also been a number of specific, individual agent-associated idiosyncratic effects. For a number of agents, these have been sufficient to cause withdrawal from investigation or the marketplace, on occasion by regulatory action. These have included:

1. *Severe phototoxicity* [99,100]. Related primarily to halogenation at the 8-position. Agents withdrawn or abandoned include Bay 3118, fleroxacin, clinafloxacin, and sparfloxacin. Incidence 5–10%.

2. *Temafloxacin syndrome* [2]. An immune-mediated hemolytic anaemia associated with renal and hepatic dysfunction (50%), and coagulopathics. Incidence approximately 0.05% of cases. In some cases, potentially related to prior quinolone/temafloxacin exposure. Withdrawn June 1992.

3. *Tosufloxacin syndromes*. A probably immune-mediated constellation of features, recognized in Japan, where regulatory warnings of severe skin eruptions, renal insufficiency, and blood dyscrasias have been issued. Remains available in Japan.

4. *Trovafloxacin hepatitis* [99]. Severe hepatic reactions including necrosis and failure requiring transplantation and causing deaths, probably immune mediated in many cases. Contributory factors including preexisting liver and other predisposing disease, coadministration of potentially hepatotoxic agents, and prior exposure to fluoroquinolones (or trovafloxacin) in at least 50% of cases. Incidence approximately 0.005%. Suspended by European Regulators June 1999; restricted in the United States.

TABLE IV   Adverse Reaction Profiles for Representative Oral Fluoroquinolones

Fluoro-quinolone	Total ADRs (%)	GI tract ADRs (%)	CNS ADRs (%)	Skin ADRs (%)	Specific warnings, etc.
1. Data obtained by standard subjective patient reporting (all dose ranges)					
Enoxacin	6.2	1.2	1.2	0.6	Interactions with xanthines, NSAIDs
Norfloxacin	9.1	3.9	4.4	0.5	None reported
Pefloxacin	8.0	5.6	0.9	2.2	Phototoxicity observed; interactions with theophylline
Ciprofloxacin	5.8	3.4	1.1	0.7	Interactions with theophylline
Ofloxacin	4.3	2.6	0.9	0.5	CNS problems at high dose and after accumulation
Levofloxacin	3.3–9.9[a]	1.8	0.5	0.2	None reported
Lomefloxacin	Not stated	5.1	5.5	2.4	High incidence of CNS and phototoxicity (FDA 1993)

[a]Up to 20% in phase IIIb/IV clinical trials.

2. Data obtained by objective questioning or by patient questionnaire					
Temafloxacin (all dose ranges)	31.5	13.4	7.3	2.4	Withdrawn 1992: hemolytic-uremic syndrome
Fleroxacin (200–400 mg)	10.4–21	5–11	6.3–9	1.5–3	High incidence of phototoxicity
Sparfloxacin (200–400 mg)	22–32	6.4–10	2→3	1.8	Phototoxicity and QT interval prolongation (see text)
Grepafloxacin (600 mg)	47	15	5	2	Withdrawn 1999: serious cardiotoxicity
Trovafloxacin (100–200 mg)	27	4–7	dizziness 12 headache 5	1	Suspended 1999: serious hepatotoxicity
Moxifloxacin (400 mg)	26	17	5	2	PMS data; no serious reports in 500,000 patients
Gatifloxacin (400 mg)	29	9	4	1	PMS data not yet available

[a]Data not yet available for gemifloxacin.

It is of note that temafloxacin, tosufloxacin, and trovafloxacin are the only compounds developed that have the 1(2,4)-difluorophenyl substituent. Their nuclear and sidechain structure is otherwise dissimilar.

Subsequently, the two fluoroquinolone class effects most frequently causing comment, sometimes associated with specific instructions from registration authorities to include special cautions and warnings in the data sheet, have been CNS effects, phototoxicity, and tendinitis, as well as QTc prolongation and associated ventricular tachyarrhythmias [99,107]

CNS effects—particularly headaches, insomnia, and dizziness—occur more commonly with ofloxacin and lomefloxacin than with other fluoroquinolones (FDA Antiinfective Advisory Committee, Open Meeting, 23 September 1993). Major psychiatric disturbances were also more common, and, in the case of lomefloxacin, convulsions have occurred significantly more frequently than with other fluoroquinolones, often with no past history or predisposing factors. However, all quinolones are contraindicated in patients with a history of convulsions.

Quinolone phototoxicity is predictably more common and potentially severe with plurally fluorinated (e.g., lomefloxacin, fleroxacin, and sparfloxacin) and, most notably 8-chloro compounds (e.g., clinafloxacin and sitafloxacin) [3,100]. It results from absorption of light by quinolones or their metabolites in tissue, following which transfer of photo energy releases oxygen radicals, allowing damage to lipids in cell membranes [102]. Differences between fluoroquinolones are dramatic: clinafloxacin and Bay 3118 were withdrawn and sparfloxacin incurred special labeling to warn of this effect, while the 8-methoxyquinolones moxifloxacin and gatifloxacin have minimal phototoxic potential [100,101, 103,104].

Skeletal problems remain a theoretical possibility in children, but tendinitis and tendon rupture have occurred in a small number of adults [105]. The effect may be more common with pefloxacin but occurs with all agents, most frequently affects the Achilles tendon, is often associated with prior corticosteroid therapy, and, although resolving spontaneously in the majority, may persist for several months in around 10% of patients.

A new effect, dose-related prolongation of the QT interval, was noted during investigation of sparfloxacin, and subsequent close surveillance of exposed populations revealed a number of ventricular arrhythmias possibly associated with therapy [106]. It has been responsible for the withdrawal of grepafloxacin, which was recognized to cause QT prolongation and subsequently reported to cause torsade de pointes (a malignant ventricular tachyrhythmia associated with QT prolongation) and seven possibly related cardiac deaths [107]. QT prolongation is a quinolone class effect and, as others, varies in degree between agents. However, all quinolones that have been tested cause QT prolongation in animals and, in sufficient quantity (far higher than human dosage), may precipitate ventricular arrhythmias, usually torsade de pointes. Very rare reports have associated sparfloxacin, grepafloxacin, and levofloxacin with ventricular arrhythmias in man, but so far no other agents have been implicated. Prolongation of the corrected (QTc) interval may be caused by other drugs, notably macrolides, antiarrhythmics, terfenadine, and cisapride, and is associated with various risk factors. These include female gender, aging, ischemic and other cardiac disease, and electrolyte disturbance. Risk factors may combine to precipitate arrhythmias [107]. All new quinolones are now labeled as causing QTc prolongation and having potential for cardiac rhythm disturbances.

INTERACTIONS WITH OTHER DRUGS

Significant interactions with other drugs have been described that reduce intestinal absorption after oral administration and may result in potentially serious problems via inhibition of various metabolic pathways, notably the cytochrome P450 system in the liver and γ-aminobutyric acid (GABA) neuroinhibitory receptors in the brain [108].

INTERACTIONS REDUCING ABSORPTION

Metallic cations significantly reduce oral absorption of fluoroquinolones by chelation in the gut. Coadministration of antacids—notably combinations of aluminum and magnesium hydroxide (Maalox)—from 2 hours before to 6 hours after dosing consistently reduces bioavailability by 30–90%. Sucralfate has similar effects. Such combinations may result in therapeutic failure [109]. Oral iron and, to a lesser extent, multivitamin–zinc complexes reduce quinolone bioavailability [110].

Although most such interactions are clinically inapparent, a study of hospital inpatients suggested that up a third receiving ciprofloxacin also received agents known to chelate the drug in the gut [111]. The possibility of therapeutic failure due to impaired absorption is clearly possible, and education of prescribers is necessary.

Coadministration of fluoroquinolones with food does not significantly reduce absorption although C_{max} values are decreased. H2 antagonists do not affect absorption except with enoxacin, for which bioavailability is decreased by 40%, but agents with effects on gastric motility (e.g., pirenzepine) may prolong the absorption phase [109].

METABOLIC AND INHIBITORY INTERACTIONS

The most clinically significant interaction between some fluoroquinolones and other drugs occurs with xanthine derivatives, most importantly with theophylline but also with caffeine. Inhibition of the cytochrome P450 system and resulting reduction in plasma clearance may cause nausea, vomiting, and, almost exclusively with enoxacin, convulsions during coadministration of theophylline [112]. The reduction in clearance is most pronounced with enoxacin and grepafloxacin, less so with pefloxacin and ciprofloxacin, and either absent or insignificant (<10%) with later derivatives [108,113,114]. Neither sparfloxacin, levofloxacin, trovafloxacin, moxifloxacin, nor gatifloxacin significantly inhibit theophylline metabolism [34]. Enoxacin must not be coadministered with theophylline, and dosage of the latter, especially the intravenous form, should either be discontinued or closely monitored (with appropriate modification) during coadministration of ciprofloxacin or pefloxacin. Fluoroquinolones also interfere with caffeine metabolism via similar mechanisms, and both resultant sleep disturbance and upper gastrointestinal symptoms may be clinically apparent [108].

Synergistic inhibition of CNS GABA receptors by fluoroquinolones and NSAIDs may cause neuroexcitatory phenomena. The effects of fluoroquinolones on the GABA receptor are dose dependent and vary between group members, the ability of which to induce convulsions in mice when combined with biphenyl acetate (the active metabolite of fenbufen) is also quite different [115]. In man, convulsions have only been reported in Japanese patients receiving both enoxacin and fenbufen [116]. The interaction between NSAIDs and other (notably, newer-generation) fluoroquinolones may be of little clinical significance [34].

CONCLUSION

The fluoroquinolone antibacterials have established a firm position in the management of moderate to severe infections, caused by a range of—mostly Gram-negative—pathogens in most of the major organ systems. In some areas (e.g., pyelonephritis, gonorrhoea, enteric fevers, oral management of osteomyelitis, and *P. aeruginosa* infections), they have become drugs of choice, often replacing parenteral therapy with cephalosporins and aminoglycosides. However, bacterial resistance has appeared not only in predictable species (e.g., staphylococci and *P. aeruginosa*) but also among organisms (e.g., *E. coli*) initially thought unlikely to be thus compromised [25,28–32].

Original fluoroquinolones were perceived to be relatively inactive against Gram-positive bacteria, and clinical failures, although in a minority, supported this view. The newer agents—including the 8-methoxyquinolones moxifloxacin and gatifloxacin, together with gemifloxacin—have greatly enhanced anti-pneumococcal potency while retaining potency similar to ciprofloxacin against the enterobacteria. Their place in RTI therapy, at a time when burgeoning multiresistance among both pneumococci and *H. influenzae* increasingly compromises therapy [117], appears ensured. However, quinolone resistance is now being reported and has clear implications for widespread use of the class, notably in sick elderly patients [118]. Considerations of potential cardiac adverse effects in this group [107], however rare, may also influence prescribing.

Other new indications may include extensions to the limited range of pediatric applications, for example, bacterial meningitis, pneumococcal and atypical pneumonias, and suppurative otitis media. These agents also exhibit potency against anaerobes and may, as did trovafloxacin [73], find a major place in intraabdominal and pelvic infection, as monotherapy replacements for cumbersome combinations.

However, the safety of the newest drugs, while established in large prelicensing studies [99–101], is only now being confirmed in uncontrolled populations. The temafloxacin debacle, the abrupt demise of trovafloxacin, and the later withdrawal of grepafloxacin convincingly argue the case for some form of statutory postmarketing surveillance. The newer agents will undoubtedly be used extensively by primary care physicians worldwide, not always appropriately [119]. The effect of the exposure of populations, perhaps including children, to such potent agents, may have at-present-unanticipated ramifications for the epidemiology and etiology of disease. It is hoped that these effects will be positive.

REFERENCES

1. Lesher, G. Y., Froelich, E. D., Gruet, M. D., *et al.* (1962). 1,8 naphthyridine derivatives. A new class of chemotherapeutic agents. *J. Med. Pharmacol. Chem.* **5**, 1063–1068.
2. Blum, M. D., Graham, D. J., and McCloskey, C. A. (1994). Temafloxacin syndrome: Review of 95 cases. *Clin. Infect. Dis.* **18**, 946–950.
3. Domagala, J. M. (1994). Structure–activity and structure–side-effect relationships for the quinolone antibacterials. *J. Antimicrob. Chemother.* **33**, 685–706.
4. Crumplin, G. C., and Smith, J. T. (1976). Nalidixic acid and bacterial chromosome replication. *Nature (London)* **260**, 643–645.
5. Gellert, M., Mizuuchi, K., O'Dea, M. H., and Nash, H. A. (1976). DNA gyrase: An enzyme that introduces superhelical turns into DAN. *Proc. Natl. Acad. Sci. U.S.A.* **73**, 3872–3876.
6. Gellert, M., Mizuuchi, K., O'Dea, M. H., *et al.* (1977). Nalidixic acid resistance: A second genetic character involved in DNA gyrase activity. *Proc. Natl. Acad. Sci. U.S.A.* **74**, 4772–4776.
7. Wang, J. C. (1985). DNA topoisomerases. *Annu. Rev. Biochem.* **54**, 665–697.
8. Gootz, T. D., and Brighty, K. E. (1996). Fluoroquinolone antibacterials: SAR, mechanism of action, resistance and clinical aspects. *Med. Res. Rev.* **16**, 433–486.

9. Shen, L. S., Mitscher, L. A., Sharma, P. N., O'Daniel, T., Chu, W. T., and Cooper, C. S. (1989). Mechanism of inhibition of DNA gyrase by quinolone antibacterials: A cooperative drug-DNA binding model. *Biochemistry* **28**, 3886–3894.

10. Neu, H. C. (1993). Synergy and antagonism of fluoroquinolones with other classes of antimicrobial agents. *Drugs* **45** (Suppl. 3), 54–58.

11. Dalhoff, A., Petersen, U., and Endermann, R. (1996). In vitro activity of Bay 12-8039, a new 8-methoxyquinolone. *Chemotherapy (Basel)* **42**, 410–425.

12. Felmingham, D., Robbins, M. J., Ingley, K., *et al.* (1997). In vitro activity of trovafloxacin, a new fluoroquinolone, against recent clinical isolates. *J. Antimicrob. Chemother.* **39** (Suppl. B), 43–49.

13. Woodcock, J. M., Andrews, J. M., Boswell, F. J., Brenwald, N. P., and Wise, R. (1997). In vitro activity of BAY 12-8039, a new fluoroquinolone. *Antimicrob. Agents Chemother.* **41**, 101–106.

14. Blondeau, J. M. (1999). A review of the comparative in vitro activities of 12 antimicrobial agents, with a focus on five new respiratory quinolones. *J. Antimicrob. Chemother.* **43** (Suppl. B), 1–11.

15. McCloskey, L., Moore, T., Niconovich, N., Donald, B., Broskey, J., Jakielaszek, C., Tittenhouse, S., and Coleman, K. (2000). The in vitro potency of gemifloxacin against a range of recent clinical isolates from the USA. *J. Antimicrob. Chemother.* **45** (Suppl. 1), 13–20.

16. Ball, P. (1994). Bacterial resistance to fluoroquinolones: Lessons to be learned. *Infection* **22** (Suppl. 2), S140–S147.

17. Cruciani, M., and Basseti, D. (1994). The fluoroquinolones as treatment for infections caused by Gram-positive bacteria. *J. Antimicrob. Chemother.* **33**, 403–417.

18. Piddock, L. J. V. (1994). New quinolones and Gram-positive bacteria. *Antimicrob. Agents Chemother.* **38**, 163–169.

19. Edelstein, P. H. (1998). Antimicrobial chemotherapy for legionnaires disease: Time for a change. *Ann. Intern. Med.* **129**, 328–330.

20. Bryan, L. E., Bedard, J., Wong, S., and Chamberland, S. (1989). Quinolone antimicrobial agents: Mechanisms of action and resistance development. *Clin. Invest. Med.* **12**, 14–19.

21. Wolfson, J. S., and Hooper, D. C. (1989). Bacterial resistance to quinolones: Mechanisms and clinical importance. *Rev. Infect. Dis.* **11** (Suppl. 5), S960–S968.

22. Kaatz, G. W., and Seo, S. M. (1995). Inducible Nor-A mediated multi-drug resistance in *Staphylococcus aureus*. *Antimicrob. Agents Chemother.* **39**, 2650–2655.

23. Janoir, C., Zeller, V., Kitzis, M. D., Moreua, N. J., and Gutmann, L. (1996). High level fluoroquinolone resistance in *Streptococcus pneumoniae* requires mutations in par C and gyr A. *Antimicrob. Agents Chemother.* **40**, 2760–2764.

24. Courvalin, P. (1990). Plasmid-mediated 4 quinolone resistance: A real or apparent absence. *Antimicrob. Agents Chemother.* **34**, 681–684.

25. Ball, P. (1990). Emergent resistance to ciprofloxacin amongst *Pseudomonas aeruginosa* and *Staphylococcus aureus*: Clinical significance and therapeutic approaches. *J. Antimicrob. Chemother.* **26** (Suppl. F), 165–179.

26. Thornsberry, C. (1994). Susceptibility of clinical bacterial isolates to ciprofloxacin in the United States. *Infection* **22** (Suppl. 2), S80–S89.

27. Kresken, M., Hafner, D., Mittermayer, H., *et al.* (1994). Prevalence of fluoroquinolone resistance in Europe. *Infection* **22** (Suppl. 2), S90–S98.

28. Oteo, J., Aracil, B., Hoyo, J. F., *et al.* (1999). Do the quinolones still constitute valid empirical therapy for community acquired urinary tract infections in Spain. *Clin. Microbiol. Infect.* **5**, 654–656.

29. Ball, P. (1994). Is resistant *Escherichia coli* bacteremia an inevitable outcome for neutropenic patients receiving a fluoroquinolone as prophylaxis. *Clin. Infect. Dis.* **20**, 560–563.

30. Muder, R. R., Brennen, C., Goetz, A. M., Wagener, M. M., and Rihs, J. D. (1991). Association with prior fluoroquinolone therapy of widespread ciprofloxacin resistance among Gram-negative isolates in a Veterans Affairs Medical Center. *Antimicrob. Agents Chemother.* **35**, 256–258.

31. Pena, C., Albareda, J. M., Pallares, R., Pujol, M., Tubau, F. E., and Ariza, J. (1995). Relationship between quinolone use and emergence of ciprofloxacin-resistant *Escherichia coli* in bloodstream infections. *Antimicrob. Agents Chemother.* **39**, 520–524.

32. Garau, J., Xercavins, M., Rodriguez-Carballeira, M., *et al.* (1999). Emergence and dissemination of quinolone-resistant *Escherichia coli* in the community. *Antimicrob. Agents Chemother.* **43**, 2736–2741.

33. Bazile Pham Khac, S., Truong, Q. C., and Lafont, J.-P., *et al.* (1996). Resistance to fluoroquinolones in *Escherichia coli* isolated from poultry. *Antimicrob. Agents Chemother.* **40**, 1504–1507.

34. Stein, G. E. (1996). Pharmacokinetics and pharmacodynamics of newer fluoroquinolones. *Clin. Infect. Dis.* **23** (Suppl. 1), S19–S24.

35. Gerding, D. N., and Hitt, J. A. (1989). Tissue penetration of the new quinolones in humans. *Rev. Infect. Dis.* **11** (Suppl. 5), S1046–S1057.

36. Decre, D., and Bergogne-Berezin, E. (1993). Pharmacokinetics of quinolones with special reference to the respiratory tree. *J. Antimicrob. Chemother.* **31**, 331–343.

37. Wise, R. (1999). A review of the clinical pharmacology of moxifloxacin, a new 8-methoxyquinolone, and its potential relation to therapeutic efficacy. *Clin. Drug Invest.* **17**, 365–387.

38. Wise, R., and Honeybourne, D. (1999). Pharmacokinetics and pharmacodynamics of fluoroquinolones in the respiratory tract. *Eur. Respir. J.* **14**, 221–229.

39. Soman, A., Honeybourne, D., Andrews, J., Jevons, G., and Wise, R. (1999). Concentrations of moxifloxacin in serum and pulmonary compartments following a single 400-mg dose in patients undergoing fibre-optic bronchoscopy. *J. Antimicrob. Chemother.* **44**, 835–838.

40. Fillastre, J. P., Leroy, A., Moulin, B., Dhib, M., Borsa-Lebas, F., and Humbert, G. (1990). Pharmacokinetics of quinolones in renal insufficiency. *J. Antimicrob. Chemother.* **26** (Suppl. B), 51–60.

41. Sorgel, F. (1989). Metabolism of gyrase inhibitors. *Rev. Infect. Dis.* **11** (Suppl. 5), S119–129.

42. Borner, K., and Lode, H. (1986). Biotransformation von ausgewahlten Gyrasehemmern. *Infection* **14** (Suppl. 1), 54–59.

43. Lode, H., Hoffken, G., Boeckk, M., Deppermann, N., Borner, K., and Koeppe, P. (1990). Quinoline pharmacokinetics and metabolism. *J. Antimicrob. Chemother.* **26** (Suppl. B), 41–49.

44. Montay, G., and Gaillot, J. (1990). Pharmacokinetics of fluoroquinolones in hepatic failure. *J. Antimicrob. Chemother.* **26** (Suppl. B), 61–67.

45. Neu, H. C. (1987). Clinical use of the quinolones. *Lancet* **2**, 1319–1322.

46. Naber, K. G. (1989). Use of quinolones in urinary tract infections and prostatitis. *Rev. Infect. Dis.* **11** (Suppl. 5), S1321–S1337.

47. Andriole, V. T. (1991). Use of quinolones in treatment of prostatitis and lower urinary tract infections. *Eur. J. Clin. Microbiol. Infect. Dis.* **10**, 343–345.

48. Fang, G., Brennen, C., Wagener, M., *et al.* (1991). Use of ciprofloxacin versus use of aminoglycosides for therapy of complicated urinary tract infection: Prospective, randomised clinical and pharmacokinetic study. *Antimicrob. Agents Chemother.* **35**, 1849–1855.

49. Ludlam, H. A., Barton, I., White, L., McMullin, C., King, A., and Phillips, I. (1990). Intraperitoneal ciprofloxacin for the treatment of peritonitis in patients receiving continuous ambulatory peritoneal dialysis (CAPD). *J. Antimicrob. Chemother.* **25**, 843–851.

50. Rose, T. F., Ellis-Pegler, R., Collins, J., and Small, M. (1990). Oral pefloxacin mesylate in the treatment of continuous ambulatory peritoneal dialysis associated peritonitis: An open, non-comparative study. *J. Antimicrob. Chemother.* **25**, 853–859.

51. Ridgway, G. L. (1993). Quinolones in sexually transmitted diseases. *Drugs* **45** (Suppl. 3), 134–138.

52. Hook, E. W., Pinson, G. B., Blalock, C. J., and Johnson, R. B. (1996). Dose-ranging study of CP 99,219 (Trovafloxacin) for treatment of uncomplicated gonorrhoea. *Antimicrob. Agents Chemother.* **40**, 1720–1721.

53. Lee, B. L., Padula, A. M., Kimbrough, R. C., Jones, S. R., Chaisson, R. E., Mills, J., and Sande, M. A. (1991). Infectious complications with respiratory pathogens despite ciprofloxacin. *New Engl. J. Med.* **325**, 520–521.

54. Ball, P. (1999). New fluoroquinolones: Real and potential roles. *Curr. Infect. Dis. Repts.* **1**, 470–479.

55. Ball, P. (2000). Future of the quinolones. *Sem. Respir. Infec.* In press.

56. File, T. M., Segreti, J., Dunbar, L., *et al.* (1997). A multicenter, randomised study comparing the efficacy and safety of intravenous and/or oral levofloxacin versus ceftriaxone and/or cefuroxime axetil in treatment of adults with community acquired pneumonia. *Antimicrob. Agents Chemother.* **41**, 1965–1972.

57. Tremolieres, F., de Kock, F., Pluck, N., and Daniel, R. (1998). Trovafloxacin versus high dose amoxicillin (1 g three times daily) in the treatment of community acquired bacterial pneumonia. *Eur. J. Clin. Microbiol. Infect. Dis.* **17**, 447–453.

58. Niederman, M., Church, D., Kaufmann, M., and Springsklee, M. (2000). Does appropriate antibiotic treatment influence outcome in community-acquired pneumonia (CAP)? *Respir. Med.* **94** (Suppl. A), A14.

59. Gallagher, K. M., L'Italien, G. J., Mauskopf, J., *et al.* (1999). Abbreviated length of stay in hospitalised patients with community acquired pneumonia treated with gatifloxacin. *Abstr. 39th Intersci. Conf. Antimicrob. Agents Chemother.*, San Francisco. Abstr. #2246.

60. Banerjee, D., and Honeybourne, D. (1999). The role of fluoroquinolones in chronic obstructive pulmonary disease. *Curr. Opin. Infect. Dis.* **12**, 543–547.

61. Chodosh, S., DeAbate, C. A., Haverstock, D., *et al.* for the Bronchitis Study Group (2000). Short-course moxifloxacin therapy for treatment of acute bacterial exacerbations of chronic bronchitis. *Respir. Med.* **94**, 18–27.

62. DeAbate, C. A., McIvor, R. A., McElvaine, P., Skuba, K., and Pierce, P. F. (1999). Gatifloxacin vs. cefuroxime axetil in patients with acute exacerbations of chronic bronchitis. *J. Respir. Dis.* **20** (Suppl. 11), S23–S29.

63. Fink, M. P., Snydman,, D. R., Niederman, M. S., *et al.* (1994). Treatment of severe pneumonia in hospitalised patients: Results of a multicenter, randomised, double blind trial comparing intravenous ciprofloxacin with imipenem-cilastatin. *Antimicrob. Agents Chemother.* **38**, 547–557.

64. Akalin, H. E. (1995). Role of quinolones in the treatment of diarrhoeal diseases. *Drugs* **49** (Suppl. 2), 128–131.

65. Gotuzzo, E., and Carrillo, C. (1994). Mini review: Quinolones in typhoid fever. *Infect. Dis. Clin. Pract.* **3**, 345–351.

66. Green, S., and Tillotson, G. (1997). Use of ciprofloxacin in developing countries. *Pediatr. Infect. Dis. J.* **16**, 150–159.

67. Bennish, M. L., Salam, M. A., and Khan, W. A. (1992). Treatment of shigellosis, III: Comparison of one or two dose ciprofloxacin with standard 5-day therapy. *A randomised, blinded trial.* *Ann. Intern. Med.* **117**, 727–734.

68. Gotuzzo, E., Seas, C., Echevarria, J., *et al.* (1995). Ciprofloxacin for the treatment of cholera: A randomised, double-blind, controlled trial of a single daily dose in Peruvian adults. *Clin. Infect. Dis.* **20**, 1485–1490.

69. Salam, I., Katelaris, P., Leigh-Smith, S., *et al.* (1994). Randomised trial of single-dose ciprofloxacin for travellers diarrhoea. *Lancet* **344**, 1537–1539.

70. Wistrom, J., and Norrby, R. (1990). Antibiotic prophylaxis of travellers' diarrhoea. *Scand. J. Infect. Dis.* **22** (Suppl. 70), 111–129.

71. Wistrom, J., and Norrby, R. (1995). Fluoroquinolones and bacterial enteritis: When and for whom. *J. Antimicrob. Chemother.* **36**, 23–39.

72. Gentry, L. O. (1991a). Review of quinolones in the treatment of infections of the skin and skin structure. *J. Antimicrob. Chemother.* **28** (Suppl. C), 97–110.

73. Weigelt, J. A., and Faro, S. (1998). Antimicrobial therapy for surgical prophylaxis and for intra-abdominal and gynecologic infections. *Am. J. Surg.* **176** (Suppl. 6A), 1S–3S.

74. Waldvogel, F. A. (1989). Use of quinolones for the treatment of osteomyelitis and septic arthritis. *Rev. Infect. Dis.* **11** (Suppl. 5), S1259–S1263.

75. Gentry, L. O. (1991b). Oral antimicrobial therapy for osteomyelitis. *Ann. Intern. Med.* **114**, 986–987.

76. Desplaces, N., Guttman, L., Carlet, J., Guibert, J., and Acar, J. F. (1986). The new quinolones and their combinations with other agents for therapy of severe infections. *J. Antimicrob. Chemother.* **17** (Suppl. A), 25–39.

77. Meunier, F., Zinner, S., Gaya, H., *et al.* (1991). Prospective randomised evaluation of ciprofloxacin versus piperacillin plus amikacin for empiric antibiotic therapy of febrile granulocytopenic cancer patients with lymphomas and solid tumours. *Antimicrob. Agents Chemother.* **35**, 873–878.

78. Davis, R., Markham, A., and Balfour, J. A. (1996). Ciprofloxacin: An updated review of its pharmacology, therapeutic efficacy and tolerability. *Drugs* **51**, 1019–1074.

79. Dekker, A., Rozenberg-Arska, M., and Verhoef, J. (1987). Infection prophylaxis in acute leukaemia: A comparison of ciprofloxacin with trimethoprim-sulfamethoxazole and colistin. *Ann. Intern. Med.* **106**, 7–12.

80. Karp, J. E., Merz, W. G., Hendricksen, C., *et al.* (1987). Oral norfloxacin for prevention of Gram-negative bacterial infections in patients with acute leukemia and granulcytopenia: A randomised, double blind, placebo-controlled trial. *Ann. Intern. Med.* **106**, 1–7.

81. Gaunt, P. N., and Lambert, B. E. (1988). Single-dose ciprofloxacin for the eradication of pharyngeal carriage of *Neisseria meningitidis*. *J. Antimicrob. Chemother.* **21**, 489–496.

82. Paladino, J. A., Sperry, H. E., Backes, J. M., *et al.* (1991). Clinical and economic evaluation of oral ciprofloxacin after an abbreviated course of intravenous antibiotics. *Am. J. Med.* **91**, 462–470.

83. Quintilliani, R., and Nightingale, C. (1994). Transitional antibiotic therapy. *Infect. Dis. Clin. Pract.* **3** (Suppl. 3), S161–S167.

84. Hamilton-Miller, J. M. T. (1996). Switch therapy: The theory and practice of early change from parenteral to non-parenteral antibiotic administration. *Clin. Microbiol. Infect.* **2**, 12–19.

85. Gentry, L. O., Rodriguez-Gomez, G., Kohler, R. B., Khan, F. A., and Rytel, M. W. (1992). Parenteral followed by oral ofloxacin for nosocomial pneumonia and community acquired pneumonia requiring hospitalisation. *Am. Rev. Respir. Dis.* **145**, 31–35.

86. Guay, D. R. (1993). Sequential antimicrobial therapy: A realistic approach to cost containment? *Pharmacoeconomics* **3**, 341–344.

87. Balfour, J. A., and Faulds, D. (1993). Oral ciprofloxacin: A pharmacoeconomic evaluation of its use in the treatment of serious infections. *Pharmacoeconomics* **3**, 389–421.

88. Paladino, J. A. (1995). Pharmacoeconomic comparison of sequential IV/oral ciprofloxacin versus ceftazidime in the treatment of nosocomial pneumonia. *Can. J. Hosp. Pharmacol.* **48**, 276–283.

89. Graham, E., Whalen, E., Smith, M. E., *et al.* (1994). Comparison of costs between ciprofloxacin and imipenem for the treatment of severe pneumonia in hospitalised patients. *Pharmacotherapy* **14**, 370–371.

90. Grossman, R., Mukherjee, J., Vaughan, D., and the Canadian Ciprofloxacin Health Economic Study Group (1998). A 1-year community-based health economic study of ciprofloxacin vs. usual antibiotic treatment in acute exacerbations of chronic bronchitis. *Chest* 113, 131–141.

91. Marrie, T. J., Lau, C. Y., Wheeler, S., Wong, C. J., Vandervoort, M. K., Feagan, B. G., and the Capital Study Investigators (2000). A controlled trial of a critical pathway for treatment of community acquired pneumonia. *JAMA* **283**, 749–755.

92. Schaad, U. B., Salam, M. A., Aujard, Y., *et al.* (1995). Use of fluoroquinolones in pediatrics: Consensus report of an International Society of Chemotherapy commission. *Pediatr. Infect. Dis. J.* **14**, 1–9.

93. Burkhardt, J. E., Walterspiel, J. N., and Schaad, U. B. (1997). Quinolone arthropathy in animals and children. *Clin. Infect. Dis.* **25**, 1196–1204.

94. Jick, S. (1997). Ciprofloxacin safety in a pediatric population. *Pediatr. Infect. Dis. J.* **16**, 130–134.

95. Hampel, B., Hullmann, R., and Schmidt, H. (1997). Ciprofloxacin in pediatrics: Worldwide clinical experience based on compassionate use—safety report. *Pediatr. Infect. Dis. J.* **16**, 127–129.

96. Grenier, B. (1989). Use of the quinolones in cystic fibrosis. *Rev. Infect. Dis.* **11** (Suppl. 5), S1245–S1252.

97. McCullers, J. A., English, B. K., and Novak, R. (2000). Isolation and characterization of vancomycin-tolerant *Streptococcus pneumoniae* from the cerebrospinal fluid of a patient who developed recrudescent meningitis. *J. Infect. Dis.* **181**, 369–373.

98. Hiramatsu, K., Hanaki, H., Ino, T., Yabuta, K., Oguri, T., and Tenover, F. C. (1997). Methicillin resistant *Staphylococcus aureus* clinical strain with reduced vancomycin susceptibility. *J. Antimicrob. Chemother.* **40**, 135–136.

99. Ball, P., Mandell, L., Niki, Y., and Tillotson, G. (1999). Comparative tolerability of the newer fluoroquinolone antibacterials. *Drug Saf.* **21**, 407–421.

100. Lipsky, B. A., and Baker, C. A. (1999). Fluoroquinolone toxicity profiles: A review focusing on newer agents. *Clin. Infect. Dis.* **28**, 352–364.

101. Breen, J., Skuba, K., and Grasela, D. (1999). Safety and tolerability of gatifloxacin, an advanced third-generation 8-methoxy fluoroquinolone. *J. Respir. Dis.* **20** (Suppl. 11), S70–S76.

102. Takayama, S., Hirohashi, M., Kato, M., and Shimada, H. (1995). Toxicity of quinolone antibacterial agents. *J. Toxicol. Environ. Health* **45**, 1–45.

103. Man, I., Murphy, J., and Ferguson, J. (1999). Fluoroquinolone phototoxicity: A comparison of moxifloxacin and lomefloxacin in normal volunteers. *J. Antimicrob. Chemother.* **43** (Suppl. B), 77–82.

104. Ferguson, J., McEwen, J., Gohler, K., Mignot, A., and Watson, D. (1998). A double-blind, placebo- and positive-controlled, randomised study to investigate the phototoxic potential of gatifloxacin, a new fluoroquinolone antibiotic. *Abstr. 6th Int. Symp. New Quinolones*, Denver.

105. Royer, R. J., Pierfitte, C., and Netter, P. (1994). Features of tendon disorders with fluoroquinolones. *Therapie* **49**, 75–76.

106. Jaillon, P., Morganroth, J., Brumpt, I., *et al.* (1996). Overview of electrocardiographic and cardiovascular safety data for sparfloxacin. *J. Antimicrob. Chemother.* **37** (Suppl. A), 161–167.

107. Ball, P. (2000). Quinolone-induced QT interval prolongation: A not so unexpected class effect. *J. Antimicrob. Chemother.* **45**, 557–559.

108. Janknegt, R. (1990). Drug interactions with quinolones. *J. Antimicrob. Chemother.* **26** (Suppl. D), 7–29.

109. Deppermann, K.-M., and Lode, H. (1993). Fluoroquinolones: Interaction profile during enteral absorption. *Drugs* **45** (Suppl. 3), 65–72.

110. Polk, R. E., Healy, D. P., Sahai, J. V., Drwal, L., and Pracht, E. (1989). Effect of ferrous sulfate and multivitamins with zinc on the absorption of ciprofloxacin in normal volunteers. *Antimicrob. Agents Chemother.* **11**, 1841–1844.

111. Lomaestro, B. M., and Lesar, T. S. (1994). Continuing problem of ciprofloxacin administered with interacting drugs. *Am. J. Hosp. Pharmacol.* **51**, 832.

112. Wijnands, W. J. A., van Heerwarden, C. L. A., and Vree, T. B. (1984). Enoxacin raises plasma theophylline concentration. *Lancet* **2**, 108–109.

113. Wijnands, W. J. A., Vree, T. B., and van Heerwarden, C. L. A. (1986). The influence of quinolone derivatives on theophylline clearance. *Br. J. Clin. Pharmacol.* **22**, 677–83.

114. Radandt, J. M., Marchbanks, C. R., and Dudley, M. N. (1992). Interactions of fluoroquinolones with other drugs: Mechanisms, variability, clinical significance and management. *Clin. Infect. Dis.* **14**, 272–284.

115. Akahane, K., Sekiguchi, M., Une, T., and Osada, Y. (1989). Structure–epileptogenic relationship of quinolones with special reference to their interaction with gamma-aminobutyric acid receptor sites. *Antimicrob. Agents Chemother.* **33**, 1704–1708.

116. Hori, S., Shimada, J., Saito, A., Matsuda, M., and Mitahara, T. (1989). Comparison of the inhibitory effects of new quinolones on gamma-aminobutyric acid receptor binding in the presence of anti-inflammatory drugs. *Rev. Infect. Dis.* **11** (Suppl. 5), 1397–1398.

117. Thornsberry, C., Jones, M. E., Hickey, M. L., Mauriz, Y., Kahn, J., and Sahm, D. (1999). Resistance surveillance of *Streptococcus pneumonia, Haemophilus influenzae* and *Moraxella catarrhalis* isolated in the Unites States, 1997–1998. *J. Antimicrob. Chemother.* **44**, 749–759.

118. Chen, D. K., McGeer, A., de Azavedo, J. C., and Low, D. E., for the Canadian Bacterial Surveillance Network (1999). Decreased susceptibility of *Streptococcus pneumoniae* to fluoro-quinolones in Canada. *New Engl. J. Med.* **341**, 233–239.

119. Frieden, T. R., and Mangi, R. J. (1990). Inappropriate use of oral ciprofloxacin. *JAMA* **264**, 1438–1440.

120. Barry, A. L., and Fuchs, P. C. (1997). Antibacterial activities of grepafloxacin, ciprofloxacin, ofloxacin and fleroxacin. *J. Chemother.* **9**, 9–16.

121. Bauernfeind, A. (1997). Comparison of the antibacterial activities of the quinolones Bay 12-8039, gatifloxacin (AM1155), trovafloxacin, clinafloxacin, levofloxacin and ciprofloxacin. *J. Antimicrob. Chemother.* **40**, 639–651.

122. Child, J., Andrews, J. M., Boswell, F., Brenwald, N., and Wise, R. (1995). The in vitro activity of CP 99,219, a new naphthyridone antimicrobial agent: A comparison with fluoroquinolone agents. *J. Antimicrob. Chemother.* **35**, 869–876.

123. Spangler, S. K., Jacobs, M. R., and Appelbaum, P. C. (1994). Activity of CP 99,219 compared with those of ciprofloxacin, grepafloxacin, metronidazole, cefoxitin, piperacillin, and piperac-illin-tazobactam against 489 anaerobes. *Antimicrob. Agents Chemother.* **38**, 2471–2476.

124. Neu, H. C., and Chin, N.-X. (1994). In vitro activity of the new fluoroquinolone CP 99,219. *Antimicrob. Agents Chemother.* **38**, 2615–2622.

125. Bremner, D. A., Dickie, A. S., and Singh, K. P. (1988). In vitro activity of fleroxacin compared to three other quinolones. *J. Antimicrob. Chemother.* **22** (Suppl. D), 19–23.

126. Haria, M., and Lamb, H. M. (1997). Trovafloxacin. *Drugs* **54**, 435–445.

127. Perry, C. M., Barman Balfour, J. A., and Lamb, H. (1999). Gatifloxacin. *Drugs* **58**, 683–696.

128. King, A., May, J., French, G., and Phillips, I. (2000). The comparative in vitro potency of gemifloxacin. *J. Antimicrob. Chemother.* **45** (Suppl. 1), 1–12.

129. Drusano, G. L. (1989). Pharmacokinetics of the quinolone antimicrobial agents. In "Quinolone Antibacterial Agents," 2nd ed. (D. C. Hooper and J. S. Wolfson, Eds.), pp. 71–105. American Society for Microbiology, Washington, DC.

130. Lode, H., Hoffken, G., Prinzing, C., *et al.* (1987). Comparative pharmacokinetics of new quinolones. *Drugs* **34** (Suppl. 1), 21–25.

131. Paton, J. H., and Reeves, D. S. (1988). Fluoroquinolone antibiotics: Microbiology, pharmacokinetics and clinical use. *Drugs* **36**, 193–228.

CHAPTER 2

Chemistry and Mechanism of Action of the Quinolone Antibacterials

KATHERINE E. BRIGHTY* and THOMAS D. GOOTZ[†]

*Department of Medicinal Chemistry and [†]*Department of Respiratory, Allergy, Immunology, Inflammation, and Infectious Diseases, Central Research Division, Pfizer, Inc., Groton, Connecticut 06340*

INTRODUCTION

Over the past fifteen years, fluoroquinolones have gained substantial prominence in the therapy of bacterial infections. Ciprofloxacin is still the most widely used agent in this class, due to its broad spectrum and excellent oral bioavailability [1]. Further development of the structure–activity relationships (SAR) in the fluoroquinolone class has produced a large number of new quinolones, many of which have been advanced to clinical testing in the last decade. Most of these new agents possess improved activity against Gram-positive pathogens compared to ciprofloxacin, and some have potent activity against anaerobes and pathogens that are resistant to many other groups of antimicrobials [2]. The myriad structural modifications that have been investigated have also led to improvements in pharmacokinetic properties and lessening of a number of adverse effects.

The mechanism of action of these new agents, however, is still inhibition of bacterial topoisomerases. The enzyme DNA gyrase was originally identified as the target of the quinolones and remains a major focus of research. The more recently discovered topoisomerase IV provides a second target for the fluoroquinolones (see the section on "Mechanism of Action").

This chapter describes the SAR that has been exploited to provide new fluoroquinolones with potent activity and favorable *in vivo* properties, and discusses the most recent advances made in our knowledge concerning the mechanism by which fluoroquinolones kill bacteria.

STRUCTURAL AND HISTORICAL BACKGROUND

Quinolone antibacterial research and development has enjoyed an enormous worldwide effort since the early 1960s. During this time, more than 10,000 structurally related agents have been described in many hundreds of patents and journal articles. The product of this wealth of research has been a continually improving progression of marketed quinolone antibacterial agents. From the early days of Gram-negative-selective agents limited to treatment of urinary tract infection, the field has matured to provide broad-spectrum drugs capable of treating not only urinary tract infections but also systemic infections caused by Gram-positive and Gram-negative pathogens at sites ranging from skin to joints to the respiratory tract. Some newer agents incorporate activity against anaerobic pathogens, making them useful in surgical and gynecological infections. The pharmacokinetic performance of these agents has also been optimized, allowing for once-daily dosing of a subset of the newer fluoroquinolones.

In the first half of this chapter, an overview of the structural evolution of the quinolone agents is presented, with emphasis on the modifications that have provided advances in therapeutic utility. For ease of discussion, the examples largely consist of marketed quinolones and those in late-stage development, including a few whose development has been halted; the general structural themes, however, are representative of the much larger arena of investigational quinolone research. The reader is referred to numerous comprehensive reviews of SAR in the quinolone field [2–5].

GENERAL STRUCTURAL FEATURES
OF THE QUINOLONES

As is evident from Figures 1 through 6, certain quinolone structural features remain constant throughout the class. Quinolone agents exhibit a bicyclic aromatic core; this can contain a carbon at the 8-position, yielding a true quinolone, or a nitrogen, which provides a ring system technically termed a naphthyridone (Figure 1). In common usage, however, both quinolone and naphthyridone structures are encompassed in the class descriptor "quinolone antibacterial agents." Antibacterial activity requires the presence of the pyridone ring on the right-hand side, as shown in a general way in Figure 1. The carboxylic

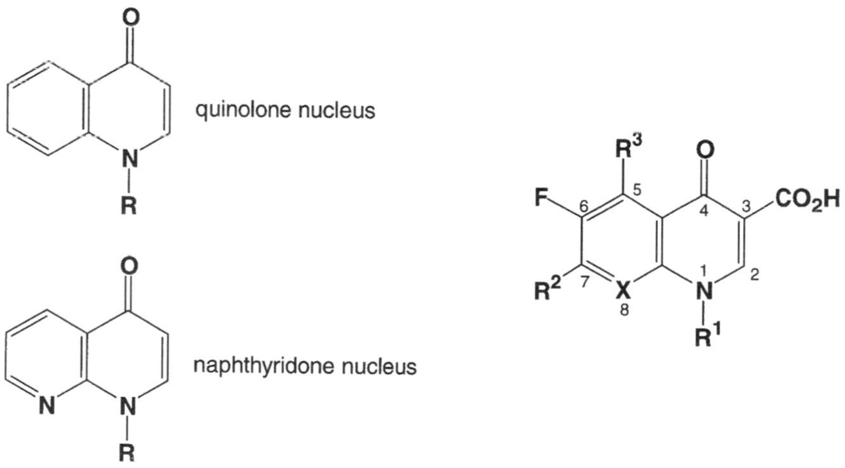

FIGURE 1   Quinolone and naphthyridone nuclei; general structural features required for antibacterial activity.

acid at the 3-position and the ketone at C-4 are required, as is the R^1-substituted nitrogen at the 1-position.[1] Substitution at C-2 is generally deleterious, although exceptions have been described in which the C-2 substituent forms a ring with R^1 (see NM394 and prulifloxacin, Figures 4 and 8). In the left-hand ring, the fluorine at C-6 is found in essentially all the modern agents; it is because of this substituent that the class is often referred to as the fluoroquinolones (but see section on "Compounds Lacking the C-6 Fluorine"). A cyclic diamine R^2 is most often present, attached through one of its nitrogens to the 7-position.[2] Some variation is permitted at C-5 and the 8-position. Although the older quinolone agents were generally unsubstituted at C-5 (R^3 = hydrogen), several more recent compounds bear small substituents such as amino or methyl at this site. At the 8-position, when X = carbon, a number of small substituents such as fluorine, chlorine, and methoxy have been found to provide improved potency.

In all the figures, structures represent racemic compounds unless they are labeled with stereochemical descriptors.

FIRST-GENERATION QUINOLONES

The first quinolone antibacterial agent had its origins in a serendipitous discovery in the early 1960s. In the course of carrying out a synthesis of chloroquine, chemists at the Sterling–Winthrop laboratories in Rensselaer, New York, isolated compound **1** (Figure 2) as a byproduct, which was found to exhibit some antibacterial activity. Iterative chemical modification, through synthesis of similar compounds and assessment of their relative potency, led to the discovery of nalidixic acid (Figure 2), an agent with moderate activity against Gram-negative organisms, and the first of the quinolone antibacterials [6]. Nalidixic acid was introduced in the United States in 1963 as a therapeutant for urinary tract infections.

---

[1]It is a fascinating aspect of the quinolone field that, over time, almost all the dogma regarding structural requirements for activity has fallen, through the ingenuity of chemists in designing new modifications (see reviews cited in [2–5]). Thus, nearly all the strict requirements outlined in the text have exceptions in the research literature (see the section on "Future Directions"). In terms of marketed and late-stage clinical agents, these structural features have held constant. However, note T-3811 in the section on "Compounds Lacking the C-6 Fluorine."

[2]These diamines are generally based on 5- and 6-membered rings:

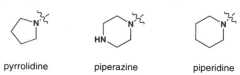

pyrrolidine   piperazine   piperidine

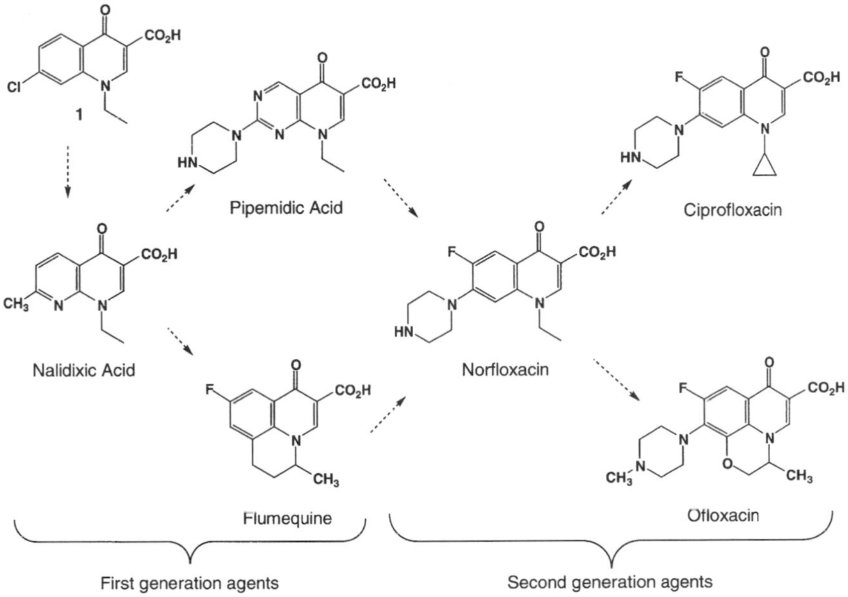

FIGURE 2   Historical evolution of quinolones.

This new class of antibacterials sparked substantial worldwide interest in preparing and testing compounds of this type. Through the 1960s and 1970s, a number of related agents were developed (Figure 3). These first-generation quinolones reflect the early experimentation with the original nalidixic acid structure. Although all these agents retain a nitrogen atom at the 1-position, the naphthyridone structure of nalidixic acid was modified by returning to the quinolone nucleus (e.g., oxolinic acid) of the original lead compound **1**. Insertion of additional nitrogen atoms into the quinolone and naphthyridone nuclei was effected at the 2-position (cinoxacin) and the 6-position (piromidic and pipemidic acids). Additional rings were fused at the 6- and 7-positions (oxolinic acid and cinoxacin) and across the 1- and 8-positions (flumequine). Addition of cyclic amines as substituents at the 7-position produced piromidic and pipemidic acids. The ethyl group on the nitrogen at the 1-position was left relatively constant; it was thought at that point that an N-1 substituent could not be larger than ethyl and retain good antibacterial potency [7].

These compounds generally displayed increased Gram-negative activity over nalidixic acid, but lacked useful activity against Gram-positive cocci (flumequine and oxolinic acid are the only first-generation agents with any substantial

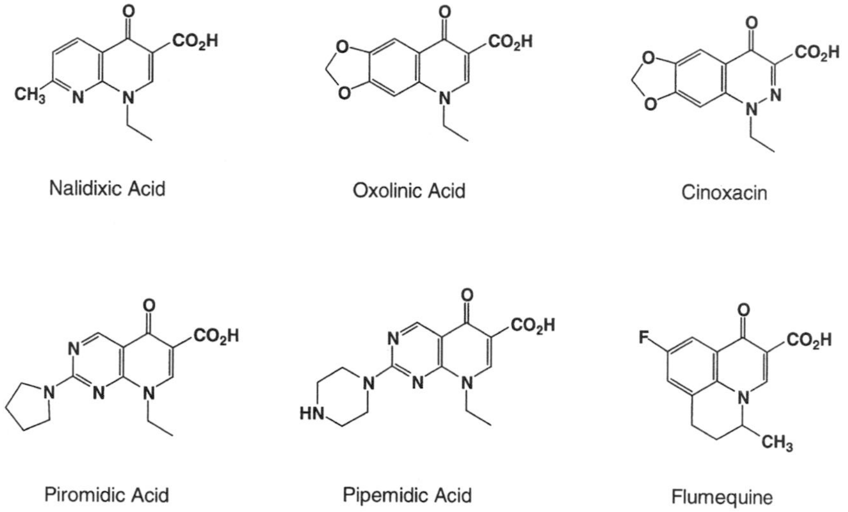

Nalidixic Acid   Oxolinic Acid   Cinoxacin

Piromidic Acid   Pipemidic Acid   Flumequine

FIGURE 3   First-generation quinolones.

Gram-positive activity), *Pseudomonas aeruginosa*, and anaerobes. They were, however, generally well absorbed after oral administration and attained high concentrations in the urinary tract, making them useful therapeutically for treatment of urinary tract infections [8,9].

SECOND-GENERATION QUINOLONES

A major advance in the quinolone field came in 1980, when chemists at the Kyorin company reported the preparation of norfloxacin, in which the cyclic diamine piperazine found in pipemidic acid is combined with the 6-fluorine found in flumequine (Figures 2 and 4) [10]. Norfloxacin exhibits some Gram-positive activity in addition to improved Gram-negative action over the earlier agents, but in practice is confined to the historical quinolone indications of urinary tract infection and treatment of sexually transmitted disease and prostatitis, due to poor serum levels and tissue distribution. Norfloxacin was the first of the fluoroquinolones, so named because of the fluorine at the 6-position. Later studies revealed that introduction of this atom serves both to increase quinolone activity against the enzyme target DNA gyrase and to facilitate penetration into the bacterial cell [11]. The utility of the 6-fluorine in enhancing potency is so substantial that it has remained essentially inviolate in the quinolones investigated since 1980 (see, however, the section on "Compounds Lacking the C-6 Fluorine").

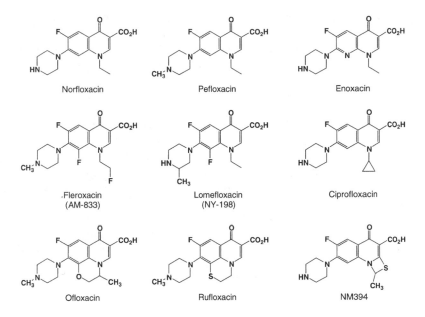

FIGURE 4 Second-generation quinolones.

Some of the modifications to the norfloxacin structure (Figure 4) seem relatively modest, yet the properties of the resulting analogues can be markedly altered, attesting to the potent influence of chemical structure on biological properties. For instance, addition of a methyl group to the distal nitrogen of the piperazine in norfloxacin yields pefloxacin, which exhibits a half-life more than twice that of norfloxacin [12]. Enoxacin, the naphthyridone analogue of norflox-acin, possesses roughly similar antibacterial activity but improved bioavailability over norfloxacin [13].

Introduction of fluorine atom(s) and addition of a methyl group onto the piperazine of norfloxacin produced fleroxacin and lomefloxacin (Figure 4). Although the antibacterial potency of these compounds is not generally improved over norfloxacin, they exhibit extended half-lives and significantly improved oral absorption [4]. Both of these compounds can be dosed once daily in the treatment of a variety of systemic infections.

Replacement of the N-1 ethyl group of norfloxacin by a cyclopropyl group yielded ciprofloxacin (Figures 2 and 4), which displays improved MIC values against Gram-positive and Gram-negative pathogens [14]. Ciprofloxacin, intro-duced in the United States in 1987 and the first of the quinolones to be useful in a variety of infections beyond the urinary tract and sexually transmitted diseases, is widely prescribed in the treatment of lower respiratory tract, skin, and joint infections.

Ofloxacin (Figure 4) has a nucleus that again borrows a feature from the first-generation quinolones: the tricyclic core is reminiscent of flumequine (Figure 2). Ofloxacin, marketed in the United States in 1991, was the second of the more broadly useful fluoroquinolone agents and has also been applied in a variety of systemic infections [15]. Rufloxacin (Figure 4) is derived from ofloxacin through replacement of the ring oxygen by a sulfur atom. Although this compound is generally less potent than norfloxacin [16], it is of note due to its unusual pharmacokinetics. The half-life of rufloxacin has been measured at >28 hr [2], significantly longer than any of the other quinolones. NM394, a later entry into the second generation, exhibits Gram-positive and Gram-negative activity similar to that of ciprofloxacin (see the section on "Activity against Gram-Negative Pathogens"). As mentioned above, this unusual structure is a departure from typical quinolones due to the C-2 substitution.

The N-1 ethyl group is present in all of these bicyclic compounds except NM394, in which the ethyl is now part of a four-membered ring, and ciprofloxacin; the cyclopropane of ciprofloxacin subsequently became the predominantly employed N-1 substituent, as can be seen by the later compounds shown in Figures 5 and 6, whereas the ethyl group has fallen almost completely out of use.

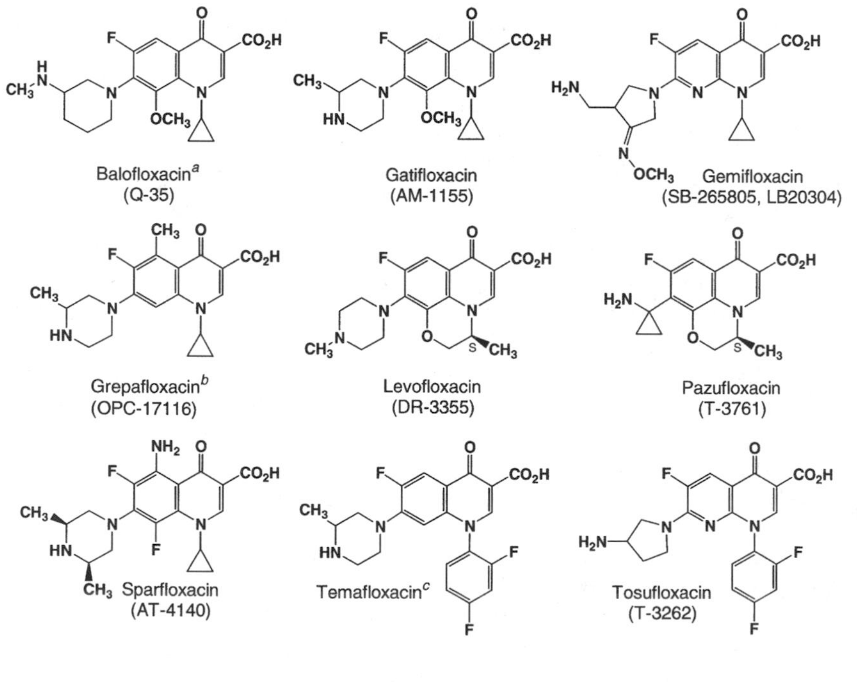

FIGURE 5   Third-generation quinolones.
Notes: [a]development discontinued; [b]withdrawn from the market in October 1999; [c]withdrawn from the market in 1992 [32].

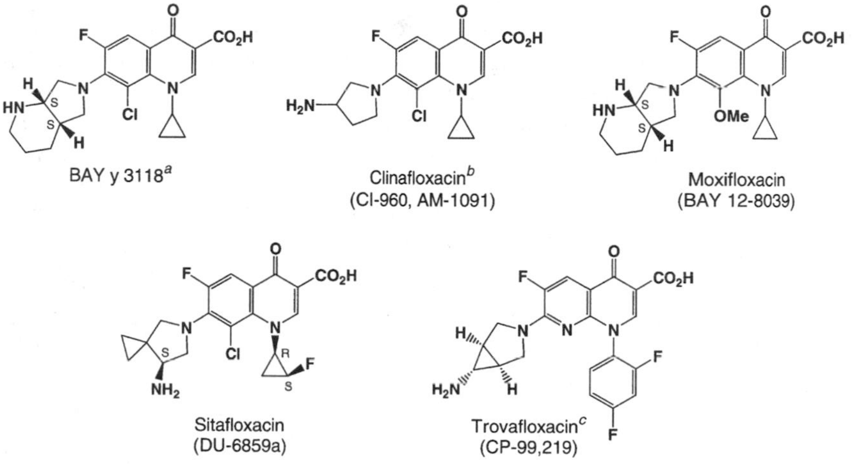

BAY y 3118[a]

Clinafloxacin[b]
(CI-960, AM-1091)

Moxifloxacin
(BAY 12-8039)

Sitafloxacin
(DU-6859a)

Trovafloxacin[c]
(CP-99,219)

FIGURE 6   Fourth-generation quinolones.
Notes: [a]development discontinued; [b]development discontinued in December 1999; [c]limited to serious infections in institutional settings as of June 1999.

In the second-generation quinolones, it is also notable that the piperazine ring remains relatively undisturbed, except for alkylation on the distal nitrogen or, less frequently, on the ring carbons. As can be seen from the later quinolones (Figures 5 and 6), use of a cyclic amino group at C-7 is almost universal. The presence of a second amine, in addition to the nitrogen bonded to C-7 of the quinolone nucleus, is not required for *in vitro* activity, but has been found to be important for good activity *in vivo* [17].[3]

These second-generation compounds are characterized by good to excellent Gram-negative activity, with ciprofloxacin exhibiting the strongest Gram-nega-

---

[3]It is interesting to note that nadifloxacin, the sole marketed modern quinolone without a distal amine, is a topical agent [18]:

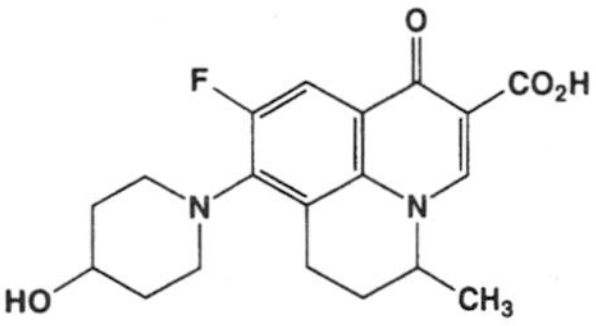

Nadifloxacin
(OPC-7251)

tive spectrum. These potency improvements are directly related to increasing potency against the enzyme target DNA gyrase. A linear correlation has been identified between the MIC against *Escherichia coli* for these agents and interaction with gyrase, as measured either by inhibition of supercoiling or cleavable complex formation [19]. The Gram-positive potency of these agents is also enhanced over that of the first-generation quinolone agents. However, these compounds are characterized by only moderate activity versus *Staphylococcus aureus*, a fact that may have contributed to the rapid rise in resistance to quinolones among methicillin-resistant *S. aureus* (MRSA) shortly after the introduction of ciprofloxacin into hospital usage [20]. Additional deficiencies in the spectrum of these agents lie in the areas of anaerobes, against which only marginal activity is observed, and the important respiratory Gram-positive pathogen *Streptococcus pneumoniae*. These agents also require multiple doses per day, with the exception of lomefloxacin, fleroxacin, and rufloxacin. While these three quinolones do offer once-daily dosing, their antibacterial potency is substantially less than that of ciprofloxacin. Fleroxacin and lomefloxacin also induce substantial photosensitivity [21]. All these deficiencies are addressed in the third generation of quinolone agents.

THIRD- AND FOURTH-GENERATION QUINOLONES

These newer compounds are characterized by increasing structural novelty and complexity (Figure 7), which has resulted in new and useful characteristics. Increased activity against Gram-positive cocci (particularly *S. pneumoniae*) over that of ciprofloxacin is the criterion applied to place agents in the third generation of quinolones, while potent activity against anaerobes was used to separate a subset of these agents into a fourth generation. In some cases, enhanced potency is combined with improved pharmacokinetics, such that the agents can be dosed once daily [22].

In this section, the structural modifications in the newer agents that have resulted in this enhanced antibacterial potency against important pathogens are highlighted. Additional characteristics that are central to the development of improved human therapeutants, such as pharmacokinetics, selectivity, and minimized potential for adverse effects, are also examined for their response to chemical modification. It is worthy of mention that, although certain substituents can impart improvements in a particular biological or chemical property, the overall characteristics of each molecule are derived from the interaction of all the substituents with each other and with the specific nucleus employed. For more detailed discussion of SAR, generally organized by position about the quinolone nucleus, the reader is referred to a number of earlier reviews (e.g., [2–5]).

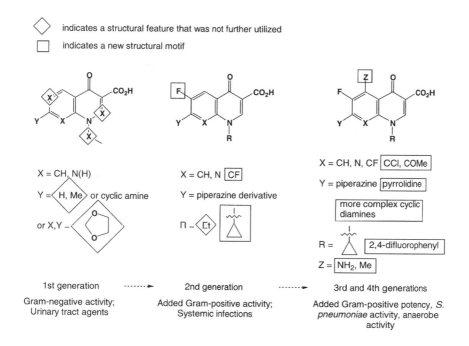

◇ indicates a structural feature that was not further utilized

▢ indicates a new structural motif

1st generation · · · · · ▶ **2nd generation** · · · · · ▶ **3rd and 4th generations**

Gram-negative activity; Urinary tract agents

Added Gram-positive activity; Systemic infections

Added Gram-positive potency, *S. pneumoniae* activity, anaerobe activity

FIGURE 7   Structural evolution of quinolones.

In vitro Potency

Overall Potency

The N-1 cyclopropyl group, which was originally described for ciprofloxacin, remains one of the most effective functionalities for providing broad-spectrum activity against aerobic organisms. Combination of the N-1 cyclopropyl with a fluorine or chlorine substituent at C-8, as in a number of newer quinolones (Figures 5 and 6), further enhances antibacterial activity [23]. Clinafloxacin, sitafloxacin, and BAY y 3118, all of which bear a chlorine atom at C-8, are among the most potent broad-spectrum agents that have been in development, and are the only compounds shown here that exhibit Gram-negative activity superior to that of ciprofloxacin [2,24,25]. Unusual SAR was found in the case of gemifloxacin (Figure 5), where the naphthyridone nucleus provided MICs improved over those of the corresponding C-8 chloroquinolone [26]. The typical potency enhancement observed on C-8 halogenation was originally suggested to result from improvement in cell penetration [11,23]. More recent work has shown, however, that the presence of a C-8 chlorine improves activity against both DNA gyrase and topoisomerase IV enzymes [27,28]. Excellent correlations were found between quinolone activity against *E. coli* DNA gyrase and MICs versus *E. coli* for a number of marketed and developmental agents. Similar correlations exist between antibacterial activity against *S. aureus* and inhibitory potency against *S. aureus* topoisomerase IV [27,28].

A C-8 methoxy group, in combination with an N-1 cyclopropane, reliably increases Gram-positive activity compared to the corresponding 8-unsubstituted quinolone, although a halogen atom can be more effective in this regard. Gram-negative potency is increased in some cases, but by less than the improvement offered by fluorine or chlorine [29]. An example is the decreased activity of moxifloxacin (Figure 6) compared to BAY y 3118 [24,30]. The only difference between these compounds is in replacement of the C-8 chlorine of the discontinued BAY y 3118 by a methoxy group in moxifloxacin, which nonetheless exhibits potent broad-spectrum activity, roughly equivalent to that of trovafloxacin [30].

The activity of the N-1 cyclopropyl C-8 substituted agents can depend further on the group at C-7. A pyrrolidine substituent in particular (see clinafloxacin, Figure 5) gives the most dramatic increase in activity on C-8 halogenation [31]. It is important to note, however, that, in addition to their potency benefits, some C-8 substituents can bring in undesirable effects, either on their own (see the section on "Phototoxicity") or in combination with an N-1 cyclopropyl group (see the section on "Selectivity").

Activity against Representative Gram-Positive Pathogens

Staphylococcus aureus

This is an area in which all of the third- and fourth-generation fluoroquinolones show improvement over ciprofloxacin [2,24,33]. As mentioned above, combination of the N-1 cyclopropane with a C-8 substituent can improve both Gram-positive and Gram-negative activity. Increasing the lipophilicity of a quinolone, however, as has been effected in many third- and fourth-generation agents, generally tends to increase potency against Gram-positive organisms while somewhat attenuating Gram-negative potency. Thus, the third- and fourth-generation compounds (Figures 5 and 6) exhibit improved activity over ciprofloxacin against *S. aureus* but, with the exception of clinafloxacin, sitafloxacin, and BAY y 3118, lesser activity against the Enterobacteriaceae [2,33]. This may arise in part through the opposing effects of hydrophobicity on penetration: increasing log D tends to enhance accumulation in *S. aureus* while decreasing penetration into Gram-negative organisms [34].

Lipophilicity can be increased by addition of one or more alkyl groups, which can be introduced at C-5 (grepafloxacin, Figure 5) and/or on the C-7 diamine sidechain (e.g., grepafloxacin, sparfloxacin, gatifloxacin, temafloxacin; see Figure 5). Surprisingly, introduction of the 5-amino group in sparfloxacin also serves to increase lipophilicity [35]. The improvement in Gram-positive activity seen for 5-amino introduction in sparfloxacin, however, is dependent on the presence of the N-1 cyclopropyl group. For most N-1 ethyl derivatives, activity is reduced by a 5-amino group [31].

Use of a 3-aminopyrrolidine sidechain at C-7 generally results in increased Gram-positive activity compared to the piperazine derivative [23,31], whereas Gram-negative potency tends to be competitive with the corresponding piperazine analogue. Clearly, many of the newer agents (e.g., clinafloxacin, sitafloxacin, BAY y 3118, moxifloxacin, tosufloxacin) take advantage of this, using pyrrolidine rings appended at C-7. Tosufloxacin (Figure 5) shows substantially more potent activity versus *S. aureus* than does the related piperazinyl quinolone temafloxacin [33]. In gemifloxacin, the core sidechain is a 3-aminomethylpyrrolidine. In this case, the methyl oxime ether moiety was added to enhance the drug's lipophilicity, improving its Gram-positive activity over that of the des-oxime analogue [26].

Although generally not providing the potency of the N-1 cyclopropyl/C-8 halogenated quinolone motif, use of the 2,4-difluorophenyl N-1 substituent (tosufloxacin, trovafloxacin, temafloxacin; see Figures 5 and 6) also enhances Gram-positive antibacterial activity over the classical ethyl substitution. This substituent, discovered independently by chemists at Abbott and Toyama [3], expanded the established SAR at the time, which held that only small N-1 substituents, similar in size to ethyl and cyclopropyl, could provide good antibacterial activity [7,36]. The 2,4-difluorophenyl and 4-fluorophenyl analogues were among the most potent of a number of substituted aryl groups [36] and have been held relatively constant in N-1 aryl compounds prepared since. Interestingly, combination of the N-1 2,4-difluorophenyl group with a C-8 halogen does not provide the enhanced potency observed for the N-1 cyclopropyl group [37].

Streptococcus pneumoniae

The new compounds, with the exception of pazufloxacin (Figure 5), all show improved activity against *S. pneumoniae* compared to ciprofloxacin. The most potent of these agents are gemifloxacin and BAY y 3118 [24,38], followed by clinafloxacin, sitafloxacin, moxifloxacin and trovafloxacin [2,39]. Balofloxacin, sparfloxacin, tosufloxacin, grepafloxacin, and gatifloxacin (Figure 5) have slightly less activity [2,40,41]. Structurally, it seems that N-1 cyclopropyl, C-8 substituted quinolones, and N-1 cyclopropyl and aryl naphthyridones can provide potent activity against *S. pneumoniae*. The relative activities of the third- and fourth-generation quinolones against *S. pneumoniae* generally mirror their performance against *S. aureus*, but in a number of cases the typical MIC_{90} for *S. pneumoniae* is two to four times higher than that for *S. aureus* [2].

The smallest improvement over ciprofloxacin is seen for levofloxacin and temafloxacin (Figure 5). The pyridobenzoxazine nucleus found in pazufloxacin and levofloxacin provides Gram-positive potency roughly equivalent to a C-8 unsubstituted N-1 cyclopropyl quinolone, as evidenced by the general similarity in Gram-positive activity of ofloxacin and ciprofloxacin [15]. For these pyridobenzoxazines, a C-7 piperazine, as in levofloxacin, is more successful at imparting *S. pneumoniae* potency than is the carbon-linked cyclopropylamine of pazufloxacin. Levofloxacin, as the more potent enantiomer of ofloxacin (see the section on "Stereochemistry"), demonstrates twice the *in vitro* activity of the racemic ofloxacin [42]. In combination with its high serum peak level, this moderate improvement in potency makes levofloxacin a clinically useful drug against *S. pneumoniae* infections.

Given the excellent activity of a number of the new quinolones against *S. pneumoniae*, and the fact that they are equally potent against sensitive and penicillin- and macrolide-resistant *S. pneumoniae* [2], these compounds have also been examined for their activity against other organisms important in respiratory tract infections. Like ciprofloxacin, essentially all the third- and fourth-generation quinolones exhibit excellent activity versus *Haemophilus influenzae* [2,43] and *Legionella pneumophila* [2,43–46]. The third- and fourth-generation agents that have been tested against *Chlamydia pneumoniae*, with the exception of temafloxacin, exhibit improved activity over second-generation quinolones. Levofloxacin, trovafloxacin, and moxifloxacin are two- to fourfold more potent than earlier agents, while grepafloxacin, gatifloxacin, gemifloxacin, sitafloxacin, and sparfloxacin are the most active, with MIC_{90}s as low as 0.03–0.06 µg/ml [43,47,48]. Overall, a number of these new agents are very promising for the empirical treatment of respiratory tract infections.

Activity against *Mycobacterium tuberculosis*

Of the second-generation quinolones, ciprofloxacin and ofloxacin have received the most examination for utility against *M. tuberculosis*. Substantially heightened *in vitro* activity against this pathogen was obtained for the more recent agents sparfloxacin, BAY y 3118, moxifloxacin, sitafloxacin, and gatifloxacin [49–54]. Each of these compounds bears the 8-substituted N-1 cyclopropyl motif. This is in agreement with SAR studies carried out around mycobacterial activity, which have shown that the N-1 cyclopropane provides better activity than the N-1 2,4-difluorophenyl group [55], and that 8-substitution is beneficial [56]. Indeed, none of the three N-aryl agents shown in Figures 5 and 6 have useful activity against *M. tuberculosis* [49,57]. Naphthyridones have been identified as a negative factor in a quantitative structure–activity relationship (QSAR) study around mycobacterial activity [58], which may account for the weak activity of gemifloxacin [59] and further contribute to the poor performance of tosufloxacin and trovafloxacin against *M. tuberculosis*. Levofloxacin, as might be expected, exhibits twofold better activity against *M. tuberculosis* than does the corresponding racemate ofloxacin [49,60].

The lesser activity of clinafloxacin, which displays *M. tuberculosis* activity similar to or just twofold improved over that of ciprofloxacin [49,61], is interesting, considering its generally equivalent activity to the highly potent sitafloxacin and BAY y 3118 against other organisms. All three compounds are built on the same 8-chloroquinolone nucleus, with the only differences residing in the 7-substituent and in the presence of a fluorine on the N-1 cyclopropane of sitafloxacin. The sidechains of sitafloxacin and BAY y 3118 can be looked at as alkylated versions of clinafloxacin, however, consistent with the observation that more highly lipophilic moieties at the 7-position confer improved antimycobacterial activity [55]. The C-7 piperazines of sparfloxacin and gatifloxacin, which are both methylated, may enhance activity in the same way.

Activity against *Mycoplasma pneumoniae*

Although the second-generation quinolones exhibited only moderate activity against *M. pneumoniae*, a number of the newer agents possess activity substantially improved over that of ciprofloxacin and ofloxacin against this pathogen. In particular, clinafloxacin, sitafloxacin, and BAY y 3118 possess very potent activity [2,62]. Sparfloxacin, trovafloxacin, gatifloxacin, moxifloxacin, grepafloxacin, and gemifloxacin have also been characterized as having excellent activity against this pathogen [63-67], whereas balofloxacin and temafloxacin are closer in activity to ciprofloxacin and ofloxacin [63,68]. These activities seem to correlate generally with the *S. aureus* and *S. pneumoniae* potencies of these agents, except for the lowered activity of balofloxacin, which may be due to its somewhat unusual piperidine sidechain.

Activity against Gram-Negative Pathogens

The activity of the newer quinolones against the Enterobacteriaceae is generally strong. Again, sitafloxacin, clinafloxacin, and BAY y 3118 are the most potent agents, outperforming ciprofloxacin against these pathogens [2,25]. Most of the third- and fourth-generation quinolones are slightly less potent than ciprofloxacin; this subset includes sparfloxacin, trovafloxacin, moxifloxacin, pazufloxacin, tosufloxacin, gatifloxacin, gemifloxacin, and levofloxacin [42,69–72]. Agents with reduced activity against the Enterobacteriaceae include balofloxacin and temafloxacin [40,73].

From this breakdown, some structural themes emerge. The 8-chloro compounds once again exhibit the highest level of activity, but 8-methoxy and 8-fluoro groups also provide potency approaching that of ciprofloxacin. Naphthyridone compounds bearing a pyrrolidine-based sidechain and an N-1 aryl group also yield good Gram-negative activity. The potent activity of the second-generation NM394 indicates that the sulfur-containing four-membered ring containing N-1 and C-2 of the quinolone nucleus can replace the N-1 cyclopropane of ciprofloxacin as far as Gram-negative *in vitro* activity is concerned [70]. Again, a correlation can be seen between the MIC against *E. coli* and the inhibition of *E. coli* gyrase [74], although additional factors such as ease of penetration into the bacterial cell also contribute to *in vitro* potency.

Versus *P. aeruginosa*, ciprofloxacin exhibits the most potent activity of the second-generation quinolones. This activity has been difficult to improve upon. Although clinafloxacin and sitafloxacin exhibit lower MICs in some studies, they, along with BAY y 3118 and the second-generation NM394, are often found to be equivalent to ciprofloxacin [2,25,75,76]. Pazufloxacin, trovafloxacin, tosufloxacin, and gemifloxacin are the next most potent agents after ciprofloxacin [57,77,78], with sparfloxacin, grepafloxacin, moxifloxacin, gatifloxacin, and levofloxacin in the following tier [40,42,79–82]. The least potent agents against *P. aeruginosa* are balofloxacin and temafloxacin [40,73].

It is interesting to note that most of the more potent derivatives against *P. aeruginosa* bear C-7 sidechains that are based on a pyrrolidine core (clinafloxacin, sitafloxacin, BAY y 3118, gemifloxacin, trovafloxacin, and tosufloxacin). This may be a reflection of the preponderance of alkylated piperazines in this group of compounds; as mentioned previously, although alkylation improves activity against Gram-positive pathogens, it generally reduces Gram-negative potency somewhat. *P. aeruginosa* clearly highlights the potency-enhancing effect of the C-8 chlorine, as evidenced by the differing activities of BAY y 3118 and moxifloxacin. Of the less commonly used sidechains, it would appear that the aminocyclopropane of pazufloxacin is more favorable for activity against *P. aeruginosa* than the piperazine found in the otherwise identical compound levofloxacin. Comparison of balofloxacin and gatifloxacin indicates that the piperidine sidechain of balofloxacin provides less effectiveness against Gram-negative organisms than does the piperazine moiety. It has been suggested that this results from lower permeation of balofloxacin into *P. aeruginosa*, as its IC_{50} against gyrase from *P. aeruginosa* is less than threefold higher than that of ciprofloxacin, while its MICs are substantially elevated [83].

Activity against Anaerobes

Activity against anaerobes such as *Bacteroides fragilis* is less widespread among these agents than is improved activity against Gram-positive pathogens. The 8-chloro quinolones clinafloxacin, sitafloxacin, and BAY y 3118, which exhibit markedly improved overall activity against aerobes, display excellent potency against anaerobes as well [2,84]. The next tier of agents includes trovafloxacin and moxifloxacin, which possess broad-spectrum anaerobe activity [85,86]. The potential for clinical application of these agents to anaerobic infections is the basis for their separation into a fourth generation of quinolones. Sparfloxacin, gatifloxacin, and grepafloxacin exhibit anaerobe activity improved over ciprofloxacin, but weaker than that of trovafloxacin, moxifloxacin, and the C-8 chloro compounds [87–89]. In a systematic study, introduction of a C-8 halogen, methyl, or methoxy group was shown to enhance activity against *B. fragilis* for both piperazine and 3-aminopyrrolidine-substituted quinolones [3]; utility of the chloro and methoxy groups is exemplified in the fourth-generation compounds. Trovafloxacin exhibits enhanced activity against anaerobes over the structurally related tosufloxacin [87,90], however, indicating a contribution for the C-7 substituent as well. Gemifloxacin exhibits potent activity against many Gram-positive anaerobes, equivalent to sitafloxacin in some cases. Versus Gram-negative anaerobes, however, its activity is variable [91].

Activity against Quinolone-Resistant Organisms

Clinafloxacin, sitafloxacin, and BAY y 3118, all of which bear a C-8 chlorine atom, exhibit potent activity against quinolone-resistant strains, particularly quinolone-resistant *S. aureus* [2,75]. In one study [92], the MICs of clinafloxacin against staphylococci, Enterobacteriaceae, and *P. aeruginosa* strains were less affected by increasing resistance to ciprofloxacin than were those of sparfloxacin and ofloxacin. Sitafloxacin, although exhibiting MIC and gyrase activity similar to those of tosufloxacin and ciprofloxacin against a quinolone-sensitive *P. aeruginosa* strain, proved much more potent than the comparative agents against a set of quinolone-resistant *P. aeruginosa* strains. Examination of sitafloxacin analogues in which either the N-1 fluorine, C-8 chlorine, or C-7 spirocyclopropane had been removed demonstrated that the C-8 chlorine, although having little effect on activity against a sensitive *P. aeruginosa* strain, imparted improved activity against quinolone-resistant strains. Measurement of the inhibitory effects of these analogues against gyrase isolated from each of these strains revealed that the heightened activity provided by the 8-chloro substituent was mediated at the level of the gyrase enzyme. For the most resistant *P. aeruginosa* strain, the gyrase supercoiling IC_{50} for sitafloxacin was 19-fold that of the quinolone-sensitive strain, whereas the corresponding increase for the des-chloro derivative was 196-fold [93].

The 8-methoxy substituent also enhances activity, although to a lesser extent, against quinolone-resistant *S. aureus*, as exemplified by gatifloxacin, moxifloxacin, and balofloxacin [94-96]. A specific role for the 8-methoxy group was originally suggested by a study [94] investigating the bactericidal activity of balofloxacin against quinolone-resistant *S. aureus*. More extensive work has been carried out examining the effects of 8-substitution on bactericidal potency as well as resistance emergence. Addition of an 8-methoxy group to ciprofloxacin increased lethal activity against wild-type *S. aureus* by a factor of 4. Against a *parC* mutant of *S. aureus*, however, the cidal activity was enhanced over ciprofloxacin by 30-fold. Interestingly, an 8-ethoxy analogue gave results similar to ciprofloxacin itself. Evidence was also obtained for an 8-methoxy group enhancing the ability to kill nongrowing cells [97]. In *E. coli*, ciprofloxacin and the same 8-methoxy analogue were shown to exhibit very different abilities to select resistant mutants: at $10 \times$ MIC, numerous colonies were obtained with ciprofloxacin from wild-type *E. coli*, and none with the 8-methoxy analogue. Using an *E. coli* strain with a preexisting *parC* mutation, however, resulted in selection of equal numbers of colonies with the two agents, indicating that topoisomerase IV in *E. coli* is involved in the ability of the C-8 methoxy group to reduce initial selection of resistant mutants [98]. Further studies examining gatifloxacin and its des-methoxy analogue against *E. coli* mutants yielded suggestions for the manner in which gatifloxacin interacts with gyrase [99] (see section on "Models of Fluoroquinolone Interactions with the Topoisomerases").

Fluoroquinolone resistance in *S. pneumoniae* remains low but is increasing in some geographical areas. Strains with decreased susceptibility to quinolones generally carry *parC* and *gyrA* mutations. Gemifloxacin, sitafloxacin, and clinafloxacin retain the highest level of potency against these strains, with MIC_{90}s 4- to 16-fold lower than those of moxifloxacin and trovafloxacin [100,101].

Quinolone resistance can also occur through efflux of drug from the bacterial cell. The most common mechanism for this in *S. aureus* is through elevated expression of the efflux system NorA. It has been noted repeatedly that the more recently developed quinolones are less affected by efflux-mediated resistance, which is frequently attributed to their lower hydrophilicity compared to older quinolones such as norfloxacin and ciprofloxacin [102]. Additional structural factors have been found to decrease interaction with NorA, including the bulkiness of the C-7 sidechain, and the hydrophobicity of the C-8 substituent [103].

As is evident from this discussion, discovery and exploitation of SAR in the quinolone area have resulted in the synthesis of increasingly potent and broad-spectrum agents. *In vitro* activity, however, is just one component of the profile necessary for successful advancement of a compound through clinical study for human use. In the following sections, the effects of structural modification on additional characteristics such as pharmacokinetics, adverse effects, and physico-chemical properties are summarized.

IN VIVO ACTIVITY

Pharmacokinetics

In a number of cases in the research literature, improved half-life and tissue penetration are observed on alkylation of a quinolone agent [2]. This may once more be a result of alkylation serving to increase the lipophilicity of the quinolones. This phenomenon is exemplified by some of the agents in Figures 5 and 6 that possess long half-lives appropriate for once-daily dosing. Grepaflox-acin can be looked at as dimethylated ciprofloxacin; this molecular modification results in substantially improved lung levels in murine studies [104] and a 2.5-fold increase in half-life in humans, to 10.3 hr [2], appropriate for once-daily administration. Sparfloxacin, which bears two alkyl groups on the C-7 piperazine and an additional C-8 fluorine compared to its parent ciprofloxacin, fits this paradigm as well, with a half-life in humans of 17.6 hr [2]. Oral efficacy in murine studies was also found to be enhanced by the presence of the two methyl groups on the piperazine [35]. In addition to its other lipophilic substituents, the 5-amino group has been found to increase the lipophilicity of the agent compared to the des-amino analogue via comparison of the octanol–water partition coefficients (log *P*) [35]. Incorporation of the methyl oxime substituent of gemifloxacin provided a nearly 10-fold improvement in oral bioavailability in rat [26].

In the case of sitafloxacin, alkylation of the C-7 pyrrolidine sidechain with the spirocyclopropane improved pharmacokinetic performance, yielding an increased C_{max} over the unsubstituted pyrrolidine in animal studies [105]. In this series, unlike some of those described previously, the alkylation did not affect antibac-terial activity.

Prulifloxacin (Figure 8) represents an interesting case of temporary alkylation, via use of a prodrug. The parent piperazine NM394 exhibited good *in vitro* activity but poor oral absorption. Addition of the *N*-(5-methyl-2-oxo-1,3-dioxol-4-yl)-methyl group, which is cleaved off to regenerate the unsubstituted piperazinyl quinolone *in vivo*, increased C_{max} and area under the curve (AUC) after oral administration by more than threefold in animal studies [106,107].

The most common position for adjustment of pharmacokinetics, as just evidenced, is on the C-7 substituent [108]. However, the naphthyridone nucleus has also been shown to yield pharmacokinetics improved over those of an 8-unsubstituted quinolone [5]. Trovafloxacin, which exhibits a half-life of 10 hr in humans [2], is one of the few newer quinolone agents that takes advantage of

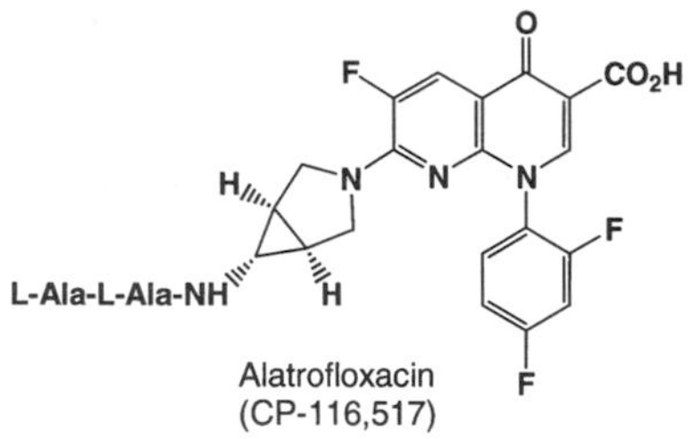

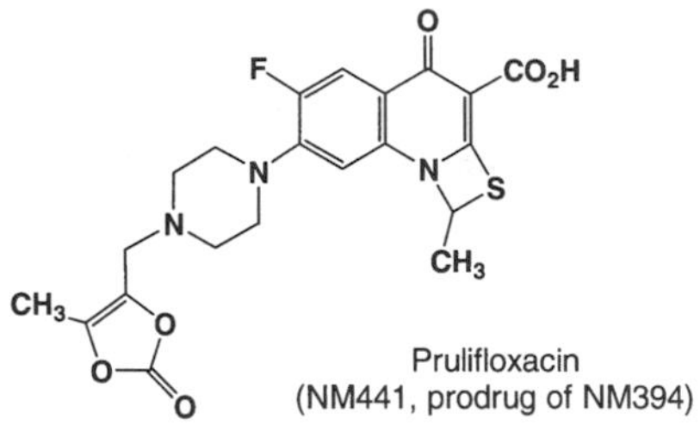

FIGURE 8 Prodrugs of quinolone agents.

this nucleus. The structurally related tosufloxacin requires twice-daily dosing, however, emphasizing the contribution of trovafloxacin's azabicyclo[3.1.0]hexane sidechain. In keeping with the information described, trovafloxacin is judged to be a relatively lipophilic quinolone by its distribution coefficient [109]. Further support for the importance of the 8-position is the fact that C-8 halogens have also been noted to improve *in vivo* activity [23].

Phototoxicity

Phototoxicity is one of the clearest examples of the effect of structure on the biological activity of quinolone agents. Introduction of halogen atoms (fluorine or chlorine) at the C-8 position of the quinolone nucleus results in compounds with an enhanced tendency to induce photosensitivity, both in humans and in animal models. In keeping with this SAR, substantial phototoxicity has been reported for fleroxacin, lomefloxacin, sparfloxacin, clinafloxacin, and BAY y 3118 [21,110,111].

In a number of the newer quinolones, the C-8 halogens have been abandoned in favor of a methoxy group at that position. This substituent also provides improved *in vitro* potency over the unsubstituted analogue (see the section on "Overall Potency"), but without the phototoxicity issues of the halogens [112]. In one example, the development of BAY y 3118 was discontinued, but the 8-methoxy analogue moxifloxacin was recently approved. Moxifloxacin and gatifloxacin have been reported to be free of phototoxicity [113,114]. Interestingly, it may not be merely removal of the halogen atom that results in an improvement in photostability. *In vitro* irradiation experiments with UV light have suggested that the 8-methoxy group in balofloxacin stabilizes the quinolone to degradation [115].

Theophylline Interactions

A number of quinolones have been shown to reduce the clearance of theophylline by inhibiting its cytochrome P450-mediated metabolism. The most significant interaction is seen with enoxacin. Ciprofloxacin, grepafloxacin, and tosufloxacin increase serum levels of theophylline also, but to a lesser extent [116,117].

No significant alteration of theophylline clearance has been seen in clinical trials with sparfloxacin, gatifloxacin, trovafloxacin, temafloxacin, moxifloxacin, levofloxacin, and balofloxacin [2,116-121]. It is notable that many of the C-8-substituted quinolones exhibit no effect on theophylline pharmacokinetics. This effect for 8-fluoro and 8-methoxy groups has been established in an SAR study [112], although in that work naphthyridones were implicated as problematic for theophylline interactions. Tosufloxacin fits this model, but again the bicyclic sidechain of trovafloxacin results in a change in activity, such that trovafloxacin does not affect theophylline pharmacokinetics. The presence of a 3-aminopyrrolidine in tosufloxacin may contribute to the interaction, as clinafloxacin, which bears the same C-7 sidechain, has been reported to increase the AUC of theophylline by two- to threefold, despite the presence of an 8-substituent [123]. Gemifloxacin does not exhibit a theophylline interaction, even though it employs a naphthyridone nucleus [124]. This may be due to the steric encumbrance provided by the methyl oxime adjacent to the aminomethyl group (*vide infra*).

The effect of methylation on the amine sidechain is a subject of debate. Increased bulk around the distal amine has been cited as a method of decreasing theophylline interactions [21]; other workers [122] have found that the position and number of methyl groups on a C-7 piperazine have little effect. Although the methylpiperazine of grepafloxacin does not distinguish it from ciprofloxacin in terms of its theophylline effects, the dimethyl substitution on sparfloxacin may contribute to its lack of interaction. In the case of balofloxacin, the presence of the methyl group on the exocyclic amine was shown to decrease the theophylline interaction compared to an unsubstituted amino group [125]. This may extend to the aminopyrrolidine sidechain: while clinafloxacin exhibits a theophylline interaction (*vide supra*), the structurally similar sitafloxacin was reported to exhibit only a small increase in serum theophylline levels [126]. In this case, the spirocyclopropane adjacent to the amino group on the pyrrolidine C-7 substituent of sitafloxacin may ameliorate the theophylline interaction.

SELECTIVITY: ACTIVITY AGAINST MAMMALIAN TOPOISOMERASE II AND GENETIC TOXICITY

Selectivity for DNA gyrase and topoisomerase IV over the related mammalian enzyme topoisomerase II is of course desirable for antibacterial therapy with quinolones. In the course of selectivity testing of the many quinolones synthesized to date, a number have been found to exhibit potent activity versus the mammalian enzyme; the potential for use of quinolone agents of this type as anticancer agents has been reviewed [127–129]. Certain structural features, most particularly those at N-1, C-7, and the 8-position, have been shown to increase activity versus topoisomerase II, which correlates with an increase in mammalian cytotoxicity and the potential for genetic toxicity [29]. In a general sense, molecular modifications that yield substantially heightened Gram-positive potency can also result in decreased selectivity for the gyrase enzyme [29]. Thus, C-7 pyrrolidines tend to show increased cytotoxicity over piperazines. Even more notable are the N-1 cyclopropyl and C-8 fluorine-, chlorine-, or methoxy-substituted quinolones. A number of studies [21] have shown that this pattern results in heightened cytotoxicity.

In several of the quinolones that have been developed, further structural manipulation has abrogated these structural tendencies, such that selective agents are generated despite the presence of the 8-substituted N-1 cyclopropyl pattern. In sparfloxacin, the two methyl groups on the piperazine ring are critical in this regard. Although sparfloxacin itself is inactive versus topoisomerase II, removal of both methyl groups results in a compound that is very potent against this enzyme. Interestingly, the *cis* stereochemistry of the methyl groups is also important: the *trans* isomer, where the methyl groups are on opposite sides of the piperazine ring, does interact with topoisomerase II [130]. The antibacterial activity of the *trans* dimethyl isomer, however, is unchanged from that of sparfloxacin itself [35].

In the case of sitafloxacin, modification of the N-1 cyclopropane was used in similar fashion. The analogue of sitafloxacin that bears an unsubstituted cyclopropane at N-1 exhibited clastogenicity and was active against topoisomerase II. Sitafloxacin, however, displays an IC_{50} of >1600 µg/ml versus topoisomerase II and displays less than one-tenth the clastogenic activity of the des-fluoro analogue [131,132]. When examined against three stereoisomers bearing enantiomeric aminopyrrolidines and/or N-1 cyclopropanes, sitafloxacin proved to be the least active against human placental topoisomerase II by as much as twofold [27]. Advancement of pazufloxacin into development was supported by its low cytotoxicity and minimal activity against topoisomerase II [133].

Thirteen marketed or late-stage quinolones that span all four generations were examined against both bacterial and mammalian topoisomerases. A good correlation was found between IC_{50}s for inhibition of *S. aureus* topoisomerase IV and inhibition of *E. coli* DNA gyrase. Importantly, neither of the bacterial enzyme activities correlated with activity against HeLa cell topoisomerase II [28].

CHEMICAL PROPERTIES

Aqueous Solubility

Fluoroquinolones as a class are generally fairly insoluble in water. All modern quinolone agents are zwitterionic in character, due to the presence of both a carboxylic acid and a basic amine; pKa values for these functional groups have been reported as 5.5–6.3 for the carboxylic acid and 7.6–9.3 for the distal amino group [134]. At low pH, both the amine and the carboxylic acid are protonated, giving the molecule an overall positive charge. Conversely, at high pH the amine is in the free base form, while the carboxyl group exists as the carboxylate anion, providing a net negative charge. Because of this, quinolones tend to be more soluble in water at acidic and basic pH, with minimum solubility expressed at neutral (physiological) pH values [135]. The crystal packing of quinolones, in which the aromatic nuclei are stacked [74], also contributes to lowered aqueous solubility; this class of agents is characterized by very high melting points, generally >200°C, indicating that the crystal forms are very stable. Extremely low solubility has been measured [136] for some quinolone agents; tosufloxacin, for example, exhibits a water solubility of 0.008 mg/ml at physiological pH [136].

The extent of aqueous solubility becomes particularly important for intravenous administration of quinolone agents. Of the more recent quinolones, an intravenous dosage form has been developed using the parent drug for ciprofloxacin, ofloxacin, fleroxacin, clinafloxacin, levofloxacin, moxifloxacin, gatifloxacin, gemifloxacin, and pazufloxacin. In cases where the intrinsic solubility of quinolones is low, prodrug strategies have been employed. The intravenous formulation for trovafloxacin consists of the highly soluble dipeptide derivative alatrofloxacin (Figure 8), which is hydrolyzed *in vivo* to provide the parent drug [137].

Chelation of Divalent and Trivalent Metal Cations

The well-known effects of antacids and certain mineral supplements in decreasing absorption and bioavailability of fluoroquinolones [138] can be traced to the β-keto-carboxylic acid functionality common to all quinolones (see Figure 1). Through the use of techniques such as infrared spectroscopy and ^{19}F and ^{13}C nuclear magnetic resonance spectroscopy, these groups have been shown to chelate divalent and trivalent metal ions [139,140]. These chemical analyses are supported by *in vivo* studies showing that concurrent administration of aluminum hydroxide affects the absorption of neither a quinolone analogue lacking the carboxylic acid group [122] nor a prodrug of ofloxacin in which the carboxylic acid is masked [141]. The strength of chelation to a quinolone varies with the metal ion, with affinity constants rising in the order $Ca^{2+} < Mg^{2+} < Fe^{3+} < Al^{3+}$ [142]. For a collection of quinolone agents, it was shown that there is a correlation between the stability constants of the quinolone–aluminum chelates and the diminution in AUC on aluminum coadministration. Two 5-amino quinolones were outliers in this analysis, suggesting that the chelate structure may be affected by the presence of a 5-substituent [122]. That the C-4 carbonyl group can interact with a 5-amino group was evidenced by the fact that the intramolecular hydrogen bond between the C-4 carbonyl oxygen and the acidic proton on the C-3 carboxylic acid in sparfloxacin is weaker than the corresponding hydrogen bond in the 5-unsubstituted pefloxacin [139]. In accord with these data, sparfloxacin has been shown to suffer less disruption of absorption on antacid coadministration than other quinolone agents [122].

The decrease in absorption of quinolones in the presence of cations is often attributed to the lower solubility of chelates in the intestinal tract. A mechanistic study [143] of the interaction of levofloxacin with aluminum hydroxide suggested that quinolones may adsorb onto aluminum hydroxide that has reprecipitated in the small intestine due to the higher pH at that site as compared to gastric fluid. It has been found in the laboratory [144] that many chelates are actually more soluble than the parent quinolones, leading to the suggestion [145] that the decrease in lipophilicity that occurs on metal chelation may be an important factor that leads to reduced bioavailability. A different effect has been invoked to explain the decrease in antibacterial activity of quinolones in the presence of high levels of magnesium ions (see the section on "Magnesium Levels").

Stereochemistry

The chemical concept of stereochemistry has become of increasing importance in making decisions regarding the advancement of agents that can exist as isomers. The three-dimensional nature of drugs and the potential for arraying four different substituents on a single carbon in two nonsuperimposable ways result in the existence of stereoisomers for any quinolone agent that has a chiral center (a carbon with four different substituents in a molecule with no mirror plane, such as ofloxacin) or substituents in different positions on a saturated ring (as in sparfloxacin).

Earlier quinolones such as flumequine, ofloxacin, and lomefloxacin were developed as racemates (1:1 mixtures of the mirror images), as are a number of the more recent agents (such as tosufloxacin, grepafloxacin, clinafloxacin, gemifloxacin, and gatifloxacin). It has been found, however, particularly for chiral centers close to the quinolone nucleus, such as the methyl group on the pyridobenzoxazine nucleus of ofloxacin, that the orientation of the substituent can be of critical importance to the compound's antibacterial activity. The (S)-methyl derivative levofloxacin, where the methyl group is designated as coming up above the plane of the page, is from 8- to 128-fold as potent as the (R)-methyl enantiomer *in vitro*, and twice as active as the racemate ofloxacin [146]. Similarly, pazufloxacin is up to 256-fold more potent than its (R) enantiomer [133]. In the case of levofloxacin, an advantage was also obtained as regards aqueous solubility, as levofloxacin was found [147] to be 10-fold more soluble in water than the racemate ofloxacin.

Although the presence or absence of the fluorine on the N-1 cyclopropane did not greatly affect the potency of sitafloxacin [148], the stereochemistry of the fluorine on a closely related series was found to be important. The *cis* orientation of nitrogen and fluorine about the cyclopropane provided more potent Gram-positive activity than did the *trans* isomer. The effect on Gram-negative activity was much smaller [149]. For the four *cis*-fluoro isomers of sitafloxacin itself (the different combinations of enantiomers at the N-1 cyclopropane and at the C-7 aminopyrrolidine), the indicated absolute stereochemistry provided the most potent Gram-positive and Gram-negative activity [105]. More recently, this heightened activity was shown to be mediated at the enzyme level, with sitafloxacin exhibiting more potent activity than its stereoisomers against *E. coli* gyrase and *S. aureus* topoisomerase IV [27].

Chiral centers at C-7 that are at some distance from the quinolone nucleus often contribute less significantly to biological activity. The enantiomers of temafloxacin [150], tosufloxacin [151], moxifloxacin [152], and gemifloxacin [153], for instance, were found to be nearly equipotent. As mentioned previously, however (see the section on "Selectivity"), the relative orientation of the methyl groups on the C-7 piperazine of sparfloxacin is important for enzyme selectivity.

FUTURE DIRECTIONS

Some important discoveries have been made that may expand the SAR of quinolone antibacterial agents into productive new areas.

COMPOUNDS LACKING THE C-6 FLUORINE

The ubiquitous C-6 fluorine, held constant for nearly two decades, has been successfully removed or replaced in a few more recent chemical series. The most advanced of these is T-3811 (Figure 9), currently in phase I clinical trials. T-3811, like the other third- and fourth-generation quinolones, exhibits Gram-positive activity improved over ciprofloxacin [154]. Its activity against penicillin-resistant *S. pneumoniae* is improved over that of trovafloxacin. Versus the Enterobacte-

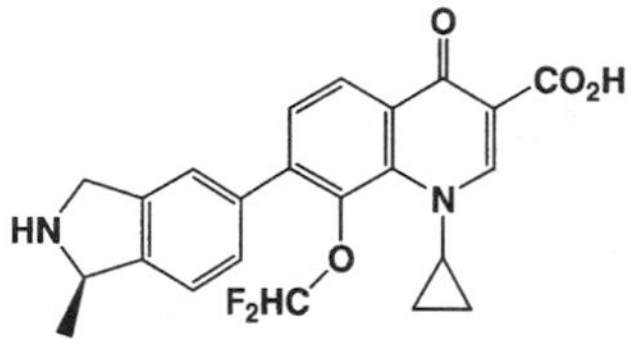

T-3811
Phase I

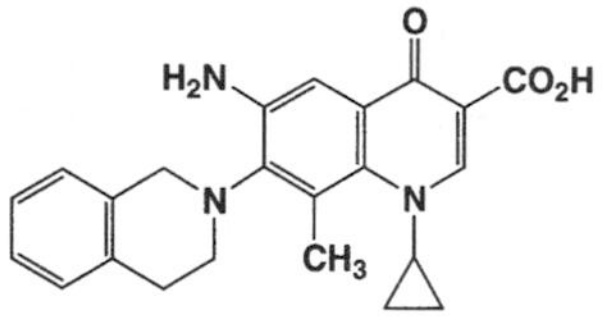

MF 5137
Investigational

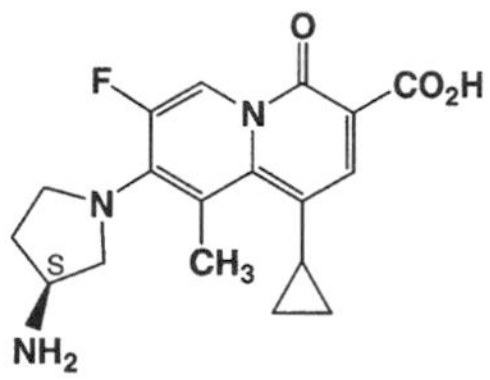

ABT-719
Investigational

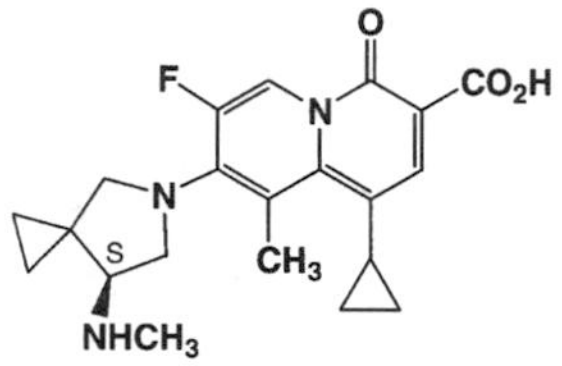

A-170568
Investigational

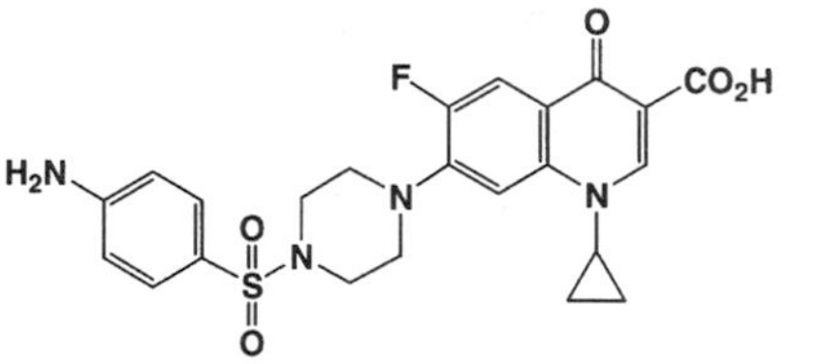

2

FIGURE 9   Selected earlier stage quinolone agents.

riaceae, T-3811 performs similarly to trovafloxacin, with activity against *P. aeruginosa* somewhat less than that of ciprofloxacin. On the basis of the limited anaerobe MIC data available, T-3811 may fall into the fourth generation of quinolones, with potent activity against key pathogens [154].

Removal of the C-6 fluorine was found to be detrimental to activity if the C-8 position is unsubstituted. For compounds bearing an 8-OMe or 8-OCHF$_2$, however, the importance of the 6-fluorine to antibacterial potency is decreased. Interestingly, in a closely related series, intravenous toxicity was decreased by removal of the 6-fluorine. T-3811 represents a departure from previously developed quinolones in additional structural aspects as well. Attachment of an aromatic group bonded directly to the C-7 carbon of the quinolone nucleus was utilized in rosoxacin in the 1970s, but compounds of this type have not progressed in a number of years. Other structural features of T-3811 were developed through toxicological examination. The 8-OCHF$_2$ decreased convulsive activity on intracerebral injection compared to the 8-methoxy derivative, as did introduction of the methyl group on the C-7 sidechain. The regiochemistry and stereochemistry of the methyl group was chosen for maximum antibacterial activity [155].

A series of 6-amino derivatives has been described that retains Gram-positive and Gram-negative activity, albeit inferior to that of ciprofloxacin [156]. It was subsequently found, however, that addition of a methyl group at the 8-position served to enhance activity, and that use of a tetrahydroisoquinoline at the 7-position provided a compound (MF 5137, Figure 9) with Gram-positive activity superior to that of ciprofloxacin [157], and an MIC_{90} against *S. pneumoniae* eightfold lower than that of ciprofloxacin [158]. MF 5137 proved as efficacious as ciprofloxacin in an *S. aureus* septicemia mouse model on oral or subcutaneous administration [157].

2-PYRIDONES

In another expansion of quinolone SAR, a series of antibacterial quinolizin-4-ones has been reported [159,160]. Generically referred to as 2-pyridones, these agents display a reorganized quinolone nucleus in which the nitrogen at the 1-position has been moved to the ring junction (see ABT-719, A-170568, Figure 9). These agents still serve to inhibit the gyrase and topoisomerase IV enzymes, however, despite this substantial structural modification [161]. The SAR of this series parallels that of the quinolones in large part, with the fluorine atom providing heightened potency against both Gram-positive and Gram-negative organisms, and a cyclopropane at the position corresponding to N-1 of the quinolone nucleus giving better activity than an ethyl group. As in the case of the quinolones, a distal amine seems to be required for *in vivo* activity. ABT-719, the most intensively examined member of this series, is an analogue of an N-1 cyclopropyl quinolone, where the cyclopropane is now bonded to a carbon atom. A methyl group at the position corresponding to C-8 of the quinolone skeleton was found to be useful in this case as well, where it proved superior to fluoro, chloro, and methoxy substituents. ABT-719 exhibits Gram-positive activity superior to that of clinafloxacin. Versus the Enterobacteriaceae, it was similar to or slightly better than ciprofloxacin and clinafloxacin, whereas *P. aeruginosa* activity was improved fourfold over ciprofloxacin. Activity against anaerobes was similar to that of clinafloxacin, and ABT-719 exhibited more potent activity than clinafloxacin against quinolone-resistant *S. aureus* and *P. aeruginosa* [162,163]. In animal models of infection, ABT-719 gave improved efficacy over ciprofloxacin against Gram-positive organisms, with Gram-negative efficacy similar to ciprofloxacin [164]. A more recent entry is A-170568, which bears a sidechain closely related to that of sitafloxacin [165,166]. While exhibiting less potent activity against *P. aeruginosa* than ABT-719, A-170568 retains potent activity against ciprofloxacin-resistant Gram-positive organisms, and excellent activity against *B. fragilis*. Importantly, this change in the sidechain structure results in a substantial decrease in the activity against the human topoisomerase II enzyme, and an increase in the murine intraperitoneal LD_{50} compared to ABT-719. While the analogue lacking the methyl on the amino group was a slightly more potent antibacterial than A-170568, it did not exhibit the same improvement in LD_{50} and topoisomerase II activities [165].

ALTERATION OF PRIMARY ENZYMATIC TARGET

Much research has been carried out to determine the primary target enzymes for fluoroquinolones, which have been found to vary between different organisms and quinolones (see section on "DNA Gyrase versus Topoisomerase IV"). Interest is high in obtaining agents with equivalent activity against both gyrase and topoisomerase IV, in the hope of minimizing the selection of resistant organisms. Sitafloxacin has been shown to have this desirable dual activity against enzymes from *S. pneumoniae* [167,168]. Some divergence in primary target in *S. pneumoniae* has been observed, with sparfloxacin and gatifloxacin reported to target gyrase, and a number of other quinolones having topoisomerase IV as primary target [169] (see [167] and the section on "DNA Gyrase versus Topoisomerase IV," however, for some inconsistencies with these conclusions).

The advanced stage quinolones that have been studied are disparate enough in structure that the SAR for enzyme selectivity is difficult to discern. One paper reports that the primary target of ciprofloxacin in *S. pneumoniae* can be converted from topoisomerase IV to gyrase through a single chemical modification [170]: addition of a 4-aminobenzenesulfonyl group to the distal nitrogen (compound **2**, Figure 9).[4] The alteration in target specificity was confirmed through examination of MIC against defined mutants, selection of first-step mutants and differential activity of ciprofloxacin and compound **2** against isolated topoisomerase IV and gyrase from *S. pneumoniae* [170]. Thus, the identity of the primary enzyme target can be altered by molecular modification solely at the C-7 substituent. Additional efforts will certainly be applied to adjust the enzymatic activity of new analogues, such that a balance of gyrase and topoisomerase IV activity can be reached.

As can be seen from this discussion, structural innovations in the quinolone area have provided agents substantially improved over ciprofloxacin, in terms of both *in vitro* potency and *in vivo* properties. These intriguing expansions in quinolone SAR suggest that continued research may yield further therapeutic advances [171].

Throughout the discovery and development of improved fluoroquinolone agents, assessment of the potency of various analogues against DNA gyrase and,

---

[4]It was shown that a sulfonamide mechanism does not contribute to the antibacterial action of compound **2** [170].

more recently, topoisomerase IV, has assisted in optimization of antibacterial activity. The following section describes mechanistic discoveries involving the action of quinolones against both DNA gyrase and topoisomerase IV.

MECHANISM OF ACTION

Classically, DNA gyrase was considered the enzymatic target of the quinolone antibacterials. Topoisomerase IV, an enzyme discovered in 1990, is now recognized as another important biochemical target in bacteria for fluoroquinolones, particularly in Gram-positive pathogens [172]. A clearer understanding of the roles played by topoisomerase IV and DNA gyrase in the replication of the bacterial chromosome has helped to elucidate the bactericidal mechanism of action of quinolones.

REPLICATION OF DNA

When considering the mechanism by which quinolones kill bacteria, much attention has been focused on the ability of these agents to inhibit the catalytic activity of DNA gyrase [173]. However, a fuller understanding of their mechanism of action can be gained by considering the implications of this enzyme inhibition on replication of the bacterial chromosome. The highly condensed nature of the bacterial chromosome makes it totally dependent on topoisomerases for managing the overall topology of this complex DNA molecule. In *E. coli*, the circular chromosome, 1100 μm in length, has to be folded inside a cell that is 1–2 μm long [174]. Relaxed DNA exists as a helical molecule, with one full turn of the helix occurring approximately every 10.4 base pairs [174]. Thus, in *E. coli* the two single strands of DNA are wrapped around each other about 400,000 times (the *E. coli* chromosome contains 4 million base pairs). In fact, however, DNA isolated from bacteria is negatively supercoiled, that is, the DNA contains slightly less than 1 helical turn per 10.4 bp [175]. It is likely that the underwound state of intracellular DNA in bacteria facilitates strand separation during DNA replication [173]. Topoisomerases are crucial enzymes for helping maintain cellular DNA in the appropriate state of supercoiling in both replicating and nonreplicating regions of the chromosome. The transcription of many genes (including those for the topoisomerases themselves) is very sensitive to the state of supercoiling of DNA [176–178]. Perhaps even more important, the process of strand separation at the replication site drastically alters the degree of supercoiling of DNA, and topoisomerases are key enzymes that adjust this shift in supercoiling both ahead of and behind the replication fork [179,180].

DNA replication in bacteria is a highly regulated process and is strictly coordinated with the growth rate of the cell [181]. In *E. coli*, replication begins at a specific sequence on the chromosome called *oriC* and proceeds along the length of the chromosome in a bidirectional manner (Figure 10). The replication forks continue around the circular chromosome until they meet at the opposite end of the molecule or encounter replication termination sequences [182]. A DNA helicase unwinds the duplex DNA substrate ahead of DNA polymerase [182,183]. Formation of the replication primosome with DNA polymerase is a highly complex process and is the subject of several other reviews [183–186]. It is relevant to the discussion of topoisomerase that the combined action of helicase and DNA polymerase introduces positive supercoils (regions of DNA with less than 10.4 bp per turn) ahead of the replication fork. If left unresolved, these positive supercoils would eventually stop progression of the replication fork [182]. It turns out that the two topoisomerases that are the biochemical targets of fluoroquinolones, DNA gyrase and topoisomerase IV, play key roles in resolving two fundamental issues involved in DNA replication. DNA gyrase works ahead

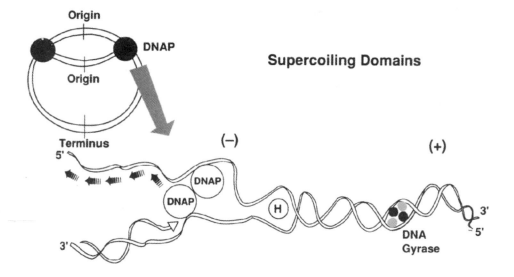

FIGURE 10 Schematic representation of the replication fork of *E. coli*. Replication of a circular chromosome initiates at a single point and proceeds in a bidirectional fashion by DNA polymerase (DNAP). Replication at the fork involves two molecules of DNA polymerase III holoenzyme and accessory proteins. The leading strand is made in a 5′-to-3′ direction, while lagging strand replication occurs through synthesis of discontinuous Okazaki fragments (represented by dashed arrows). A 5′-to-3′ helicase (H) unwinds the DNA to allow fork progression. The positive supercoils created ahead of the replication fork are relieved by the negative supercoiling activity of DNA gyrase.

of the replication fork [183] to remove excess positive supercoils, and topoisomerase IV conducts separation of the linked daughter DNA molecules [183] after replication is complete (Figure 10). These two topoisomerases are absolutely essential in permitting successful replication and cell partitioning of DNA molecules. Since the chromosome of rapidly growing bacterial cells contains multiple replication forks, it is easy to appreciate the significance of the coordinated activities of DNA gyrase and topoisomerase IV [187]. It is important to understand the properties of these two topoisomerases to understand how fluoroquinolones so effectively inhibit their normal function in the bacterial cell.

BACTERIAL TOPOISOMERASES

Classification

From a mechanistic point of view, all topoisomerases are classified as either type I or type II enzymes. Topoisomerases catalyze the passage of one DNA strand through another; type I enzymes perform DNA passage after creating a single strand break, and type II enzymes catalyze the passage of a double-strand region of DNA through a double-strand break in the helix [74,188]. For both classes of topoisomerase, strand passage is accomplished by a transient single (type I) or double (type II) strand break followed by a resealing step, both of which are mediated by the enzyme. In bacteria, four DNA topoisomerases have been characterized [74] in terms of their biochemical mechanism of strand passage (Table I). The type I enzymes consist of topoisomerase I (ω protein) and topoisomerase III. The type II enzymes include the major intracellular targets of fluoroquinolones, DNA gyrase and topoisomerase IV.

TABLE I   Classification of Bacterial Topoisomerases

Topoisomerase	Type	Designation	Predominant function in cell
I	I	ω protein	Relaxes negatively supercoiled DNA
II	II	DNA gyrase	Introduces negative supercoils into DNA
III	I	–	Decatenation of replication intermediate
IV	II	–	Chromosome partitioning

Topoisomerase I was first isolated in 1969 from *E. coli* [189]. This enzyme is a monomer of 110 kDa that is encoded by the *topA* gene in *E. coli*. Topoisomerase I catalyzes the relaxation or removal of negative supercoils from DNA in the absence of adenosine triphosphate (ATP) [189]. Topoisomerase I, an essential enzyme in *E. coli*, functions to counterbalance the activity of DNA gyrase in the bacterial cell [173]. Topoisomerase III can also remove negative supercoils in DNA, but it is more efficient at decatenation of nicked daughter DNA molecules of linked plasmids following their replication [190]. Neither topoisomerase I nor topoisomerase III is very sensitive to inhibition by fluoroquinolones [191]. It remains clear that type II enzymes are the principal targets of these antimicrobials.

DNA Gyrase

Early studies pointed to DNA gyrase as being the principal target of nalidixic and oxolinic acids [192,193]. Although the initial studies characterizing DNA gyrase were performed with *E. coli*, gyrase has been isolated from numerous other species [173]. Unlike the type I enzymes, the type II topoisomerases share a significant degree of homology at the protein level. DNA gyrase possesses amino acid motifs [194] that are conserved in type II enzymes isolated from phage and eukaryotes.

DNA gyrase has a tetrameric A_2B_2 structure (Table II) [192,193]. The enzyme in *E. coli* consists of two GyrA (97 kDa) and two GyrB (90 kDa) subunits that are encoded by the *gyrA* and *gyrB* genes, respectively. The structural genes from DNA gyrase are unlinked and reside at 48 min (*gyrA*) and 83 min (*gyrB*) on the *E. coli* chromosome [195]. The intact holoenzyme has a mass of 353 kDa, as determined by small-angle neutron scattering [196]. Gyrase introduces negative supercoils into DNA in the presence of ATP and is the only topoisomerase able to perform this activity [74,175]. The DNA-binding domain of gyrase is extremely important for imparting site recognition with DNA. A specific segment of double-stranded DNA, about 120 bp in length, comes in contact with gyrase. The DNA is actually wrapped around the enzyme surface in an ordered way so as to permit intramolecular strand passage. It is this ordered wrapping of the DNA that favors introduction of negative supercoils, the fundamental reaction of DNA gyrase. DNA gyrase is also able to decatenate linked molecules of DNA but with less efficiency than topoisomerase IV. Double-strand DNA passage occurs following creation of a transient cleavage intermediate; if the passage of a double-stranded section of DNA through the transient break introduces a negative supercoil, the hydrolysis of ATP is required to drive this process. This energy transduction process is mediated by the B subunits of DNA gyrase, which conduct the hydrolysis of ATP [194]. The ATP-binding domain is located in the N-terminal half of GyrB [194]. In the absence of ATP, gyrase relaxes supercoiled DNA,

TABLE II   Properties of DNA Gyrase and Topoisomerase IV

Property	DNA Gyrase		Topoisomerase IV	
	E. coli	S. aureus	E. coli	S. aureus
Subunits	A_2/B_2	A_2/B_2	$(ParC)_2$ $(ParE)_2$	$(ParC)_2$ $(ParE)_2$
MW subunits (kDa)	97/90	105/75	84/70	90/79
Gene	gyrA/gyrB	gyrA/gyrB	parC/parE	parC/parE
Contiguous genes	No	Yes	No	Yes
Major in vitro Catalytic function	DNA super-coiling	DNA super-coiling	Decatenation	Decatenation
Cellular function	Negative super-coiling and elimination of (+) supercoils at replication fork	Negative super-coiling and elimination of (+) supercoils at replication fork	Decatenation of linked daughter DNA molecules	Decatenation of linked daughter DNA molecules

although it does this less efficiently [175]. Since all type II topoisomerases share significant sequence homology, the functional domains present in these enzymes have been found to correlate with specific sequences of the structural genes [194]. The GyrA subunit can be divided into two functional domains [74]. Following cleavage with trypsin, the 875-aa residue GyrA can be divided into a 64-kDa fragment and a 33-kDa fragment. The DNA breakage and reunion domain resides in the 64-kDa part of the molecule, while the 33-kDa piece contains the functional domain for A/B subunit interaction and DNA binding [74]. The N-terminal portion of GyrA contains the Tyr-122 residue that participates in the breakage–reunion reaction with DNA [74,194]. This occurs through a transesterification that results in attachment of the 5′-phosphoryl end of the cleaved DNA backbone to the hydroxyl group of Tyr-122. Breaks occur on opposite strands of DNA through bond formation with the two A subunits contained in a single A_2B_2 tetramer of gyrase, resulting in a 4-bp staggered break on opposite strands of DNA. Thus, Tyr-122 is considered to be within the active site of the gyrase enzyme [74,194]. The transient complex created by bonding of the GyrA Tyr-122 to DNA is referred to as the cleavable complex. It can be demonstrated in the laboratory by adding protein denaturants such as sodium dodecyl sulfate (SDS) to the cleavage reaction and submitting the reaction products to electrophoresis in agarose, which shows the cleavage product of DNA. It is known that fluoroquinolones stabilize the cleavable complex, trapping this intermediate in a form that is readily detectable in the laboratory using cell-free systems or whole cells [193]. Thus, fluoroquinolones do not induce DNA cleavage; rather, they enhance gyrase-mediated DNA cleavage.

Models of Fluoroquinolone Interactions with the Topoisomerases

Numerous observations have pointed to the importance of fluoroquinolones for inhibiting the normal functions of DNA gyrase and topoisomerase IV. However, little direct information exists describing the basic interaction of these agents at the active site of these enzymes. Questions concerning how quinolones bind to topoisomerases and produce their inhibitory effects have resulted in the development of several models to fit the available data.

Although the original resistance mutation studies in *E. coli* pointed to the importance of GyrA in mediating the interaction with quinolones, subsequent binding studies by Shen and Pernet [197] implicated direct binding of quinolones to DNA. Shen's initial publication showed no binding of labeled norfloxacin to GyrA, GyrB, or the holoenzyme, but rather binding to DNA alone. A later study [198] illustrated the ability of gyrase to enhance the binding of quinolones to double-stranded DNA. Shen's model suggests that quinolone molecules bind directly to the single-stranded DNA regions created by gyrase during formation of the cleavable complex. The quinolones are thought to interact with the DNA bases via hydrogen bonding through the 3-carboxy and 4-oxo groups. Drug binding is proposed to be cooperative, with four molecules binding at the pocket created by the action of gyrase on the DNA substrate [74]. Shen [74] further proposes that the four drug molecules undergo self-association via molecular stacking of the aromatic rings and hydrophobic interactions between the N-1 substituents. In this model, the C-7 substituent on the fluoroquinolone is proposed to interact with GyrB.

However, the model as envisioned by Shen has drawn considerable controversy. Much of the controversy has stemmed from the emphasis the model places on quinolones binding to DNA only. Results obtained by Willmott and Maxwell [199], in contrast to Shen's data, show that radiolabeled norfloxacin does not bind to DNA gyrase or DNA separately. Using a spin column technique, drug was shown to bind efficiently only to the complex of gyrase and DNA. These investigators did not detect drug binding to isolated gyrase or DNA alone as observed by Shen. Using ciprofloxacin and a mutant gyrase containing a serine replacement at Tyr-122 (a mutation that does not permit cleavage of DNA), similar amounts of labeled drug were bound as were measured for wild-type gyrase [200]. This indicates that DNA cleavage and single-strand generation is not a prerequisite for quinolone binding to the gyrase–DNA complex as proposed by Shen.

Several additional investigations have further defined the active domains of DNA gyrase. Studies show that treatment of the 97-kDa GyrA protein with trypsin generates fragments of 64 and 33 kDa [201]. The smaller fragment (C-terminal piece) consists of amino-acid residues 572 to 875 and is responsible for binding DNA in a positive superhelical conformation. However, this fragment lacks all catalytic activity [202]. The N-terminal 64-kDa fragment contains the active site tyrosine, and studies show that homologous fragments in the size range of 58–64 kDa demonstrate catalytic activity [203]. When these N-terminal GyrA fragments are combined with GyrB, the resulting truncated enzyme can perform ATP-dependent relaxation and enhanced decatenation, but not supercoiling [204]. The 33-kDa C-terminal portion of GyrA, which binds DNA, evidently plays an essential role in the positive wrapping of DNA that confers the unique property of negative supercoiling of DNA gyrase [204]. The crystal structure of the 59-kDa GyrA fragment (GyrA59) has been determined to 2.8-Å resolution [205], and the structure suggests a mechanism explaining the DNA breakage–reunion activity of DNA gyrase. A new GyrA dimer contact was identified that forms a concave docking groove that accepts the "G" segment of DNA [205]. This "G," or gate segment of the DNA, is the duplex segment that is completely cut by DNA gyrase. The active site tyrosine (residue 122) of each GyrA protein attacks one phosphodiester backbone of the DNA molecule, forming a transient, covalent intermediate in which both strands of the DNA are cleaved. This crucial intermediate step in the formation of the cleavable complex stabilizes the broken ends of the DNA G segment, preventing the generation of broken DNA ends that would be cytotoxic to the cell. In this model, the transport piece, or "T" segment of duplex DNA, is shuttled through the gap created by GyrA in the stabilized G DNA segment (Figure 11). This G segment is then released from the Tyr-122 tethers on both GyrA subunits, resealed, and the translocated T segment is released from gyrase. Eukaryotic topoisomerase II appears to have a comparable "DNA opening platform," but the quaternary changes that occur in that topoisomerase appear to be quite different from the protein subunit movements that drive DNA double-strand passage in bacterial DNA gyrase [205,206].

This strand-passage mechanism takes advantage of the fact that the concave region formed by the GyrA dimer from *E. coli* gyrase contains numerous basic amino-acid residues (Arg-121 on the Tyr-122 monomer, as well as His-80, Arg-32, and Lys-42 on the opposite GyrA monomer) that can function to anchor the noncovalently bound 3′-end of the cleaved DNA [205]. The translocation of the T-DNA segment is coupled to ATP hydrolysis, and may involve the cooperative interaction of multiple gate forms generated within the gyrase-DNA complex.

Evidence supporting the direct interaction of fluoroquinolones in stabilizing the gyrase–DNA complex has come from proteolytic fingerprint studies conducted with truncated forms of *E. coli* GyrB. Conformational changes in gyrase

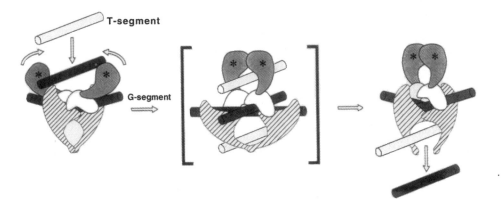

FIGURE 11 A model for the double-strand DNA transport by type II topoisomerases based on crystallographic and electron microscopic data. The ATPase domains shown in light gray on the top of the molecule dimerize after binding ATP (asterisk) around the T-segment of DNA. The T-segment (transport) is then passed through the G-segment of DNA. The transiently cleaved G-segment is stabilized by the enzyme during double-strand passage. After passage of the double-strand T-segment, the G-segment of DNA is religated and the T-segment released from the enzyme complex. Reprinted with permission from J. M. Berger [207].

following quinolone binding involve specific, conserved residues near the active site of the enzyme. Such conserved domains of proteins are often very resistant to attack by endopeptidases compared with less structured regions of the protein [205]. Binding of fluoroquinolone can induce conformational changes that alter susceptibility to proteolytic attack of the domain near Tyr-122. Elegant studies by Maxwell's group indicate that preincubation of DNA and the 47-kDa domain of GyrB (complex III) with 100 μM ciprofloxacin protects this domain from proteolytic attack by trypsin [204]. It is hypothesized that ciprofloxacin binding to the gyrase–DNA complex induces a conformational change that is detected by a shift from trypsin sensitivity to resistance. Tests using gyrase altered at the active site (Tyr-122 to Ser) retained trypsin resistance. However, a drug-resistant gyrase (GyrA containing Trp-83) failed to demonstrate the characteristic protective effect with ciprofloxacin against trypsin attack [204].

Such results underscore the interdependence of both GyrA and GyrB subunits in terms of mediating catalysis of DNA cleavage strand passage and strand resealing by gyrase. In addition, studies with *E. coli* DNA gyrase suggest that binding of ATP during catalysis promotes dimerization of the two GyrB subunits. This molecular dimerization captures the DNA T segment and helps direct it through the double-strand break in the G DNA segment. This double-strand passage process is stabilized by specific residues in GyrA [204]. Subsequent hydrolysis of the ATP cofactor allows the poststrand passage equilibrium of gyrase and DNA to reestablish native enzyme and a DNA molecule with a linking number (supercoiled state) changed by a factor of one.

The conformational changes in gyrase that catalyze the double-strand DNA cleavage–religation reaction have been characterized in recent publications. However, the precise molecular interactions of fluoroquinolones within the cleavable complex remain poorly understood. Results from several investigators indicate that fluoroquinolones bind to a localized single-strand region of DNA, generated in the cleavable complex by gyrase [208]. Gyrase itself plays a major role in quinolone binding to the complex, since specific mutations in the QRDR of gyrase that are associated with drug resistance decrease quinolone binding [199]. More recent evidence shows that quinolone binding to the cleavable complex of gyrase and DNA induces a conformational change that inhibits the supercoiling activity of the enzyme [209]. Through measurement of the kinetic rates of ATP hydrolysis by gyrase before and after quinolone binding, it was discerned that quinolone binding and drug-induced cleavage occur in two distinguishable steps. In addition, as in the case with topoisomerase IV, DNA cleavage within the complex does not need to occur for the quinolone to bind with high affinity to the cleavable complex [209].

Structure–activity relationships of some new fluoroquinolones have been described that attempt to explain their enhanced potency against topoisomerases. Fluoroquinolones containing the C-8 methoxy moiety are reported to have high antibacterial potency and greater activity relative to desmethoxy derivatives against *E. coli* containing known *gyrA* mutations [98,99]. The methoxy analogues also selected quinolone-resistant mutants from *E. coli in vitro* with a lower frequency than their desmethoxy counterparts [98] (see section on "Activity against Quinolone-Resistant Organisms"). It has been hypothesized that the presence of the C-8 methoxy group confers greater efficiency in promoting the release of broken DNA fragments following formation of the ternary cleavable complex of quinolone–gyrase–DNA. The C-8 methoxy derivative gatifloxacin was compared to its desmethoxy derivative and with ciprofloxacin in terms of potency against *E. coli* K-12 mutants with known mutations in GyrA and ParC [99]. Gatifloxacin retained a relatively greater degree of potency against GyrA mutants that contained alterations mapping within the α-helix 4 domain, thought to play a critical role in binding DNA during double-strand passage. The inference from this MIC data was that gatifloxacin may interact with a specific region of the cleavable complex, with a higher degree of affinity than the other quinolones tested. Unfortunately, no direct biochemical data measuring formation of the cleavable complex between gatifloxacin analogues and DNA gyrase were included in this study with which to address this hypothesis. This potential property of gatifloxacin is evidently not limited to the C-8 methoxy moiety, since several other new fluoroquinolones without this substituent are considerably more potent than gatifloxacin against both the Enterobacteriaceae and numerous Gram-positive pathogens [210].

All of the more recent data appear to point to the key role played by the new fluoroquinolones in increasing the formation of cleavage intermediates within the cleavable complex formed by gyrase, DNA, and drug. This dynamic interaction has been studied extensively at the biochemical level in the case of eukaryotic topoisomerase II enzymes and anticancer agents [211] but is only beginning to be addressed mechanistically in the case of bacterial gyrase and the fluoroquinolones [209,212]. It is important to remember that all of the initial mechanism-of-action studies were conducted with DNA gyrase purified from *E. coli*. As with other members of the Enterobacteriaceae, DNA gyrase is the primary or more sensitive enzyme target for fluoroquinolones. Interestingly, this is generally not the case for Gram-positive pathogens such as *S. aureus* and *S. pneumoniae*, where topoisomerase IV is often shown to be the more sensitive topoisomerase II target.

Several amino-acid residues around the Tyr-122 of GyrA are important for mediating resistance to fluoroquinolones. The region spanning Ala-67 to Gln-106 is termed the quinolone resistance-determining region (QRDR). The most important residue in *E. coli* GyrA is Ser-83, which is the most frequently mutated site conferring quinolone resistance [213–216]. The free hydroxyl at Ser-83 and the small size of this residue appear to be important, since substitution to Tyr or Leu confers resistance. This switch to a larger, nonpolar amino acid appears to weaken the interaction between the fluoroquinolone and the gyrase–DNA complex [214,216,217]. It is also interesting to note that some organisms, such as *Campylobacter jejuni* and *P. aeruginosa*, normally contain a threonine in place of serine at position 83 of GyrA. These organisms are approximately 10-fold less susceptible to fluoroquinolones than are wild-type strains of *E. coli* [194], underscoring the importance of the amino acid at position 83.

Topoisomerase IV

It has been 10 years since the discovery of topoisomerase IV in *E. coli* [172]. While this type II topoisomerase was initially characterized by its relative insensitivity to all fluoroquinolones, much new information has been generated with this important enzyme over the past decade. This second enzymatic target of fluoroquinolones shares several properties with DNA gyrase. As shown in Table II, topoisomerase IV also has a tetrameric structure, and the respective A and B subunits from both enzymes share significant homology. The subunits of topoisomerase IV are encoded by the *parC* and *parE* genes. In *E. coli*, the *parC* gene shares 36% identity and 60% similarity with *gyrA* at the amino-acid level

[172,194,218]. A homologue of *gyrB*, *parE* shares 42% identity and 62% similarity [172,194,218].

The *parC* gene was first identified in cells demonstrating a partitioning defect. Such cells grew in an elongated fashion with the nucleoid enlarged. These and subsequent observations indicated that topoisomerase IV is involved with decatenation of linked DNA molecules. Topoisomerase IV can decatenate DNA before completion of a round of replication, whereas DNA gyrase can decatenate only after a round of replication [219]. The principal enzyme for separating replicated DNA molecules in the bacterial cell is believed to be topoisomerase IV. The decatenation activity of topoisomerase IV from *E. coli* is approximately fivefold greater than its relaxation activity *in vitro* [218]. Unlike gyrase, topoisomerase IV does not wrap DNA around itself. Therefore, intermolecular strand passage is favored, leading to its important role in separating two linked DNA molecules [220,221]. Both enzymes have evolved to perform specialized functions in the cell, and both are essential for cell growth. They therefore represent two potential lethal targets for fluoroquinolones.

TOPOISOMERASE SENSITIVITY TO FLUOROQUINOLONES

DNA Gyrase versus Topoisomerase IV

In many ways, the discovery of topoisomerase IV in 1990 has complicated our understanding of how fluoroquinolones kill bacteria. Originally it was thought that DNA gyrase was the primary target of these agents. In *E. coli*, primary resistance mutations were mapped to DNA gyrase rather than to the newly discovered topoisomerase IV [215–217]. Such data were consistent with the notion that gyrase was the primary target in the cell. In addition, early reports indicated that gyrase supercoiling was several times more sensitive to inhibition by fluoroquinolones *in vitro* than was the decatenation activity of topoisomerase IV [218,222]. However, more recent reports have found this difference to be only two- to threefold [223,224]. In contrast, reports with *S. aureus* mutants selected in a stepwise fashion with ciprofloxacin indicated that mutation to resistance occurred first in *parC* rather than in *gyrA* [225,226]. These observations, contrary to what was observed in Gram-negative bacteria, suggested that topoisomerase IV may in fact be the primary target of ciprofloxacin in some Gram-positive species of bacteria. This was also found to be the case in several subsequent reports [227,228] in which ciprofloxacin was used to select resistance with strains of *S. pneumoniae*. In these cases, the first step of resistance selection was associated with mutations in ParC, usually consisting of substitution at Ser-79. These observations with ParC in Gram-positives do not completely explain the situation, however. One report [229] indicates that stepwise selected mutants obtained with sparfloxacin in *S. pneumoniae* demonstrate changes in *gyrA* first, rather than *parC*. Clearly, the interactions of fluoroquinolones with DNA gyrase and topoisomerase IV are complex: the most sensitive topoisomerase target may vary between species and with respect to the particular quinolone in question.

Observations made with mutant selection using whole cells have been complemented by studies with cell-free topoisomerases. A 1996 study [230] compared the sensitivities to fluoroquinolones of DNA gyrase and topoisomerase IV isolated from *E. coli* and *S. aureus*. *Escherichia coli* DNA gyrase supercoiling activity was approximately fivefold more sensitive to ciprofloxacin, sparfloxacin, and norfloxacin than was topoisomerase IV decatenation activity. A different response was observed with both enzymes isolated from *S. aureus*, since IC_{50} values for topoisomerase IV decatenation were twofold (sparfloxacin) to eightfold lower than those obtained for DNA gyrase supercoiling inhibition. Thus, biochemical results with these enzymes generally agree with mutant selection studies indicating that differential sensitivity to quinolones is observed between the topoisomerases of *S. aureus* and *E. coli*. However, IC_{50} values for *E. coli* gyrase supercoiling inhibition were 10-fold lower than those obtained for inhibition of *S. aureus* topoisomerase IV decatenation, consistent with the greater overall susceptibility of *E. coli* to these fluoroquinolones [230].

Reports have shown that topoisomerase IV in Gram-positive bacteria serves as a lethal target for many fluoroquinolones, much in the same manner as DNA gyrase in Gram-negatives [231]. For example, with topoisomerase IV isolated from *E. coli*, norfloxacin was shown to stabilize a cleavable complex formed between DNA and the enzyme. Binding of norfloxacin to DNA induced structural alterations in the molecule that were enhanced in the presence of topoisomerase IV [232]. The generation of cleavage product from these ternary complexes could, in theory, be lethal to the cell in the example of formation of a single DNA double-strand break [231,232]. The rate of collision between the replication fork and the stable DNA adduct would influence the efficiency of cell killing.

Newly published studies have furthered our understanding of the biochemical mechanism by which fluoroquinolones stabilize the cleavable complex. The action of ciprofloxacin on the individual steps in the *E. coli* topoisomerase IV catalytic cycle has been examined in careful detail [233]. Topoisomerase IV was 10-fold more active than eukaryotic topoisomerase II in establishing a DNA cleavage equilibrium (for DNA and the enzyme) in the absence of drug [233]. Furthermore, in agreement with results from other studies [231,232], norfloxacin and ciprofloxacin were relatively potent at stimulating topoisomerase IV-mediated DNA cleavage [233]. Ciprofloxacin stimulated generation of DNA cleavage product both by increasing the forward rate of DNA cleavage, as well as inhibiting religation of broken DNA held in the topoisomerase IV–DNA complex. This observation underscores the importance of topoisomerase IV as a lethal target in some bacterial species. While DNA gyrase in Gram-negative organisms is significantly more sensitive to cleavage complex stabilization by quinolones, both gyrase and topoisomerase IV appear to share a common enzymatic mechanism resulting in lethal cleavage complex formation. Since this mechanism is a fundamental property of both type II topoisomerases, it is not surprising that topoisomerase IV could be the primary or more sensitive enzyme target in some species. In the Gram-positives *S. aureus* and *S. pneumoniae*, it is cleavable complex formation that correlates with lethality, not inhibition of catalytic activity in the cell [231–233]. In contrast, inhibition of the catalytic activity of type II topoisomerases (supercoiling or decatenation) seems to be primarily the result of interfering with enzyme-ATP utilization [233].

Some newer fluoroquinolones such as sitafloxacin, clinafloxacin, trovafloxacin, gatifloxacin, gemifloxacin, and moxifloxacin possess significantly improved activity compared to ciprofloxacin against many Gram-positive pathogens. This observation has stimulated several more recent studies aimed at understanding the specific interaction of new agents with DNA gyrase and topoisomerase IV isolated from these organisms.

Osheroff and colleagues [234] purified topoisomerase IV from *S. aureus* and compared its sensitivity to quinolones *in vitro* to that of *E. coli* topoisomerase IV. These investigators found that the *S. aureus* enzyme was more active at forming DNA cleavage product with ciprofloxacin than the *E. coli* enzyme. Concentrations of ciprofloxacin required to double the level of DNA cleavage product (over that obtained with enzyme and DNA alone) were 150 and 500 n*M* for topoisomerase IV from *S. aureus* and *E. coli*, respectively. Careful studies that exploited the intrinsic differences between the temperature optima for the forward and reverse DNA cleavage reactions showed that ciprofloxacin both stimulated the forward reaction of cleavage product formation and inhibited religation of DNA [234]. Two mutant topoisomerase IV enzymes tested containing GrlA changes in either S80F or E84K were 20–27 times less sensitive to ciprofloxacin than wild-type topoisomerase IV in these cleavage experiments.

Additional studies from these researchers demonstrated that the newer fluoroquinolones levofloxacin and trovafloxacin were 1.8- and 7-fold more potent than ciprofloxacin in stimulating *S. aureus* topoisomerase IV-mediated DNA cleavage [235]. The greater degree of potency with trovafloxacin was hypothesized to result from greater kinetic affinity of this fluoroquinolone for the enzyme–DNA complex. Ciprofloxacin, levofloxacin, and trovafloxacin produced qualitatively similar cleavage patterns with topoisomerase IV in experiments with radiolabeled DNA substrate. However, trovafloxacin generated considerably greater amounts of cleavage product at selected cleavage sites in the DNA. Trovafloxacin was also more potent at inhibiting poststrand passage DNA religation than ciprofloxacin or levofloxacin [235]. These quantitative differences in potency against purified topoisomerase IV from *S. aureus* are thought to be reflective of the comparatively lower MICs observed with trovafloxacin against many Gram-positive bacteria.

Additional studies further characterize the potent activity of structurally novel fluoroquinolones against Gram-positive bacteria. A single mutation in both topoisomerase IV (S80F or S80Y) and DNA gyrase (S84L) in *S. aureus* elevated the MIC of trovafloxacin from 0.03 µg/ml to 1.0 µg/ml. Such *S. aureus* double mutants had MICs to ciprofloxacin and levofloxacin of ≥8 µg/ml [236,237]. Ciprofloxacin lost all bactericidal activity against the double mutants even when tested at concentrations four- and eightfold above the elevated MIC. In a collection of *S. aureus* clinical isolates with reduced quinolone susceptibility, MICs to ciprofloxacin were generally reduced at least fourfold by addition of the NorA efflux inhibitor reserpine, while the greater activity of levofloxacin, sparfloxacin, or trovafloxacin was not increased further by this agent [236].

The 2-pyridones, an interesting new class of agents related to the fluoroquinolones (see section on "2-Pyridones"), were also tested against *S. aureus* DNA gyrase and topoisomerase IV [161]. As with results obtained with ciprofloxacin, trovafloxacin, and clinafloxacin, the 2-pyridone ABT-719 was twice as potent in stimulating topoisomerase IV-mediated DNA cleavage than cleavage with gyrase. In agreement with other published biochemical data, most of the potent new fluoroquinolones are more active against topoisomerase IV than DNA gyrase from Gram-positive species examined thus far.

Studies have described new fluoroquinolones that appear to possess equivalent potency against both DNA gyrase and topoisomerase IV. This concept seems appealing, as compounds with such dual-target activity would select resistant mutants only at very low frequency. The relative sensitivities of DNA gyrase and topoisomerase IV to new quinolones have been studied most extensively in *S. pneumoniae*. Mutation data generated with quinolone-susceptible cells indicate that resistance to clinafloxacin occurs in a stepwise fashion at a very low frequency ($5–8.5 \times 10^{-10}$). The authors speculated that this infrequent resistance selection rate with clinafloxacin could be attributed to its high bactericidal potency against pneumococci, as well as a potential to attack both topoisomerase II targets equally [238]. Despite the dual targeting mechanism proposed for this compound, high-level clinafloxacin-resistant mutants (MICs 64 µg/ml) were obtained *in vitro* after four steps of selection. The mutants contained changes in both GyrA and ParC. Careful studies utilizing highly purified topoisomerases in DNA cleavage assays have added key information to this question. First, Pan and Fisher demonstrated that ciprofloxacin, sparfloxacin, and clinafloxacin are 25 to 80 times more potent at inducing *S. pneumoniae* topoisomerase IV-mediated DNA cleavage *in vitro* than DNA gyrase-mediated cleavage [239]. Clinafloxacin was 10-fold more potent at stimulating DNA cleavage with topoisomerase IV than ciprofloxacin or sparfloxacin. While this more recent biochemical data showing a preference for topoisomerase IV seems somewhat at odds with the stepwise mutant selection data, both procedures can be affected by several experimental parameters. These include the effect of adding potassium glutamate to enhance enzyme activity, differences in cellular penetration of drug to each enzyme, and the presence of other physiological and DNA repair processes present in the whole cell that do not come into play in cell-free assays [239].

Chemical modifications made to new fluoroquinolones continue to provide information useful in solving the puzzle of target selection. An extremely potent agent, sitafloxacin, was shown to possess equivalent potency against DNA gyrase and topoisomerase IV in *S. pneumoniae* [167]. Other studies illustrate that modifications made at the C-7 position of ciprofloxacin appear to redirect target sensitivity from topoisomerase IV to DNA gyrase [170] (see section on "Alteration of Primary Enzymatic Target"). Additional data generated by mutant selection in pneumococcus suggest that gatifloxacin and sparfloxacin preferentially target DNA gyrase, while ciprofloxacin, levofloxacin, and trovafloxacin preferentially target topoisomerase IV [169]. The new agent gemifloxacin appears to retain considerable potency against pneumococcal isolates that are highly resistant to ciprofloxacin (MIC of 64 µg/ml) that contained both reserpine-sensitive efflux resistance as well as mutations in ParC, Par E, and GyrB [240]. Further studies in *S. aureus* suggest that moxifloxacin preferentially targets topoisomerase IV [241]. Thus, the available data indicate that the chemical moieties placed on the fluoroquinolone nucleus play an important role in determining the sensitivity of the target topoisomerase.

KILLING OF BACTERIAL CELLS BY FLUOROQUINOLONES

Stabilization of the Cleavable Complex and Subsequent Events

The available data indicate that the hallmark of the interaction between fluoroquinolones and DNA gyrase is stabilization of the cleavable complex. The ternary complex between drug, enzyme, and DNA is formed via a reversible process and can dissociate to form the original active components. Because fluoroquinolones stabilize the topoisomerase–DNA complex, the lethal event in the cell has been presumed to result from stabilization of the covalent bond between gyrase and DNA. Newer data, however, suggest that the lethal event in the cell occurs in a subsequent step, which comes about as a result of fluoroquinolone stabilization of covalent bond formation between gyrase and DNA.

It is also interesting that several studies in the literature suggest that fluoroquinolones possess additional mechanisms of cell killing, termed mechanisms A, B, and C [242,243]. Mechanism A, thought to be common to all quinolones, is blocked by inhibitors of RNA or protein synthesis and is active against growing cells [243]. The second mechanism of killing (mechanism B) occurs at high quinolone concentrations against nongrowing cells and is not inhibited by preventing protein synthesis. The third mechanism (mechanism C) is proposed to be active against nongrowing cells but does require active protein or RNA synthesis. One of the interesting and yet unresolved issues is whether these additional mechanisms are in fact unique or whether they are simply different manifestations of the bactericidal outcome resulting from drug stabilization of the cleavable complex mentioned previously.

Some of the most fundamental observations made with respect to the mechanism of action of quinolones were noted with nalidixic acid in 1965 by William Goss and coworkers [244]. These investigators found that sublethal concentrations of nalidixic acid (3.0 μg/ml) inhibited DNA synthesis in *E. coli* 15TAU by approximately 40%. This level of drug was sufficient to stop growth of the cells as a result of inhibition of DNA synthesis. At 10 μg/ml of nalidixic acid, DNA synthesis was inhibited by 72% and the cells began to lose viability. Washing of cells that had been exposed to this level of drug for 75 min restored cell viability, indicating that the lethal effect was reversible. The lethal effect of nalidixic acid was prevented when RNA and protein synthesis were blocked in the cells, which was described later as mechanism A [244]. Although protein synthesis inhibition blocked cell killing by nalidixic acid, it had little effect on inhibition of DNA synthesis [244]. These studies were the first to show that significant inhibition of DNA synthesis by a quinolone could occur without causing lethality, suggesting that some additional event was required for cell death.

Thus, inhibition of DNA synthesis alone is insufficient to explain how quinolones kill bacteria; other events after formation of the cleavable complex appear to lead to cell death. One potential explanation for the lethal action of quinolones is manifested in the "poison hypothesis." This hypothesis suggests that, because gyrase normally removes positive supercoils ahead of the replication fork, stabilization of the cleavable complex by quinolones causes the replication fork to collide with the complex, leading to sudden and lethal cessation of DNA replication. Indeed, results from pulse-labeling studies [245] show that DNA gyrase is concentrated near replication forks. Although this hypothesis is supported by evidence [246], the exact lethal mechanism elicited by quinolones against the bacterial cell is not completely understood.

Cleavage complexes are also formed with quinolones and topoisomerase IV [218]. The interaction of fluoroquinolone with topoisomerase IV was shown to produce a slow inhibition of DNA synthesis in *E. coli* cells containing *gyrA* resistance mutations [223]. Since topoisomerase IV does not exert its activity ahead of the replication fork, it might be concluded that stabilization of cleavable complexes with this enzyme does not lead to fork arrest. A study from Marians's group [180] shows that this is not the case. These investigators constructed three different mutants of *parC* in topoisomerase IV from *E. coli*. Mutant alleles in ParC were constructed at Ser-80 to Leu, Tyr-120 to Phe, and the Ser-80/Leu, Tyr-120/Phe double mutant. The corresponding subunits were reconstituted with the wild-type ParE subunit. Given the nature of these mutations in ParC, none of the mutant enzymes would be expected to form a stabilized cleavable complex in the presence of a quinolone. Using an *in vitro oriC* DNA replication system, the group showed that none of the three mutant enzymes could block replication fork progression in the presence of norfloxacin. The wild-type enzyme formed a measurable cleavable complex with norfloxacin and potently arrested replication fork progression in the presence of drug [180]. Because the mutant topoisomerase IV alleles could not form a cleavable complex with norfloxacin, it was concluded that DNA strand cleavage in the ternary complex of DNA–topoisomerase IV–norfloxacin was a prerequisite to replication fork arrest. This event was not sufficient to cause measurable DNA breakage, however, because a second step to denature the topoisomerase was required to generate double-strand breakage of the DNA. These experiments establish that, at least *in vitro*, a quinolone-stabilized cleavable complex formed between DNA and topoisomerase IV causes replication fork arrest. Thus, in the cell, topoisomerase IV may be a lethal target of quinolones by a mechanism similar to that described for DNA gyrase. These experiments also suggest that collision of a replication fork with a quinolone-stabilized cleavable complex may not be sufficient to cause double-strand breaks in DNA that kill the cell. Some lethal event beyond blockage of the replication fork appears to account for the killing action of fluoroquinolones.

A number of investigators have observed the occurrence of DNA strand breaks in cells treated with quinolones [179]. Nucleoids from cells treated with bactericidal concentrations of oxolinic acid sedimented more slowly than those isolated from untreated cells [247]. This indicated that the DNA isolated from treated cells was less negatively supercoiled. Further characterization of the DNA suggested that it contained free DNA ends, apparently resulting from double-strand breaks derived by formation of the cleavable complex with drug. In considering the mechanism of production of such free DNA ends, it was postulated that a protein, yet to be identified, catalyzed their release. The effect of chloramphenicol on the killing action of oxolinic acid was studied further by Drlica and colleagues [247]. These investigators found that inhibition of protein synthesis by chloramphenicol not only antagonized the killing action of oxolinic acid but also prevented the typical DNA strand breaks from occurring in the cell. It is this process of DNA end release, and not inhibition of DNA synthesis, that is thought to produce the bactericidal effect of these agents. This process may not function to the same degree with all quinolones, however, because the lethal action of the newer potent fluoroquinolones is only partially blocked by protein and RNA synthesis inhibitors [242]. This alternative mechanism could still involve the release of free DNA ends from the quinolone–gyrase–DNA complex; it has been shown that treatment of cells with ciprofloxacin disrupts the ability of chromosomal DNA to maintain normal supercoiling even in the presence of chloramphenicol [247].

Another property of fluoroquinolones may help to explain how such free DNA ends could be generated from the ternary complex. Quinolones have been shown to stimulate illegitimate recombination and deletions that may result from the dissociation–reassociation of the gyrase–DNA complex. Also, oxolinic acid stimulated formation of λ biotransducing phage by two to three orders of magnitude via illegitimate recombination [248]. The production of phage stimulated by oxolinic acid was prevented in bacterial host cells containing a mutation in *gyrA* that conferred quinolone resistance. The ability of quinolones to induce illegitimate recombination may provide a mechanism by which the same ternary complex could produce free DNA ends on the bacterial chromosome, which would result in lethality.

As reviewed by Drlica [179], all of these properties of quinolones could be consistent with earlier results describing the multiple mechanisms of bacterial cell killing as outlined by Smith and Lewin [242,243]. The first mechanism of cell killing (mechanism A) is common to many quinolones and is inhibited by chloramphenicol [243]. This mechanism is consistent with the removal of the gyrase–quinolone complexes formed with DNA, creating free DNA ends. An as-yet-undiscovered protein is responsible for this removal of the complexes, thus accounting for the sensitivity of this mechanism of cell killing to RNA and protein synthesis inhibitors. The second mechanism is not susceptible to chloramphenicol and could result from the reversible process of gyrase subunit dissociation while the enzyme is complexed to DNA. The end result of this opening of the complex would be creation of the free DNA ends that can be lethal to the cell. Because this mechanism has been shown to occur at high quinolone concentrations, the suggestion has been made that such subunit dissociation may be favored by stacking of drug molecules at the active site of DNA gyrase [179,247]. Such drug stacking has been proposed by Shen [197,198] in his mechanistic models of quinolone action. A final mechanism outlined by Smith and Lewin involves the action of norfloxacin and ciprofloxacin against nongrowing bacterial cells, such as in tests with cells suspended in saline. Nalidixic acid does not kill nongrowing cells. Because mutations in *parC* of topoisomerase IV confer resistance to ciprofloxacin and norfloxacin but not to nalidixic acid, it has been hypothesized [179,223,247,249] that this last mechanism may involve topoisomerase IV.

The SOS Response

Whether the actual mechanism of cell killing by fluoroquinolones involves replication fork arrest or the drug–gyrase–DNA interactions described previously, the resulting damage to the bacterial chromosome is likely to stimulate repair attempts by the cell. The fluoroquinolones are known to induce the multigene cluster known as the SOS system [250–252]. Much has been written about the role of the SOS system associated with quinolones, but no clear pathway to cell death via this repair pathway has emerged. Induction of the SOS system involves three proteins: RecA, RecBCD, and LexA. LexA is the repressor of the SOS regulon, and this protein is cleaved by the RecA protein when RecA is induced by small nucleic acids. This may involve short oligonucleotides and/or single-stranded DNA. Once induced, the RecBCD enzyme requires the presence of a double-stranded DNA end. Available data [253] suggest that this situation occurs at the replication fork. The double-strand breaks created by the ternary complex of topoisomerase–DNA–quinolone may also provide access for RecBCD to the chromosome [179]. RecBCD induction leads to an increase in quinolone-associated mutagenesis [254,255] as well as increased cell survival in the presence of quinolone. Because *recA* and *recBC* mutants are more susceptible to the bactericidal action of quinolones, these genes are likely responsible for repair of the damage caused to DNA [255]. A number of other genes might be involved in the repair of DNA lesions caused by quinolones [179,255,256]. The importance of the various systems for repairing the damage caused by the different fluoroquinolones will be the subject of future investigations.

Factors That Affect the Bactericidal Activity of Quinolones

Magnesium Levels

A number of physiological conditions and growth medium parameters affect the bactericidal activity of quinolones. It is well known that cations, particularly aluminum and magnesium, cause decreased absorption of quinolones from the gastrointestinal tract [257] (see the section on "Chelation of Divalent and Trivalent Metal Cations"). The MICs of quinolones are also negatively affected by elevated levels of magnesium, resulting in 2- to 16-fold increases in MICs [139,258,259]. Magnesium levels in urine often reach 8–10 mM, and these concentrations can raise the MIC to quinolones in some bacteria up to 64-fold [258,260]. Magnesium is an important cofactor for several of the topoisomerases [261]; however, high levels are thought to antagonize the penetration of fluoroquinolones into the bacterial cell [262]. In the case of Gram-negative cells, which contain an outer membrane, the more hydrophobic quinolones are thought to permeate into the cells via the self-promoted pathway, in which they chelate the magnesium ions that stabilize the structure of the outer membrane [263].

Magnesium decreases quinolone activity against such cells by antagonizing the accumulation of compound into the cell. Because hydrophobic quinolones, such as sparfloxacin, utilize the self-promoted pathway, excess magnesium antagonizes the Gram-negative activity of these quinolones to the greatest degree [262]. Because magnesium plays an important role in determining the antibacterial activity of quinolones, studies have attempted to characterize the physicochemical interaction of Mg^{2+} with the quinolone nucleus. Using the technique of infrared spectroscopy, it was shown [139] that Mg^{2+} interacts with the ketone and carboxylic acid moieties of the pyridone ring. Different analogues display different affinity constants for Mg^{2+}, however, as assessed by ^{19}F nuclear magnetic resonance spectroscopy, with sparfloxacin binding the least ($K_a = 10.1 \pm 0.6 \times 10^2$ M^{-1}) and pefloxacin binding Mg^{2+} more avidly ($K_a = 21 \pm 1.2 \times 10^2$ M^{-1}). A 1:1 stoichiometry was assigned to these complexes [139]. One study [264] has determined the intracellular concentration of Mg^{2+} in *E. coli* to be approximately 100 mM. The intracellular concentration of quinolone was determined to be 0.1 mM [139]; taken together with the affinity constants given above, it can be assumed that quinolones are complexed with Mg^{2+} inside the bacterial cell. The active component in forming the cleavable complex with DNA and gyrase, therefore, is quinolone–Mg^{2+}, as hypothesized by several investigators [139,199,260,265]. Although the interaction with magnesium is important at several different levels in the cell, any inhibition of killing activity with quinolones by this cation is likely a result of decreased drug penetration to its lethal target.

Effects of pH

The killing activity of some quinolones has also been shown to be influenced by the pH and oxygen tension of the medium. At pH levels below 6.8, the inhibitory activity of quinolones is antagonized, raising MICs several-fold [266]. This is relevant to treating infections of the urinary tract, where urine pH values can be in the acidic range. This effect, coupled with the high concentrations of magnesium in urine, can cause decreased killing of some bacteria by fluoroquinolones in the urinary tract.

Effects of Anaerobiosis

The activity of currently available quinolones against anaerobic pathogens is highly variable [2,267] (see section on "Activity against Anaerobes"). Much has been written about the role of oxygen in the killing of bacteria by quinolones [268,269]. Most of these observations come from studies [268] with *E. coli* KL16 and *S. aureus* E3T grown at high and low inoculum. At an inoculum of 1.0×10^{10} cfu/ml, the killing activities of ciprofloxacin and ofloxacin were greatly diminished compared with tests performed at 1.0×10^{6} cfu/ml [268]. This led investigators to conclude that decreased oxygen tension in cultures at the high inoculum interfered with the killing activity of these fluoroquinolones. These results are subject to other interpretations [270], because crowding of cells at such high densities may also decrease cell division, leading to decreased killing activity of quinolones. Experiments designed to test these parameters and to characterize the proposed effect of oxygen on the killing activity of quinolones have not been thoroughly conducted.

Data for the new fluoroquinolones in fact suggest that they are highly bactericidal in an anaerobic environment. For example, studies [271] of trovafloxacin against a wide variety of anaerobes grown in the absence of oxygen show that cells were killed at drug concentrations equal to or only twofold above MIC values. Trovafloxacin was also highly efficacious in a rat abscess model with a mixed infection of anaerobes and facultative organisms [272]. Furthermore, the newer quinolones have been shown [273] to decrease the viable counts of facultative organisms in the anaerobic environment of the human gastrointestinal tract following oral dosing.

Thus, the effect of oxygen on the bactericidal activity of fluoroquinolones is unclear. Many of the newer agents have potent activity against anaerobes as well as facultative organisms grown in an anaerobic environment. If the absence of oxygen in susceptibility test medium antagonizes killing by the older quinolones, this property does not appear to be a limitation of the newer agents.

CONCLUSION

It would serve us well to remember that the mechanistic basis of any class of antimicrobials against broad groups of pathogenic bacteria requires years of intensive research to understand. Perhaps the issue of the dual targeting of novel fluoroquinolones against both type II topoisomerases is only of academic interest. While the frequency of high-level ciprofloxacin resistance in pneumococci is currently at very low levels, similar resistance to this agent in staphylococci is quite high globally [274]. The reason for this dichotomy in clinical resistance is undoubtedly related to several factors. The intrinsic potency against type II topoisomerases, optimum cell permeability of drug, as well as the judicious use of new fluoroquinolones, will all play important roles in determining the future clinical utility of these important agents.

REFERENCES

1. Neu, H. C. (1994). Major advances in antibacterial quinolone therapy. *Adv. Pharmacol.* **29**, 227–262.

2. Gootz, T. D., and Brighty, K. E. (1996). Fluoroquinolone antibacterials: SAR, mechanism of action, resistance, and clinical aspects. *Med. Res. Rev.* **16**, 433–486.

3. Asahina, Y., Ishizaki, T., and Suzue, S. (1992). Recent advances in structure–activity relationships in new quinolones. *Prog. Drug Res.* **38**, 57–106.

4. Chu, D. T. W., and Fernandes, P. B. (1991). Recent developments in the field of quinolone antibacterial agents. *Adv. Drug Res.* **21**, 39–144.

5. Rosen, T. (1990). The fluoroquinolone antibacterial agents. *Prog. Med. Chem.* **27**, 236–295.

6. Lesher, G. Y., Froelich, E. J., Gruett, M. D., Bailey, J. H., and Brundage, R. P. (1962). 1,8-Naphthyridine derivatives: A new class of chemotherapeutic agents. *J. Med. (Pharm.) Chem.* **5**, 1063–1065.

7. Albrecht, R. (1977). Development of antibacterial agents of the nalidixic acid type. *Prog. Drug Res.* **21**, 9–104.

8. Moellering Jr., R. C. (1996). The place of quinolones in everyday clinical practice. *Chemotherapy (Basel)* **42** (Suppl. 1), 54–61.

9. Rádl, S. (1996). From chloroquine to antineoplastic drugs? The story of antibacterial quinolones. *Arch. Pharmacol.* **329**, 115–119.

10. Koga, H., Itoh, A., Murayama, S., Suzue, S., and Irikura, T. (1980). Structure–activity relationships of antibacterial 6,7- and 7,8-disubstituted 1-alkyl-1,4-dihydro-4-oxoquinoline-3-carboxylic acids. *J. Med. Chem.* **23**, 1358–1363.

11. Domagala, J. M., Hanna, L. D., Heifetz, C. L., Hutt, M. P., Mich, T. F., Sanchez, J. P., and Solomon, M. (1986). New structure–activity relationships of the quinolone antibacterials using the target enzyme: The development and application of a DNA gyrase assay. *J. Med. Chem.* **29**, 394–404.

12. Wise, R., Lister, D., McNulty, C. A. M., Griggs, D., and Andrews, J. M. (1986). The comparative pharmacokinetics of five quinolones. *J. Antimicrob. Chemother.* **18** (Suppl. D), 71–81.

13. Hooper, D. C., and Wolfson, J. S. (1985). The fluoroquinolones: Pharmacology, clinical uses, and toxicities in humans. *Antimicrob. Agents Chemother.* **28**, 716–721.

14. Wolfson, J. S., and Hooper, D. C. (1985). The fluoroquinolones: Structures, mechanisms of action and resistance, and spectra of activity *in vitro*. *Antimicrob. Agents Chemother.* **28**, 581–586.

15. Monk, J. P., and Campoli-Richards, D. M. (1987). Ofloxacin: A review of its antibacterial activity, pharmacokinetic properties and therapeutic use. *Drugs* **33**, 346–391.

16. Wise, R., Andrews, J. M., Matthews, R., and Wolstenholme, M. (1992). The *in vitro* activity of two new quinolones: Rufloxacin and MF 961. *J. Antimicrob. Chemother.* **29**, 649–660.

17. Culbertson, T. P., Domagala, J. M., Hagen, S. E., Hutt, M. P., Nichols, J. B., Mich, T. F., Sanchez, J. P., Schroeder, M. C., Solomon, M., and Worth, D. F. (1989). Structure-activity relationships of the quinolone antibacterials: The nature of the C_7-side chain. In "International Telesymposium on Quinolones" (P. B. Fernandes, ed.), pp. 47–71. J. R. Prous Science Publishers, Barcelona.

18. Kurokawa, I., Akamatsu, H., Nishijima, S., Asada, Y., and Kawabata, S. (1991). Clinical and bacteriologic evaluation of OPC-7251 in patients with acne: A double-blind group comparison study versus cream base. *J. Am. Acad. Dermatol.* **25**, 674–681.

19. Crumplin, G. C. (1990). Molecular effects of 4-quinolones upon DNA gyrase: DNA systems. In "The 4-Quinolones" (G. C. Crumplin, ed.), pp. 53–68. Springer, New York.

20. Blumberg, H. M., Rimland, D., Carroll, D. J., Terry, P., and Wachsmuth, I. K. (1991). Rapid development of ciprofloxacin resistance in methicillin-susceptible and -resistant *Staphylococcus aureus*. *J. Infect. Dis.* **163**, 1279–1285.

21. Domagala, J. M. (1994). Structure–activity and structure–side-effect relationships for the quinolone antibacterials. *J. Antimicrob. Chemother.* **33**, 685–706.

22. Ball, P., Fernald, A., and Tillotson, G. (1998). Therapeutic advances of new fluoroquinolones. *Expert Opin. Invest. Drugs* **7**, 761–783.

23. Sanchez, J. P., Domagala, J. M., Hagen, S. E., Heifetz, C. L., Hutt, M. P., Nichols, J. B., and Trehan, A. K. (1988). Quinolone antibacterial agents: Synthesis and structure–activity relationships of 8-substituted quinoline-3-carboxylic acids and 1,8-naphthyridine-3-carboxylic acids. *J. Med. Chem.* **31**, 983–991.

24. Wise, R., Andrews, J. M., and Brenwald, N. (1993). The *in vitro* activity of BAY y 3118, a new chlorofluoroquinolone. *J. Antimicrob. Chemother.* **31**, 73–80.

25. Bauernfeind, A. (1993). Comparative *in vitro* activities of the new quinolone, BAY y 3118, and ciprofloxacin, sparfloxacin, tosufloxacin, CI-960 and CI-990. *J. Antimicrob. Chemother.* **31**, 505–522.

26. Hong, C. Y., Kim, Y. K., Chang, J. H., Kim, S. H., Choi, H., Nam, D. H., Kim, Y. Z., and Kwak, J. H. (1997). Novel fluoroquinolone antibacterial agents containing oxime-substituted (aminomethyl) pyrrolidines: Synthesis and antibacterial activity of 7-(4-(aminomethyl)-3-(methoxyimino)pyrrolidin-1-yl)-1-cyclopropyl-6-fluoro-4-oxo-1,4-dihydro[1,8]naphthyridine-3-carboxylic acid (LB20304). *J. Med. Chem.* **40**, 3584–3593.

27. Akasaka, T., Kurosaka, S., Uchida, Y., Tanaka, M., Sato, K., and Hayakawa, I. (1998). Antibacterial activities and inhibitory effects of sitafloxacin (DU-6859a) and its optical isomers against type II topoisomerases. *Antimicrob. Agents Chemother.* **42**, 1284–1287.

28. Takei, M., Fukuda, H., Yasue, T., Hosaka, M., and Oomori, Y. (1998). Inhibitory activities of gatifloxacin (AM-1155), a newly developed fluoroquinolone, against bacterial and mammalian type II topoisomerases. *Antimicrob. Agents Chemother.* **42**, 2678–2681.

29. Suto, M. J., Domagala, J. M., Roland, G. E., Mailloux, G. B., and Cohen, M. A. (1992). Fluoroquinolones: Relationships between structural variations, mammalian cell cytotoxicity and antimicrobial activity. *J. Med. Chem.* **35**, 4745–4750.

30. Woodcock, J. M., Andrews, J. M., Boswell, F. J., Brenwald, N. P., and Wise, R. (1997). *In vitro* activity of BAY 12-8039, a new fluoroquinolone. *Antimicrob. Agents Chemother.* **41**, 101–106.

31. Domagala, J. M., Bridges, A. J., Culbertson, T. P., Gambino, L., Hagen, S. E., Karrick, G., Porter, K., Sanchez, J. P., Sesnie, J. A., Spense, G., Szotek, D., and Wemple, J. (1991). Synthesis and biological activity of 5-amino- and 5-hydroxyquinolones, and the overwhelming influence of the remote N_1-substituent in determining the structure–activity relationship. *J. Med. Chem.* **34**, 1142–1154.

32. Blum, M. D., Graham, D. J., and McCloskey, C. A. (1994). Temafloxacin syndrome: Review of 95 cases. *Clin. Infect. Dis.* **18**, 946–950.

33. Barry, A. L., and Jones, R. N. (1989). *In vitro* activities of temafloxacin, tosufloxacin (A-61827) and five other fluoroquinolone agents. *J. Antimicrob. Chemother.* **23**, 527–535.

34. Bazile, S., Moreau, N., Bouzard, D., and Essiz, M. (1992). Relationships among antibacterial activity, inhibition of DNA gyrase, and intracellular accumulation of 11 fluoroquinolones. *Antimicrob. Agents Chemother.* **36**, 2622–2627.

35. Miyamoto, T., Matsumoto, J.-I., Chiba, K., Egawa, H., Shibamori, K.-I., Minamida, A., Nishimura, Y., Okada, H., Kataoka, M., Fujita, M., Hirose, T., and Nakano, J. (1990). Synthesis and structure-activity relationships of 5-substituted 6,8-difluoroquinolones, including sparfloxacin, a new quinolone antibacterial agent with improved potency. *J. Med. Chem.* **33**, 1645–1656.

36. Chu, D. T. W., Fernandes, P. B., Claiborne, A. K., Pihuleac, E., Nordeen, C. W., Maleczka Jr., R. E., and Pernet, A. G. (1985). Synthesis and structure–activity relationships of novel arylfluoroquinolone antibacterial agents. *J. Med. Chem.* **28**, 1558–1564.

37. Chu, D. T. W., Fernandes, P. B., Maleczka Jr., R. E., Nordeen, C. W., and Pernet, A. G. (1987). Synthesis and structure-activity relationship of 1-aryl-6,8-difluoroquinolone antibacterial agents. *J. Med. Chem.* **30**, 504–509.

38. Johnson, D. M., Jones, R. N., and Erwin, M. E. (1999). Anti-streptococcal activity of SB-265805 (LB20304), a novel fluoronaphthyridone, compared with five other compounds, including quality control guidelines. *Diag. Microbiol. Infect. Dis.* **33**, 87–91.

39. Biedenbach, D. J., Barrett, M. S., Croco, M. A. T., and Jones, R. N. (1998). BAY 12-8039, a novel fluoroquinolone: Activity against important respiratory tract pathogens. *Diag. Microbiol. Infect. Dis.* **31**, 45–50.

40. Ito, T., Otsuki, M., and Nishino, T. (1992). *In vitro* antibacterial activity of Q-35, a new fluoroquinolone. *Antimicrob. Agents Chemother.* **36**, 1708–1714.

41. Hoellman, D. B., Lin, G., Jacobs, M. R., and Appelbaum, P. C. (1999). Anti-pneumococcal activity of gatifloxacin compared with other quinolone and non-quinolone agents. *J. Antimicrob. Chemother.* **43**, 645–649.

42. Davis, R., and Bryson, H. M. (1994). Levofloxacin: A review of its antibacterial activity, pharmacokinetics and therapeutic efficacy. *Drugs* **47**, 677–700.

43. Blondeau, J. M. (1999). A review of the comparative *in vitro* activities of 12 antimicrobial agents, with a focus on five new respiratory quinolones. *J. Antimicrob. Chemother.* **43** (Suppl. B), 1–11.

44. Gaja, M. (1992). *In vitro* and *in vivo* antibacterial activity of four newly developed quinolone agents against *Legionella* infection. *Chemotherapy (Tokyo)* **40**, 1–10.

45. Edelstein, P. H., Edelstein, M. A. C., Lehr, K. H., and Ren, J. (1996). *In vitro* activity of levofloxacin against clinical isolates of *Legionella* spp., its pharmacokinetics in guinea pigs, and use in experimental *Legionella pneumophila* pneumonia. *J. Antimicrob. Chemother.* **37**, 117–126.

46. Felmingham, D., Robbins, M., Dencer, C., Salman, H., Mathias, I., and Ridgway, G. (1999). *In vitro* activity of gemifloxacin against *Streptococcus pneumoniae*, *Haemophilus influenzae*, *Moraxella catarrhalis*, *Legionella pneumophila* and *Chlamydia* spp. *Abstr. 21st Int. Cong. Chemother.*, Birmingham, UK. Abstr. #P408.

47. Soejima, R., Niki, Y., Kishimoto, T., Miyashita, N., Kubota, Y., and Nakata, K. (1995). *In vitro* and *in vivo* activities of sparfloxacin and reference drugs against *Chlamydia pneumoniae*. *J. Infect. Chemother.* **1**, 107–111.

48. Hammerschlag, M. R. (1999). Activity of quinolones against *Chlamydia pneumoniae*. *Drugs* **58** (Suppl. 2), 78–81.

49. Yew, W. W., Piddock, L. J. V., Li, M. S. K., Lyon, D., Chan, C. Y., and Cheng, A. F. B. (1994). *In vitro* activity of quinolones and macrolides against mycobacteria. *J. Antimicrob. Chemother.* **34**, 343–351.

50. Sirgel, F. A., Venter, A., and Heilmann, H.-D. (1995). Comparative *in vitro* activity of BAY y 3118, a new quinolone, and ciprofloxacin against *Mycobacterium tuberculosis* and *Mycobacterium avium* complex. *J. Antimicrob. Chemother.* **35**, 349–351.

51. Saito, H., Tomioka, H., Sato, K., and Dekio, S. (1994). *In vitro* and *in vivo* antimycobacterial activities of a new quinolone, DU-6859a. *Antimicrob. Agents Chemother.* **38**, 2877–2882.

52. Tomioka, H., Saito, H., and Sato, K. (1993). Comparative antimycobacterial activities of the newly synthesized quinolone AM-1155, sparfloxacin, and ofloxacin. *Antimicrob. Agents Chemother.* **37**, 1259–1263.

53. Gillespie, S. H., and Billington, O. (1999). Activity of moxifloxacin against mycobacteria. *J. Antimicrob. Chemother.* **44**, 393–395.

54. Gillespie, S. H. (1999). The activity of moxifloxacin and other fluoroquinolones against *Mycobacterium tuberculosis* and other mycobacteria. In "Moxifloxacin In Practice" (D. Adam and R. Finch, eds.), Vol. 1, pp. 71–79. Maxim Medical, Oxford.

55. Renau, T. E., Sanchez, J. P., Gage, J. W., Dever, J. A., Shapiro, M. A., Gracheck, S. J., and Domagala, J. M. (1996). Structure–activity relationships of the quinolone antibacterials against mycobacteria: Effect of structural changes at N-1 and C-7. *J. Med. Chem.* **39**, 729–735.

56. Renau, T. E., Gage, J. W., Dever, J. A., Roland, G. E., Joannides, E. T., Shapiro, M. A., Sanchez, J. P., Gracheck, S. J., Domagala, J. M., Jacobs, M. R., and Reynolds, R. C. (1996). Structure–activity relationships of quinolone agents against mycobacteria: Effect of structural modifications at the 8 position. *Antimicrob. Agents Chemother.* **40**, 2363–2368.

57. Child, J., Andrews, J., Boswell, F., Brenwald, N., and Wise, R. (1995). The *in vitro* activity of CP-99,219, a new naphthyridone antimicrobial agent: A comparison with fluoroquinolone agents. *J. Antimicrob. Chemother.* **35**, 869–876.

58. Jacobs, M. R. (1995). Activity of quinolones against mycobacteria. *Drugs* **49** (Suppl. 2), 67–75.

59. Ruiz-Serrano, M. J., Alcalá, L., Martínez, L., Díaz, M. S., Marín, M., González Abad, M. J., and Bouza, E. (1999). *In vitro* activity of six quinolones against clinical isolates of *Mycobacterium tuberculosis* susceptible and resistant to first-line antituberculous drugs. *Abstr. 39th Intersci. Conf. Antimicrob. Agents Chemother.*, San Francisco. Abstr. #1492.

60. Mor, N., Vanderkolk, J., and Heifets, L. (1994). Inhibitory and bactericidal activities of levofloxacin against *Mycobacterium tuberculosis in vitro* and in human macrophages. *Antimicrob. Agents Chemother.* **38**, 1161–1164.

61. Wise, R., Ashby, J. P., and Andrews, J. M. (1988). *In vitro* activity of PD 127,391, an enhanced-spectrum quinolone. *Antimicrob. Agents Chemother.* **32**, 1251–1256.

62. Renaudin, H., and Bébéar, C. (1995). *In vitro* susceptibility of mycoplasmas to a new quinolone, BAY y 3118. *Drugs* **49** (Suppl. 2), 243–245.

63. Kenny, G. E., and Cartwright, F. D. (1993). Susceptibilities of *Mycoplasma hominis*, *Mycoplasma pneumoniae*, and *Ureaplasma urealyticum* to a new quinolone, OPC 17116. *Antimicrob. Agents Chemother.* **37**, 1726–1727.

64. Kenny, G. E., and Cartwright, F. D. (1996). Susceptibilities of *Mycoplasma pneumoniae*, *Mycoplasma hominis*, and *Ureaplasma urealyticum* to a new quinolone, trovafloxacin (CP-99,219). *Antimicrob. Agents Chemother.* **40**, 1048–1049.

65. Ishida, K., Kaku, M., Irifune, K., Mizukane, R., Takemura, H., Yoshida, R., Tanaka, H., Usui, T., Tomono, K., Suyama, N., Koga, H., Kohno, S., and Hara, K. (1994). *In vitro* and *in vivo* activity of a new quinolone, AM-1155, against *Mycoplasma pneumoniae*. *J. Antimicrob. Chemother.* **34**, 875–883.

66. Hannan, P. C. T., and Woodnutt, G. (1999). Comparative activities of gemifloxacin, other fluoroquinolones, erythromycin and doxycycline against human mycoplasmas and ureaplasmas and *in vitro* development of resistance to certain of these agents in *Mycoplasma pneumoniae*. *Abstr. 39th Intersci. Conf. Antimicrob. Agents Chemother.*, San Francisco. Abstr. #2295.

67. Bébéar, C. M., Renaudin, H., Boudjadja, A., and Bébéar, C. (1998). *In vitro* activity of BAY 12-8039, a new fluoroquinolone, against mycoplasmas. *Antimicrob. Agents. Chemother.* **42**, 703–704.

68. Gohara, Y., Arai, S., Akashi, A., Kuwano, K., Tseng, C.-C., Matsubara, S., Matumoto, M., and Furudera, T. (1993). *In vitro* and *in vivo* activities of Q-35, a new fluoroquinolone, against *Mycoplasma pneumoniae*. *Antimicrob. Agents Chemother.* **37**, 1826–1830.

69. King, A., Bethune, L., and Phillips, I. (1991). The *in vitro* activity of tosufloxacin, a new fluorinated quinolone, compared with that of ciprofloxacin and temafloxacin. *J. Antimicrob. Chemother.* **28**, 719–725.

70. Yoshida, T., and Mitsuhashi, S. (1993). Antibacterial activity of NM394, the active form of prodrug NM441, a new quinolone. *Antimicrob. Agents Chemother.* **37**, 793–800.

71. Hohl, A. F., Frei, R., Pünter, V., von Graevenitz, A., Knapp, C., Washington, J., Johnson, D., Jones, R. N. (1998). International multicenter investigation of LB20304, a new fluoronaphthyridone. *Clin. Microbiol Infect.* **4**, 280–284.

72. Bauernfeind, A. (1997). Comparison of the antibacterial activities of the quinolones Bay 12-8039, gatifloxacin (AM 1155), trovafloxacin, clinafloxacin, levofloxacin and ciprofloxacin. *J. Antimicrob. Chemother.* **40**, 639–651.

73. Nye, K., Shi, Y. G., Andrews, J. M., Ashby, J. P., and Wise, R. (1989). The *in vitro* activity, pharmacokinetics and tissue penetration of temafloxacin. *J. Antimicrob. Chemother.* **24**, 415–424.

74. Shen, L. L., and Chu, D. T. W. (1996). Type II DNA topoisomerases as antibacterial targets. *Curr. Pharmaceut. Design* **2**, 195–208.

75. Bremm, K. D., Petersen, U., Metzger, K. G., and Endermann, R. (1992). *In vitro* evaluation of BAY y 3118, a new full-spectrum fluoroquinolone. *Chemotherapy (Basel)* **38**, 376–387.

76. Gootz, T. D., and McGuirk, P. R. (1994). New quinolones in development. *Expert Opin. Invest. Drugs* **3**, 93–114.

77. Muratani, T., Inoue, M., and Mitsuhashi, S. (1992). *In vitro* activity of T-3761, a new fluoroquinolone. *Antimicrob. Agents Chemother.* **36**, 2293–2303.

78. Cormican, M. G., and Jones, R. N. (1997). Antimicrobial activity and spectrum of LB20304, a novel fluoronaphthyridone. *Antimicrob. Agents Chemother.* **41**, 204–211.

79. Jolley, A., Andrews, J. M., Brenwald, N., and Wise, R. (1993). The *in vitro* activity of a new highly active quinolone, DU-6859a. *J. Antimicrob. Chemother.* **32**, 757–763.

80. Neu, H. C., Fang, W., Gu, J.-W., and Chin, N.-X. (1992). *In vitro* activity of OPC-17116. *Antimicrob. Agents Chemother.* **36**, 1310–1315.

81. Hosaka, M., Kinoshita, S., Toyama, A., Otsuki, M., and Nishino, T. (1995). Antibacterial properties of AM-1155, a new 8-methoxy quinolone. *J. Antimicrob. Chemother.* **36**, 293–301.

82. Dalhoff, A., Petersen, U., and Endermann, R. (1996). *In vitro* activity of BAY 12-8039, a new 8-methoxyquinolone. *Chemotherapy* **42**, 410–425.

83. Ito, T., Kojima, K., Koizumi, K., Nagano, H., and Nishino, T. (1994). Inhibitory activity on DNA gyrase and intracellular accumulation of quinolones: Structure-activity relationship of Q-35 analogs. *Biol. Pharmacol. Bull.* **17**, 927–930.

84. Aldridge, K. E. (1994). Increased activity of a new chlorofluoroquinolone, BAY y 3118, compared with activities of ciprofloxacin, sparfloxacin, and other antimicrobial agents against anaerobic bacteria. *Antimicrob. Agents Chemother.* **38**, 1671–1674.

85. MacGowan, A. P., Bowker, K. E., Holt, H. A., Wootton, M., and Reeves, D. S. (1997). Bay 12-8039, a new 8-methoxy-quinolone: Comparative *in vitro* activity with nine other antimicrobials against anaerobic bacteria. *J. Antimicrob. Chemother.* **40**, 503–509.

86. Betriu, C., Gómez, M., Palau, M. L., Sánchez, A., and Picazo, J. J. (1999). Activities of new antimicrobial agents (trovafloxacin, moxifloxacin, sanfetrinem, and quinupristin-dalfopristin) against *Bacteroides fragilis* group: Comparison with the activities of 14 other agents. *Antimicrob. Agents Chemother.* **43**, 2320–2322.

87. Appelbaum, P. C. (1995). Quinolone activity against anaerobes: Microbiological aspects. *Drugs* **49** (Suppl. 2), 76–80.

88. Hecht, D. W., and Wexler, H. M. (1996). *In vitro* susceptibility of anaerobes to quinolones in the United States. *Clin. Infect. Dis.* **23** (Suppl. 1), S2–S8.

89. Kato, N., Kato, H., Tanaka-Bandoh, K., Watanabe, K., and Ueno, K. (1997). Comparative *in vitro* and *in vivo* activity of AM-1155 against anaerobic bacteria. *J. Antimicrob. Chemother.* **40**, 631–637.

90. Aldridge, K. E., Ashcraft, D., and Bowman, K. A. (1997). Comparative *in vitro* activities of trovafloxacin (CP-99,219) and other antimicrobials against clinically significant anaerobes. *Antimicrob. Agents Chemother.* **41**, 484–487.

91. Goldstein, E. J. C., Citron, D. M., Warren, Y., Tyrrell, K., and Merriam, C. V. (1999). *In vitro* activity of gemifloxacin (SB 265805) against anaerobes. *Antimicrob. Agents Chemother.* **43**, 2231–2235.

92. Thomson, K. S., Sanders, C. C., and Hayden, M. E. (1991). *In vitro* studies with five quinolones: Evidence for changes in relative potency as quinolone resistance rises. *Antimicrob. Agents Chemother.* **35**, 2329–2334.

93. Kitamura, A., Hoshino, K., Kimura, Y., Hayakawa, I., and Sato, K. (1995). Contribution of the C-8 substituent of DU-6859a, a new potent fluoroquinolone, to its activity against DNA gyrase mutants of *Pseudomonas aeruginosa*. *Antimicrob. Agents Chemother.* **39**, 1467–1471.

94. Ito, T., Matsumoto, M., and Nishino, T. (1995). Improved bactericidal activity of Q-35 against quinolone-resistant staphylococci. *Antimicrob. Agents Chemother.* **39**, 1522–1525.

95. Fukuda, H., Hori, S., and Hiramatsu, K. (1998). Antibacterial activity of gatifloxacin (AM-1155, CG5501, BMS-206584), a newly developed fluoroquinolone, against sequentially acquired quinolone-resistant mutants and the *norA* transformant of *Staphylococcus aureus*. *Antimicrob. Agents Chemother.* **42**, 1917–1922.

96. Schedletzky, H., Wiedemann, B., and Heisig, P. (1999). The effect of moxifloxacin on its target topoisomerases from *Escherichia coli* and *Staphylococcus aureus*. *J. Antimicrob. Chemother.* **43** (Suppl. B), 31–37.

97. Zhao, X., Wang, J.-Y., Xu, C., Dong, Y., Zhou, J., Domagala, J., and Drlica, K. (1998). Killing of *Staphylococcus aureus* by C-8 methoxy fluoroquinolones. *Antimicrob. Agents Chemother.* **42**, 956–958.

98. Zhao, X., Xu, C., Domagala, J., and Drlica, K. (1997). DNA topoisomerase targets of the fluoroquinolones: A strategy for avoiding bacterial resistance. *Proc. Natl. Acad. Sci. U.S.A.* **94**, 13991–13996.

99. Lu, T., Zhao, X., and Drlica, K. (1999). Gatifloxacin activity against quinolone-resistant gyrase: Allele-specific enhancement of bacteriostatic and bactericidal activities by the C-8 methoxy group. *Antimicrob. Agents Chemother.* **43**, 2969–2974.

100. Jones, M. E., Sahm, D. F., Martin, N., Scheuring, S., Heisig, P., Thornsberry, C., Köhrer, K., and Schmitz, F.-J. (2000). Prevalence of *gyrA*, *gyrB*, *parC*, and *parE* mutations in clinical isolates of *Streptococcus pneumoniae* with decreased susceptibilities to different fluoroquinolones and originating from worldwide surveillance studies during the 1997–1998 respiratory season. *Antimicrob. Agents Chemother.* **44**, 462–466.

101. Chen, D. K., McGeer, A., de Azavedo, J. C., and Low, D. E. (1999). Decreased susceptibility of *Streptococcus pneumoniae* to fluoroquinolones in Canada. *New Engl. J. Med.* **341**, 233–239.

102. Yamada, H., Kurose-Hamada, S., Fukuda, Y., Mitsuyama, J., Takahata, M., Minami, S., Watanabe, Y., and Narita, H. (1997). Quinolone susceptibility of *norA*-disrupted *Staphylococcus aureus*. *Antimicrob. Agents Chemother.* **41**, 2308–2309.

103. Takenouchi, T., Tabata, F., Iwata, Y., Hanzawa, H., Sugawara, M., and Ohya, S. (1996). Hydrophilicity of quinolones is not an exclusive factor for decreased activity in efflux-mediated resistant mutants of *Staphylococcus aureus*. *Antimicrob. Agents Chemother.* **40**, 1835–1842.

104. Imada, T., Miyazaki, S., Nishida, M., Yamaguchi, K., and Goto, S. (1992). *In vitro* and *in vivo* antibacterial activities of a new quinolone, OPC-17116. *Antimicrob. Agents Chemother.* **36**, 573–579.

105. Kimura, Y., Atarashi, S., Kawakami, K., Sato, K., and Hayakawa, I. (1994). (Fluorocyclopropyl)quinolones, 2: Synthesis and stereochemical structure-activity relationships of chiral 7-(7-amino-5-azaspiro[2.4]heptan-5-yl)-1-(2-fluorocyclopropyl) quinolone antibacterial agents. *J. Med. Chem.* **37**, 3344–3352.

106. Segawa, J., Kitano, M., Kazuno, K., Matsuoka, M., Shirahase, I., Ozaki, M., Matsuda, M., Tomii, Y., and Kise, M. (1992). Studies on pyridonecarboxylic acids, 1: Synthesis and antibacterial evaluation of 7-substituted-6-halo-4-oxo-4*H*-[1,3]thiazeto[3,2-*a*]quinoline-3-carboxylic acids. *J. Med. Chem.* **35**, 4727–4738.

107. Ozaki, M., Matsuda, M., Tomii, Y., Kimura, K., Segawa, J., Kitano, M., Kise, M., Shibata, K., Otsuki, M., and Nishino, T. (1991). *In vivo* evaluation of NM441, a new thiazeto-quinoline derivative. *Antimicrob. Agents Chemother.* **35**, 2496–2499.

108. Mitscher, L. A., Devasthale, P., and Zavod, R. (1993). Structure-activity relationships. *In* "Quinolone Antimicrobial Agents," 2nd ed. (D. C. Hooper and J. S. Wolfson, eds.), pp. 3–51. American Society for Microbiology, Washington, DC.

109. Brighty, K. E., and Gootz, T. D. (1997). The chemistry and biological profile of trovafloxacin. *J. Antimicrob. Chemother.* **39** (Suppl. B), 1–14.

110. Tack, K. J., McGuire, N. M., and Eiseman, I. A. (1995). Initial clinical experience with clinafloxacin in the treatment of serious infections. *Drugs* **49** (Suppl. 2), 488–491.

111. Schmidt, U., and Schluter, G. (1996). Studies on the mechanism of phototoxicity of BAY y 3118 and other quinolones. In "Biological Reactive Intermediates V" (R. Snyder, ed.), pp. 117–120. Plenum, New York.

112. Sanchez, J. P., Gogliotti, R. D., Domagala, J. M., Gracheck, S. J., Huband, M. D., Sesnie, J. A., Cohen, M. A., and Shapiro, M. A. (1995). The synthesis, structure–activity, and structure–side effect relationships of a series of 8-alkoxy- and 5-amino-8-alkoxyquinolone antibacterial agents. *J. Med. Chem.* **38**, 4478–4487.

113. Man, I., Murphy, J., and Ferguson, J. (1999). Fluoroquinolone phototoxicity: A comparison of moxifloxacin and lomefloxacin in normal volunteers. *J. Antimicrob. Chemother.* **43** (Suppl. B), 77–82.

114. Ferguson, J., McEwen, J., Goehler, K., and Mignot, A. (1998). A double-blind, placebo- and positive-controlled randomized study to investigate the phototoxic potential of gatifloxacin, a new fluoroquinolone antibiotic. *Abstr. 38th Intersci. Conf. Antimicrob. Agents Chemother.*, San Diego. Abstr. #A-78.

115. Matsumoto, M., Kojima, K., Nagano, H., Matsubara, S., and Yokota, T. (1992). Photostability and biological activity of fluoroquinolones substituted at the 8 position after UV irradiation. *Antimicrob. Agents Chemother.* **36**, 1715–1719.

116. Sörgel, F., and Kinzig, M. (1993). Pharmacokinetics of gyrase inhibitors, Part 2: Renal and hepatic elimination pathways and drug interactions. *Am. J. Med.* **94** (Suppl. 3A), 56S–69S.

117. Niki, Y., Hashiguchi, K., Okimoto, N., and Soejima, R. (1992). Quinolone antimicrobial agents and theophylline. *Chest* **101**, 881.

118. Niki, Y., Hashiguchi, K., Miyashita, N., Nakajima, M., Matsushima, T. (1999). Influence of gatifloxacin, a new quinolone antibacterial, on pharmacokinetics of theophylline. *J. Infect. Chemother.* **5**, 156–162.

119. Hashiguchi, K., Nakabayashi, M., Yoshida, K., Miyashita, N., Nakajima, M., Niki, Y., and Soejima, R. (1995). Effect of balofloxacin on the serum concentration of theophylline. *Nippon Kagaku Ryoho Gakkai Zasshi* **43** (Suppl. 5), 168–173.

120. Vincent, J., Teng, R., Dogolo, L. C., Willavize, S. A., and Friedman, H. L. (1997). Effect of trovafloxacin, a new fluoroquinolone antibiotic, on the steady-state pharmacokinetics of theophylline in healthy volunteers. *J. Antimicrob. Chemother.* **39** (Suppl. B), 81–86.

121. Wise, R. (1999). A review of the clinical pharmacology of moxifloxacin, a new 8-methoxyquinolone, and its potential relation to therapeutic efficacy. *Clin. Drug Invest.* **17**, 365–387.

122. Mizuki, Y., Fujiwara, I., and Yamaguchi, T. (1996). Pharmacokinetic interactions related to the chemical structures of fluoroquinolones. *J. Antimicrob. Chemother.* **37** (Suppl. A), 41–55.

123. Randinitis, E. J., Koup, J. R., Rausch, G., and Vassos, A. B. (1999). Effect of clinafloxacin on the pharmacokinetics of theophylline and caffeine. *Drugs* **58** (Suppl. 2), 248–249.

124. Davy, M., Allen, A., Bird, N., Rost, K. L., and Fuder, H. (1999). Lack of effect of gemifloxacin on the steady-state pharmacokinetics of theophylline in healthy volunteers. *Abstr. 21st Int. Cong. Chemother.*, Birmingham, UK, Abstr. #P419.

125. Nabuchi, Y., Yano, K., Asoh, Y., Tanaka, K., and Takatoh, M. (1993). Effect of Q-35, a new pyridone carboxylic acid, on theophylline metabolism in rat liver microsomes. *Yakubutsu Dotai* **8**, 239–245.

126. Niki, Y., Itokawa, K., and Okazaki, O. (1998). Effects of sitafloxacin, a new quinolone antimicrobial, on theophylline metabolism in *in vitro* and *in vivo* studies. *Antimicrob. Agents Chemother.* **42**, 1751–1755.

127. Barrett, J. F. (1996). Quinolone antibacterials and derivatives as antineoplastic agents. *Expert Opin. Invest. Drugs* **5**, 1021–1031.

128. Rádl, S., and Dax, S. (1994). Quinolone congeners as mammalian topoisomerase-II inhibitors. *Curr. Med. Chem.* **1**, 262–270.

129. Xia, Y., Yang, Z.-Y., Morris-Natschke, S. L., and Lee, K.-H. (1999). Recent advances in the discovery and development of quinolones and analogs as antitumor agents. *Curr. Med. Chem.* **6**, 179–194.

130. Gootz, T. D., McGuirk, P. R., Moynihan, M. S., and Haskell, S. L. (1994). Placement of alkyl substituents on the C-7 piperazine ring of fluoroquinolones: Dramatic differential effects on mammalian topoisomerase II and DNA gyrase. *Antimicrob. Agents Chemother.* **38**, 130–133.

131. Hoshino, K., Sato, K., Kitamura, A., Hayakawa, I., Sato, M., and Osada, Y. (1991). Inhibitory effects of DU-6859, a new fluorinated quinolone, on type II topoisomerases. *Abstr. 31st Intersci. Conf. Antimicrob. Agents Chemother.*, Chicago. Abstr. #1506.

132. Shimada, H., and Itoh, S. (1991). Effects of DU-6859 and the related quinolone antibacterial agents on mammalian chromosomes. *Abstr. 31st Intersci. Conf. Antimicrob. Agents Chemother.*, Chicago. Abstr. #1507.

133. Todo, Y., Takagi, H., Iino, F., Fukuoka, Y., Takahata, M., Okamoto, S., Saikawa, I., and Narita, H. (1994). Pyridonecarboxylic acids as antibacterial agents, IX: Synthesis and structure–activity relationship of 3-substituted 10-(1-aminocyclopropyl)-9-fluoro-7-oxo-2,3-dihydro-7*H*-pyrido-[1,2,3-*de*]-1,4-benzoxazine-6-carboxylic acids and their 1-thio and 1-aza analogues. *Chem. Pharm. Bull.* **42**, 2569–2574.

134. Sörgel, F., and Kinzig, M. (1993). Pharmacokinetics of gyrase inhibitors, Part 1: Basic chemistry and gastrointestinal disposition. *Am. J. Med.* **94** (Suppl. 3A), 44S–55S.

135. Riley, C. M., Kindberg, C. G., and Stella, V. J. (1989). The physicochemical properties of quinolone antimicrobials variously substituted at C-7. Implications in the development of liquid dosage forms. In "International Telesymposium on Quinolones" (P. B. Fernandes, ed.), pp. 21–36. J. R. Prous Science Publishers, Barcelona.

136. Rosen, T., Chu, D. T. W., Lico, I. M., Fernandes, P. B., Marsh, K., Shen, L., Cepa, V. G., and Pernet, A. G. (1988). Design, synthesis and properties of (4*S*)-7-(4-amino-2-substituted-pyrrolidin-1-yl)quinolone-3-carboxylic acids. *J. Med. Chem.* **31**, 1598–1611.

137. Brighty, K. E., Gootz, T. D., Girard, A., Shanker, R., Castaldi, M. J., Girard, D., Miller, S. A., and Faiella, J. (1994). Prodrugs of CP-99,219 for IV administration: Synthesis and evaluation resulting in identification of CP-116,517. *Abstr. 34th Intersci. Conf. Antimicrob. Agents Chemother.*, Orlando, Florida. Abstr. #F28.

138. Lomaestro, B. M., and Bailie, G. R. (1995). Absorption interactions with fluoroquinolones, 1995 update. *Drug Saf.* **12**, 314–333.

139. Lecomte, S., Baron, M. H., Chenon, M. T., Coupry, C., and Moreau, N. J. (1994). Effect of magnesium complexation by fluoroquinolones on their antibacterial properties. *Antimicrob. Agents Chemother.* **38**, 2810–2816.

140. Shimada, J., Shiba, K., Oguma, T., Miwa, H., Yoshimura, Y., Nishikawa, T., Okabayashi, Y., Kitagawa, T., and Yamamoto, S. (1992). Effect of antacid on absorption of the quinolone lomefloxacin. *Antimicrob. Agents Chemother.* **36**, 1219–1224.

141. Maeda, Y., Omoda, K., Konishi, T., Takahashi, M., Kihira, K., Hibino, S., and Tsukiai, S. (1993). Effects of aluminium-containing antacid on bioavailability of ofloxacin following oral administration of pivaloyloxymethyl ester of ofloxacin as prodrug. *Biol. Pharmacol. Bull.* **16**, 594–599.

142. Ross, D. L., and Riley, C. M. (1994). Dissociation and complexation of the fluoroquinolone antimicrobials—an update. *J. Pharm. Biomed. Anal.* **12**, 1325–1331.

143. Tanaka, M., Kurata, T., Fujisawa, C., Ohshima, Y., Aoki, H., Okazaki, O., and Hakusui, H. (1993). Mechanistic study of inhibition of levofloxacin absorption by aluminum hydroxide. *Antimicrob. Agents Chemother.* **37**, 2173–2178.

144. Ross, D. L., and Riley, C. M. (1992). Physicochemical properties of the fluoroquinolone antimicrobials, III: Complexation of lomefloxacin with various metal ions and the effect of metal ion complexation on aqueous solubility. *Int. J. Pharm.* **87**, 203–213.

145. Ross, D. L., Elkinton, S. K., Knaub, S. R., and Riley, C. M. (1993). Physicochemical properties of the fluoroquinolone antimicrobials, VI: Effect of metal–ion complexation on octan-1-ol-water partitioning. *Int. J. Pharm.* **93**, 131–138.

146. Hayakawa, I., Atarashi, S., Yokohama, S., Imamura, M., Sakano, K.-I., and Furukawa, M. (1986). Synthesis and antibacterial activities of optically active ofloxacin. *Antimicrob. Agents Chemother.* **29**, 163–164.

147. Une, T., Fujimoto, T., Sato, K., and Osada, Y. (1988). *In vitro* activity of DR-3355, an optically active ofloxacin. *Antimicrob. Agents Chemother.* **32**, 1336–1340.

148. Hayakawa, I., Atarashi, S., Kimura, Y., Kawakami, K., Saito, T., Yafune, T., Sato, K., Une, T., and Sato, M. (1991). Design and structure–activity relationship of new N₁-*cis*-2-fluorocyclopropyl quinolones. *Abstr. 31st Intersci. Conf. Antimicrob. Agents Chemother.*, Chicago. Abstr. #1504.

149. Atarashi, S., Imamura, M., Kimura, Y., Yoshida, A., and Hayakawa, I. (1993). Fluorocyclopropyl quinolones, 1: Synthesis and structure-activity relationships of 1-(2-fluorocyclopropyl)-3-pyridonecarboxylic acid antibacterial agents. *J. Med. Chem.* **36**, 3444–3448.

150. Chu, D. T. W., Nordeen, C. W., Hardy, D. J., Swanson, R. N., Giardina, W. J., Pernet, A. G., and Plattner, J. J. (1991). Synthesis, antibacterial activities, and pharmacological properties of enantiomers of temafloxacin hydrochloride. *J. Med. Chem.* **34**, 168–174.

151. Rosen, T., Chu, D. T. W., Lico, I. M., Fernandes, P. B., Shen, L., Borodkin, S., and Pernet, A. G. (1988). Asymmetric synthesis and properties of the enantiomers of the antibacterial agent 7-(3-aminopyrrolidin-1-yl)-1-(2,4-difluorophenyl)-1,4-dihydro-6-fluoro-4-oxo-1,8-naphthyridine-3-carboxylic acid hydrochloride. *J. Med. Chem.* **31**, 1586–1590.

152. Petersen, U., Bremm, K.-D., Dalhoff, A., Endermann, R., Heilmann, W., Krebs, A., and Schenke, T. (1999). The synthesis and *in vitro* and *in vivo* antibacterial activity of moxifloxacin (BAY

12-8039), a new 8-methoxyquinolone. In "Moxifloxacin In Practice" (D. Adam and R. Finch, eds.), Vol. 1, pp. 13–26. Maxim Medical, Oxford.

153. Allen, A., Bygate, E., Coleman, K., McAllister, P., and Teillol-Foo, M. (1999). *In vitro* activity and single-dose pharmacokinetics of the (+)- and (–)-enantiomers of gemifloxacin in volunteers. *Abstr. 21st Int. Cong. Chemother.*, Birmingham, UK. Abstr. #P449.

154. Takahata, M., Mitsuyama, J., Yamashiro, Y., Yonezawa, M., Araki, H., Todo, Y., Minami, S., Watanabe, Y., and Narita, H. (1999). *In vitro* and *in vivo* antimicrobial activities of T-3811ME, a novel des-F(6)-quinolone. *Antimicrob. Agents Chemother.* **43**, 1077–1084.

155. Hayashi, K., Todo, Y., Hamamoto, S., Ojima, K., Yamada, M., Kito, T., Takahata, M., Watanabe, Y., and Narita, H. (1997). T-3811, a novel des-F(6)-quinolone: Synthesis and *in vitro* activity of 7-(isoindolin-5-yl) derivatives. *Abstr. 37th Intersci. Conf. Antimicrob. Agents Chemother.*, Toronto. Abstr. #F-158.

156. Cecchetti, V., Clementi, S., Cruciani, G., Fravolini, A., Pagella, P. G., Savino, A., and Tabarrini, O. (1995). 6-Aminoquinolones: A new class of quinolone antibacterials? *J. Med. Chem.* **38**, 973–982.

157. Cecchetti, V., Fravolini, A., Lorenzini, M. C., Tabarrini, O., Terni, P., and Xin, T. (1996). Studies on 6-aminoquinolones: Synthesis and antibacterial evaluation of 6-amino-8-methylquinolones. *J. Med. Chem.* **39**, 436–445.

158. Wise, R., Pagella, P. G., Cecchetti, V., Fravolini, A., and Tabarrini, O. (1995). *In vitro* activity of MF 5137, a new potent 6-aminoquinolone. *Drugs* **49** (Suppl. 2), 272–273.

159. Li, Q., Chu, D. T. W., Claiborne, A., Cooper, C. S., Lee, C. M., Raye, K., Berst, K. B., Donner, P., Wang, W., Hasvold, L., Fung, A., Ma, Z., Tufano, M., Flamm, R., Shen, L. L., Baranowski, J., Nilius, A., Alder, J., Meulbroek, J., Marsh, K., Crowell, D., Hui, Y., Seif, L., Melcher, L. M., Henry, R., Spanton, S., Faghih, R., Klein, L. L., Tanaka, S. K., and Plattner, J. J. (1996). Synthesis and structure–activity relationships of 2-pyridones: A novel series of potent DNA gyrase inhibitors as antibacterial agents. *J. Med. Chem.* **39**, 3070–3088.

160. Ma, Z., Chu, D. T. W., Cooper, C. S., Li, Q., Fung, A. K. L., Wang, S., Shen, L. L., Flamm, R. K., Nilius, A. M., Alder, J. D., Meulbroek, J. A., and Or, Y. S. (1999). Synthesis and antimicrobial activity of 4*H*-4-oxoquinolizine derivatives: Consequences of structural modification at the C-8 position. *J. Med. Chem.* **42**, 4202–4213.

161. Saiki, A. Y. C., Shen, L. L., Chen, C.-M., Baranowski, J., and Lerner, C. G. (1999). DNA cleavage activities of *Staphylococcus aureus* gyrase and topoisomerase IV stimulated by quinolones and 2-pyridones. *Antimicrob. Agents Chemother.* **43**, 1574–1577.

162. Flamm, R. K., Vojtko, C., Chu, D. T. W., Li, Q., Beyer, J., Hensey, D., Ramer, N., Clement, J. J., and Tanaka, S. K. (1995). *In vitro* evaluation of ABT-719, a novel DNA gyrase inhibitor. *Antimicrob. Agents Chemother.* **39**, 964–970.

163. Eliopoulos, G. M., Wennersten, C. B., Cole, G., Chu, D., Pizzuti, D., and Moellering Jr., R. C. (1995). *In vitro* activity of A-86719.1, a novel 2-pyridone antimicrobial agent. *Antimicrob. Agents Chemother.* **35**, 850–853.

164. Alder, J., Clement, J., Meulbroek, J., Shipkowitz, N., Mitten, M., Jarvis, K., Oleksijew, A., Hutch Sr., T., Paige, L., Flamm, B., Chu, D., and Tanaka, K. (1995). Efficacies of ABT-719 and related 2-pyridones, members of a new class of antibacterial agents, against experimental bacterial infections. *Antimicrob. Agents Chemother.* **39**, 971–975.

165. Armiger, Y. L., Chu, D. T. W., Fung, A. K. L., Li, Q., Wang, A., Nilius, A., Alder, J., Ewing, P., Stone, G., Meulbroek, J., Bui, M., Shen, L. L., Paige, L., Or, Y. S., and Plattner, J. J. (1998). The discovery of A-165753 and 170568, two potent broad spectrum antimicrobial agents. *Abstr. 38th Intersci. Conf. Antimicrob. Agents Chemother.*, San Diego. Abstr. #F86.

166. Fung, A. K. L., and Shen, L. L. (1999). The 2-pyridone antibacterial agents: 8-position modifications. *Curr. Pharmaceut. Design* **5**, 515–543.

167. Morrissey, I., and John, G. (1999). Activities of fluoroquinolones against *Streptococcus pneumoniae* type II topoisomerases purified as recombinant proteins. *Antimicrob. Agents Chemother.* **43**, 2579–2585.
168. Onodera, Y., Uchida, Y., Tanaka, M., and Sato, K. (1999). Dual inhibitory activity of sitafloxacin (DU-6859a) against DNA gyrase and topoisomerase IV of *Streptococcus pneumoniae*. *J. Antimicrob. Chemother.* **44**, 533–536.
169. Fukuda, H., and Hiramatsu, K. (1999). Primary targets of fluoroquinolones in *Streptococcus pneumoniae*. *Antimicrob. Agents Chemother.* **43**, 410–412.
170. Alovero, F. L., Pan, X.-S., Morris, J. E., Manzo, R. H., and Fisher, L. M. (2000). Engineering the specificity of antibacterial fluoroquinolones: Benzenesulfonamide modifications at C-7 of ciprofloxacin change its primary target in *Streptococcus pneumoniae* from topoisomerase IV to gyrase. *Antimicrob. Agents Chemother.* **44**, 320–325.
171. Bryskier, A. (1997). Novelties in the field of fluoroquinolones. *Expert Opin. Invest. Drugs* **6**, 1227–1245.
172. Kato, J., Nishimura, Y., Imamura, R., Niki, H., Hiraga, S., and Suzuki, H. (1990). New topoisomerase essential for chromosome segregation in *E. coli*. *Cell* **63**, 393–404.
173. Hooper, D. C., and Wolfson, J. S. (1993). Mechanisms of quinolone action and bacterial killing. In "Quinolone Antimicrobial Agents," 2nd ed. (D. C. Hooper and J. S. Wolfson, eds.), pp. 53–75. American Society for Microbiology, Washington, DC.
174. Cairns, J. (1963). The chromosome of *Escherichia coli*. *Cold Spring Harbor Symp. Quant. Biol.* **28**, 43–46.
175. Gellert, M. (1981). DNA topoisomerases. *Annu. Rev. Biochem.* **50**, 879–910.
176. Kreuzer, K. N., and Cozzarelli, N. R. (1979). *Escherichia coli* mutants thermosensitive for DNA gyrase subunit A: Effects on DNA replication, transcription, and bacteriophage growth. *J. Bacteriol.* **140**, 424–435.
177. Menzel, R., and Gellert, M. (1983). Regulation of the genes for *E. coli* DNA gyrase: Homoeostatic control of DNA supercoiling. *Cell* **34**, 105–113.
178. Menzel, R., and Gellert, M. (1987). Modulation of transcription by DNA supercoiling: A deletion analysis of the *E. coli* gyrA and gyrB promoters. *Proc. Natl. Acad. Sci. U.S.A.* **84**, 4185–4189.
179. Drlica, K., and Zhao, X. (1997). DNA gyrase, topoisomerase IV, and the 4-quinolones. *Microbiol. Mol. Biol. Rev.* **61**, 377–392.
180. Hiasa, H., Yousef, D. O., and Marians, K. J. (1996). DNA strand cleavage is required for replication fork arrest by a frozen topoisomerase–quinolone–DNA ternary complex. *J. Biol. Chem.* **271**, 26424–26429.
181. Marians, K. J. (1992). Prokaryotic DNA replication. *Annu. Rev. Biochem.* **61**, 673–719.
182. McHenry, C. S. (1992). DNA replication. In "Emerging Targets in Antibacterial and Antifungal Chemotherapy" (J. Sutcliffe and N. Georgopapadakou, eds.), pp. 37–67. Chapman and Hall, New York.
183. Marians, K. J. (1996). Replication fork progression. In "*E. coli* and *Salmonella* Cellular and Molecular Biology," 2nd ed. (F. C. Neidhardt, ed.), Vol. 1, pp. 749–763. American Society for Microbiology, Washington, DC.
184. McHenry, C. S., and Kornberg, A. (1977). DNA polymerase III holoenzyme of *Escherichia coli*: Purification and resolution into subunits. *J. Biol. Chem.* **252**, 6478–6484.
185. Kornberg, A., and Baker, T. A. (1992). "DNA Replication." W. H. Freeman and Co., New York.
186. Hill, T. M. (1996). Features of the chromosomal terminus region. In "*Escherichia coli* and *Salmonella* Cellular and Molecular Biology" (F. Neidhardt, R. Curtis, J. L. Ingraham, E. C. C. Lin, K. B. Low, B. Magasanik, W. Reznikoff, M. Riley, M. Schaechter, and H. E. Umbarger, eds.), Vol. 2, pp. 1602–1614. American Society for Microbiology, Washington, DC.

187. Helmstetter, C. E. (1996). Timing of synthetic activities in the cell cycle. In "*Escherichia coli and Salmonella* Cellular and Molecular Biology" (F. Neidhardt, R. Curtis, J. L. Ingraham, E. C. C. Lin, K. B. Low, B. Magasanik, W. Reznikoff, M. Riley, M. Schaechter, and H. E. Umbarger, eds.), Vol. 2, pp. 1627–1639. American Society for Microbiology, Washington, DC.

188. Lewis, R. J., Tsai, F. T. F., and Wigley, D. B. (1996). Molecular mechanisms of drug inhibition of DNA gyrase. *Bioessays* **18**, 661–671.

189. Wang, J. C. (1971). Interaction between DNA and an *Escherichia coli* protein omega. *J. Mol. Biol.* **55**, 523–533.

190. DiGate, R. J., and Marians, K. J. (1988). Identification of a potent decatenating enzyme from *E. coli*. *J. Biol. Chem.* **263**, 13366–13373.

191. Moreau, N. J., Robaux, H., Baron, L., and Tabary, X. (1990). Inhibitory effects of quinolones on prokaryotic and eukaryotic DNA topoisomerases I and II. *Antimicrob. Agents Chemother.* **34**, 1955–1960.

192. Gellert, M., Mizuuchi, K., O'Dea, M. H., Itoh, T., and Tomizawa, J. (1977). Nalidixic acid resistance: A second genetic character involved in DNA gyrase activity. *Proc. Natl. Acad. Sci. U.S.A.* **74**, 4772–4776.

193. Sugino, A., Peebles, C. L., Kruezer, K. N., and Cozzarelli, N. R. (1977). Mechanism of action of nalidixic acid: Purification of *Escherichia coli nalA* gene product and its relationship to DNA gyrase and a novel nicking-closing enzyme. *Proc. Natl. Acad. Sci. U.S.A.* **74**, 4767–4771.

194. Huang, W. M. (1996). Bacterial diversity based on type II DNA topoisomerase genes. *Annu. Rev. Genet.* **30**, 79–107.

195. Bachmann, B. J. (1990). Linkage map of *Escherichia coli* K12, edition 8. *Microbiol. Rev.* **54**, 130–197.

196. Krueger, S., Zuccai, G., Wlodawer, A., Langowski, J., O'Dea, M., Maxwell, A., and Gellert, M. (1990). Neutron and light-scattering studies of DNA gyrase and its complex with DNA. *J. Mol. Biol.* **211**, 211–220.

197. Shen, L., and Pernet, A. G. (1985). Mechanism of inhibition of DNA gyrase by analogues of nalidixic acid: The target of the drugs is DNA. *Proc. Natl. Acad. Sci. U.S.A.* **82**, 307–311.

198. Shen, L., Kohlbrenner, W. E., Weigl, D., and Baranowski, J. (1989). Mechanism of quinolone inhibition of DNA gyrase. *J. Biol. Chem.* **264**, 2973–2978.

199. Willmott, C. J. R., and Maxwell, A. (1993). A single point mutation in the DNA gyrase A protein greatly reduces binding of fluoroquinolones to the gyrase DNA complex. *Antimicrob. Agents Chemother.* **37**, 126–127.

200. Critchlow, S. E., and Maxwell, A. (1996). DNA cleavage is not required for binding of quinolone drugs to the DNA gyrase-DNA complex. *Biochemistry* **35**, 7387–7393.

201. Reece, R. J., and Maxwell, A. (1989). Tryptic fragments of the *Escherichia coli* DNA gyrase A protein. *J. Biol. Chem.* **264**, 19648–19653.

202. Reece, R. J., and Maxwell, A. (1991). The C-terminal domain of the *Escherichia coli* DNA gyrase A subunit is a DNA-binding protein. *Nucleic Acids Res.* **19**, 1399–1405.

203. Reece, R. J., and Maxwell, A. (1991). Probing the limits of the DNA breakage-reunion domain of the *Escherichia coli* DNA gyrase A protein. *J. Biol. Chem.* **266**, 3540–3546.

204. Kampranis, S. C., and Maxwell, A. (1998). Conformational changes in DNA gyrase revealed by limited proteolysis. *J. Biol. Chem.* **273**, 22606–22614.

205. Cabral, J. H. M., Jackson, A. P., Smith, C. V., Shikotra, N., Maxwell, A., and Liddington, R. C. (1997). Crystal structure of the breakage–reunion domain of DNA gyrase. *Nature* **388**, 903–906.

206. Fass, D., Bogden, C. E., and Berger, J. M. (1999). Quaternary changes in topoisomerase II may direct orthogonal movement of two DNA strands. *Nature Struc. Biol.* **6**, 322–326.

207. Berger, J. M. (1998). Type II DNA topoisomerases. *Curr. Opin. Struct. Biol.* **8**, 26–32.

208. Hooper, D. C. (1999). Mode of action of fluoroquinolones. *Drugs* **58** (Suppl. 2), 6–10.

209. Kampranis, S. C., and Maxwell, A. (1998). The DNA gyrase–quinolone complex. *J. Biol. Chem.* **273**, 22615–22626.

210. Andrews, J., Ashby, J., Jevons, G., Marshall, T., Lines, N., and Wise, R. (2000). A comparison of antimicrobial resistance rates in Gram-positive pathogens isolated in the UK from October 1996 to January 1997 and October 1997 to January 1998. *J. Antimicrob. Chemother.* **45**, 285–293.

211. Gootz, T. D., and Osheroff, N. (1993). Quinolones and eukaryotic topoisomerases. In "Quinolone Antimicrobial Agents," 2nd ed (D. C. Hooper and J. S. Wolfson, eds.), pp. 139–160, American Society for Microbiology, Washington, DC.

212. Scheirer, K. E., and Higgins, N. P. (1997). The DNA cleavage reaction of DNA gyrase. *J. Biol. Chem.* **272**, 27202–27209.

213. Yoshida, H., Bogaki, M., Nakamura, M., and Nakamura, S. (1990). Quinolone resistance-determining region in the DNA gyrase gene of *Escherichia coli. Antimicrob. Agents Chemother.* **34**, 1271–1272.

214. Cullen, M. E., Wyke, A. W., Kuroda, R., and Fisher, L. M. (1989). Cloning and characterization of a DNA gyrase A gene from *Escherichia coli* that confers clinical resistance to 4-quinolones. *Antimicrob. Agents Chemother.* **33**, 886–894.

215. Oram, M., and Fisher, L. M. (1991). 4-Quinolone resistance mutations in the DNA gyrase of *Escherichia coli* clinical isolates identified by using the polymerase chain reaction. *Antimicrob. Agents Chemother.* **35**, 387–389.

216. Maxwell, A. (1992). The molecular basis of quinolone action. *J. Antimicrob. Chemother.* **30**, 409–414.

217. Hallett, P., and Maxwell, A. (1991). Novel quinolone resistance mutations of the *Escherichia coli* DNA gyrase A protein: Enzymatic analysis of mutant proteins. *Antimicrob. Agents Chemother.* **35**, 335–340.

218. Peng, H., and Marians, K. (1993). *E. coli* topoisomerase IV: Purification, characterization, subunit structure and subunit interactions. *J. Biol. Chem.* **268**, 24481–24490.

219. Peng, H., and Marians, K. (1993). Decatenation activity of topoisomerase IV during *oriC* and pBR322 DNA replication *in vitro. Proc. Natl. Acad. Sci. U.S.A.* **90**, 8571–8575.

220. Zechiedrich, E. L., and Cozzarelli, N. R. (1995). Roles of topoisomerase IV and DNA gyrase in DNA unlinking during replication of *Escherichia coli. Genes Dev.* **9**, 2859–2869.

221. Peng, H., and Marians, K. (1995). The interaction of *Escherichia coli* topoisomerase IV with DNA. *J. Biol. Chem.* **270**, 25286–25290.

222. Kato, J.-I., Suzuki, H., and Ikeda, H. (1992). Purification and characterization of DNA topoisomerase IV in *Escherichia coli. J. Biol. Chem.* **267**, 25676–25684.

223. Khodursky, A. B., Zechdiedrich, E. L., and Cozzarelli N. R. (1995). Topoisomerase IV is a target of quinolones in *Escherichia coli. Proc. Natl. Acad. Sci. U.S.A.* **92**, 11801–11805.

224. Hoshino, K., Kitamura, A., Morrissey, I., Sato, K., Kato, J.-I., and Ikeda, H. (1994). Comparison of inhibition of *Escherichia coli* topoisomerase IV by quinolones with DNA gyrase inhibition. *Antimicrob. Agents Chemother.* **38**, 2623–2627.

225. Ferrero, L., Cameron, B., and Crouzet, J. (1995). Analysis of *gyrA* and *grlA* mutations in stepwise-selected ciprofloxacin-resistant mutants of *Staphylococcus aureus. Antimicrob. Agents Chemother.* **39**, 1554–1558.

226. Ferrero, L., Cameron, B., Manse, B., Lagneaux, D., Crouzet, J., Famechon, A., and Blanche, F. (1994). Cloning and primary structure of *Staphylococcus aureus* DNA topoisomerase IV: A primary target of fluoroquinolones. *Mol. Microbiol.* **13**, 641–653.

227. Pan, X.-S., Ambler, J., Mehtar, S., and Fisher, M. L. (1996). Involvement of topoisomerase IV and DNA gyrase as ciprofloxacin targets in *Streptococcus pneumoniae*. *Antimicrob. Agents Chemother.* **40**, 2321–2326.

228. Gootz, T. D., Zaniewski, R., Haskell, S., Schmieder, B., Tankovic, J., Girard, D., Courvalin, P., and Polzer, R. (1996). Activity of the new fluoroquinolone trovafloxacin (CP-99,219) against DNA gyrase and topoisomerase IV mutants of *Streptococcus pneumoniae*. *Antimicrob. Agents Chemother.* **40**, 2691–2697.

229. Pan, X.-S., and Fisher, M. L. (1997). Targeting of DNA gyrase in *Streptococcus pneumoniae* by sparfloxacin: Selective targeting of gyrase or topoisomerase IV by quinolones. *Antimicrob. Agents Chemother.* **41**, 471–474.

230. Blanche, F., Cameron, B., Bernard, F.-X., Maton, L., Manse, B., Ferrero, L., Ratet, N., Lecog, C., Goniot, A., Bisch, D., and Crouzet, J. (1996). Differential behaviors of *Staphylococcus aureus* and *Escherichia coli* type II DNA topoisomerases. *Antimicrob. Agents Chemother.* **40**, 2714–2720.

231. Khodursky, A. B., and Cozzarelli, N. R. (1998). The mechanism of inhibition of topoisomerase IV by quinolone antibacterials. *J. Biol. Chem.* **273**, 27668–27677.

232. Marians, K. J., and Hiasa, H. (1997). Mechanism of quinolone action: A drug induced structural perturbation of the DNA precedes strand cleavage by topoisomerase IV. *J. Biol. Chem.* **272**, 9401–9409.

233. Anderson, V. E., Gootz, T. D., and Osheroff, N. (1998). Topoisomerase IV catalysis and the mechanism of quinolone action. *J. Biol. Chem.* **273**, 17879–17885.

234. Anderson, V. E., Zaniewski, R. P., Kaczmarek, F. S., Gootz, T. D., and Osheroff, N. (1999). Quinolones inhibit DNA religation mediated by *Staphylococcus aureus* topoisomerase IV. *J. Biol. Chem.* **274**, 35927–35932.

235. Anderson, V. E., Zaniewski, R. P., Kaczmarek, F. S., Gootz, T. D., and Osheroff, N. (2000). Action of quinolones against *Staphylococcus aureus* topoisomerase IV: Basis for DNA cleavage enhancement. *J. Biochem.* **39**, 2726–2732.

236. Gootz, T. D., Zaniewski, R. P., Haskell, S. L., Kaczmarek, F. S., and Maurice, A. E. (1999). Activities of trovafloxacin compared with those of other fluoroquinolones against purified topoisomerases and *gyrA* and *grlA* mutants of *Staphylococcus aureus*. *Antimicrob. Agents Chemother.* **43**, 1845–1855.

237. Fitzgibbons, J. E., John, J. F., Delucia, J. L., and Dubin, D. T. (1998). Topoisomerase mutations in trovafloxacin-resistant *Staphylococcus aureus*. *Antimicrob. Agents Chemother.* **42**, 2122–2124.

238. Pan, X.-S., and Fisher, L. M. (1998). DNA gyrase and topoisomerase IV are dual targets of clinafloxacin action in *Streptococcus pneumoniae*. *Antimicrob. Agents Chemother.* **42**, 2810–2816.

239. Pan, X.-S., and Fisher, L. M. (1999). *Streptococcus pneumoniae* DNA gyrase and topoisomerase IV: Overexpression, purification, and differential inhibition by fluoroquinolones. *Antimicrob. Agents Chemother.* **43**, 1129–1136.

240. Heaton, V. J., Goldsmith, C. E., Ambler, J. E., and Fisher, L. M. (1999). Activity of gemifloxacin against penicillin-and ciprofloxacin-resistant *Streptococcus pneumoniae* displaying topoisomerase- and efflux-mediated resistance mechanisms. *Antimicrob. Agents Chemother.* **43**, 2998–3000.

241. Aras, I. R., and Hooper, D. C. (1998). Mechanisms and frequency of resistance to moxifloxacin in comparison to ciprofloxacin in *Staphylococcus aureus*. *Abstr. 6th Int. Sym. New Quinolones*, Denver.

242. Lewis, C., Howard, B., and Smith, J. (1991). Protein- and RNA-synthesis independent bactericidal activity of ciprofloxacin that involves the A subunit of DNA gyrase. *J. Med. Microbiol.* **34**, 19–22.

243. Smith, J. T., and Lewin, C. S. (1988). Chemistry and mechanisms of action of the quinolone antibacterials. In "The Quinolones" (V. T. Andriole, ed.), pp. 23–82. Academic Press, San Diego.

244. Goss, W. A., Deitz, W. H., and Cook, T. M. (1965). Mechanism of action of nalidixic acid on *Escherichia coli. J. Bacteriol.* **89**, 1068–1074.

245. Drlica, K., Manes, S. H., and Engle, E. C. (1980). DNA gyrase on the bacterial chromosome: Possibility of two levels of action. *Proc. Natl. Acad. Sci. U.S.A.* **77**, 6879–6883.

246. Willmott, C. J. R., Critchlow, S. E., Eperon, I. C., and Maxwell, A. (1994). The complex of DNA gyrase and quinolone drugs with DNA forms a barrier to transcription by RNA polymerase. *J. Mol. Biol.* **242**, 351–363.

247. Chen, C.-R., Malik, M., Snyder, M., and Drlica, K. (1996). DNA gyrase and topoisomerase IV on the bacterial chromosome: Quinolone-induced DNA cleavage. *J. Mol. Biol.* **258**, 627–637.

248. Shimizu, H., Yamaguchi, H., and Ikeda, H. (1995). Molecular analysis of λ biotransducing phage produced by oxolinic acid-induced illegitimate recombination *in vivo. Genetics* **140**, 889–896.

249. Deguchi, T., Yasuda, M., Nakano, M., Ozeki, S., Ezaki, T., Saito, I., and Kawada, Y. (1996). Quinolone-resistant *Neisseria gonorrhoeae*: Correlation of alteration in the GyrA subunit of DNA gyrase and the ParC subunit of topoisomerase IV with antimicrobial susceptibility profiles. *Antimicrob. Agents Chemother.* **40**, 1020–1023.

250. Gudas, L. J., and Pardee, A. B. (1976). DNA synthesis inhibition and the induction of protein X in *Escherichia coli. J. Mol. Biol.* **101**, 459–477.

251. Phillips, I., Culebras, E., Moreno, F., and Baquero, F. (1987). Induction of the SOS response by new 4-quinolones. *J. Antimicrob. Chemother.* **20**, 631–638.

252. Piddock, L., and Wise, R. (1987). Induction of the SOS response in *Escherichia coli* by 4-quinolone antimicrobial agents. *FEMS Microbiol. Lett.* **41**, 289–294.

253. Stahl, F. W., Kobayashi, I., and Stahl, M. M. (1983). Chi is activated by a variety of routes. In "Mechanisms of DNA Replication and Recombination" (N. R. Cozzarelli, ed.), pp. 773–783. Alan R. Liss, New York.

254. Power, R., and Phillips, I. (1993). Correlation between *umuC* induction and *Salmonella* mutagenicity assay for quinolone antimicrobial agents. *FEMS Microbiol. Lett.* **112**, 251–254.

255. McDaniel, L. S., Rogers, L. H., and Hill, W. E. (1978). Survival of recombination-deficient mutants of *Escherichia coli* during incubation with nalidixic acid. *J. Bacteriol.* **134**, 1195–1198.

256. McCoy, E., Petriello, L., and Rosenkranz, J. (1980). Non-mutagenic genotoxicants: Novobiocin and nalidixic acid, two inhibitors of DNA gyrase. *Mutat. Res.* **79**, 33–43.

257. Flor, S., Gudy, D., Opsal, J., Tack, K., and Matske, G. (1990). Effect of magnesium-aluminum hydroxide and calcium carbonate antacids on bioavailability of ofloxacin. *Antimicrob. Agents Chemother.* **34**, 2436–2438.

258. Chin, N.-X., and Neu, H. C. (1983). *In vitro* activity of enoxacin, a quinolone carboxylic acid, compared with those of norfloxacin, new beta-lactams, aminoglycosides, and trimethoprim. *Antimicrob. Agents Chemother.* **24**, 754–763.

259. Neu, H. C., Novelli, A., and Chin, N.-X. (1989). Comparative *in vitro* activity of a new quinolone, AM-1091. *Antimicrob. Agents Chemother.* **33**, 1036–1041.

260. Hirschhorn, L., and Neu, H. C. (1986). Factors influencing the *in vitro* activity of two new aryl-fluoroquinolone antimicrobial agents, difloxacin (A-56619) and A-56620. *Antimicrob. Agents Chemother.* **30**, 143–146.

261. Sutcliffe, J. A., Gootz, T. D., and Barrett, J. F. (1989). Biochemical characteristics and physiological significance of major DNA topoisomerases. *Antimicrob. Agents Chemother.* **33**, 2027–2033.

262. Chapman, J. S., and Georgopapadakou, N. H. (1988). Routes of quinolone permeation in *Escherichia coli. Antimicrob. Agents Chemother.* **32**, 438–442.

263. Timmers, K., and Sternglanz, R. (1978). Ionization and divalent cation dissociation constants of nalidixic and oxolinic acids. *Bioinorg. Chem.* **9**, 145–155.

264. Snavely, M. D. (1990). Magnesium transport in prokaryotic cells. In "Metal Ions in Biological Systems" (H. Siegel, ed.), Vol. 26, pp. 155–175. Marcel Dekker, New York.

265. Palu, G., Valisena, S., Ciarrocchi, G., Gatto, B., and Palumbo, M. (1992). Quinolone binding to DNA is mediated by magnesium ions. *Proc. Natl. Acad. Sci. U.S.A.* **89**, 9671–9675.

266. Bauernfeind, A., and Petermuller, C. (1983). *In vitro* activity of ciprofloxacin, norfloxacin, and nalidixic acid. *Eur. J. Clin. Microbiol.* **2**, 111–115.

267. Aldridge, K. E., and Ashcraft, D. S. (1997). Comparison of the *in vitro* activities of BAY 12-8039, a new quinolone, and other antimicrobials against clinically important anaerobes. *Antimicrob. Agents Chemother.* **41**, 709–711.

268. Morrissey, I., and Smith, J. T. (1994). The importance of oxygen in the killing of bacteria by ofloxacin and ciprofloxacin. *Microbios* **79**, 43–53.

269. Morrissey, I., and Smith, J. T. (1990). Ofloxacin and ciprofloxacin are not bactericidal under anaerobic conditions. *Abstr. 3rd Int. Symp. New Quinolones*, Vancouver, Canada. Abstr. #155.

270. Cooper, M. A., Andrews, J. M., and Wise, R. (1991). Bactericidal activity of sparfloxacin and ciprofloxacin under anaerobic conditions. *J. Antimicrob. Chemother.* **28**, 399–405.

271. Spangler, S. K., Jacobs, M. R., and Appelbaum, P. C. (1997). Time-kill study of the activity of trovafloxacin compared to ciprofloxacin, sparfloxacin, metronidazole, cefoxitin, piperacillin, and piperacillin/tazobactam against six anaerobes. *J. Antimicrob. Chemother.* **39** (Suppl. B), 23–27.

272. Onderdonk, A. B. (1996). Efficacy of trovafloxacin (CP-99,219), a new fluoroquinolone, in an animal model for intraabdominal sepsis. *Infect. Dis. Clin. Prac.* **5** (Suppl. 3), S117–S119.

273. Korten, U., and Murray, B. E. (1993). Impact of the fluoroquinolones on gastrointestinal flora. *Drugs* **45**, 125–133.

274. Hershberger, E., and Rybak, M. J. (2000). Activities of trovafloxacin, gatifloxacin, clinafloxacin, sparfloxacin, levofloxacin, and ciprofloxacin against penicillin-resistant *Streptococcus pneumoniae* in an *in vitro* infection model. *Antimicrob. Agents Chemother.* **44**, 598–601.

CHAPTER 3

Comparative In-Vitro Properties of the Quinolones

IAN PHILLIPS, ANNA KING, and KEVIN SHANNON

Department of Microbiology, United Medical and Dental School of Guy's and St. Thomas' Hospital, London, SE1 7EH, United Kingdom

---

Introduction
Gram-Negative Aerobes
   Enterobacteriaceae
   Other Gram-Negative Aerobes
Gram-Positive Aerobes
Anaerobes
Miscellaneous Organisms
Conclusion
References

INTRODUCTION

The spectrum of *in-vitro* activity of the quinolones has evolved considerably since the introduction of the first member of the group, nalidixic acid, with its essentially narrow range of activity against some Gram-negative species. At first, improvements were largely in pharmacological properties, and the activity of cinoxacin, flumequine, pipemidic acid, and oxolinic acid against nalidixic acid-susceptible enterobacteria does not differ much from that of nalidixic acid itself [1], but resistance is rather less common. Acrosoxacin is more active, but less so than most of the other newer 4-quinolones, but may be useful against *Neisseria gonorrhoeae*. Staphylococci and streptococci are resistant to the early quinolones. Table I summarizes the *in-vitro* findings for these older agents.

The Quinolones, Third Edition

The members of the next generation of quinolones have considerably greater activity in terms of potency than most of the older agents. They also have an increasingly broad range of activity, first against Gram-negative aerobic organisms other than the Enterobacteriaceae (e.g., norfloxacin), then, in addition, against Gram-positive aerobic organisms (e.g., ciprofloxacin and ofloxacin, and, even more, many of the newer agents), and most recently against anaerobes (e.g., clinafloxacin). Although directed spectra of activity may have been the goal, the newest agents have as broad a range of activity as any currently available antibacterial agents. Since the first edition of this book, many new quinolones have been investigated, but few have progressed to the point of clinical use. In this edition we consider several newer compounds that have been developed to clinical-trial stage, including some with side effects that currently appear to preclude their general clinical use.

There have been many reports, and a number of reviews (e.g., [2–4]), of the *in-vitro* activity of the newer quinolones. Our results, to be discussed in detail below, do not differ from the consensus of the many reports by others [5]. We have published our results on norfloxacin [6], ciprofloxacin [7], enoxacin and ofloxacin [8], pefloxacin [9], clinafloxacin (PD 127,391, AM-1091, CI-960) [10], temafloxacin (TA 167, A 62254) [11], tosufloxacin (A 61827), T3262) [12], and gemifloxacin, moxifloxacin, and trovafloxacin [13], and we have also studied fleroxacin, amifloxacin, lomefloxacin, sparfloxacin (AT-4140, PD 131501, CI 978, PR 64206), rufloxacin (MF 934), and grepafloxacin (OPC 17116). For two drugs that we have

TABLE I The *In-Vitro* Activity of Older Quinolones[a]

	Compound	MIC_{50}	MIC_{90}	MIC_{100}
Enterobacteria	Nalidixic acid	4	128	>128
	Cinoxacin			
	Fluemquine	2–4	8–32	3–>128
	Pipemidic acid			
	Oxolonic acid			
Pseudomonas	Nalidixic acid	64	>128	>128
aeruginosa	Cinoxacin	>128	>128	>128
	Fluemquine			
	Pipemidic acid	4–16	8–64	32–>128
	Oxolinic acid			
Staphylococcus	Nalidixic acid			
aureus	Pipemidic acid	64	64–>128	128–>128
	Cinoxacin			
Streptococci	Nalidixic acid			
	Cinoxacin	>128	>128	>128
	Pipemidic acid			
	Oxolinic acid			

[a]Adapted from Shannon and Phillips (1985) [1].

not studied, levofloxacin and gatifloxacin, we include tabulated results from other investigators, including their results for ciprofloxacin as a reference point. However, we shall use only our own results for the organisms that we have studied because we have information on individual isolates and can, therefore, calculate geometrical mean MICs and percentage susceptibilities for the various compounds, as a demonstration of their relative activity. These clinical isolates have been collected over the past fifteen years. We have included isolates resistant to nalidixic acid but, with few exceptions, not strains resistant to the newer quinolones for which ciprofloxacin has been the marker. This has enabled us to make valid comparisons of the *in-vitro* activity of the different drugs on the same set of isolates. Resistance rates among the organisms in our collection are therefore emphatically not those encountered in our clinical material at any one time. Thus, in most instances, we can, with some confidence, relate at least the MIC_{50} to the basal susceptible population of each species we have studied. We have, however, made some separate comparisons of the activity of newer quinolones on some more common species that have now acquired ciprofloxacin resistance.

For assessing percentage susceptibilities, we have used the breakpoints for susceptibility and for moderate susceptibility defined by the British Society for Antimicrobial Chemotherapy (BSAC) [14], except for nalidixic acid, for which the NCCLS breakpoint for susceptibility was used [15]. The BSAC breakpoints are often one concentration lower for each susceptibility category (S, I, or R). The actual breakpoints used are listed in Tables II, V, VI, and VIII.

Geometrical mean MICs were calculated by finding the arithmetic mean of logarithmic values of the MICs ($\log_2$ MIC + 21) and then calculating the antilogarithm. Confidence intervals for the mean were calculated as described by Gardner and Altman [16], also on logarithmic values for which the antilogarithms were then found. For the few organisms for which upper endpoints of the MIC had not been determined, MICs were taken as twice the highest concentration tested for the purposes of calculating mean MICs and also for the calculation of linear correlation coefficients between MICs of pairs of compounds. Weighted averages of MIC_{50} and MIC_{90} values are presented in the tables for levofloxacin and gatifloxacin, which we have not studied, in comparison with ciprofloxacin as a reference compound.

The susceptibility of bacteria to quinolones is affected by pH, but whereas norfloxacin, ciprofloxacin, and ofloxacin, for example, are less active at pH 5.6 than at pH 7.4, nalidixic acid, flumequine, oxolinic acid, and cinoxacin are more active at pH 5.6 than at pH 7.4 [17]; at pH 5.6 the MICs of ciprofloxacin and nalidixic acid were 0.2 and 1 mg/liter, respectively, for *E. coli* KL16 in contrast to 0.004 and 3 mg/liter at pH 7.4. However, the activity of trovafloxacin (CP 99,219) is little affected by pH [18]. An increase in magnesium concentration from 0.2 to 5.6 m*M* reduces quinolone activity at all pH values [17]. The finding that magnesium antagonizes quinolone activity was confirmed by Auckenthaler and his colleagues [19]; calcium antagonizes ofloxacin and pefloxacin but not ciprofloxacin, and zinc does not antagonize any of the quinolones.

The quinolones are usually bactericidal. Auckenthaler and colleagues [19] found the average minimum bactericidal concentration (MBC)/MIC ratio for norfloxacin, pefloxacin, and enoxacin to be between 1 and 2 for the majority of organisms and between 2 and 3 for *Streptococcus agalactiae* and *Enterococcus faecalis*; ciprofloxacin had higher MBC/MIC ratios than these three quinolones for *Pseudomonas* and most staphylococci, but lower ratios for enterobacteria, *Strep. agalactiae*, and *Ent. faecalis*. Smith [20] reported that the "most bactericidal concentration" (at which there is the greatest degree of killing in 3 hr), and which we prefer to call the "optimum bactericidal concentration," is about 30 times greater than the MIC, at least against the laboratory strain of *E. coli* tested (0.15 mg/liter compared to an MIC of 0.004 mg/liter for ciprofloxacin; 0.9:0.03 mg/liter for ofloxacin; 1.5:0.04 mg/liter for norfloxacin, and 90:3 mg/liter for nalidixic acid). At their optimum bactericidal concentrations, ciprofloxacin and ofloxacin killed 90% of the *E. coli* in 19 minutes, whereas others of the older quinolones took at least twice as long. It must be remembered that all measurements of bactericidal activity depend on the implicit definition as dead of a bacterium incapable of continued division to produce a colony. Such "dead" organisms may possess continuing metabolic activity, and may even continue to grow for a period after exposure [21].

GRAM-NEGATIVE AEROBES

ENTEROBACTERIACEAE

Table II summarizes the activity of the 4-quinolones against the enterobacteria. All the compounds are intrinsically highly active. Strains susceptible to nalidixic acid (MICs ≤16 mg/liter) have MIC_{50} (and mean MIC) values appreciably lower than those for resistant (nalidixic acid MICs ≥32 mg/liter) strains (Table II). The results that we used for gatifloxacin and levofloxacin [22,23] were not related to nalidixic acid susceptibility. However, the ciprofloxacin MIC_{50} corresponds to that for our nalidixic acid-susceptible organisms, and the MIC_{90} to that for resistant organisms (although the range is much greater than ours), demonstrating that both of these newer drugs are marginally less active than ciprofloxacin against enterobacteria. This difference in susceptibilities is reflected in the high degree of correlation between the MICs of all pairs of 4-quinolones assessed (Table III); we found that the highest correlation coefficient was 0.94 for sparfloxacin/temafloxacin and the lowest 0.497 for nalidixic acid/sparfloxacin.

On the basis of the MIC_{25} to MIC_{75} range calculated for the group as a whole, except gatifloxacin and levofloxacin, clinafloxacin is clearly the most active (Figure 1), followed by ciprofloxacin. There was a gradual reduction in average activity for the other compounds, with the MIC_{25} to MIC_{75} ranges overlapping. All of the enterobacteria that we studied were susceptible to clinafloxacin, and 90% or more were susceptible to the other compounds (Table II).

TABLE II The *in-Vitro* Activity of Quinolones against Enterobacteriaceae

	Nalidixic acid MICs ≤16 mg/l (260 isolates)			Nalidixic acid MICs ≥32 mg/l (40 isolates)			All isolates	
	Range of MICs	MIC_{50}	MIC_{90}	Range of MICs	MIC_{50}	MIC_{90}	Susceptible[b] (%)	Mod. susceptible[c] (%)
Clinafloxacin	0.001–0.125	0.016	0.03	0.016–0.25	0.06	0.25	100	0
Ciprofloxacin	0.002–1	0.016	0.06	0.03–2	0.25	2	98.3	1.7
Gemifloxacin	0.001–1	0.03	0.125	0.03–2	0.25	1	93.6	5.4
Tosufloxacin	0.004–1	0.06	0.125	0.03–2	0.25	1	99.7	0.3
Grepafloxacin	0.001–4	0.06	0.25	0.06–2	0.5	2	97.7	2.3
Trovafloxacin	0.002–2	0.06	0.25	0.03–2	0.5	2	98	2
Norfloxacin	0.016–4	0.06	0.25	0.125–8	0.5	4	94.3	5
Moxifloxacin	0.004–2	0.125	0.25	0.06–2	0.5	1	98.6	1.4
Sparfloxacin	0.002–2	0.125	0.5	0.06–2	1	2	98	2.0
Ofloxacin	0.03–2	0.06	0.25	0.125–8	1	4	98.3	1.7
Fleroxacin	0.03–1	0.125	0.25	0.125–8	1	4	95.3	4.3
Enoxacin	0.06–2	0.125	0.5	0.25–32	2	4	93	6
Lomefloxacin	0.03–2	0.125	0.5	0.5–8	2	4	91.3	7.7
Pefloxacin	0.03–2	0.125	0.5	0.25–16	2	4	90.3	9
Temafloxacin	0.008–4	0.25	1	0.125–4	1	4	93.3	6.7
Nalidixic acid	1–16	4	8	32–>128	>128	>128	86.6	–
Ciprofloxacin[a]	0.002–	0.03		–128		2		
Gatifloxacin[a]	0.004–	0.06		–128		1		
Levofloxacin[a]	0.004–	0.06		->128		4		

[a] 1192 isolates with nalidixic acid MICs not reported [22,23].

[b] Upper limits of susceptibility: 2 mg/liter of ofloxacin, 16 mg/liter of nalidixic acid, 0.25 mg/liter of gemifloxacin, 1 mg/liter of other compounds.

[c] Moderately susceptible: MICs 4 to 8 mg/liter of ofloxacin, 0.5–1 mg/liter of gemifloxacin, 2 to 4 mg/liter of other compounds, apart from nalidixic acid for which no moderately susceptible category is defined.

There are differences between enterobacterial species in susceptibility to the quinolones, as shown in Figure 2 for five compounds including ciprofloxacin, the most active compound in general clinical use, and clinafloxacin, which has the greatest *in-vitro* activity, and other compounds chosen to illustrate a range of activities. *Hafnia alvei* is the most susceptible to ciprofloxacin (mean MIC 0.007 mg/liter), followed by the two *Citrobacter* species. *Escherichia coli*, *Klebsiella*, and *Proteus mirabilis*, the enterobacteria isolated most frequently from clinical specimens, although highly susceptible in absolute terms, are among the least susceptible to ciprofloxacin (mean MICs 0.0260.047 mg/liter), followed only by *Serratia* and *Providencia stuartii*. Clinafloxacin is usually more active than ciprofloxacin; this is most marked for *E. coli*, which is the third most susceptible species to clinafloxacin. Gemifloxacin, moxifloxacin, and ofloxacin are notably less active than ciprofloxacin or clinafloxacin. The order of activity for the most active drugs—clinafloxacin > ciprofloxacin > gemifloxacin > moxifloxacin > ofloxacin—is maintained against almost all species, although the mean MIC of ciprofloxacin is very slightly lower than that of clinafloxacin for *Citrobacter*

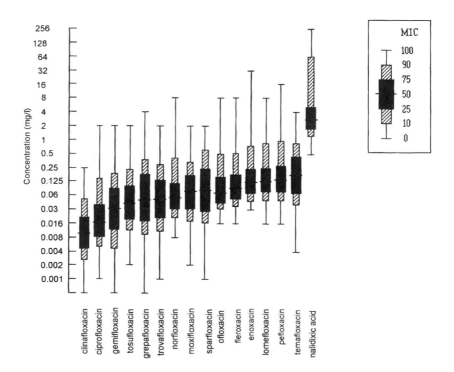

FIGURE 1   The *in-vitro* activity of 4-quinolones against Enterobacteriaceae.

TABLE III Correlation Coefficients for MICs of Quinolones against Enterobacteriaceae

	Clina-floxacin	Cipro-floxacin	Gemi-floxacin	Tosu-floxacin	Grepa-floxacin	Trova-floxacin	Nor-floxacin	Moxi-floxacin	Spar-floxacin	Ofloxacin	Fler-oxacin	Enox-acin	Lome-floxacin	Pe-floxacin	Tema-floxacin
Ciprofloxacin	0.850														
Gemifloxacin	0.807	0.754													
Tosufloxacin	0.854	0.803	0.882												
Grepafloxacin	0.785	0.707	0.869	0.885											
Trovafloxacin	0.793	0.743	0.867	0.908	0.891										
Norfloxacin	0.713	0.888	0.601	0.639	0.527	0.592									
Moxifloxacin	0.821	0.743	0.876	0.885	0.878	0.888	0.591								
Sparfloxacin	0.825	0.734	0.877	0.922	0.905	0.888	0.535	0.848							
Ofloxacin	0.805	0.881	0.706	0.748	0.644	0.712	0.861	0.726	0.663						
Fleroxacin	0.852	0.863	0.704	0.753	0.674	0.710	0.790	0.752	0.682	0.851					
Enoxacin	0.803	0.881	0.712	0.742	0.662	0.695	0.879	0.727	0.655	0.894	0.879				
Lomefloxacin	0.850	0.891	0.739	0.782	0.687	0.715	0.808	0.747	0.706	0.847	0.897	0.896			
Pefloxacin	0.843	0.893	0.742	0.786	0.693	0.713	0.836	0.762	0.708	0.906	0.887	0.901	0.884		
Temafloxacin	0.822	0.729	0.867	0.924	0.889	0.848	0.543	0.887	0.940	0.668	0.711	0.676	0.714	0.709	
Nalidixic acid	0.693	0.749	0.540	0.586	0.512	0.550	0.776	0.589	0.497	0.752	0.830	0.832	0.822	0.795	0.536

freundii, and the mean MIC of gemifloxacin is lower than that of ciprofloxacin for *Citrobacter koseri* and *E. coli*, and the same or very slightly higher for *Enterobacter aerogenes*, *Enterobacter cloacae*, *Klebsiella* spp. and *Providencia stuartii*. The new compounds moxifloxacin and gemifloxacin are notably less active against *Proteus* spp., and the mean MIC of ofloxacin is lower than that of either of these two drugs against *Proteus vulgaris* and lower than that of moxifloxacin against *Proteus mirabilis*.

Salmonella and *Shigella* also are, in the absence of acquired resistance, highly susceptible to the quinolones [24–26], as is *Yersinia enterocolitica* (MIC_{50} of ciprofloxacin 0.01 mg/liter) [2].

Levofloxacin (L-ofloxacin) is about twice as active as ofloxacin (mixture) against many bacteria, including enterobacteria [23,25]. Gatifloxacin has similar activity [22,23]. Rufloxacin has relatively poor activity against enterobacteria, being less active than norfloxacin [27].

Table IV shows a comparison of $MICs_{50}$ and MIC ranges for Enterobacteriaceae that are resistant to ciprofloxacin. Although clinafloxacin, gemifloxacin,

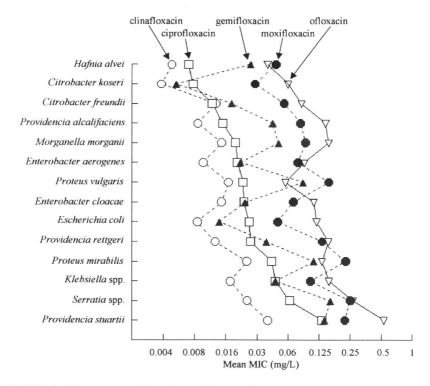

FIGURE 2 The *in-vitro* activity of ciprofloxacin (□), clinafloxacin (○), gemifloxacin (▲) moxifloxacin (●), and ofloxacin (▽) against Enterobacteriaceae.

and moxifloxacin are more active than ciprofloxacin, MICs are clearly considerably elevated.

OTHER GRAM-NEGATIVE AEROBES

Taking ciprofloxacin as a standard for comparison, *Neisseria gonorrhoeae* and *Aeromonas* spp. are the most susceptible (mean MICs 0.002–0.004 mg/liter), and *Haemophilus influenzae* and *Moraxella catarrhalis* are also more susceptible than the enterobacteria. *Acinetobacter* is somewhat and *Pseudomonas* and related species are appreciably less susceptible. *Gardnerella vaginalis*, with a mean ciprofloxacin MIC of 1 mg/liter, is the least susceptible. Clinafloxacin is usually the most active of all the drugs, followed by ciprofloxacin and the newer quinolones, the order very much depending on species.

The order of activity of the 4-quinolones against *Acinetobacter* is different from that against the enterobacteria (Table V). Gemifloxacin, clinafloxacin, and trovafloxacin are most active, and sparfloxacin, grepafloxacin, moxifloxacin, and tosufloxacin are all slightly more active than ciprofloxacin or ofloxacin. None of the isolates tested were resistant to most of the quinolones (Table V), but 11% were resistant to norfloxacin. Rufloxacin has relatively poor activity (MIC$_{50}$ 2 mg/liter) [27].

TABLE IV   The *in-Vitro* Activity of Quinolones against Ciprofloxacin-Resistant (MICs >4 mg/liter) Gram-Negative Isolates[a]

Compound	Enterobacteriaceae (87)[b]		*Pseudomonas aeruginosa* (13)	
	Range of MICs	MIC$_{50}$	Range of MICs	MIC$_{50}$
Clinafloxacin	0.5–16	2	2–16	4
Gemifloxacin	1->128	16	4->128	64
Moxifloxacin	2–128	16	2->128	64
Ciprofloxacin	8->128	16	8->128	32
Trovafloxacin	8->128	32	2->128	128
Grepafloxacin	8->128	32	4->128	64
Ofloxacin	8–128	32	32->128	128

[a]Data from [13] and unpublished observations of A. King, K. P. Shannon and I. Phillips.

[b]*Escherichia coli* (42), *Klebsiella* spp. (24), *Enterobacter cloacae* (6), *E. aerogenes* (6), *Serratia* spp. (5), *Citrobacter freundii* (3), *Morganella morganii* (1).

TABLE V The *in-Vitro* Activity of Quinolones against *Acinetobacter, Aeromonas*, pseudomonads and *Campylobacter*[a]

Organism (no. of isolates)	Compound	Range of MICs (mg/l)	MIC$_{50}$	MIC$_{90}$	Mean MIC[b]	Suscept-ible[c] (%)	Moder. suscept.[d] (%)	Refer-ences
Acinetobacter spp. (27)	Gemifloxacin	0.001–0.125	0.001	0.125	0.0043	100	0	
	Trovafloxacin	0.001–0.125	0.004	0.03	0.0062	100	0	
	Clinafloxacin	0.001–0.125	0.004	0.06	0.0077	100	0	
	Sparfloxacin	0.002–0.125	0.008	0.06	0.009	100	0	
	Grepafloxacin	0.001–0.125	0.016	0.06	0.0107	100	0	
	Moxifloxacin	0.001–0.25	0.008	0.125	0.013	100	0	
	Tosufloxacin	0.002–0.25	0.008	0.125	0.015	100	0	
	Temafloxacin	0.004–0.5	0.008	0.25	0.017	100	0	
	Ciprofloxacin	0.008–0.5	0.016	0.25	0.029	100	0	
	Ofloxacin	0.008–0.5	0.06	0.25	0.052	100	0	
	Pefloxacin	0.03–1	0.06	0.5	0.125	100	0	
	Fleroxacin	0.03–2	0.125	0.5	0.142	96.3	3.7	
	Lomefloxacin	0.03–1	0.125	0.5	0.150	100	0	
	Enoxacin	0.06–4	0.25	2	0.340	85.2	14.8	
	Norfloxacin	0.06–8	1	8	0.663	66.7	22.2	
	Nalidixic acid	1–16	2	8	2.86	100	–	
(140)	Ciprofloxacin	0.008–4	0.125	0.5				[23]
	Gatifloxacin	0.002–2	0.03	0.125				
	Levofloxacin	0.008–2	0.06	0.25				
Aeromonas spp. (13)	Clinafloxacin	0.001–0.004	0.002	0.004	0.0022	100	0	
	Ciprofloxacin	0.004–0.016	0.004	0.016	0.0063	100	0	
	Gemifloxacin	0.001–0.06	0.03	0.03	0.0087	100	0	
	Pefloxacin	0.008–0.03	0.016	0.03	0.0142	100	0	
	Norfloxacin	0.008–0.03	0.016	0.016	0.0140	100	0	
	Fleroxacin	0.008–0.03	0.016	0.03	0.0163	100	0	
	Tosufloxacin	0.004–0.03	0.016	0.03	0.0165	100	0	
	Ofloxacin	0.016–0.03	0.016	0.03	0.0183	100	0	
	Trovafloxacin	0.008–0.06	0.016	0.06	0.0186	100	0	
	Enoxacin	0.016–0.03	0.03	0.03	0.0239	100	0	
	Grepafloxacin	0.016–0.06	0.03	0.06	0.0274	100	0	

Organism (n)	Antibiotic	Range						Ref
	Sparfloxacin	0.008–0.06	0.03	0.06	0.0287	100	0	
	Lomefloxacin	0.016–0.03	0.03	0.03	0.0281	100	0	
	Temafloxacin	0.008–0.125	0.06	0.125	0.0482	100	0	
	Moxifloxacin	0.016–0.125	0.06	0.125	0.0526	100	0	
	Nalidixic acid	0.008–0.12	0.12	0.12	0.094	100	–	
(32)	Ciprofloxacin	0.002–0.016	0.004	0.008				[23]
	Gatifloxacin	0.008–0.06	0.016	0.03				
	Levofloxacin	0.004–0.06	0.016	0.03				
Pseudomonas aeruginosa (40)	Clinafloxacin	0.03–4	0.125	0.5	0.162	92.5	7.5	
	Ciprofloxacin	0.06–16	0.125	4	0.229	87.5	7.5	
	Tosufloxacin	0.125–32	0.25	4	0.457	84.6	10.3	
	Grepafloxacin	0.125–16	0.5	4	0.555	77.5	12.5	
	Gemifloxacin	0.125–32	0.5	4	0.618	47.2	30.5	
	Trovafloxacin	0.125–64	0.5	4	0.745	75.0	12.5	
	Enoxacin	0.25–>128	0.5	16	0.822	74.3	12.8	
	Norfloxacin	0.25–64	0.5	16	0.883	69.2	17.9	
	Temafloxacin	0.5–64	1	8	1.31	64.1	23.1	
	Ofloxacin	0.25–64	1	16	1.37	72.5	15.0	
	Sparfloxacin	0.25–64	1	16	1.48	64.1	23.1	
	Pefloxacin	1–8	1	8	1.84	52.9	26.5	
	Lomefloxacin	0.25–128	1	32	2.07	56.4	23.1	
	Moxifloxacin	0.25–64	2	8	2.22	40.0	40.0	
	Fleroxacin	0.5–>128	1	16	2.35	58.9	17.9	
	Nalidixic acid	64–>512	64	>512	121	0	–	
(100)	Ciprofloxacin	0.06–32	1	8				[22,23]
	Gatifloxacin	0.25–128	4	32				
	Levofloxacin	0.25–64	2	32				
Pseudomonads (18)[c]	Clinafloxacin	0.008–0.25	0.06	0.125	0.034	100	0	
	Gemifloxacin	0.008–0.5	0.125	0.5	0.092	72.2	27.8	
	Grepafloxacin	0.016–1	0.125	1	0.106	100	0	
	Ciprofloxacin	0.016–0.5	0.125	0.25	0.111	100	0	
	Trovafloxacin	0.016–2	0.125	1	0.135	94.4	5.6	
	Tosufloxacin	0.016–2	0.125	0.5	0.152	94.4	5.6	
	Moxifloxacin	0.004–4	0.25	2	0.170	77.8	22.2	

(continued)

TABLE V (continued)

Organism (no. of isolates)	Compound	Range of MICs (mg/l)	MIC$_{50}$	MIC$_{90}$	Mean MIC[b]	Susceptible[c] (%)	Moder. suscept.[d] (%)	References
	Sparfloxacin	0.03–2	0.25	2	0.223	83.3	16.7	
	Enoxacin	0.03–2	0.25	1	0.354	94.4	5.6	
	Ofloxacin	0.03–2	0.5	2	0.397	100	0	
	Temafloxacin	0.03–8	0.5	2	0.412	83.3	11.1	
	Lomefloxacin	0.125–2	0.5	2	0.412	83.3	16.7	
	Fleroxacin	0.06–2	0.5	2	0.463	83.3	16.7	
	Norfloxacin	0.03–2	1	2	0.707	83.3	16.7	
	Pefloxacin	0.06–4	1	4	0.850	52.9	47.1	
Burkolderia cepacia (20)	Trovafloxacin	0.03–0.5	0.125	0.25				[18]
	Sparfloxacin	0.06–1	0.125	0.25				
	Tosufloxacin	0.06–0.5	0.125	0.25				
	Ciprofloxacin	0.12–2	0.25	0.5				
(54)	Ciprofloxacin	0.03–256	2	256				[23]
	Clinafloxacin	0.016–128	1	128				
	Levofloxacin	0.125–512	1	128				
	Trovafloxacin	0.03–256	2	256				
	Gatifloxacin	0.03–256	2	256				
	Moxifloxacin	0.03–512	4	256				
Stenotrophomonas maltophilia (13)	Clinafloxacin	0.03–1	0.125	0.25	0.125	100	0	
	Moxifloxacin	0.03–2	0.125	1	0.163	92.3	7.7	
	Sparfloxacin	0.03–2	0.25	0.5	0.213	92.3	7.7	
	Grepafloxacin	0.06–2	0.25	0.5	0.250	92.3	7.7	
	Trovafloxacin	0.06–2	0.25	1	0.278	92.3	7.7	
	Tosufloxacin	0.06–4	0.25	1	0.278	92.3	7.7	
	Gemifloxacin	0.125–4	0.5	2	0.500	38.5	46.2	
	Temafloxacin	0.125–8	1	2	0.852	69.2	23.1	
	Ofloxacin	0.5–4	1	4	1.38	84.6	15.4	
	Fleroxacin	0.5–16	2	2	1.45	46.2	46.2	
	Ciprofloxacin	0.25–8	2	4	1.53	46.2	46.2	
	Lomefloxacin	0.5–4	2	4	1.80	30.8	70.2	
	Enoxacin	1–8	4	8	3.60	7.7	69.2	

(60)							[22,23]
Ciprofloxacin	0.5	0.25–128	16			0	
Gatifloxacin	0.25	0.06–32	4			0	
Levofloxacin	0.25	0.125–64	8			0	
Campylobacter coli/jejuni (20)							
Clinafloxacin	0.008	0.008–0.03	0.016	0.011	100	0	
Temafloxacin	0.03	0.016–0.06	0.03	0.027	100	0	
Sparfloxacin	0.03	0.016–0.06	0.06	0.032	100	0	
Tosufloxacin	0.03	0.016–0.06	0.03	0.032	100	0	
Grepafloxacin	0.03	0.016–0.25	0.06	0.044	100	0	
Ciprofloxacin	0.125	0.06–0.5	0.125	0.102	100	0	
Ofloxacin	0.125	0.06–0.5	0.25	0.134	100	0	
Fleroxacin	0.25	0.125–0.5	0.25	0.189	100	0	
Lomefloxacin	0.25	0.125–1	0.25	0.250	100	0	
Pefloxacin	0.25	0.125–1	0.5	0.277	100	0	
Norfloxacin	0.25	0.125–1	0.5	0.308	100	0	
Enoxacin	0.5	0.25–1	0.5	0.392	100	0	
C. jejuni (18)							[23]
Moxifloxacin	0.03	0.03–0.125	0.125				
Trovafloxacin	0.06	0.03–0.125	0.125				
Gatifloxacin	0.125	0.06–0.25	0.25				
Clinafloxacin	0.06	0.06–0.25	0.25				
Levofloxacin	0.125	0.06–0.5	0.5				
Ciprofloxacin	0.25	0.125–1	1				
Helicobacter pylori (14)							[23]
Moxifloxacin	0.06	0.06–0.125	0.125				
Trovafloxacin	0.06	0.06–0.125	0.125				
Clinafloxacin	0.06	0.06–0.125	0.125				
Gatifloxacin	0.125	0.125–0.25	0.25				
Levofloxacin	0.25	0.125–0.5	0.5				
Ciprofloxacin	0.25	0.25–0.5	0.5				

[a] Data from [6–13] and unpublished observations of A. King, K. P. Shannon, and I. Phillips, except where indicated.

[b] Geometric mean MIC (calculated from $\log_2$ MIC + 21).

[c] Upper limits of susceptibility: 2 mg/liter of ofloxacin, 16 mg/liter of nalidixic acid, 0.25 mg/liter of gemifloxacin, 1 mg/liter of other compounds.

[d] Moderately susceptible: MICs 4 to 8 mg/liter of ofloxacin, 0.5–1 mg/liter of gemifloxacin, 2 to 4 mg/liter of other compounds, apart from nalidixic acid, for which no moderately susceptible category is defined.

[e] *Burkholderia cepacia* (1), *Comamonas acidovorans* (7), *Pseudomonas fluorescens* (2), *Pseudomonas putida* (8), *P. stutzeri* (1).

The few strains of *Aeromonas* that we tested were extremely susceptible to all the quinolones, with no MICs higher than 0.12 mg/liter (Table V). Clinafloxacin and ciprofloxacin have the greatest activity. *Aeromonas* is also extremely susceptible to gatifloxacin and levofloxacin (Table V).

Vibrio spp., including *Vibrio cholerae*, both O1 and non-O1, and *V. parahaemolyticus*, are susceptible to ciprofloxacin, trovafloxacin, tosufloxacin, temafloxacin, moxifloxacin, and norfloxacin (MICs ≤0.015–0.25 mg/liter) [26,28–30], and somewhat less susceptible to rufloxacin (MICs 0.06–1 mg/liter) [31]. *V. vulnificus* is also susceptible to norfloxacin (MICs –0.25 mg/liter) [29].

Clinafloxacin is once again the most active *in vitro* against *Campylobacter* spp. (Table IV), and ciprofloxacin is less active than many of the newer agents. Rufloxacin has reasonably good activity against quinolone-susceptible campylobacters (MIC$_{50}$ 1 mg/liter) [31]. *Helicobacter pylori* is usually susceptible to ciprofloxacin, but many of the newer drugs are more active (Table V). Fleroxacin and lomefloxacin (MICs 0.5–8 mg/liter) and, even more, pefloxacin, norfloxacin (MICs 1–16 mg/liter), and enoxacin (MICs 1–32 mg/liter) are less active [32–34].

Pseudomonas aeruginosa is appreciably less susceptible to the quinolones than are the enterobacteria or *Acinetobacter* (Table V). The highest activity is shown by clinafloxacin, with a mean MIC of 0.115 mg/liter, about 10 times higher than for the enterobacteria. Lomefloxacin is the least active of the agents that we have studied, but gatifloxacin appears even less active (Table V). None of our isolates of *Ps. aeruginosa* was resistant to clinafloxacin, but 6% were resistant to ciprofloxacin, the second most active compound, and 22% were resistant to lomefloxacin, the least active. Levofloxacin has been reported to be about twofold more active than ofloxacin (mixture) against *Ps. aeruginosa* [25], and the results in Table V suggesting the opposite should be interpreted with caution since the comparison is indirect. Rufloxacin has poor activity [26].

Table IV demonstrates that the mechanisms that lead to ciprofloxacin resistance in *Ps. aeruginosa* also mediate resistance to the other drugs, although the MICs may be lower.

Pseudomonads other than *Ps. aeruginosa* are intrinsically susceptible to the quinolones (Table V). Although differences in susceptibility are small, *Ps. fluorescens* and *Comomonas acidovorans* are the most susceptible to quinolones, followed by *Ps. putida*, with *Burkholderia cepacia* and *Stenotrophomonas maltophilia* the least susceptible. Levofloxacin is reported to be about twofold more active than ofloxacin (mixture) against pseudomonads [25,35], whereas D-ofloxacin has poorer activity [35]. The relative activity depends on the mixture of species. For example, trovafloxacin was more active than ciprofloxacin and approximately equal in activity to sparfloxacin and tosufloxacin against *B. cepacia* in the studies of Neu and Chin [18] (Table IV). Since Bauernfeind *et al.* [23] (Table V) included many more resistant isolates in their study of *B. cepacea* (Table V), affecting even the MIC$_{50}$, it is difficult to make comparisons. On the basis of range, clinafloxacin may be the most active drug. Against *S. maltophilia*, clinafloxacin is again the most active drug, and over 90% of isolates are susceptible to moxifloxacin, sparfloxacin, grepafloxacin, trovafloxacin, and tosufloxacin. Ciprofloxacin is among the least active. Gatifloxacin and levofloxacin appear to be in the middle range, taking into account the inclusion of more resistant strains by Bauernfeind *et al.* (Table V).

Alcaligenes spp. are usually susceptible to ciprofloxacin (MICs <0.12–4 mg/liter, MIC_{50} 0.5. MIC_{90} 4 mg/liter), but resistance to norfloxacin is common (MICs <0.12–32 mg/liter, MIC_{50} 4, MIC_{90} 32 mg/liter) [36]. However, *Alcaligenes denitrificans* subsp. *xylosoxidans* is relatively resistant to quinolones (MICs 0.03–2 mg/liter of clinafloxacin, 0.5–4 mg/liter of fleroxacin, 0.5–8 mg/liter of ciprofloxacin and sparfloxacin, 0.5–16 mg/liter of temafloxacin, and 1–16 mg/liter of enoxacin) [37]. The MICs of moxifloxacin are 2–16 mg/liter, gatifloxacin 4–16 mg/liter, trovafloxacin 2–32 mg/liter, and levofloxacin 4–16 mg/liter [23].

All the quinolones are active against *Haemophilus influenzae*, *Moraxella catarrhalis*, and *Neisseria gonorrhoeae* (Table VI). As against most Gram-negative aerobes, clinafloxacin is the most active, followed closely by many of the newer drugs as well as ciprofloxacin (Table VI), but rufloxacin is less so [27]. *Neisseria meningitidis* is highly susceptible to ciprofloxacin, moxifloxacin, grepafloxacin, levofloxacin, gemifloxacin, and trovafloxacin (MIC_{50} <0.03 mg/liter), and also to norfloxacin, enoxacin, and ofloxacin [27,38–40], although rufloxacin is somewhat less active (MICs 0.12 mg/liter) [27]. *Moraxella* spp. other than *M. catarrhalis* are usually susceptible to ciprofloxacin and norfloxacin (MICs <0.12–8, MIC_{90} values <0.12 mg/liter of norfloxacin, 0.25 mg/liter of ciprofloxacin) [36]. *Haemophilus ducreyi* is highly susceptible to ciprofloxacin (MICs <0.03–2 mg/liter, MIC_{50} <0.03 mg/liter) but less so to norfloxacin and ofloxacin (MICs <0.03-8 mg/liter, MIC_{50} 0.5 mg/liter) [41].

Gardnerella vaginalis is less susceptible to all the quinolones (Table VI), with clinafloxacin (mean MIC 0.16 mg/liter) the most active. However, many of the newer drugs have mean MICs of less than 2 mg/liter. Most isolates of *G. vaginalis* are resistant to lomefloxacin, norfloxacin, and enoxacin (Table V).

Bordetella pertussis and *B. parapertussis* are susceptible to ciprofloxacin, ofloxacin, and temafloxacin (MIC_{90} 0.06–0.12 mg/liter) [42]. Bauernfeind found that *B. pertussis* was even more susceptible to ciprofloxacin, as well as moxifloxacin, gatifloxacin, trovafloxacin, clinafloxacin, and levofloxacin [23]. *Bordetella bronchiseptica* is susceptible to ciprofloxacin (MICs 0.25–0.5 mg/liter) and usually to norfloxacin (MICs 0.25–4 mg/liter) [36].

Brucella melitensis has been reported to be susceptible to ciprofloxacin (MICs 0.12–0.5 mg/liter) [43]. However, Garcia-Rodriguez *et al.* [44] found quinolones to be less active against *Brucella* at pH 5 than at pH 7 and also found an increase in MICs with larger inoculum sizes; *B. abortus* was more resistant than *B. melitensis*. *Pasteurella multocida* is susceptible to ciprofloxacin, enoxacin, and ofloxacin (MICs ≤0.03–0.5 mg/liter), with ciprofloxacin the most active [45]. *Agrobacter* is susceptible to ciprofloxacin (MICs 0.03–0.06 mg/liter), enoxacin, norfloxacin, pefloxacin, and ofloxacin (MICs 0.12–1 mg/liter) [19].

The susceptibility of *Legionella pneumophila* to quinolones is much greater in a liquid medium than on buffered charcoal yeast extract agar [46]; for example, the

TABLE VI The *in-Vitro* Activity of Quinolones against *Haemophilus influenzae, Moraxella catarrhalis, Neisseria gonorrhoeae,* and *Gardnerella vaginalis*[a]

Organism (no. of isolates)	Compound	Range of MICs (mg/l)	MIC$_{50}$	MIC$_{90}$	Mean MIC[b]	Suscept- ible[c] (%)	Moder. suscept.[d] (%)	Refer- ences
Haemophilus influenzae (28)	Clinafloxacin	0.001–0.008	0.002	0.008	0.0020	100	0	
	Gemifloxacin	0.001–0.06	0.002	0.016	0.0034	100	0	
	Sparfloxacin	0.002–0.06	0.008	0.016	0.0068	100	0	
	Trovafloxacin	0.001–0.125	0.008	0.03	0.0075	100	0	
	Tosufloxacin	0.002–0.06	0.008	0.03	0.0107	100	0	
	Grepafloxacin	0.001–0.125	0.008	0.06	0.0090	100	0	
	Ciprofloxacin	0.004–0.016	0.016	0.016	0.0110	100	0	
	Temafloxacin	0.008–0.25	0.016	0.06	0.0225	100	0	
	Moxifloxacin	0.001–0.25	0.03	0.06	0.0249	100	0	
	Ofloxacin	0.016–0.125	0.03	0.03	0.0294	100	0	
	Pefloxacin	0.008–0.06	0.03	0.06	0.0302	100	0	
	Lomefloxacin	0.016–0.25	0.06	0.125	0.0548	100	0	
	Norfloxacin	0.03–0.125	0.06	0.125	0.0625	100	0	
	Fleroxacin	0.03–0.125	0.06	0.125	0.0670	100	0	
	Enoxacin	0.06–0.5	0.125	0.25	0.130	100	0	
	Nalidixic acid	0.5–4	2	4	1.83	100	–	
(74)	Ciprofloxacin	0.002–0.016	0.008	0.016				[23]
	Gatifloxacin	0.008–0.03	0.008	0.016				
	Levofloxacin	0.008–0.06	0.03	0.06				
Moraxella catarrhalis (20)	Clinafloxacin	0.008–0.016	0.008	0.016	0.0110	100	0	
	Gemifloxacin	0.004–0.03	0.016	0.03	0.0173	100	0	
	Ciprofloxacin	0.002–0.03	0.016	0.03	0.0173	100	0	
	Trovafloxacin	0.016–0.03	0.016	0.03	0.0213	100	0	
	Grepafloxacin	0.008–0.03	0.03	0.03	0.0221	100	0	
	Tosufloxacin	0.008–0.03	0.03	0.03	0.0229	100	0	

	Sparfloxacin	0.016–0.03	0.03	0.03	0.0254	100	0
	Temafloxacin	0.03–0.06	0.06	0.06	0.0604	100	0
	Ofloxacin	0.06–0.125	0.06	0.125	0.0769	100	0
	Moxifloxacin	0.016–0.125	0.125	0.25	0.105	100	0
	Lomefloxacin	0.06–0.25	0.125	0.125	0.121	100	0
	Enoxacin	0.03–0.25	0.125	0.25	0.144	100	0
	Pefloxacin	0.125–0.25	0.125	0.25	0.145	100	0
	Fleroxacin	0.125–0.25	0.125	0.25	0.165	100	0
	Norfloxacin	0.03–0.25	0.25	0.25	0.196	100	0
	Nalidixic acid	4–8	4	8	4.46	100	–
(60)							[23]
	Ciprofloxacin	0.004–0.03	0.016	0.03			
	Gatifloxacin	0.004–0.03	0.03	0.03			
	Levofloxacin	0.016–0.03	0.016	0.03			
Neisseria gonorrhoeae (30)	Clinafloxacin	0.001–0.008	0.001	0.001	0.0011	100	0
	Gemifloxacin	0.001–0.008	0.001	0.004	0.0014	100	0
	Trovafloxacin	0.001–0.008	0.002	0.004	0.0022	100	0
	Moxifloxacin	0.001–0.016	0.001	0.016	0.0025	100	0
	Ciprofloxacin	0.002–0.008	0.002	0.004	0.0025	100	0
	Sparfloxacin	0.001–0.008	0.002	0.008	0.0025	100	0
	Tosufloxacin	0.001–0.008	0.004	0.008	0.0030	100	0
	Temafloxacin	0.002–0.016	0.004	0.016	0.0056	100	0
	Ofloxacin	0.004–0.03	0.004	0.016	0.0066	100	0
	Lomefloxacin	0.008–0.06	0.016	0.06	0.0203	100	0
	Norfloxacin	0.016–0.06	0.016	0.06	0.0206	100	0
	Fleroxacin	0.016–0.06	0.016	0.06	0.0229	100	0
	Pefloxacin	0.016–0.125	0.016	0.06	0.0242	100	0
	Enoxacin	0.016–0.06	0.03	0.06	0.0254	100	0
	Nalidixic acid	0.5–2	1	2	1.02	100	–

(continued)

TABLE VI (continued)

Organism (no. of isolates)	Compound	Range of MICs (mg/l)	MIC$_{50}$	MIC$_{90}$	Mean MIC[b]	Suscept-ible[c] (%)	Moder. suscept.[d] (%)	References
(34)	Ciprofloxacin	0.002–03	0.008	0.008				[23]
	Gatifloxacin	0.002–03	0.008	0.016				
	levofloxacin	0.004–0.03	0.016	0.016				
Gardnerella vaginalis (20)	Clinafloxacin	0.125–0.25	0.125	0.25	0.165	100	0	
	Moxifloxacin	0.06–1	0.25	0.5	0.308	100	0	
	Gemifloxacin	0.06–1	0.25	0.5	0.33	60	40	
	Sparfloxacin	0.5–0.5	0.5	0.5	0.500	100	0	
	Temafloxacin	0.5–1	0.5	1	0.555	100	0	
	Tosufloxacin	0.5–1	1	1	0.901	100	0	
	Grepafloxacin	0.5–2	1	1	1.00	90	10	
	Trovafloxacin	1–1	1	1	1	100	0	
	Ciprofloxacin	0.5–2	1	2	1.37	50	50	
	Ofloxacin	1–2	1	2	1.41	100	0	
	Pefloxacin	2–8	4	8	4.00	0	85	
	Fleroxacin	4–8	4	8	5.46	0	55	
	Lomefloxacin	4–8	8	8	6.96	0	20	
	Norfloxacin	8–32	16	16	13.5	0	0	
	Enoxacin	8–32	16	32	16.0	0	0	
	Nalidixic acid	64–512	256	512	246.0	0	–	
(18)	Ciprofloxacin	3.13–6.25	3.13	6.25				[60]
	Gatifloxacin	1.56	1.56	1.56				

[a] Data from [6–13] and unpublished observations of A. King, K. P. Shannon, and I. Phillips, except where indicated.

[b] Geometric mean MIC (calculated from log$_2$ MIC + 21).

[c] Upper limits of susceptibility: 2 mg/liter of ofloxacin, 16 mg/liter of nalidixic acid, 0.25 mg/liter of gemifloxacin, 1 mg/liter of other compounds.

[d] Moderately susceptible: MICs 4 to 8 mg/liter of ofloxacin, 0.5–1 mg/liter of gemifloxacin, 2 to 4 mg/liter of other compounds, apart from nalidixic acid, for which no moderately susceptible category is defined.

MIC_{50} of ciprofloxacin was 0.01 mg/liter in a liquid medium but 0.4 mg/liter on a solid medium. Saito and his colleagues [47] have reported standard reference strains of *L. pneumophila* and other species of *Legionella* to be susceptible to ofloxacin (MICs <0.002–0.03), ciprofloxacin (MICs 0.008–0.03), and enoxacin and norfloxacin (MICs <0.002–0.25 mg/liter) when tested on buffered starch yeast extract agar; the non-*pneumophila* legionellae tended to be the most susceptible. Trovafloxacin tends to be slightly more active than ciprofloxacin against legionellae [27]. While pefloxacin has approximately equal activity to ciprofloxacin and ofloxacin against legionellae [48], temafloxacin appears to be a little more active than ciprofloxacin against *L. pneumophila* [42]. A comprehensive comparative study [49] reported trovafloxacin to be the most active quinolone, closely followed by levofloxacin, grepafloxacin, moxifloxacin, and gemifloxacin for *Legionella pneumophila*, with similar results for other *Legionalla* species.

GRAM-POSITIVE AEROBES

The quinolones are less active against staphylococci and streptococci than against the aerobic Gram-negative rods; nonetheless, many of the newer agents are highly active (Table VII), with gemifloxacin marginally in the lead for both (Figure 3a,b). For staphylococci and streptococci, the lowest mean MIC of ciprofloxacin is against coagulase-negative staphylococci. *Staph. aureus* and *Staph. saprophyticus* come next, followed by β-hemolytic streptococci (Lancefield groups A, C, and G), *Streptococcus agalactiae*, and enterococci, with alpha- and nonhemolytic streptococci and *Strep. pneumoniae* the least susceptible. Many of the newer agents are roughly 10-fold more active than ciprofloxacin.

Gemifloxacin, moxifloxacin, clinafloxacin, and tosufloxacin, followed by trovafloxacin, sparfloxacin, and grepafloxacin, were the most active against *Staph. aureus* (Table VII). All our isolates, including 10 methicillin-resistant strains, were susceptible to these compounds and also to ofloxacin, pefloxacin, and fleroxacin, but one was only moderately susceptible to ciprofloxacin. Gatifloxacin and levofloxacin are active against ciprofloxacin-susceptible strains (Table VII). The activity of the quinolones against coagulase-negative staphylococci is broadly similar to that against *Staph. aureus*, but *Staph. saprophyticus* is slightly less susceptible to most of the drugs (Table VII).

Levofloxacin is about twofold more active than ofloxacin (mixture) against staphylococci [25,50,51], whereas D-ofloxacin has poorer activity [51]. Rufloxacin has poor activity against staphylococci, being in general less active than norfloxacin [27].

Strep. pneumoniae is almost equally susceptible to gemifloxacin, trovafloxacin, and clinafloxacin, and only marginally less so to moxifloxacin, sparfloxacin, and tosufloxacin, than to grepafloxacin and temafloxacin, but about half of our isolates were only moderately susceptible to ciprofloxacin, and most isolates were resistant to pefloxacin, fleroxacin, norfloxacin, lomefloxacin, and enoxacin (Table VII).

TABLE VII The *in-Vitro* Activity of Quinolones Against Staphylococci and Streptococci[a]

Organism (no. of isolates)	Compound	Range of MICs (mg/l)	MIC$_{50}$	MIC$_{90}$	Mean MIC[b]	Suscept-ible[c] (%)	Moder. suscept.[d] (%)	References
Staphylococcus aureus (40)	Gemifloxacin	0.004–0.06	0.03	0.06	0.025	100	0	
	Moxifloxacin	0.016–0.06	0.03	0.06	0.031	100	0	
	Clinafloxacin	0.016–0.06	0.03	0.06	0.035	100	0	
	Tosufloxacin	0.016–0.125	0.03	0.06	0.040	100	0	
	Trovafloxacin	0.016–0.25	0.06	0.06	0.046	100	0	
	Sparfloxacin	0.03–0.125	0.06	0.125	0.067	100	0	
	Grepafloxacin	0.03–0.125	0.06	0.125	0.071	100	0	
	Temafloxacin	0.06–0.5	0.125	0.25	0.162	100	0	
	Ciprofloxacin	0.125–2	0.25	0.5	0.330	97.5	2.5	
	Ofloxacin	0.125–1	0.25	0.5	0.347	100	0	
	Pefloxacin	0.25–1	0.5	0.5	0.435	100	0	
	Fleroxacin	0.25–1	0.5	1	0.555	100	0	
	Lomefloxacin	0.5–2	1	1	0.871	92.5	7.5	
	Enoxacin	0.5–2	1	2	1.00	77.5	22.5	
	Norfloxacin	0.5–4	1	2	1.17	67.5	32.5	
	Nalidixic acid	32–128	64	64	52.0	0	–	
(90)	Ciprofloxacin	0.125–0.5	0.25	0.5		100		[23]
	Gatifloxacin	0.03–0.25	0.06	0.125		100		
	Levofloxacin	0.06–0.25	0.125	0.25		100		
Coagulase-negative staphylococci (30)[e]	Gemifloxacin	0.004–0.06	0.016	0.03	0.0192	100	0	
	Clinafloxacin	0.004–0.06	0.03	0.06	0.0198	100	0	
	Tosufloxacin	0.016–0.06	0.03	0.06	0.0418	100	0	
	Moxifloxacin	0.03–0.125	0.06	0.06	0.0499	100	0	
	Trovafloxacin	0.016–0.125	0.06	0.125	0.073	100	0	
	Grepafloxacin	0.03–0.25	0.06	0.125	0.0807	100	0	
	Sparfloxacin	0.03–0.25	0.125	0.25	0.106	100	0	
	Temafloxacin	0.06–0.5	0.25	0.25	0.180	100	0	
	Ciprofloxacin	0.06–1	0.25	0.5	0.228	100	0	
	Ofloxacin	0.125–1	0.25	0.5	0.323	100	0	
	Pefloxacin	0.125–2	0.5	1	0.500	92.1	7.9	

Organism (no. of strains)	Drug	MIC range	MIC₅₀	MIC₉₀	Mean	%S	%R	Ref
	Enoxacin	0.25–4	0.5	2	0.747	89.5	10.5	
	Fleroxacin	0.25–8	0.5	2	0.761	89.5	7.9	
	Lomefloxacin	0.25–2	1	1	0.775	92.1	7.9	
	Norfloxacin	0.25–8	1	2	1.00	76.3	18.4	
	Nalidixic acid	32–256	64	128	71.0	0	–	
(20)	Ciprofloxacin	0.125–8	0.25	4				[22]
	Gatifloxacin	0.06–2	0.06	2				
Staphylococcus saprophyticus (21)	Gemifloxacin	0.008–0.06	0.016	0.03	0.022	100	0	
	Clinafloxacin	0.03–0.125	0.06	0.06	0.065	100	0	
	Tosufloxacin	0.06–0.25	0.125	0.125	0.121	100	0	
	Moxifloxacin	0.125–0.5	0.125	0.125	0.129	100	0	
	Trovafloxacin	0.125–0.25	0.125	0.125	0.134	100	0	
	Grepafloxacin	0.06–0.25	0.125	0.25	0.134	100	0	
	Sparfloxacin	0.125–0.25	0.125	0.25	0.163	100	0	
	Temafloxacin	0.25–1	0.5	0.5	0.468	100	0	
	Ciprofloxacin	0.25–0.5	0.5	0.5	0.484	100	0	
	Ofloxacin	0.5–1	1	1	0.968	100	0	
	Lomefloxacin	2–4	2	4	2.44	0	100	
	Pefloxacin	1–4	2	4	2.44	4.8	95.2	
	Enoxacin	2–4	4	4	3.17	0	100	
	Fleroxacin	2–4	4	4	3.62	0	100	
	Norfloxacin	2–8	4	4	3.87	0	95.2	
(30)	Ciprofloxacin	0.25–0.5	0.5	0.5				[22]
	Gatifloxacin	0.125–0.5	0.25	0.25				
Streptococcus pneumoniae (20)	Gemifloxacin	0.03–0.125	0.06	0.125	0.072	100	0	
	Trovafloxacin	0.03–0.125	0.125	0.125	0.088	100	0	
	Clinafloxacin	0.06–0.25	0.125	0.125	0.121	100	0	
	Moxifloxacin	0.125–0.25	0.25	0.25	0.196	100	0	
	Sparfloxacin	0.125–0.5	0.25	0.5	0.258	100	0	
	Tosufloxacin	0.125–0.5	0.25	0.5	0.285	100	0	
	Grepafloxacin	0.25–1	0.5	1	0.534	100	0	
	Temafloxacin	0.5–1	1	1	0.794	100	0	

(continued)

TABLE VII (continued)

Organism (no. of isolates)	Compound	Range of MICs (mg/l)	MIC$_{50}$	MIC$_{90}$	Mean MIC[b]	Suscept-ible[c] (%)	Moder. suscept.[d] (%)	References
	Ciprofloxacin	0.5–2	1	2	1.30	52.4	47.6	
	Ofloxacin	1–2	2	2	1.74	100	0	
	Pefloxacin	4–16	8	8	7.21	0	20	
	Fleroxacin	4–16	8	8	7.49	0	14.3	
	Norfloxacin	4–16	8	16	8.00	0	15	
	Lomefloxacin	4–16	8	16	8.57	0	5	
	Enoxacin	4–16	8	16	9.19	0	10	
	Nalidixic acid	128–>512	>512	>512	–	0	–	[23]
(65)	Ciprofloxacin	0.25–4	1	4				
	Gatifloxacin	0.06–1	0.25	1				
	Levofloxacin	0.25–2	1	2				
alpha- and non-hemolytic streptococci (19)	Gemifloxacin	0.016–0.25	0.06	0.125	0.063	100	0	
	Clinafloxacin	0.06–0.125	0.125	0.125	0.100	100	0	
	Trovafloxacin	0.06–0.5	0.125	0.5	0.150	100	0	
	Moxifloxacin	0.25–0.5	0.25	0.5	0.308	100	0	
	Tosufloxacin	0.125–1	0.25	0.5	0.311	100	0	
	Sparfloxacin	0.25–1	0.5	1	0.645	100	0	
	Grepafloxacin	0.25–2	1	2	0.747	89.5	10.5	
	Ciprofloxacin	0.5–2	1	2	1.16	73.7	26.3	
	Temafloxacin	0.5–4	1	4	1.16	78.9	21.0	
	Ofloxacin	1–4	2	4	2.00	88.9	11.1	
	Norfloxacin	4–16	8	16	7.71	0	31.6	
	Lomefloxacin	4–32	8	32	10.3	0	5.3	
	Fleroxacin	8–64	8	32	12.9	0	5.3	
	Pefloxacin	8–>16	16	>16	16.0	0	0	
	Enoxacin	4–>32	16	32	17.2	0	5.3	
	Nalidixic acid	128–>512	512	>512				[22]
(29)	Ciprofloxacin	0.25–2	0.5	1				
	Gatifloxacin	0.125–0.5	0.25	0.5				

	Range	MIC₅₀	MIC₉₀	Mean	%S	%R
β-haemolytic streptococci (40)						
Gemifloxacin	0.03–0.125	0.06	0.06	0.057	100	0
Clinafloxacin	0.06–0.125	0.06	0.125	0.071	100	0
Moxifloxacin	0.06–0.5	0.25	0.5	0.25	100	0
Trovafloxacin	0.25–0.5	0.25	0.5	0.312	100	0
Sparfloxacin	0.06–1	0.5	0.5	0.254	100	0
Grepafloxacin	0.25–1	0.5	0.5	0.420	100	2.5
Ciprofloxacin	0.06–2	0.5	1	0.399	97.5	2.5
Temafloxacin	0.25–4	0.5	1	0.626	97.5	2.5
Ofloxacin	0.5–2	1	2	0.785	97.5	2.5
Norfloxacin	1–4	2	4	1.68	2.5	95
Lomefloxacin	1–16	4	8	2.98	0	50
Fleroxacin	2–32	4	8	5.76	0	50
Enoxacin	2–32	8	16	6.39	0	32.5
Pefloxacin	4–>16	8	16	9.51	0	10
Nalidixic acid	128–>512	>512	>512	9.68	0	10
(77)						[23]
Ciprofloxacin	0.25–2	1	1			
Gatifloxacin	0.06–1	0.25	0.5			
Levofloxacin	0.25–1	1	1			
***Streptococcus agalactiae* (25)**						
Gemifloxacin	0.03–0.125	0.06	0.06	0.057	100	0
Clinafloxacin	0.06–0.125	0.125	0.125	0.103	100	0
Moxifloxacin	0.06–0.5	0.25	0.5	0.25	100	0
Trovafloxacin	0.25–0.5	0.25	0.5	0.312	100	0
Sparfloxacin	0.25–0.5	0.5	0.5	0.369	100	0
Grepafloxacin	0.125–1	0.5	0.5	0.379	100	0
Tosufloxacin	0.25–0.5	0.5	0.5	0.401	100	0
Ciprofloxacin	0.5–2	1	2	0.871	88	12
Temafloxacin	0.5–2	2	2	1.21	64	36
Ofloxacin	1–2	2	2	1.84	100	0
Norfloxacin	4–8	4	8	5.43	0	56
Lomefloxacin	4–16	8	8	6.77	0	28
Fleroxacin	4–16	8	8	7.78	0	8
Enoxacin	8–16	16	16	14.7	0	8
Pefloxacin	8–>16	16	>16	>16	0	0
Nalidixic acid	128–>512	>512	>512		0	0

(continued)

TABLE VII (continued)

Organism (no. of isolates)	Compound	Range of MICs (mg/l)	MIC$_{50}$	MIC$_{90}$	Mean MIC[b]	Suscept-ible[c] (%)	Moder. suscept.[d] (%)	References
(38)	Ciprofloxacin	0.25–2	1	2				[23]
	Gatifloxacin	0.06–1	0.25	0.5				
	Levofloxacin	0.5–1	0.5	1				
Enterococci (25)	Gemifloxacin	0.008–1	0.06	0.25	0.076	92	8	
	Clinafloxacin	0.06–0.5	0.125	0.25	0.144	100	0	
	Trovafloxacin	0.06–2	0.25	0.5	0.230	96	4	
	Moxifloxacin	0.125–1	0.25	0.5	0.279	100	0	
	Grepafloxacin	0.06–2	0.25	1	0.339	92	8	
	Tosufloxacin	0.125–4	0.5	1	0.401	92	8	
	Sparfloxacin	0.125–1	0.5	1	0.460	100	0	
	Ciprofloxacin	0.5–4	1	2	1.06	80	20	
	Temafloxacin	0.5–8	1	2	1.21	60	36	
	Ofloxacin	1–8	2	4	2.11	84	16	
	Fleroxacin	2–8	4	4	3.39	0	92	
	Norfloxacin	2–8	4	8	3.58	0	92	
	Lomefloxacin	2–8	4	8	3.89	0	88	
	Pefloxacin	2–8	4	8	4.00	0	85	
	Enoxacin	2–16	8	8	5.58	0	48	
	Nalidixic acid	128–>512	>512	>512				
(145)	Ciprofloxacin	0.25–32	2	8				[23]
	Gatifloxacin	0.125–8	1	2				
	Levofloxacin	0.25–32	1	4				

[a] Data from [6–13] and unpublished observations of A. King, K. P. Shannon, and I. Phillips, except where indicated.

[b] Geometric mean MIC (calculated from log$_2$ MIC + 21).

[c] Upper limits of susceptibility: 2 mg/liter of ofloxacin, 16 mg/liter of nalidixic acid, 0.25 mg/liter of gemifloxacin, 1 mg/liter of other compounds.

[d] Moderately susceptible: MICs 4 to 8 mg/liter of ofloxacin, 0.5–1 mg/liter of gemifloxacin, 2 to 4 mg/liter of other compounds, apart from nalidixic acid, for which no moderately susceptible category is defined.

[e] Staphylococcus epidermidis (25), S. warneri (1), S. xylosus (1), S. simulans (2), S. haemolyticus (5), S. hominis (3), S. cohnii (1).

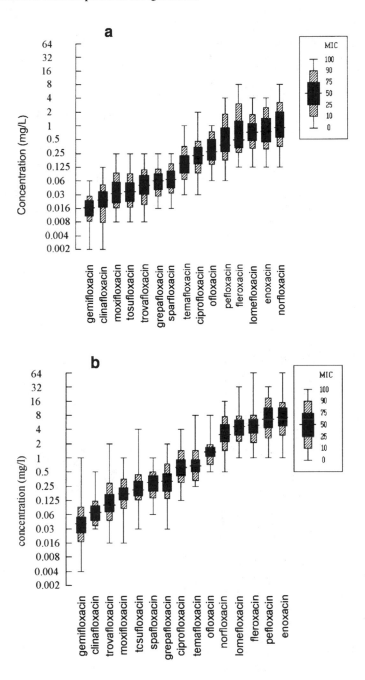

FIGURE 3 The *in-vitro* activity of quinolones against (**a**) staphylococci and (**b**) streptococci.

Gatifloxacin is also among the more active drugs as judged by its range (from 0.06 mg/liter). All of our isolates of alpha- and nonhemolytic streptococci, β-hemolytic streptococci (Lancefield groups A, C, and G), and *Strep. agalactiae* were highly susceptible to gemifloxacin and clinafloxacin, followed by moxifloxacin or trovafloxacin, then tosufloxacin and sparfloxacin, and at least moderately susceptible to grepafloxacin, ciprofloxacin, temafloxacin, and ofloxacin. However, except for members of Lancefield groups A, C, and G, resistance to norfloxacin, lomefloxacin, fleroxacin, pefloxacin, and enoxacin is the rule. Gatifloxacin is also among the more active drugs against streptococci (Table VII), but rufloxacin has poor activity (MICs 8–32 mg/liter) [27].

All our isolates of enterococci were susceptible to gemifloxacin, clinafloxacin, moxifloxacin, and sparfloxacin, and at least moderately susceptible to trovafloxacin, grepafloxacin, tosufloxacin, ciprofloxacin, and ofloxacin (Table VII). Gatifloxacin is more active than ciprofloxacin (Table VII).

Table VIII shows that, in contrast to the Enterobacteriaceae, ciprofloxacin-resistant Gram-positive bacteria may be much more susceptible to clinafloxacin, gemifloxacin, trovafloxacin, and moxifloxacin than to ciprofloxacin, some strains being within the conventional susceptible range.

Listeria monocytogenes is susceptible to ciprofloxacin (MICs 0.25–1 mg/liter) but less susceptible to ofloxacin (MICs 0.5–2 mg/liter), and norfloxacin, pefloxacin, and enoxacin (MICs 2–16 mg/liter) [19,52]. Sparfloxacin and levofloxacin have similar activity to ciprofloxacin, but clinafloxacin (MICs 0.06–0.25 mg/liter) and trovafloxacin (MICs 0.06–1 mg/liter) are more active against this organism

TABLE VIII   The *in-Vitro* Activity of Quinolones against Ciprofloxacin-Resistant (MICs >4 mg/liter) Gram-Positive Isolates[a]

Compound	Staphylococci (33)[b]		Enterococci (24)		Streptococcus pneumoniae (8)	
	Range of MICs	MIC$_{50}$	Range of MICs	MIC$_{50}$	Range of MICs	MIC$_{50}$
Clinafloxacin	0.5–4	1	1–4	4	0.25–1	1
Gemifloxacin	0.5–8	2	1–64	8	0.125–1	0.5
Trovafloxacin	0.5–8	2	2–32	16	0.06–4	4
Moxifloxacin	2–8	4	2–32	16	0.25–8	4
Grepafloxacin	16–32	32	16–32	32	0.25–16	8
Ofloxacin	16->128	16	16->128	>128	4->128	32
Ciprofloxacin	32->128	128	16->128	128	8–128	64

[a]Data from [13] and unpublished observations of A. King, K. P. Shannon, and I. Phillips.
[b]*Staphylococcus aureus* (18), coagulase-negative staphylococci (15).

[18,25,53], as are gemifloxacin, moxifloxacin, and gatifloxacin [54]. *Corynebacterium jeikeium* is intrinsically susceptible to ciprofloxacin (MICs 0.12–1 mg/liter), ofloxacin (MICs 0.25–2 mg/liter), and norfloxacin (MICs 0.5–4 mg/liter) [52], and also to sparfloxacin and fleroxacin [55,56]. Trovafloxacin (MIC_{50} 2 mg/liter, MIC_{90} 8 mg/liter) is reported to be about 16-fold more active than ciprofloxacin in a study that found poor activity of the latter compound against *C. jeikeium* [26]. Group D2 corynebacteria have been reported to be mostly susceptible to ciprofloxacin (MICs <0.12–4 mg/liter, MIC_{90} 1 mg/liter), ofloxacin (MICs <0.12–8 mg/liter, MIC_{90} 0.5 mg/liter), and norfloxacin (MICs 0.25–>16 mg/liter, MIC_{50} 1 mg/liter, MIC_{90} 8 mg/liter) [57], but a more recent study reported them to be mostly resistant to norfloxacin, enoxacin, pefloxacin, ofloxacin, ciprofloxacin, temafloxacin, lomefloxacin, fleroxacin, and sparfloxacin [58]. Gemifloxacin appears to be about 4- to 10-fold more active than ciprofloxacin against a variety of corynebacteria [54]. Activity very much depends on species [59]. The corynebacteria illustrate particularly well the problems of making comparisons of activity based on different studies, particularly for organisms with a high incidence of acquired resistance.

ANAEROBES

Among the anaerobes, *Bacteroides ureolyticus*, *Mobiluncus*, and peptostreptococci are the most susceptible, with the *Bacteroides fragilis* group usually the least susceptible. Clinafloxacin is overall the most active compound, but the order for the rest varies for the different genera.

Clinafloxacin and trovafloxacin are the only compounds to which all isolates in the *B. fragilis* group are susceptible, but more than 90% are at least moderately susceptible to tosufloxacin, gemifloxacin, sparfloxacin, moxifloxacin, grepafloxacin, and temafloxacin [60] (Table IX). Differences between species in the *B. fragilis* group are minor, but *B. fragilis* is among the most susceptible and *B. ovatus* and *B. uniformis* among the less susceptible species, as was found also with ciprofloxacin for a larger number of *B. fragilis* group organisms [61]. Our finding of reasonable activity for trovafloxacin against *Bacteroides fragilis* (Table IX) does not agree with that of Gooding and Jones [62], who reported higher MICs (1–>8 mg/liter, MIC_{50} >8 mg/liter). Rufloxacin has poor activity (MICs 16–32 mg/liter) against *Bacteroides* [27].

The order of activity of the quinolones against the *Prevotella/Porphyromonas* group is much the same as against the *B. fragilis* group, but the organisms are generally more susceptible. *P. bivia* and *P. oralis* are often slightly less susceptible than other members of this group (Table IX).

B. ureolyticus is uniquely susceptible to all the quinolones, and exquisitely susceptible to clinafloxacin and gemifloxacin (Table IX).

TABLE IX The *in-Vitro* Activity of Quinolones Against Anaerobes[a]

Organism (no. of isolates)	Compound	Range of MICs (mg/l)	MIC$_{50}$	MIC$_{90}$	Mean MIC[b]	Suscept-ible[c] (%)	Moder. suscept.[d] (%)	References
Bacteroides fragilis group[e] (57)	Clinafloxacin	0.03–1	0.06	0.25	0.091	100	0	
	Trovafloxacin	0.125–1	0.5	0.5	0.448	100	0	
	Tosufloxacin	0.5–4	1	2	0.833	84.2	25.8	
	Gemifloxacin	0.25–16	1	2	1.02	5.2	78.9	
	Sparfloxacin	0.5–16	1	2	1.17	66.7	31.6	
	Moxifloxacin	0.5–8	1	2	1.26	52.6	43.9	
	Grepafloxacin	1–8	2	4	1.84	31.6	61.4	
	Temafloxacin	0.5–16	2	4	1.95	31.6	64.9	
	Ofloxacin	1–64	4	8	3.63	13.9	47.4	
	Ciprofloxacin	1–64	4	32	6.91	1.8	43.9	
	Fleroxacin	0.125–64	8	32	8.61	1.8	29.8	
	Lomefloxacin	4–128	8	32	8.82	0	31.6	
	Enoxacin	4–>32	16	>32	22.2	0	1.8	
	Norfloxacin	4–>128	64	128	63.2	0	1.8	
(20)	Ciprofloxacin	2–32	8	8				[23]
	Gatifloxacin	0.25–8	0.5	1				
	Levofloxacin	2–8	2	2				
Prevotella Porphyromonas (40)[f]	Clinafloxacin	0.016–0.25	0.03	0.06	0.034	100	0	
	Moxifloxacin	0.125–1	0.25	0.25	0.210	100	0	
	Trovafloxacin	0.125–2	0.5	1	0.564	97.5	2.5	
	Tosufloxacin	0.125–2	0.5	1	0.619	97.5	2.5	
	Gemifloxacin	0.06–16	1	2	0.886	10	62.5	
	Temafloxacin	0.125–8	1	2	0.933	77.5	20.0	
	Ofloxacin	0.5–4	1	2	1.09	97.5	2.5	
	Ciprofloxacin	0.5–8	1	2	1.13	67.5	30.0	
	Sparfloxacin	0.25–8	2	4	1.52	37.5	60.0	
	Grepafloxacin	1–8	2	4	2.42	12.5	85.0	
	Fleroxacin	0.5–8	2	4	2.42	5	90.0	
	Lomefloxacin	2–32	4	8	4.84	0	62.5	
	Norfloxacin	1–64	4	8	4.92	2.5	62.5	
	Enoxacin	1–16	1	16	5.86	2.5	47.5	

Organism (ref.)	Drug	Range						Ref.
(94)	Ciprofloxacin	1.56–50	6.25	12.5		100	0	
	Gatifloxacin	0.05–6.25	1.56	3.13		100	0	
B. ureolyticus (10)	Clinafloxacin	0.002–0.004	0.002	0.004	0.0026	100	0	[60]
	Gemifloxacin	0.002–0.008	0.004	0.008	0.0039	100	0	
	Moxifloxacin	0.016–0.06	0.016	0.03	0.021	100	0	
	Tosufloxacin	0.016–0.06	0.03	0.06	0.0335	100	0	
	Ciprofloxacin	0.016–0.06	0.03	0.06	0.0359	100	0	
	Trovafloxacin	0.03–0.125	0.03	0.03	0.036	100	0	
	Ofloxacin	0.06–0.125	0.125	0.125	0.0947	100	0	
	Grepafloxacin	0.03–0.25	0.125	0.008	0.095	100	0	
	Temafloxacin	0.06–0.5	0.06	0.25	0.109	100	0	
	Norfloxacin	0.06–0.25	0.125	0.25	0.125	100	0	
	Lomefloxacin	0.125–0.5	0.25	0.5	0.218	100	0	
	Pefloxacin	0.12–0.5	0.25	0.5	0.218	100	0	
	Enoxacin	0.25–0.5	0.25	0.25	0.268	100	0	
	Sparfloxacin	0.125–1	0.25	1	0.330	100	0	
	Nalidixic acid	32–128	32	128	64.0	0	0	
Fusobacterium spp. (10)[g]	Clinafloxacin	0.016–0.06	0.03	0.06	0.0385	100	0	
	Gemifloxacin	0.03–0.5	0.06	0.25	0.0846	93.7	6.3	
	Moxifloxacin	0.06–1	0.125	1	0.185	100	0	
	Tosufloxacin	0.125–0.5	0.25	0.5	0.308	100	0	
	Trovafloxacin	0.125–1	0.5	0.5	0.369	100	0	
	Temafloxacin	0.5–1	0.5	1	0.707	100	0	
	Sparfloxacin	0.5–2	1	2	0.933	80.0	20.0	
	Ciprofloxacin	1–2	1	2	1.23	70.0	30.0	
	Ofloxacin	0.5–4	2	4	1.87	70.0	30.0	
	Grepafloxacin	0.5–8	4	8	3.48	20.0	50.0	
	Lomefloxacin	2–8	8	8	5.66	0	40.0	
	Fleroxacin	2–16	8	16	7.46	0	20.0	
	Norfloxacin	8–16	16	16	12.1	0	0	
	Pefloxacin	4–64	8	32	14.9	0	10.0	
	Enoxacin	16–32	16	32	22.6	0	0	
	Nalidixic acid	128–512	256	512	315	0	0	[60]
(13)	Ciprofloxacin	0.05–1.56	1.56	1.56				
	Gatifloxacin	0.05–0.39	0.2	0.39				

(continued)

TABLE IX (continued)

Organism (no. of isolates)	Compound	Range of MICs (mg/l)	MIC$_{50}$	MIC$_{90}$	Mean MIC[b]	Suscept-ible[c] (%)	Moder. suscept.[d] (%)	Refer-ences
Mobiluncus (19)	Clinafloxacin	0.03–0.06	0.06	0.06	0.045	100	0	
	Gemifloxacin	0.008–0.06	0.03	0.03	0.026	100	0	
	Sparfloxacin	0.06–0.25	0.125	0.25	0.112	100	0	
	Grepafloxacin	0.06–0.5	0.125	0.5	0.161	100	0	
	Trovafloxacin	0.125–0.25	0.125	0.25	0.177	100	0	
	Moxifloxacin	0.125–0.5	0.25	0.5	0.203	100	0	
	Tosufloxacin	0.125–0.5	0.25	0.5	0.289	100	0	
	Ciprofloxacin	0.03–1	0.5	1	0.387	100	0	
	Temafloxacin	0.25–1	0.5	1	0.579	100	0	
	Ofloxacin	0.5–2	1	2	1.29	100	0	
	Lomefloxacin	2–4	4	4	3.10	0	100	
	Fleroxacin	2–8	4	8	4.00	0	84.21	
	Norfloxacin	1–8	4	8	4.30	10.53	47.37	
	Enoxacin	2–8	8	8	5.36	0	42.11	
	Pefloxacin	4–16	8	16	7.17	0	26.32	
	Nalidixic acid	128–256	256	256	187	0		
(18)	Ciprofloxacin	0.05–0.78	0.39	0.78	0.39			[60]
	Gatifloxacin	0.1–0.2	0.2	0.2	0.2			
Peptostrepto-coccus spp. (39)[h]	Gemifloxacin	0.004–0.06	0.06	6.06	0.0359	100	0	
	Clinafloxacin	0.008–0.25	0.03	0.125	0.0462	100	0	
	Moxifloxacin	0.016–0.25	0.125	0.25	0.125	100	0	
	Trovafloxacin	0.03–0.5	0.125	0.5	0.134	100	0	
	Tosufloxacin	0.03–0.5	0.25	0.5	0.166	100	0	
	Sparfloxacin	0.03–4	0.25	1	0.309	97.4	2.6	
	Grepafloxacin	0.03–2	0.5	1	0.383	94.8	5.1	
	Temafloxacin	0.125–1	0.5	1	0.390	100	0	
	Ciprofloxacin	0.125–8	0.5	2	0.500	84.6	12.8	
	Ofloxacin	0.25–16	0.5	4	1.00	74.4	23.1	
	Norfloxacin	0.5–16	2	8	2.19	35.9	46.1	
	Fleroxacin	0.5–64	2	8	2.43	33.3	43.6	
	Lomefloxacin	0.5–16	2	8	2.71	17.9	48.7	
	Pefloxacin	0.25–32	4	16	3.41	35.9	15.5	

Organism (n)	Compound							Ref.
	Enoxacin	2–8	8	8	5.51	0	38.5	[60]
	Nalidixic acid	64–512	256	512	304	0		
(85)	Ciprofloxacin	0.05–6.25	0.78	1.56				
	Gatifloxacin	0.06–8	0.39	1.56				
Clostridium spp. (25)[i]	Clinafloxacin	0.03–1	0.25	1	0.184	100	0	
	Gemifloxacin	0.008–1	0.25	1	0.188	59.3	40.7	
	Trovafloxacin	0.06–8	0.5	4	0.500	85.2	7.4	
	Tosufloxacin	0.06–16	1	8	0.794	66.7	20.8	
	Sparfloxacin	0.03–16	2	8	1.12	41.7	37.5	
	Moxifloxacin	0.25–16	1	8	1.17	55.6	33.3	
	Grepafloxacin	0.06–16	2	16	1.68	41.7	20.8	
	Temafloxacin	0.125–64	4	32	2.31	41.7	37.5	
	Ciprofloxacin	0.125–>32	8	32	2.87	40.0	8.0	
	Ofloxacin	0.25–>32	8	32	3.48	40.0	40.0	
	Fleroxacin	0.5–128	16	128	7.13	25.0	20.8	
	Lomefloxacin	0.5–128	16	64	7.57	24.0	20.0	
	Pefloxacin	0.5–64	16	64	8.22	24.0	16.0	
	Enoxacin	0.5–>32	16	32	8.94	24.0	16.0	
	Norfloxacin	0.25–>32	32	>32	9.71	20.0	20.0	
(15)	Ciprofloxacin	0.25–8	0.25	4				[22,23]
	Gatifloxacin	0.06–1	0.25	1				

[a] Data from [6–13] and unpublished observations of A. King, K. P. Shannon, and I. Phillips, except where indicated.

[b] Geometric mean MIC (calculated from log$_2$ MIC + 21).

[c] Upper limits of susceptibility: 2 mg/liter of ofloxacin, 0.25 mg/liter of gemifloxacin, 16 mg/liter of nalidixic acid, 1 mg/liter of other compounds.

[d] Moderately susceptible: MICs 4–8 mg/liter of ofloxacin, 0.5–1 mg/liter of gemifloxacin, 2–4 mg/liter of other compounds, apart from nalidixic acid, for which no moderately susceptible category is defined.

[e] *Bacteroides fragilis* (9), *B. distasonis* (8), *B. ovatus* (10), *B. thetaiotaomicron* (10), *B. vulgatus* (10), *B. uniformis* (10).

[f] *Prevotella bivia* (5), *P. melaninogenica* (5), *P. disiens* (7), *P. oralis* (8), *P. intermedia* (5), *P. oris* (6), *Porphyromonas asaccharolytica* (4).

[g] *Fusobacterium necrophorum* (5), *F. nucleatum* (5).

[h] *Peptostreptococcus anaerobius* (19), *P. asaccharolyticus* (7), *P. magnus* (7), *P. prevotii* (6).

[i] *Clostridium perfringens* (6), *C. ramosum* (5), *C. difficile* (5), *C. clostridiiforme* (5), *C. butyricum* (4).

All the fusobacteria are susceptible to clinafloxacin, gemifloxacin, moxiflox-acin, gatifloxacin, tosufloxacin, trovafloxacin, and temafloxacin, in that order, and at least moderately susceptible to sparfloxacin, ciprofloxacin, and ofloxacin (Table IX). All isolates of *Mobiluncus* are susceptible to the same drugs plus sparfloxacin, grepafloxacin, and ofloxacin, but most are resistant to enoxacin and pefloxacin (Table IX).

Peptostreptococci are most susceptible to gemifloxacin, clinafloxacin, moxi-floxacin, trovafloxacin, tosufloxacin, sparfloxacin, grepafloxacin, and temaflox-acin (Table IX). Gatifloxacin has similar activity to ciprofloxacin. *Peptostrepto-coccus magnus* is usually more susceptible than the other organisms.

Clostridia show a wide range of susceptibilities to quinolones; all are susceptible to clinafloxacin but only 20–85% to the other compounds (Table IX). *Clostridium perfringens* (ciprofloxacin MICs 0.12–1 mg/liter) and *C. butyricum* (ciprofloxacin MICs 0.5 mg/liter) are more susceptible than *C. ramosum*, *C. difficile*, or *C. clostridiforme* (ciprofloxacin MICs 4–16, 8, and 16–64 mg/liter, respectively). Rufloxacin has poor activity (MICs 4–32 mg/liter) [27]. In a study of 100 isolates, Delmee and Avesani [63] found *Clostridium difficile* to be resistant to nearly all the earlier quinolones, including ofloxacin (MICs 8–16 mg/liter), ciprofloxacin (MICs 8–32 mg/liter), norfloxacin (MICs 32–128 mg/liter), peflox-acin (MICs (64–128 mg/liter), and enoxacin and nalidixic acid (MICs 64–256 mg/liter). They did not report results for clinafloxacin, but we found MICs of this compound to be 0.25 mg/liter for all our isolates of *C. difficile*; tosufloxacin, moxifloxacin, trovafloxacin, and gemifloxacin (MICs 1–2 mg/liter) were the next most active compounds.

MISCELLANEOUS ORGANISMS

Mycobacterium tuberculosis has been reported susceptible to ciprofloxacin and ofloxacin (MICs 0.25–1 mg/liter), and pefloxacin (MICs 0.3–2.5 mg/liter), but less so to norfloxacin (MICs 2–8 mg/liter) and enoxacin (MICs 0.3–>5 mg/liter) [64–66]. Sparfloxacin and moxifloxacin have similar activity to ciprofloxacin [67]. Members of the *M. avium complex* are less susceptible (ciprofloxacin MICs 0.5–>16 mg/liter), as are *M. intracellulare*, *M. cheloni*, *M. fortuitum*, and *M. kansasii* [64,65]. The newer fluoroquinolones usually have similar activity to ciprofloxacin [68]. Trovafloxacin appears to lack useful activity against most mycobacteria [26], and gemifloxacin against *Mycobacterium tuberculosis* [69].

Nocardia asteroides is relatively insusceptible to quinolones, with MIC_{50} values of 4–8 mg/liter of ciprofloxacin and ofloxacin, 32 mg/liter of norfloxacin, enoxacin, and pefloxacin, 64 mg/liter of amifloxacin, and >128 mg/liter of nalidixic acid [19,70]. Yazawa *et al.* [71] reported tosufloxacin (MIC_{70} 7.5

mg/liter) to be more active than ciprofloxacin (MIC_{70} 12.1 mg/liter). Other species of *Nocardia* generally had fairly similar susceptibilities, but *N. farcina* was more susceptible (ciprofloxacin MIC_{70} 0.96 mg/liter; tosufloxacin MIC_{70} <0.39 mg/liter) [71].

Chlamydia trachomatis is resistant to enoxacin and norfloxacin (MICs 8–16 mg/liter) but susceptible to sparfloxacin (MICs 0.06 mg/liter), and often to ciprofloxacin (MICs 0.5–2 mg/liter), lomefloxacin, and ofloxacin (MICs 1–4 mg/liter) [72–75]. Ofloxacin at a concentration of 1 mg/liter was reported to be completely lethal to one strain of *C. trachomatis* in monolayers of McCoy cells [75]. Gemifloxacin and trovafloxacin appear to be highly active against *C. trachomatis*, with MICs mostly around 0.03–0.06 mg/liter [76,77], and grepafloxacin is only slightly less active [78]. Against *Chlamydia pneumoniae*, gemifloxacin and grepafloxacin are more active than levofloxacin, moxifloxacin, trovafloxacin, and ofloxacin [78,79].

The older quinolones lack useful activity against *Ureaplasma ureolyticum*; ofloxacin (MICs 1–16 mg/liter, MIC_{50} 4 mg/liter) is the most active of those tested by Aznar *et al.* [73], and the MICs of ciprofloxacin, norfloxacin, and enoxacin are in the range 4–>64 mg/liter. Perea *et al.* [74] reported lower MICs (0.5–8 mg/liter) of ciprofloxacin and found lomefloxacin and sparfloxacin to be slightly more active than ciprofloxacin. *U. urealyticum* is most susceptible to gemifloxacin (MICs 0.06–0.25 mg/liter), trovafloxacin (MICs 0.06–0.5 mg/liter), and moxifloxacin (MIC 0.06 mg/liter), compared with sparfloxacin, levofloxacin, or grepafloxacin (0.25–1 mg/liter), ciprofloxacin (0.5–8 mg/liter), and ofloxacin (1–4 mg/liter) [26,80–82].

Mycoplasma pneumoniae is not particularly susceptible to quinolones, with MIC_{50}/MIC_{90} values of 1.6/1.6 for ofloxacin, 3.1/6.3 for enoxacin, and 6.3/12 for norfloxacin [83,84]. It is as susceptible to trovafloxacin (MIC 0.25 mg/liter) as to sparfloxacin and fourfold less susceptible to ofloxacin [80]. Higher activity of trovafloxacin has been reported (MICs 0.03–0.12 mg/liter compared to 0.5–2 mg/liter of ciprofloxacin) [26]. More recent studies suggest that gemifloxacin and grepafloxacin are most active, closely followed by trovafloxacin, with levofloxacin somewhat less active [85].

Ciprofloxacin (5 mg/liter) is effective in eliminating *Coxiella burnetii* from persistently infected fibroblasts [86]. Sparfloxacin (1 mg/liter) cures cells recently infected with *C. burnetii* within 4 to 9 days and cures multiplying, persistently infected cells within 10 days [87]. MICs of pefloxacin (assessed in a microplate assay) have been reported to be 0.5 mg/liter for *Rickettsia conorii* and 1 mg/liter for *R. rickettsii* [88]; ciprofloxacin MICs were 0.25 mg/liter for *R. conorii* and 1 mg/liter for *R. rickettsii* [89]; ofloxacin MICs were 1 mg/liter for both *R. conorii* and *R. rickettsii* [90]; sparfloxacin MICs were 0.25–0.5 mg/liter for *R. conorii* and 0.12–0.25 mg/liter for *R. rickettsii* [87].

CONCLUSION

Many quinolones have been developed and investigated. Useful activity against Gram-positive organisms and anaerobes has become more common. However, in terms of activity on a weight basis, clinafloxacin, which was consistently the most active of the drugs considered in the first edition, is still the most active against nearly all organisms. Nevertheless, it should not be forgotten that other factors, considered elsewhere in this book, are also involved in determining which of the quinolones are most useful in clinical practice.

REFERENCES

1. Shannon, K. P., and Phillips, I. (1985). The antimicrobial spectrum of the quinolones. *Res. Clin. Forums* **7**, 29–36.
2. Wolfson, J. S., and Hooper, D. C. (1985). The fluoroquinolones: structures, mechanisms of action and resistance, and spectra of activity in vitro. *Antimicrob. Agents Chemother.* **28**, 581–586.
3. Eliopoulos, G. M. (1986). In vitro activity of new quinolone antimicrobial agents. In "Microbiology—1986" (L. Leive, ed.), pp. 219–221. American Society for Microbiology, Washington DC.
4. Wiedemann, B., and Grimm, H. (1996). Susceptibility to antibiotics: Species incidence and trends. In "Antibiotics in Laboratory Medicine" (V. Lorian, ed.), pp 900–1168. Williams & Wilkins, Baltimore.
5. Phillips, I., and King, A. (1988). The comparative activity of the 4-quinolones. *Rev. Infect. Dis.* **10** (Suppl. 1), S70–S76.
6. King, A., Warren, C., Shannon, K., and Phillips, I. (1982). In vitro antibacterial activity of norfloxacin (MK-0366) *Antimicrob. Agents Chemother.* **21**, 604–607.
7. King, A., Shannon, K., and Phillips, I. (1984). The in-vitro activity of ciprofloxacin compared with that of norfloxacin and nalidixic acid. *J. Antimicrob. Chemother.* **13**, 325–331.
8. King, A., Shannon, K., and Phillips I. (1985). The in-vitro activities of enoxacin and ofloxacin compared with that of ciprofloxacin. *J. Antimicrob. Chemother.* **15**, 551–558.
9. King, A., and Phillips, I. (1986). The comparative in-vitro activity of pefloxacin. *J. Antimicrob. Chemother.* **17** (Suppl. B), 1–10.
10. King, A., Boothman, C., and Phillips, I. (1988). The in-vitro activity of PD127,391, a new quinolone. *J. Antimicrob. Chemother.* **22**, 135–141.
11. King, A., Bethune, L., and Phillips, I. (1991a). The in-vitro activity of temafloxacin compared with other antimicrobial agents. *J. Antimicrob. Chemother.* **27**, 769–779.
12. King, A., Bethune, L., and Phillips, I. (1991b). The in-vitro activity of tosufloxacin, a new fluorinated quinolone, compared with that of ciprofloxacin and temafloxacin. *J. Antimicrob. Chemother.* **28**, 719–725.
13. King, A., May, J., French, G., and Phillips, I. (2000). Comparative in-vitro potency of gemifloxacin. *J. Antimicrob. Chemother.* **45**, (Suppl. S1), 1–12.
14. Working Party on Antibiotic Sensitivity Testing of the British Society for Antimicrobial Chemotherapy (1991). A guide to sensitivity testing. *J. Antimicrob. Chemother.* **27** (Suppl. D), 1–48.

15. National Committee for Clinical Laboratory Standards (2000). "Methods for Dilution Antimicrobial Susceptibility Tests for Bacteria That Grow Aerobically," 5th ed. Approved Standard M7-A5, Supplemental Tables M100-S10. National Committee for Clinical Laboratory Standards, Villanova, PA.

16. Gardner, M. J., and Altman, D. G. (1986). Confidence intervals rather than P values: Estimation rather than hypothesis testing. *Br. Med. J.* **292**, 746–750.

17. Smith, J. T., and Ratcliffe, N. T. (1986). Effect of pH and magnesium on the in vitro activity of ciprofloxacin. In "Proceedings of the 1st International Ciprofloxacin Workshop" (H. C. Neu and H. Weuta, eds.), pp. 12–16. Excerpta Medica, Amsterdam.

18. Neu, H. C., and Chin, N.-X. (1994). In vitro activity of the new fluoroquinolone CP-99,219. *Antimicrob. Agents Chemother.* **38**, 2615–2622.

19. Auckenthaler, R., Michea-Hamzehpour, and M., Pechère, J. C. (1986). In-vitro activity of newer quinolones against aerobic bacteria. *J. Antimicrob. Chemother.* **17** (Suppl. B), 29–39.

20. Smith, J. T. (1986). The mode of action of 4-quinolones and possible mechanisms of resistance. *J. Antimicrob. Chemother.* **18** (Suppl. D), 21–29.

21. Mason, D. J., Power, E. G. M., Talsania, H., Phillips, I., and Gant, V. A. (1995). Antibacterial action of ciprofloxacin. *Antimicrob. Agents Chemother.* **39**, 2752–2758.

22. Wise, R., Brenwald, N. P., Andrews, J. M., and Boswell, F. (1997). The activity of the methylpiperazinyl fluoroquinolone CG 5501: A comparison with other fluoroquinolones. *J. Antimicrob. Chemother.* **39**, 447–452.

23. Bauernfeind, A. (1997). Comparison of the antibacterial activities of the quinolones Bay 12-8039, gatifloxacin (AM 1155), trovafloxacin, clinafloxacin, levofloxacin and ciprofloxacin. *J. Antimicrob. Chemother.* **40**, 639–651.

24. Reeves, D. S., Bywater, M. J., Holt, H. A., and White, L. O. (1984). In-vitro studies with ciprofloxacin, a new 4-quinolone compound. *J. Antimicrob. Chemother.* **13**, 333–346.

25. Fu, K. P., Lafredo, S. C., Foleno, B., Isaacson, D. M., Barrett, J. F., Tobia, A. J., and Rosenthale M. E. (1992). In vitro and in vivo antibacterial activities of levofloxacin (L-ofloxacin), an optically active ofloxacin. *Antimicrob. Agents Chemother.* **36**, 860–866.

26. Felmingham, D., Robbins, M. J., Ingley, K., Mathias, I., Bhogal, II., Leakey, A., Ridgway, G. L., and Grüneberg, R. N. (1997). In-vitro activity of trovafloxacin, a new fluoroquinolone, against recent clinical isolates. *J. Antimicrob. Chemother.* **39** (Suppl. B), 43–49.

27. Wise, R., Andrews, J. M., Matthews, R., and Wolstenholme, M. (1992). The in-vitro activity of two new quinolones: Rufloxacin and MF 961. *J. Antimicrob. Chemother.* **29**, 649–660.

28. Morris, J. G., Tenney, J. H., and Drusano, G. L. (1985). In vitro susceptibility of pathogenic vibrio species to norfloxacin and six other antimicrobial agents. *Antimicrob. Agents Chemother.* **28**, 442–445.

29. Bryan, J. P., Waters, C., Sheffield, J., Krieg, R. E., Perine, P. L., and Wagner K. (1990). In vitro activities of tosufloxacin, temafloxacin, and A-56620 against pathogens of diarrhea. *Antimicrob. Agents Chemother.* **34**, 368–370.

30. Felmingham, D., Robbins, M. J., Leakey, A., *et al.* (1997). In vitro activity of Bay 12-8039. *J. Clin. Microbiol. Infect. Dis.* **3** (Suppl. 2), 285.

31. Soriano, F., Fernández-Roblas, R., López, J. C., García-Corbeira, P., and Aguilar, L. (1994). Comparative in-vitro activity of rufloxacin with five other antimicrobial agents against bacterial enteric pathogens. *J. Antimicrob. Chemother.* **34**, 157–160.

32. McNulty, C. A. M., Dent, J., and Wise, R. (1985). Susceptibility of clinical isolates of *Campylobacter pyloridis* to 11 antimicrobial agents. *Antimicrob. Agents Chemother.* **28**, 837–838.

33. Lambert, T., Megraud, F., Gerbaud, G., and Courvalin, P. (1986). Susceptibility of *Campylobacter pyloridis* to 20 antimicrobial agents. *Antimicrob. Agents Chemother.* **30**, 510–511.

34. Simor, A. E., Ferro, S., and Low, D. E. (1989). Comparative in vitro activities of six new fluoroquinolones and other oral antimicrobial agents against *Campylobacter pylori. Antimicrob. Agents Chemother.* **33**, 108–109.

35. Spangler, S. K., Visalli, M. A., Jacobs, M. R., and Appelbaum, P. C. (1996). Susceptibilities of non-*Pseudomonas aeruginosa* Gram-negative nonfermentative rods to ciprofloxacin, ofloxacin, levofloxacin, D-ofloxacin, sparfloxacin, ceftazidime, piperacillin, piperacillin-tazobactam, trimethoprim-sulfamethoxazole, and imipenem. *Antimicrob. Agents Chemother.* **40**, 772–775.

36. Appelbaum, P. C., Spangler, S. K., and Sollenberger, L. (1986). Susceptibility of non-fermentative Gram-negative bacteria to ciprofloxacin, norfloxacin, amifloxacin, pefloxacin and cefpirome. *J. Antimicrob. Chemother.* **18**, 675–679.

37. Rolston, K. V., and Messer, M. (1990). The in-vitro susceptibility of *Alcaligenes denitrificans* subsp. *xylosoxidans* to 40 antimicrobial agents. *J. Antimicrob. Chemother.* **26**, 857–860.

38. Barry, A. L., Thornsberry, C., and Jones, R. N. (1986). In vitro evaluation of A-56619 and A-56620, two new quinolones. *Antimicrob. Agents Chemother.* **29**, 40–43.

39. de la Fuente, L., Giménez, M. J., and Berrón, B. (in press). In vitro activity of gemifloxacin and 13 other antimicrobials against 400 Spanish isolates of *Neisseria meningitidis* collected between 1998 and 1999. *Abstr. 3rd Eur. Cong. Chemother.*, Madrid.

40. Woodcock, J. M., Andrews, J. M., Boswell, F. J., Brenwald, N. P., and Wise, R. (1997). In vitro activity of BAY 12-8039, a new fluoroquinolone. *Antimicrob. Agents Chemother.* **41**, 101–106.

41. Liebowitz, L. D., Saunders, J., Fehler, G., Ballard, R. C., and Koornhof, H. J. (1986). In vitro activity of A-56619 (difloxacin), A-56620, and other new quinolone antimicrobial agents against genital pathogens. *Antimicrob. Agents Chemother.* **30**, 948–950.

42. Hardy, D. J. (1991). In vitro activity of temafloxacin against Gram-negative bacteria: An overview. *Am. J. Med.* **91** (Suppl. 6a), 19S–23S.

43. Bosch, J., Linares, J., Lopez de Goicoechea, M. J., Ariza, J., Cisnal, M. C., and Martin R. (1986). In-vitro activity of ciprofloxacin, ceftriaxone and five other antimicrobial agents against 95 strains of *Brucella melitensis. J. Antimicrob. Chemother.* **17**, 459–461.

44. García-Rodriguez, J. A., García Sanchez, J. E., and Trujillano, I. (1991a). Lack of effective bactericidal activity of new quinolones against *Brucella* spp. *Antimicrob. Agents Chemother.* **35**, 756–759.

45. Goldstein, E. J., and Citron, D. M. (1988). Comparative activities of cefuroxime, amoxicillin-clavulanic acid, ciprofloxacin, enoxacin, and ofloxacin against aerobic and anaerobic bacteria isolated from bite wounds. *Antimicrob. Agents Chemother.* **32**, 143–1148.

46. Pohlod, D. J., and Saravolatz, L. D. (1986). Activity of quinolones against Legionellaceae. *J. Antimicrob. Chemother.* **17**, 540–541.

47. Saito, A., Koga, H., Shigeno, H., Watanabe, K., Mori, K., Kohno, S., Shigeno, Y., Suzuyama, Y., Yamaguchi, K., Hirota, M., and Hara, K. (1986). The antimicrobial activity of ciprofloxacin against *Legionella* species and the treatment of experimental *Legionella* pneumonia in guinea pigs. *J. Antimicrob. Chemother.* **18**, 251–260.

48. Deforges, L. P., Fournet, M. P., Sossy, C. J., Dournon, E., and Duval, J. R. (1985). In vitro susceptibility of *Legionella pneumophila* to 21 antimicrobial agents. In "Proceedings of the 14th International Congress of Chemotherapy, Kyoto, 1985," pp. 594–550. University of Tokyo Press.

49. Dubois, J., and St. Pierre, C. (1999). Comparative in vitro activity and postantibiotic effect of gemifloxacin against *Legionella* spp. *J. Antimicrob. Chemother.* **44** (Suppl. A), 136.

50. Eliopoulos, G. M., Wennersten, C. B., and Moellering Jr., R. C. (1996). Comparative in vitro activity of levofloxacin and ofloxacin against Gram-positive bacteria. *Diag. Microbiol. Infect. Dis.* **25**, 35–41.

51. von Eiff, C., and Peters, G. (1996). In-vitro activity of ofloxacin, levofloxacin and D-ofloxacin against staphylococci. *J. Antimicrob. Chemother.* **38**, 259–263.

52. Mandell, W., and Neu, H. C. (1986). In vitro activity of CI-934, a new quinolone, compared with that of other quinolones and other antimicrobial agents. *Antimicrob. Agents Chemother.* **29**, 852–857.

53. Boisivon, A., Dhoyen, N., and Carbon, C. (1995). Activity of CI-960 alone and in combination with amoxycillin against *Listeria monocytogenes*, and comparison with other quinolones. *J. Antimicrob. Chemother.* **36**, 527–530.

54. Martinéz-Martinéz, L., Joyanes, P., Suárez, A. I., and Perea, E. J. (1999). Activity of gemifloxacin against clinical isolates of *Listeria monocytogenes* and coryneform bacteria. *Abstr. 39th Intersci. Conf. Antimicrob. Agents Chemother.*, San Francisco. Abstr. #P1504.

55. Rolston, K. V., Nguyen, H., Messer, M., LeBlanc, B., Ho, D. H., and Bodey, G. P. (1990). In vitro activity of sparfloxacin (CI-978; AT-4140) against clinical isolates from cancer patients. *Antimicrob. Agents Chemother.* **34**, 2263–2266.

56. Louie, A., Baltch, A. L., Ritz, W. J., and Smith, R. P. (1991). In vitro activity of sparfloxacin and six reference antibiotics against Gram-positive bacteria. *Chemotherapy* **37**, 275–282.

57. Fernandez-Roblas, R., Prieto, S., Santamaria, M., Ponte, C., and Soriano, F. (1987). Activity of nine antimicrobial agents against Corynebacterium group D2 strains isolated from clinical specimens and skin. *Antimicrob. Agents Chemother.* **31**, 821–822.

58. García-Rodriguez J. A., García Sanchez, J. E., Munoz Bellido, J. L., Nebreda Mayoral, T., García Sanchez, E., and García García, I. (1991b). In vitro activity of 79 antimicrobial agents against Corynebacterium group D2. *Antimicrob. Agents Chemother.* **35**, 2140–2143.

59. Martinéz–Martinéz, L., Pascual, A., Suárez, A.I., and Perea, E.J. (1999). In vitro activity of levofloxacin, ofloxacin and D–ofloxacin against coryneform bacteria and *Listeria monocytogenes*. *J. Antimicrob. Chemother.* **43** (Suppl. C), 27–32.

60. Kato, N., Kato, H., Tanaka-Bandoh, K., Watanabe, K., and Ueno, K. (1997). Comparative in-vitro activity of AM-1155 against anaerobic bacteria. *J. Antimicrob. Chemother.* **40**, 631–637.

61. Phillips, I., King, A., Nord, C.-E., and Hoffstedt, B. (1992). Antibiotic sensitivity of the *Bacteroides fragilis* group in Europe. *Eur. J. Clin. Microbiol. Infect. Dis.* **11**, 292–304.

62. Gooding, B. B., and Jones, R. N. (1993). In vitro antimicrobial activity of CP-99,219, a novel azabicyclo-naphthyridone. *Antimicrob. Agents Chemother.* **37**, 349–53.

63. Delmee, M., and Avesani, V. (1986). Comparative in vitro activity of seven quinolones against 100 clinical isolates of *Clostridium difficile*. *Antimicrob. Agents Chemother.* **29**, 374–375.

64. Gay, J. D., DeYoung, D. R., and Roberts, G. D. (1984). In vitro activities of norfloxacin and ciprofloxacin against *Mycobacterium tuberculosis*, *M. avium complex*, *M. cheloni*, *M. fortuitum*, and *M. kansasii*. *Antimicrob. Agents Chemother.* **26**, 94–96.

65. Fenlon, C. H., and Cynamon, M. H. (1986). Comparative in vitro activities of ciprofloxacin and other 4-quinolones against *Mycobacterium tuberculosis* and *Mycobacterium intracellulare*. *Antimicrob. Agents Chemother.* **29**, 386–388.

66. Davies, S., Sparham, P. D., and Spencer, R. C. (1987). Comparative in-vitro activity of five fluoroquinolones against mycobacteria. *J. Antimicrob. Chemother.* **19**, 605–609.

67. Rastogi, N., and Goh, K. S. (1991). In vitro activity of the new difluorinated quinolone sparfloxacin (AT-4140) against *Mycobacterium tuberculosis* compared with activities of ofloxacin and ciprofloxacin. *Antimicrob. Agents Chemother.* **35**, 1933–1936.

68. Gillespie, S. H. (1999). The activity of moxifloxacin and other fluoroquinolones against *Mycobacterium tuberculosis* and other mycobacteria. In "Moxifloxacin in Practice," Vol. 1. (D. Adam and R. Finch, eds.), pp. 71–79. R. Maxim Medical, Oxford.

69. Ruiz-Serrano, M. J., Alcalá, L., Martínez, L., Díaz, M. S., Marín, M., Gonzaléz Abad, M. J., and Bouza, E. (1999). In vitro activity of six quinolones against clinical isolates of *Mycobacterium tuberculosis* susceptible and resistant to first-line antituberculosis drugs. *Abstr. 39th Intersci. Conf. Antimicrob. Agents Chemother.*, San Francisco. Abstr. #P1492.

70. Gombert, M. E., Aulicinio, T. M., Du Bouchet, L., and Berkowitz, L. R. (1987). Susceptibility of *Nocardia asteroides* to new quinolones and beta-lactams. *Antimicrob. Agents Chemother.* **31**, 2013–2014.

71. Yazawa, K., Mikami, Y., and Uno, J. (1989). In vitro susceptibility of *Nocardia* spp. to a new fluoroquinolone, tosufloxacin (T-3262). *Antimicrob. Agents Chemother.* **33**, 2140–2141.

72. Heesen, F. W., and Muytjens, H. L. (1984). In vitro activities of ciprofloxacin, norfloxacin, pipemidic acid, cinoxacin, and nalidixic acid against *Chlamydia trachomatis*. *Antimicrob. Agents Chemother.* **25**, 123–124.

73. Aznar, J., Caballero, M. C., Lozano, M. C., de Miguel, C., Pallomares, J. C., and Perea, E. J. (1985). Activities of new quinolone derivatives against genital pathogens. *Antimicrob. Agents Chemother.* **27**, 76–78.

74. Perea, E. J., Aznar, J., Garcia-Iglesias, M. C., and Pascual, A. (1996). Comparative in-vitro activity of sparfloxacin against genital pathogens. *J. Antimicrob. Chemother.* **37** (Suppl. A), 19–25.

75. Bailey, J. M. G., Heppleston, C., and Richmond, S. J. (1984). Comparison of the in vitro activities of ofloxacin and tetracycline against *Chlamydia trachomatis* as assessed by indirect immunofluorescence. *Antimicrob. Agents Chemother.* **26**, 13–16.

76. Felmingham, D., Robbins, M., Dencer, C., Salman, H., Mathias, I., and Ridgway, G. (1999). In vitro activity of gemifloxacin against *Streptococcus pneumoniae*, *Haemothilus influenzae*, *Neisseria catarrhalis*, *Legionella pneumophila* and *Chlamydia* spp. *J. Antimicrob. Chemother.* **44** (Suppl. A), 131.

77. Jones, R. B., Van Der Pol, B., and Johnson, R. B. (1997). Susceptibility of *Chlamydia trachomatis* to trovafloxacin. *J. Antimicrob. Chemother.* **39** (Suppl. B), 63–65.

78. Ridgway, G. L., Salman, H., Robbins, M. J., Dencer, C., and Felmingham, D. (1997). In vitro activity of grepafloxacin against *Chlamydia* spp., *Mycoplasma* spp., *Ureaplasma urealyticum* and *Legionella* spp. *J. Antimicrob. Chemother.* **40** (Suppl. A), 31–34.

79. Roblin, P. M., Reznik, T., Kutlin, A., and Hammerschlag, M. R. (1999). In vitro activity of gemifloxacin against recent clinical isolates of *Chlamydia pneumoniae*. *Abstr. 39th Intersci. Conf. Antimicrob. Agents Chemother.*, San Francisco. Abstr. #P2312.

80. Kenny, G. E., and Cartwright, F. D. (1996). Susceptibilities of *Mycoplasma pneumoniae*, *Mycoplasma hominis*, and *Ureaplasma urealyticum* to a new quinolone, trovafloxacin (CP-99,219). *Antimicrob. Agents Chemother.* **40**, 1048–1049.

81. Hannan, P. C. T., and Woodnutt, G., (1999). Comparative activities of bemifloxacin, othe fluoroquinolones, erythromycin and doxycycline against human mycoplasmas and ureaplasmas (Mollicutes) and in vitro development of resistance to certain of these agents. *Abstr. 39th Intersci. Conf. Antimicrob. Agents Chemother.*, San Francisco. Abstr. #P2295.

82. Felmingham, D., Robbins, M. J., Leakey, A., Salman, H., Dencer, C., Clark, S., Ridgway, G. L., and Grüneberg, R. N. (1996). In vitro activity of Bay 12-8039 against bacterial respiratory tract pathogens, mycoplasmas and obligate anaerobic bacteria. *Abstr. 36th Intersci. Conf. Antimicrob. Agents Chemother.*, New Orleans. Abstr. #PF8.

83. Osada, Y., and Ogawa, H. (1983). Antimycoplasmal activity of ofloxacin (DL-8280). *Antimicrob. Agents Chemother.* **23**, 509–511.

84. Nakamura, S., Minami, A., Katae, H., Inoue, S., Yamagishi, J., Talase, Y., and Shimizu, M. (1983). In vitro antibacterial properties of AT-2266, a new pyridonecarboxylic acid. *Antimicrob. Agents Chemother.* **23**, 641–648.

85. Duffy, L. B., Crabb, D., Searcey, K., and Kempf, M. C. (1999). Comparative activity of gemifloxacin and new quinolones, macrolides, tetracycline and clindamycin against *Mycoplasma* species. *Abstr. 39th Intersci. Conf. Antimicrob. Agents Chemother.*, San Francisco. Abstr. #1500.

86. Yeaman, M. R., Mitscher, L. A., and Baca, O. G. (1987). In vitro susceptibility of *Coxiella burnetii* to antibiotics, including several quinolones. *Antimicrob. Agents Chemother.* **31**, 1079–1084.

87. Raoult, D., Bres, P., Drancourt, M., and Vestris, G. (1991). In vitro susceptibilities of *Coxiella burnetii*, *Rickettsia rickettsii*, and *Rickettsia conorii* to the fluoroquinolone sparfloxacin. *Antimicrob. Agents Chemother.* **35**, 88–91.

88. Raoult, D., Roussellier, P., Vestris, G., Galicher, V., Perez, R., and Tamalet, J. (1987). Susceptibility of *Rickettsia conorii* and *R. rickettsii* to pefloxacin *in vitro* and *in ovo*. *J. Antimicrob. Chemother.* **19**, 303–305.

89. Raoult, D., Roussellier, P., Galicher, V., Perez, R., and Tamalet, J. (1986). Susceptibility of *Rickettsia conorii* to ciprofloxacin as determined by suppressing lethality in chicken embryos and by plaque assay. *Antimicrob. Agents Chemother.* **29**, 424–425.

90. Raoult, D., Yeaman, M., and Baca, O. (1989). Susceptibility of *Rickettsia* and *Coxiella burnetii* to quinolones. *Rev. Infect. Dis.* **11** (Suppl. 5), S896.

CHAPTER 4

Bacterial Resistance to Quinolones

Mechanisms and Clinical Implications

THILO KÖHLER and JEAN-CLAUDE PECHÈRE

Department of Genetics and Microbiology, University of Geneva, CH-1211 Geneva, Switzerland

INTRODUCTION

Quinolones are excellent antibiotics that have proven to be helpful in a number of clinical indications. In the years following launch, they became extremely popular, and their consumption increased rapidly, both in human medicine and, unfortunately, in animal food preparations. This chapter describes the two main mechanisms of bacterial resistance to quinolones and their prevalence among medically relevant bacteria. The impact of the resistance emerging during quinolone therapy is discussed.

MECHANISMS OF QUINOLONE RESISTANCE

Bacteria can become resistant to quinolones by mutations in the target molecules, that is, the topoisomerases II and IV, or by active efflux. Earlier observations of plasmid-mediated resistance [1,2] have been confirmed [3], but quinolone resistance determinants seem essentially chromosome encoded in both mechanisms.

Regarding the target alterations in Gram-negative bacteria, the gyrase protein (topoisomerase II) is the primary target for quinolones, in particular the *gyrA* subunit. In addition, mutations in the topoisomerase IV can further increase the level of resistance. In Gram-positive bacteria, both topoisomerase II and IV can be the primary targets, depending on the bacterial species and the compound (Table I).

Active efflux is not fully documented in every bacterial species, but seems to be widespread, if not universal, in clinically relevant bacteria. Active efflux is responsible for low-level resistance that might act as a first step in resistance selection. Outer membrane permeability contributes to the intrinsic level of resistance to quinolones in some species, but its role in acquired resistance remains unclear because porin mutations do not significantly alter quinolone MICs.

GRAM-NEGATIVE BACTERIA

ESCHERICHIA COLI

The major target for mutations in *E. coli* is the *gyrA* gene. Most of the mutations identified so far are located in a small region, called the quinolone resistance-determining region (QRDR), encoding amino acids 67 to 106 [4], the commonest substitution being Ser83 replaced by Leu, followed by Ser83Val and Ser83Ala

TABLE I   Overview of Resistance Mechanisms to Quinolones

Organism	Primary targets	Secondary targets	Efflux	References
Gram negatives				
Escherichia coli	GyrA	GyrB, ParC, ParE	AcrAB	[4–21]
Salmonella typhimurium	GyrA	GyrB		[22–24]
Klebsiella	GyrA	ParC	*ramA*	[28–32]
Pseudomonas aeruginosa	GyrA	GyrB	MexAB–OprM MexCD–OprJ MexEF–OprN MexXY–OprM	[33–35,42,43] [44] [40,45] [46,47]
Neisseria gonorrhoeae	GyrA	ParC		[55–57]
Campylobacter	GyrA		No designation	[58–62]
Helicobacter pylori	GyrA			[63,64]
Gram positives				
Staphylococcus aureus	GrlA	GyrA, GyrB	NorA	[72–78]
Enterococcus faecalis	GyrA		No designation	[90–92]
Streptococcus pneumoniae	Depends on quinolone molecule (see text)		PmrA	[82–88] [89]
Mycobacteria	GyrA	GyrB	LfrA	[94–100]

[5]. This results in a 40-fold increase in ciprofloxacin MICs. Higher increases are conferred by a double mutation at residues Ser83 and Asp87 [6]. Not all *gyrA* mutations confer resistance to all quinolones. For example, mutations Asp82Gly or Gly81Asp alone lead to a low-level resistance to fluoroquinolones but not to nalidixic acid. However, when both mutations were present, resistance to all tested quinolones was found [7].

The resistance phenotype can be reversed by introduction of a wild-type *gyrA* gene that is dominant over the mutated allele. Due to DNA homologies, this complementation assay can be used in numerous bacterial species to confirm the existence of mutations in the gyrase gene. Only few cases have been reported [8] where mutations in *gyrB*, the second subunit of the gyrase protein, caused low-level quinolone resistance.

Topoisomerase IV has been identified as an additional target for quinolone action [9]. Similarly to the gyrase, this enzyme is composed of two subunits, *parC* and *parE*. Among 15 clinical isolates for which ciprofloxacin MICs were lower than 1 mg/liter, 8 showed a change in the serine residue at position 80, 4 showed a change in Glu84, and 3 showed changes in both amino acids. No mutations were detected in 12 clinical isolates for which ciprofloxacin MICs were lower than 0.25 mg/liter [10]. Apparently, *parC* mutations occur mostly in highly quinolone-resistant strains and probably only in conjunction with *gyrA* mutations [11,12].

The *nfxD* conditional resistance locus was identified as a mutant allele of *parE*, coding for the second subunit of topoisomerase IV [13]. The mutation in *parE* at codon 445 (Leu to His) is in a region that is homologous to the region of *gyrB* in which quinolone-resistance mutations have been identified. These findings suggest that *parC* and *parE* from *E. coli* are secondary targets that contribute to decreased fluoroquinolone susceptibility.

Several efflux systems have been characterized in *E. coli*. The multiple antibiotic resistance (*mar*) locus is responsible for resistance to fluoroquinolones and other structurally unrelated antibiotics [14]. Mutations in the *marR* regulator gene exist in quinolone-resistant clinical *E. coli* isolates that all contain a deletion and a point mutation in *marR* [15]. However, mutations in the *mar* genes have pleiotropic effects, including decreased expression of the outer-membrane protein OmpF [16], which could affect uptake of quinolones. However, *ompF* deletion mutants show only a moderate twofold increase in quinolone MICs [11,16–18], suggesting that the *acrAB* efflux system, which is overexpressed in *mar* mutants, plays the major role in decreasing quinolone accumulation [19]. In good agreement, gyrase mutations failed to produce significant levels of quinolone resistance when the *acrAB* locus is inactivated [20]

SALMONELLA SPP.

Quinolone-resistant isolates of *Salmonella* spp. of clinical or veterinary origin exhibited *gyrA* mutations analogous to those found in *E. coli* (Ser83Phe, Asp87Gly, or Asp87Tyr) or a single novel mutation outside of the QRDR resulting in an Ala119Glu change [21]. As in *E. coli*, *gyrB* is also a target for quinolones. A clinical isolate of *S. typhimurium* with a ciprofloxacin MIC at 32 mg/liter showed mutations in both *gyrA* and *gyrB* [6]. In another study [22], among 11 quinolone-resistant clinical isolates tested, only 1 presented a point mutation in *gyrB* (Ser463Tyr), suggesting that, as in *E. coli*, *Salmonella* mutations in *gyrB* occur less frequently than in *gyrA*.

Analysis of nalidixic acid-resistant clinical isolates of *S. typhimurium* showed no differences in outer-membrane protein or lipopolysaccharide (LPS) composition. The MICs for ciprofloxacin were 0.25 mg/liter and for nalidixic acid 1024 mg/liter. Although all isolates presented mutations in GyrA (Ser83Phe), no changes were observed in the ParC protein [23].

Decreased accumulation of quinolones was found in isolates from a ciprofloxacin-treated patient, suggesting active efflux as a mechanism of resistance. Isolates lacking OmpF porin, however, showed no decrease in quinolone accumulation [24]. Whether the *mar* operon of *Salmonella* [25] also confers resistance to fluoroquinolones remains to be determined.

KLEBSIELLA SPP.

The *gyrA* gene of *K. pneumoniae* shares 90% amino-acid identity with its *E. coli* counterpart [26]. GyrA is the primary target of quinolones and is responsible, in association with *parC* mutations, for high-level quinolone resistance [27,28]. Decreased accumulation of fluoroquinolones has been observed in one posttreatment isolate of *K. pneumoniae*, suggesting a role for antibiotic efflux in low-level fluoroquinolone resistance [28]. Resistant mutants selected *in vitro* on chloramphenicol also showed cross-resistance to other antibiotics, including nalidixic acid and norfloxacin [29]. *RamA*, a regulator gene associated with this phenotype in *Klebsiella*, was able to confer multidrug resistance when expressed in *E. coli* [29].

PSEUDOMONAS AERUGINOSA

As for most of the Gram-negative bacteria, mutations in *P. aeruginosa gyrA* are responsible for high-level resistance to fluoroquinolones [30]. The *gyrA* gene of *P. aeruginosa* has been cloned [31], and the deduced amino-acid sequence was found to share 67% identity with the *E. coli* GyrA protein. Mutations were located in the same DNA region as in the *E. coli* gene, causing the following alterations: Asp87Asn, Asp87Tyr, and Thr83Ile. Three different combinations of double mutations at positions 83 and 87 of *gyrA* have been identified in clinical isolates of *P. aeruginosa* [32]. They all confer high-level resistance (> 100 mg/liter) to ofloxacin and ciprofloxacin. One quinolone-resistant mutant isolated from urinary tract infection was shown by complementation to have a mutation in *gyrB* [33]. However, the strain was also cross-resistant to carbenicillin, chloramphenicol, and novobiocin, implying that other mutations might have occurred.

Several quinolone-resistant mutants of *P. aeruginosa* revealed increased expression of outer-membrane protein(s) in the range of 45–50 kDa [34–36]. Because accumulation of quinolones was reduced compared to a susceptible wild-type strain, it was concluded that these proteins constitute a permeability barrier to quinolone penetration. The mutations, called *nfxB* [34], *nfxC* [37], and *nalB* [38], were, however, associated with cross-resistance to nonquinolone agents—namely, carbenicillin and tetracycline (*nalB*), chloramphenicol (*nfxB*, *nfxC*), and imipenem (*nfxC*). In 1993 it became clear that the overexpressed outer-membrane proteins did not affect permeability but were actually part of multidrug efflux systems with broad substrate specificity. The MexA–MexB–OprM efflux system [39], overexpressed in *NalB*-type mutants, confers resistance to nalidixic acid and fluoroquinolones [40]. Three (so far) further antibiotic efflux systems identified in *P. aeruginosa* share a similar genetic organization. The MexC–MexD–OprJ efflux system, which confers resistance to quinolones, erythromycin, zwitterionic cephems, and chloramphenicol, was shown to be overexpressed in *NfxB*-type mutants [41,42]. A third multidrug efflux system, called MexE–MexF–OprN, specifying resistance to all quinolones and to chloramphenicol, was characterized [43] and seems to be overexpressed in *NfxC*-type mutants of *P. aeruginosa* [44]. A fourth efflux system affecting the activity of fluoroquinolones is MexXY, which also contributes to the natural resistance of *P. aeruginosa* to aminoglycosides [45,46]

NalB-type mutants have been isolated from fluoroquinolone-treated patients and shown to contain mutations in MexR, the repressor of the MexA–MexB–OprM efflux system [47,48]. Mutants overexpressing the MexC–MexD–OprJ efflux system were found among clinical isolates that were shown by complementation to carry mutations in the *nfxB* regulator gene [42]. A clinical isolate from a norfloxacin-treated patient presented mutations in *gyrA* as well as an *nfxC* mutation [49]. In mice infected with *P. aeruginosa* and treated with pefloxacin, *nfxB*- and *nfxC*-type mutants occurred [50]. These studies demonstrate that quinolones are excellent substrates for efflux systems that can produce fluoroquinolone resistance in clinical isolates.

The increase in MICs depends on the quinolone and the particular efflux system. Although the older quinolones (nalidixic, pipemidic, and oxolinic acid) show a two- to fourfold increase in MIC in the different efflux mutants, the fluoroquinolones are in general better substrates, with a three- to eightfold increase in MIC [51].

Conflicting results have been reported regarding which resistance mechanism is preferentially selected by *P. aeruginosa* in response to quinolone exposure. At concentrations close to the MIC, efflux-type mechanisms were selected almost exclusively in the laboratory strain PAO1. The gyrase type mutations appeared only at quinolone concentrations above 4× MIC [51]. However, in another *in vitro* study [52], *gyrA* mutants were selected first and subsequently efflux-type mutants occurred.

NEISSERIA GONORRHOEAE

Genes homologous to the *E. coli gyrA* and *parC* genes have been identified in *N. gonorrhoeae* [53]. Sequential selection of ciprofloxacin-resistant mutants *in vitro* showed mutations in *gyrA* at positions 91 (Ser–Phe) and 95 (Asp–Asn), and subsequently in *parC* at positions 88 (Ser–Pro) and 91 (Glu–Lys), resulting in a final high increase in ciprofloxacin MICs [53]. Clinical isolates from Japan also presented mutations in *gyrA* and in *parC* [54]. So far only one efflux system, composed of the three proteins MtrC, MtrD, and MtrE, has been identified in *N. gonorrhoeae*. It affects resistance to hydrophobic antibiotics. However, overexpression or deletion of this system did not affect ciprofloxacin MICs [55].

CAMPYLOBACTER SPP.

GyrA genes have been cloned and sequenced from *C. jejuni* [56] and from *C. fetus* [57]. A ciprofloxacin-resistant clinical isolate and an *in-vitro*-selected mutant of *C. fetus* both showed the same mutation at position 91 (Asp–Tyr), resulting in MICs of 8 to 16 mg/liter. In *C. jejuni*, mutations occurred at position 86 (Thr–Ile) in clinical isolates and at amino acids 86 (Thr–Ile), 90 (Asp–Ala), and 70 (Ala–Thr) in *in-vitro*-selected strains [56,58]. Cross-resistance to fluoroquinolones was observed in nalidixic acid-selected mutants, which were shown to have gyrase proteins 100-fold less susceptible to quinolones [59]. *In-vitro*-selected pefloxacin-resistant mutants of *C. jejuni* have been isolated and shown to display decreased accumulation of pefloxacin and ciprofloxacin compared to the sensitive parental strain. The mutants were also cross-resistant to nonquinolone agents [60]. These results, together with the presence of outer-membrane proteins overexpressed in the multidrug-resistant (MDR) strains, suggest the existence of an antibiotic efflux system involved in quinolone resistance.

HELICOBACTER PYLORI

Closely related to *C. jejuni* (76.5% amino-acid identity), the *gyrA* gene of *H. pylori* was cloned [61] and shown to be responsible for resistance to ciprofloxacin. The mutations identified occurred at positions 87 (Asn–Lys), 88 (Ala–Val), and 91 (Asp–Gly, –Asn, or –Tyr). Among 11 ciprofloxacin-resistant mutants of *H. pylori*, only 1 did not present changes in the *gyrA* gene, which seems therefore to be the primary target specifying quinolone resistance. The existence of antibiotic efflux systems has been suggested in *H. pylori* [62], but their involvement in quinolone resistance remains to be determined.

MISCELLANEOUS

In *Coxiella burnetii*, low-level fluoroquinolone-resistant strains did not show GyrA alterations, whereas in high-level resistant strains a point mutation was identified in the *gyrA* gene [63]. Gyrase-associated quinolone resistance has been demonstrated in *Serratia marcescens* [64], and *Morganella morganii* and *Proteus mirabilis* [65], and efflux-mediated fluoroquinolone resistance was found in *Proteus mirabilis* [66] and *Burkholderia cepacia* [67]. One efflux system, NorM, has been shown to affect the activity of norfloxacin in *Vibrio parahaemolyticus* [69].

GRAM-POSITIVE BACTERIA

Several new fluoroquinolone compounds, such as sparfloxacin, moxifloxacin, gatifloxacin, gemifloxacin, and clinafloxacin have been developed on the basis of improved activity against Gram-positive bacteria. It was then possible to observe that the elective topoisomerase target was drug dependent in a given Gram-positive species. In addition, a first topoisomerase mutation able to increase the MIC of older quinolones such as ciprofloxacin over the susceptibility breakpoint affects to a lesser degree the newer drugs, so that their MICs may remain within the susceptibility range. However, selection of a second topoisomerase mutation generally generates strains actually resistant to the most potent compounds. The consequences of these observations are double. First, the first mutation can be missed by susceptibility testing of the new compounds: rattlesnakes without rattles. Second, once primary mutations have been selected after the extensive use of ancient-generation fluoroquinolones, there is an actual risk of selecting a second-step mutation with the new compounds, leading to resistance to all fluoroquinolones.

STAPHYLOCOCCUS AUREUS

DNA gyrase GyrA mutations were the first alteration to be discovered in ciprofloxacin-resistant strains of *S. aureus* [69], where a QRDR similar to that from *E. coli* has been identified. Changes have been found in Ser84 to Leu or Ala, Ser85 to Pro, and Glu88 to Lys [69,70]. DNA gyrase *gyrB* can also be altered in quinolone-resistant isolates, with Asp437 to Asn or Arg458 to Gln [70]. Some isolates with high levels of quinolone resistance displayed combined mutations in both *S. aureus* and *gyrB* genes [70].

However, further analysis [71] showed that mutations in the QRDR of GyrA were not present in isolates with a low level of resistance, which in turn had GrlA alterations (Ser83 of *E. coli* to Phe or Tyr). It was also observed that mutations in GrlA were present in isolates with a high level of quinolone resistance [71]. Altogether, these experiments suggest that the DNA topoisomerase IV is a primary target of fluoroquinolones in *S. aureus*. This idea was supported by stepwise selection experiments (see below) and by the fact that quinolone-resistant *S. aureus* mutants were easily isolated from an *S. aureus* harboring a plasmid with the mutated *grlA* gene, but not from the same strain lacking the plasmid [72].

Contribution to fluoroquinolone resistance in *S. aureus* is also provided by the chromosome-encoded membrane protein NorA [73], which acts as a reserpine-susceptible multidrug efflux transporter [74]. NorA takes energy from the transmembrane proton gradient and actively pumps out of the bacterial cell a number of structurally unrelated compounds, such as norfloxacin and several other quinolones, rhodamine, ethidium bromide, acridine orange, tetracycline, and chloramphenicol [75]. However, NorA affects moxifloxacin, sparfloxacin, or trovafloxacin to a lesser degree than ciprofloxacin or levofloxacin [75].

Stepwise selection of *S. aureus* on increasing concentrations of ciprofloxacin indicated that the first-step mutants exhibited *grlA* alterations (ciprofloxacin MIC 2 mg/liter); the second-step mutants (ciprofloxacin MIC 32 mg/liter) exhibited in addition reduced accumulation of norfloxacin suggestive of active efflux. Mutations in *gyrA* were found only in the third-step mutants, that is, after selection of *grlA* alteration, in highly resistant strains (ciprofloxacin MIC at 128 mg/liter), confirming that DNA topoisomerase IV is actually the primary target of ciprofloxacin in *S. aureus* [76]. The combined role of efflux and DNA gyrase alterations was also shown in highly quinolone-resistant MRSA [77]. Multiple mutations conferring high ciprofloxacin resistance demonstrated long-term stability in antibiotic free environment [78]. A newly discovered gene, *recG*, probably involved in DNA repair, also affects quinolone activity [79].

STREPTOCOCCUS PNEUMONIAE

Selection of the primary target is drug dependent. In both laboratory and clinical settings, ciprofloxacin-resistant isolates show most commonly ParC alterations at Ser79 to Tyr or Phe, at Ala84 to Thr, Asp83 to Tyr, Lys137 to Asn, Asp83 to His [82–84]. These strains have ciprofloxacin MICs between 8 and 64 mg/liter. Less frequently, ParE alterations have also been found (Asp435Asn), with ciprofloxacin MICs at 8 or 16 mg/liter [83]. It is only after repeated exposure to ciprofloxacin that some mutants with high-level ciprofloxacin resistance (MICs ≥64 mg/liter) exhibit, in addition to the ParC or ParE alterations, changes in GyrA

[80–82,84]. These mutations in *S. aureus* replace Ser84 by Tyr or Phe, or Glu88 by Lys. With ciprofloxacin, mutation in *parC* appears to be a prerequisite before mutation in *gyrA* can augment the resistance level [80,85]. In the same context of repeated exposure to ciprofloxacin and selection of high-level resistance, mutations in GyrB were found at Asp435 substituted by Asn [81,83]. These observations suggest that, as in *S. aureus*, the mutations in *parC* precede those in *gyrA*, and that topoisomerase IV is a primary target for ciprofloxacin in *S. pneumoniae*. However, substitutions in the quinolone molecule, in particular modifications at C-7, may change the primary target [86]. If ciprofloxacin, trovafloxacin, gemifloxacin, and norfloxacin select first a *parC* mutation, the primary target of moxifloxacin and gatifloxacin is *gyrA* (personal unpublished data).

The multidrug transporter PmrA is involved in low-level resistance to quinolones [87]. As in other Gram-positive bacteria where such pumps have been identified, the multidrug transporter of *S. pneumoniae* is sensitive to reserpine. PmrA activation is associated with MICs of ciprofloxacin around 1–3 mg/liter, that is, remaining in the susceptible range. More recent data have shown that the activity of PmrA depends on the quinolone, affecting more hydrophilic (ciprofloxacin, norfloxacin) than hydrophobic (sparfloxacin, moxifloxacin) fluoroquinolones.

ENTEROCOCCUS FAECALIS

Heterologous DNA gyrase subunit complementation first showed that a mutation in the *S. aureus* gene was the major contributor to fluoroquinolone resistance in *E. faecalis* [88]. Ciprofloxacin mutants contained a change from Ser83 to Arg or to Ile, or from Glu87 to Lys or Gly (*E. coli gyrA* coordinates) [89,90]. Interestingly, the same DNA *gyrA* region did not seem to be altered in ciprofloxacin-resistant *E. faecium*, suggesting that other mechanisms of fluoroquinolone resistance may be found in some enterococci [88].

Studies indicated that an energy-dependent efflux was able to pump out norfloxacin in *E.faecalis* and *E. faecium* strains [91]. The genetic determinants of these efflux systems remain to be identified.

MYCOBACTERIA

Point mutations in *S. aureus* were also observed in clinical isolates of *Mycobacterium tuberculosis* [92,93]. *In-vitro*-selected ofloxacin resistant mutants had either mutations in *S. aureus* and/or *gyrB* or presented an efflux phenotype, the latter conferring only low-level resistance [94]. The DNA sequences obtained from fluoroquinolone-resistant mutants of *M. smegmatis* exhibited nucleotide modifications in the *gyrA* gene at positions 83 (Ala to Val), or 87 (Asp to Gly), or both [95]. The LfrA efflux pump has been shown to confer fluoroquinolone resistance when expressed on multicopy plasmids [96] by decreasing drug accumulation [97]. Ciprofloxacin-resistant mutants obtained *in vitro* showed a 64-fold increase in MIC, presented an altered GyrA, and probably also expressed the LfrA efflux pump [98].

CLINICAL IMPACT OF BACTERIAL RESISTANCE TO QUINOLONES

PREVALENCE OF QUINOLONE RESISTANCE

In the domain of quinolone resistance, great variations exist between bacterial species, clinical settings, and local epidemiology. A major trend does exist, however. Resistance is much more commonly encountered in hospital practice (notably among the nonfermenters, the enterococci, and, above all, MRSA strains) than in community-acquired infections. However, increasing resistance in *N. gonorrhoeae* and *S. pneumoniae* is a growing concern.

FLUOROQUINOLONE RESISTANCE IN HOSPITAL PRACTICE

Before launch, most of the nosocomial pathogens were susceptible to fluoroquinolones, but their use in the therapy of hospital infections has been followed by a marked increase of resistant isolates both in the United States and in Europe (Table II).

Gram-Positive Cocci

For still-unknown reasons, quinolone resistance in staphylococci depends on susceptibility to methicillin. If in most studies less than 10% of methicillin-susceptible isolates are resistant to quinolones, the resistance is notably more prevalent in the methicillin-resistant strains [99–102]. The rapid emergence of fluoroquinolone resistance in staphylococci after launch has been underlined on several occasions [99,102–106]. Typing analysis has repeatedly indicated that methicillin–quinolone double mutants belong to a number of different clones, and not to special mutants [100,101,107], but the dissemination of an unique methicillin- and quinolone-resistant strain over several hospitals has also been documented [108]. No scientific explanation has been found so far to link fluoroquinolone and methicillin resistance, but a surprising synergism has been found between oxacillin and quinolone in *S. aureus* strains exhibiting the double resistance [109].

TABLE II   Rates of Resistance to Ciprofloxacin in Clinical Isolates from Hospital Origin

Bacterial species (no. of strains)	Location	Period	Percent resistant	Reference
Gram-positive cocci				
S. aureus (17,978)	USA	1990–91	9.1	[104]
S. aureus (2849)	Europe	1990	10.5	[152]
S. aureus				
Oxa-S (1256)	USA	1993	7	[106]
Oxa-R (620)			93	
CN[a] staphylococci (9129)	USA	1990–91	19.4	[104]
CN staphylococci (1694)	Europe	1990	21	[152]
E. faecalis (100)	France	1986	0	[99]
E. faecalis (100)		1993	14	
E. faecalis (1488)	Europe	1990	10.3	[152]
E. faecalis (2551)	USA	1990–91	8.1	[104]
Enterobacteriaceae				
E. coli (200)	USA	1983	0	[106]
E. coli (2833)		1993	0	
E. coli (28805)	USA	1990–91	1.6	[104]
E. coli (2,928)	Europe	1990	0.6	[152]
K. pneumoniae (118)	USA	1983	0	[106]
K. pneumoniae (1016)	USA	1993	6	[106]
K. pneumoniae (9774)	USA	1990–91	3.4	[106]
K. pneumoniae (763)	Europe	1990	3.5	[104]
E. cloacae (57)	USA	1983	0	[106]
E. cloacae (483)			5	
E. cloacae (5170)	USA	1990–91	1.1	[104]
E. cloacae (514)	Europe	1990	1.2	[152]
S. marcescens (41)	USA	1983	0	[106]
S. marcescens(221)		1993	5	
S. marcescens (2846)	USA	1990–91	3.7	[104]
P. stuartii (46)	USA	1993	54	[106]
P. stuartii (536)	USA	1990–91	5.1	[104]
P. stuartii (45)	Europe	1990	26.7	[152]
Other Gram-negative bacilli				
P. aeruginosa (102)	USA	1983	3	[106]
P. aeruginosa (1249)		1993	16	
P. aeruginosa (16,206)	USA	1990–91	7.8	[104]
P. aeruginosa (1,887)	Europe	1990	13	[152]
S. maltophilia (25)	USA	1983	64	[106]
S. maltophilia (250)		1993	56	
S. maltophilia (540)	USA	1990–91	32.4	[104]

[a]CN = coagulase-negative.

Many enterococci are naturally resistant to fluoroquinolones, but some of the newer compounds seem to be more active. Rapid emergence of resistance may compromise this hope (Table II). The role of cross-infection in the emergence of resistance is strongly suggested by molecular typing [110]. For example, in clinical isolates of *E. faecalis* from a French hospital the percentage of resistance passed from 0% in 1986 to 24 and 14%, respectively, in 1992 and 1993; further analysis suggested that this increase was due to the spread of a single clone [111].

Enterobacteriaceae

Even in hospital practice, and with the exception of a few centers, *E. coli* and *Proteus* spp. are susceptible to fluoroquinolones in a great majority of the cases. In most institutions, resistant rates remain below 20% in *Klebsiella* spp., *E. cloacae*, and *Serratia* spp., but, for unclear reasons, they can be notably higher in *Providencia stuartii* (Table II). However, fluoroquinolone-resistant Enterobacteriaceae can spread within a short time, resistant strains arising from susceptible strains [112].

Other Gram-Negative Rods

Not surprisingly, resistance is frequently encountered in *P. aeruginosa* and other *Pseudomonas* spp. (*P. paucimobilis* is generally susceptible), *S. maltophilia*, *Acinetobacter* spp. (with the exception of *A. lwoffii*), and *Alcaligenes* spp. (Table II).

FLUOROQUINOLONE RESISTANCE IN COMMUNITY-ACQUIRED INFECTIONS

Acquired resistance is still relatively rare among the common pathogens causing infections in the community, but the recent rise in resistance rates is concerning. This should be put into the perspective of a more extensive use of fluoroquinolone drugs both in humans and in animal food. Overall, there is a trend suggesting that resistance levels are higher in developing than in developed countries [113].

Respiratory Pathogens

The emergence of penicillin-resistant *S. pneumoniae* clinical isolates has led to an increased trend to prescribe fluoroquinolones in respiratory infections, especially the new molecules with augmented anti-Gram-positive potency. However, reports have documented emergence of resistance to quinolones in *S. pneumoniae* (Table III). Initially and contrary to other antibiotic classes, this resistance appeared independent of penicillin resistance [114,115], but more recent reports

TABLE III Rates of Quinolone Resistance in Clinical Isolates from Common Community-Acquired Infections

Bacterial species (no. of strains)	Location	Period	Reference drug	Percent resistant	Reference
Respiratory pathogens					
S. pneumoniae					
peni. S (1406)	Western Europe, USA	1992–93	Ciprofloxacin	12.1	[115]
peni. I (228)				16.7	
peni. R (222)				7.7	
S. pneumoniae (7551)	Canada	1993	Ciprofloxacin	0	[117]
		1998		1.7	
S. pyogenes (240)	Europe	1993–94	Ciprofloxacin	12.1	[167]
H. influenzae (2718)	Western Europe, USA	1992–93	Ciprofloxacin, ofloxacin	0	[119]
H. influenzae (300)	Japan	1994	Ciprofloxacin	8.7	[118]
H. parainfluenzae (183)	Western Europe, USA	1992–93	Ciprofloxacin, ofloxacin	0	[120]
M. catarhalis (818)	Western Europe, USA	1992–93	Ciprofloxacin, ofloxacin	0	[132]
C. pneumoniae (25)	Japan	1993–96	Sparfloxacin	0	[127]
M. pneumoniae (50)	Japan	Not shown	Ciprofloxacin, ofloxacin	0	[168]
M. pneumoniae (40)	USA	1963–76	Trovafloxacin, sparfloxacin	0	[123]

Pathogen	Country	Year	Drug	%	Ref.
Genital pathogens					
N. gonorrhoeae (977)	UK	1989	Ciprofloxacin	2.3	[179]
N. gonorrhoeae (2141)	Australia	1984–90	Ciprofloxacin	2.0	[132]
N. gonorrhoeae (4086)	Hong Kong	1992	Ofloxacin	0.5	[128]
		1994		10.4	
M. hominis (40)	France	1990	Sparfloxacin	0	[133]
M. hominis (42)	USA	1963–90	Trovafloxacin, sparfloxacin	0	[123]
U. urealyticum (40)	France	1990	Sparfloxacin	0	[133]
U. urealyticum (46)	USA	1963–90	Trovafloxacin, sparfloxacin	0	[123]
C. trachomatis (27)	USA	1988	Ofloxacin	0	[134]
Digestive pathogens					
Salmonella spp. (903)	USA	1990–91	Ciprofloxacin	0	[104]
Salmonella spp. (27,693)	UK	1991	Ciprofloxacin	0.3	[141]
Salmonella spp. (31,147)	UK	1994	Ciprofloxacin	2.1	[141]
Shigella spp. (252)	USA	1985–89	Nalidixic acid	0.4	[170]
Shigella spp. (223)	USA	1990–91	Ciprofloxacin	0	[104]
C. jejuni (102)	Finland	1978–80	Ciprofloxacin	0	[148]
C. jejuni (100)		1990		9	
Urinary pathogens					
E. coli (1710)	Europe	1990	Ciprofloxacin	0.8	[152]
E. coli (304)	Spain	1988	Norfloxacin	0	[135]
E. coli (824)		1991		4.36	

unfortunately contradicted the first observation [116]. Resistance also occurs in *S. pyogenes*, but, in any case, quinolones are not recommended for the treatment of group A streptococci pharyngitis. Quinolone resistance in *H. influenzae* has been documented, notably in Japan, independent of amoxicillin activity [117], but such resistance remains uncommon [118]. Quinolone resistance is rare or absent in *H. parainfluenzae* [119] and *Moraxella catarrhalis* [120].

No resistance has been found in clinical isolates of *Mycoplasma pneumoniae* [121–123], despite the possibility to select this resistance *in vitro* [124], or in *Legionella pneumophila* [125]. *Chlamydia pneumoniae* is regularly sensitive to the newest fluoroquinolones, but a few strains are borderline with ciprofloxacin (MIC at 2 mg/liter) and ofloxacin (MIC at 1 mg/liter) [126].

Genital Pathogens

The emergence of resistance to antibiotics is a major obstacle in the control of gonorrhea. Fluoroquinolone drugs are now a well-established therapy for the disease, but resistance has emerged in *N. gonorrhoeae* very sharply in some areas. In Hong Kong, for instance, the frequency of resistant strains passed from 0.5% in 1992 to 10.4% in late 1994 [127] and is even higher in other Asian regions. A majority of quinolone-resistant strains exhibit cross-resistance to penicillin, tetracycline, or both [128]. Monitoring for fluoroquinolone resistance obviously has become critical for ensuring efficient therapy [129], but the criteria for interpreting fluoroquinolone resistance, based on treatment outcome, had to be set because of multiplication of strains with "diminished susceptibility" of unknown significance. An expert consensus proposed that the strains with MICs ≥ 2.0 mg/liter for ofloxacin and ≥ 1 mg/liter for ciprofloxacin should be considered resistant [130]. Fluoroquinolone underdosing in patients with gonorrhea should be avoided in order to limit the risk of resistance selection [131]. The newer quinolones, such as moxifloxacin, gatifloxacin, and sparfloxacin, are regularly active against *Ureaplasma urealyticum*, *Mycoplasma hominis*, and *Chlamydia trachomatis* [122,132,133]. No quinolone is recommended for treating syphilis.

Urinary Pathogens

A majority of community-acquired urinary tract infections are caused by Enterobacteriaceae, mostly *E. coli*, with less than 1% of quinolone resistance. More resistance can be found in some areas (e.g., Spain [135,136]) where emergence of resistance has been correlated with fluoroquinolone consumption [134].

Digestive Pathogens

Quinolones have several potential advantages in the management of bacterial diarrhea [136,137], notably because of the low prevalence of resistance in most areas. Until the early 1990s, quinolone resistance in salmonellas was rare or nonexistent. Fluoroquinolones appear especially useful in enteric fever caused by multiresistant *S. typhi* [138,139]. Unfortunately, this favorable situation may change; a trend toward resistance increase is now observed in some areas: from 0.3 to 2.1% between 1991 and 1994 in England and Wales in nontyphi salmonellas, with an even incidence at 39.6% in *Salmonella hadar* in 1994 [140]. In Romania, 8% of isolated salmonella isolates were resistant to quinolones [141].

Quinolones are very helpful in severe shigellosis caused by multiresistant bacteria, but some cases of quinolone resistance are now recognized, notably in Asia [142,143] and Africa [144]. *Campylobacter jejuni* and *C. coli* are naturally susceptible to quinolones, but emergence of resistance during therapy has been documented in several occasions [145,146]. In Finland, no resistance to ciprofloxacin was found in campylobacters isolated between 1978 and 1980, when 9% of strains identified in 1990 were resistant [147]. Quinolone resistance has been described in *Helicobacter pylori* [148], but these compounds are not currently used for *H. pylori* infection [149,150].

QUINOLONE USE AND EMERGENCE OF RESISTANCE

As suggested by some of the data from Tables II and III, a relationship seems to exist between quinolone use and subsequent emergence of resistance, especially in hospital settings. When the first fluoroquinolone (norfloxacin) was launched in Europe in 1984, an increasing usage of these drugs was rapidly observed. Resistance to quinolones was also augmented in some bacterial species isolated from hospitalized patients. Resistance rates were 0.7, 1.0, 3.8, and 7.0% in *P. aeruginosa*, 0, 0.5, 6.6, and 6.8% in *S. aureus*, and 2.2, 0.7, 4.9, and 7.7% in *E. faecalis* for the years 1983, 1986, 1989, and 1990, respectively [151]. By contrast, in the same study, the prevalence of resistant Enterobacteriaceae strains remained stable between 1983 and 1990. A correlation between ciprofloxacin resistance and fluoroquinolone use has also been observed in Spain with *E. coli* bacteremia in nonneutropenic patients [152]. However, the data clearly linking community use of fluoroquinolones with resistance emergence are not straightforward even in the species at risk, such as staphylococci and *P. aeruginosa* [154]. A few exceptions exist, however, and such species as *Campylobacter* [147] and *N. gonorrhoeae* [128], as discussed above, are more directly exposed to resistance selection during therapy.

Quinolone resistance is sometimes observed during the monitoring of quinolone-treated patients. According to a review of 173 articles [154], this occurred in 4.7% of 3417 patients treated in Europe or the United States. Emergence of resistance was responsible for clinical failure in more than 80% of these cases. Quinolones are not the only antibiotic class selecting resistance during therapy. By comparison, emergence of resistance was more frequent during therapy with penicillin (6.4%) and aminoglycoside (5.5%), whereas cephalosporins and imipenem appeared less prone to select resistance (3.4 and 2.8%, respectively) [154]. Infections most often associated with quinolone resistance during therapy included cystic fibrosis, endocarditis, osteomyelitis, prostatitis, and lung abscesses (i.e., infections in which pathogens may be exposed to quinolone concentrations below the MIC) [154–157]. Confounding factors, such as the presence of pus or indwelling devices, or interactions that reduce quinolone absorption from the gastrointestinal tract, have also to be considered [155]. Along the same lines, animal models and clinical practice suggest that resistance may result from underdosing [50,158]. The bacterial species most prone to produce resistance are those with higher-than-average initial MICs, particularly *P. aeruginosa* and the staphylococci. Resistance is most commonly documented in patients staying in intensive care units or receiving mechanical ventilation, and in studies carried out in university or teaching hospitals [154]. The risk of acquisition of fluoroquinolone-resistant isolates of *P. aeruginosa* is strongly associated with prior receipt of a fluoroquinolone [159,160]. Prophylactic use of fluoroquinolones in patients with profound neutropenia also predisposes to emergence of fluoroquinolone-resistant *E. faecalis* bacteremia [156,161].

However, the relationship between quinolone use and quinolone resistance is not straightforward, and other factors have to be considered. The problem of resistance selection during therapy is largely confined to certain bacterial species, infecting certain hospitalized patients. In addition, quinolone use is not necessarily associated with emergence of resistance [162]. Horizontal spread of resistant clones certainly plays a significant role in the diffusion of resistance [163], well illustrated by the quinolone-resistant MRSA strains and multidrug-resistant *E. faecalis*. Well-defined antibiotic policies, good hygiene measures, and strong infection control programs are key points for limiting the spread of antibiotic resistance.

REFERENCES

1. Munshi, M. H., Sack, D. A., Haider, K., Ahmed, Z. U., Rahaman, M. M., and Morshed, M. G. (1987). Plasmid-mediated resistance to nalidixic acid in *Shigella dysenteriae* type 1. *Lancet* **2**, 419–421.

2. Panhotra, B. R., Desai, B., and Sharma, P. L. (1985). Nalidixic-acid-resistant *Shigella dysenteriae* I [letter]. *Lancet* **1**, 763.

3. Martinez-Martinez, L., Pascual, A., and Jacoby, G. A. (1998). Quinolone resistance from a transferable plasmid. *Lancet* **351**, 797–799.

4. Yoshida, H., Bogaki, M., Nakamura, M., and Nakamura, S. (1990). Quinolone resistance-determining region in the DNA gyrase *gyrA* gene of *Escherichia coli*. *Antimicrob. Agents Chemother.* **34**, 1271–1272.

5. Tavio, M., Vila, J., Ruiz, J., Martin-Sanchez, A. M., and de Anta, M. T. (1999). Mechanisms involved in the development of resistance to fluoroquinolones in *Escherichia coli* isolates. *J. Antimicrob. Chemother.* **44**, 735–742.

6. Heisig, P. (1993). High-level fluoroquinolone resistance in a *Salmonella typhimurium* isolate due to alterations in both *gyrA* and *gyrB* genes. *J. Antimicrob. Chemother.* **32**, 367–377.

7. Truong, Q. C., Ouabdesselam, S., Hooper, D. C., Moreau, N. J., and Soussy, C. J. (1995). Sequential mutations of *gyrA* in *Escherichia coli* associated with quinolone therapy. *J. Antimicrob. Chemother.* **36**, 1055–1059.

8. Yoshida, H., Bogaki, M., Nakamura, M., Yamanaka, L. M., and Nakamura, S. (1991). Quinolone resistance-determining region in the DNA gyrase *gyrB* gene of *Escherichia coli*. *Antimicrob. Agents Chemother.* **35**, 1647–1650.

9. Khodursky, A. B., Zechiedrich, E. L., and Cozzarelli, N. R. (1995). Topoisomerase IV is a target of quinolones in *Escherichia coli*. *Proc. Natl. Acad. Sci. U.S.A.* **92**, 11801–11805.

10. Vila, J., Ruiz, J., Goni, P., and De Anta, M. T. (1996). Detection of mutations in *parC* in quinolone-resistant clinical isolates of *Escherichia coli*. *Antimicrob. Agents Chemother.* **40**, 491–493.

11. Heisig, P. (1996). Genetic evidence for a role of *parC* mutations in development of high-level fluoroquinolone resistance in *Escherichia coli*. *Antimicrob. Agents Chemother.* **40**, 879–885.

12. Kumagai, Y., Kato, J. I., Hoshino, K., Akasaka, T., Sato, K., and Ikeda, H. (1996). Quinolone-resistant mutants of *Escherichia coli* DNA topoisomerase IV *parC* gene. *Antimicrob. Agents Chemother.* **40**, 710–714.

13. Breines, D. M., Ouabdesselam, S., Ng, E. Y., Tankovic, J., Shah, S., Soussy, C. J., and Hooper, D. C. (1997). Quinolone resistance locus *nfxD* of *Escherichia coli* is a mutant allele of the *parE* gene encoding a subunit of topoisomerase IV. *Antimicrob. Agents Chemother.* **41**, 175–179.

14. Cohen, S. P., McMurry, L. M., Hooper, D. C., Wolfson, J. S., and Levy, S. B. (1989). Cross-resistance to fluoroquinolones in multiple-antibiotic-resistant (Mar) *Escherichia coli* selected by tetracycline or chloramphenicol: Decreased drug accumulation associated with membrane changes in addition to OmpF reduction. *Antimicrob. Agents Chemother.* **33**, 1318–1325.

15. Maneewannakul, K., and Levy, S. B. (1996). Identification for *mar* mutants among quinolone-resistant clinical isolates of *Escherichia coli*. *Antimicrob. Agents Chemother.* **40**, 1695–1698.

16. Chapman, J. S., and Georgopapadakou, N. H. (1988). Routes of quinolone permeation in *Escherichia coli*. *Antimicrob. Agents Chemother.* **32**, 438–442.

17. Kotera, Y., Inoue, M., and Mitsuhashi, S. (1990). Activity of KB-5246 against outer membrane mutants of *Escherichia coli* and *Salmonella typhimurium*. *Antimicrob. Agents Chemother.* **34**, 1323–1325.

18. Mitsuyama, J., Itoh, Y., Takahata, M., Okamoto, S., and Yasuda, T. (1992). In vitro antibacterial activities of tosufloxacin against and uptake of tosufloxacin by outer membrane mutants of *Escherichia coli*, *Proteus mirabilis*, and *Salmonella typhimurium*. *Antimicrob. Agents Chemother.* **36**, 2030–2036.

19. Okusu, H., Ma, D., and Nikaido, H. (1996). AcrAB efflux pump plays a major role in the antibiotic resistance phenotype of *Escherichia coli* multiple-antibiotic-resistance (Mar) mutants. *J. Bacteriol.* **178**, 306–308.

20. Oethinger, M., Kern, W. V., Jellen-Ritter, A. S., McMurry, L. M., and Levy, S. B. (2000). Ineffectiveness of topoisomerase mutations in mediating clinically significant fluoroquinolone resistance in *Escherichia coli* in the absence of the AcrAB efflux pump. *Antimicrob. Agents Chemother.* **44**, 10–13.

21. Griggs, D. J., Gensberg, K., and Piddock, L. J. (1996). Mutations in *gyrA* gene of quinolone-resistant *Salmonella serotypes* isolated from humans and animals. *Antimicrob. Agents Chemother.* **40**, 1009–1013.

22. Gensberg, K., Jin, Y. F., and Piddock, L. J. (1995). A novel *gyrB* mutation in a fluoroquinolone-resistant clinical isolate of *Salmonella typhimurium*. *FEMS Microbiol. Lett.* **132**, 57–60. [Erratum appears in *FEMS Microbiol. Lett.*, 1996, **137**(2–3), 293.]

23. Ruiz, J., Castro, D., Goni, P., Santamaria, J. A., Borrego, J. J., and Vila, J. (1997). Analysis of the mechanism of quinolone resistance in nalidixic acid-resistant clinical isolates of *Salmonella* serotype *Typhimurium*. *J. Med. Microbiol.* **46**, 623–628

24. Piddock, L. J., Griggs, D. J., Hall, M. C., and Jin, Y. F. (1993). Ciprofloxacin resistance in clinical isolates of *Salmonella typhimurium* obtained from two patients. *Antimicrob. Agents Chemother.* **37**, 662–666.

25. Sulavik, M. C., Dazer, M., and Miller, P. F. (1997). The *Salmonella typhimurium mar* locus: Molecular and genetic analyses and assessment of its role in virulence. *J. Bacteriol.* **179**, 1857–1866.

26. Dimri, G. P., and Das, H. K. (1990). Cloning and sequence analysis of *gyrA* gene of *Klebsiella pneumoniae*. *Nucleic Acids Res.* **18**, 151–156.

27. Deguchi, T., Fukuoka, A., Yasuda, M., Nakano, M., Ozeki, S., Kanematsu, E., Nishino, Y., Ishihara, S., Ban, Y., and Kawada, Y. (1997). Alterations in the GyrA subunit of DNA gyrase and the ParC subunit of topoisomerase IV in quinolone-resistant clinical isolates of *Klebsiella pneumoniae*. *Antimicrob. Agents Chemother.* **41**, 699–701.

28. Deguchi, T., Kawamura, T., Yasuda, M., Nakano, M., Fukuda, H., Kato, H., Kato, N., Okano, Y., and Kawada, Y. (1997). In vivo selection of *Klebsiella pneumoniae* strains with enhanced quinolone resistance during fluoroquinolone treatment of urinary tract infections. *Antimicrob. Agents Chemother.* **41**, 1609–1611.

29. George, A. M., Hall, R. M., and Stokes, H. W. (1995). Multidrug resistance in *Klebsiella pneumoniae*: A novel gene, *ramA*, confers a multidrug resistance phenotype in *Escherichia coli*. *Microbiology* **141**, 1909–1920.

30. Cambau, E., Perani, E., Dib, C., Petinon, C., Trias, J., and Jarlier, V. (1995). Role of mutations in DNA gyrase genes in ciprofloxacin resistance of *Pseudomonas aeruginosa* susceptible or resistant to imipenem. *Antimicrob. Agents Chemother.* **39**, 2248–2252.

31. Kureishi, A., Diver, J. M., Beckthold, B., Schollaardt, T., and Bryan, L. E. (1994). Cloning and nucleotide sequence of *Pseudomonas aeruginosa* DNA gyrase *gyrA* gene from strain PAO1 and quinolone-resistant clinical isolates. *Antimicrob. Agents Chemother.* **38**, 1944–1952.

32. Yonezawa, M., Takahata, M., Matsubara, N., Watanabe, Y., and Narita, H. (1995). DNA gyrase *gyrA* mutations in quinolone-resistant clinical isolates of *Pseudomonas aeruginosa*. *Antimicrob. Agents Chemother.* **39**, 1970–1972.

33. Yoshida, T., Muratani, T., Iyobe, S., and Mitsuhashi, S. (1994). Mechanisms of high-level resistance to quinolones in urinary tract isolates of *Pseudomonas aeruginosa*. *Antimicrob. Agents Chemother.* **38**, 1466–1469.

34. Hirai, K., Suzue, S., Irikura, T., Iyobe, S., and Mitsuhashi, S. (1987). Mutations producing resistance to norfloxacin in *Pseudomonas aeruginosa*. *Antimicrob. Agents Chemother.* **31**, 582–586.

35. Legakis, N. J., Tzouvelekis, L. S., Makris, A., and Kotsifaki, H. (1989). Outer membrane alterations in multiresistant mutants of *Pseudomonas aeruginosa* selected by ciprofloxacin. *Antimicrob. Agents Chemother.* **33**, 124–127.

36. Masuda, N., Sakagawa, E., and Ohya, S. (1995). Outer membrane proteins responsible for multiple drug resistance in *Pseudomonas aeruginosa*. *Antimicrob. Agents Chemother.* **39**, 645–649.

37. Fukuda, H., Hosaka, M., Hirai, K., and Iyobe, S. (1990). New norfloxacin resistance gene in *Pseudomonas aeruginosa* PAO. *Antimicrob. Agents Chemother.* **34**, 1757–1761.

38. Rella, M., and Haas, D. (1982). Resistance of *Pseudomonas aeruginosa* PAO to nalidixic acid and low levels of β-lactam antibiotics: Mapping of chromosomal genes. *Antimicrob. Agents Chemother.* **22**, 242–249.

39. Poole, K., Krebes, K., McNally, C., and Neshat, S. (1993). Multiple antibiotic resistance in *Pseudomonas aeruginosa*: Evidence for involvement of an efflux operon. *J. Bacteriol.* **175**, 7363–7372.

40. Li, X. Z., Nikaido, H., and Poole, K. (1995). Role of *mexA–mexB–oprM* in antibiotic efflux in *Pseudomonas aeruginosa*. *Antimicrob. Agents Chemother.* **39**, 1948–1953.

41. Poole, K., Gotoh, N., Tsujimoto, H., Zhao, Q., Wada, A., Yamasaki, T., Neshat, S., Yamagishi, J., Li, X. Z., and Nishino, T. (1996). Overexpression of the *mexC–mexD–oprJ* efflux operon in *nfxB*-type multidrug-resistant strains of *Pseudomonas aeruginosa*. *Mol. Microbiol.* **21**, 713–724.

42. Jakics, E. B., Iyobe, S., Hirai, K., Fukuda, H., and Hashimoto, H. (1992). Occurrence of the *nfxB* type mutation in clinical isolates of *Pseudomonas aeruginosa*. *Antimicrob. Agents Chemother.* **36**, 2562–2565.

43. Köhler, T., Michéa-Hamzehpour, M., Henze, U., Gotoh, N., Curty, L. K., and Pechère, J. C. (1997). Characterization of MexE-MexF-OprN, a positively regulated multidrug efflux system of *Pseudomonas aeruginosa*. *Mol. Microbiol.* **23**, 345–354.

44. Fukuda, H., Hosaka, M., Iyobe, S., Gotoh, N., Nishino, T., and Hirai, K. (1995). *nfxC*-type quinolone resistance in a clinical isolate of *Pseudomonas aeruginosa*. *Antimicrob. Agents Chemother.* **39**, 790–792.

45. Aires, J. R., Köhler, T., Nikaido, H., and Plésiat, P. (1999). Involvement of an active efflux system in the natural resistance of *Pseudomonas aeruginosa* to aminoglycosides. *Antimicrob. Agents Chemother.* **43**, 2624–2628.

46. Westbrock-Wadman, S., Sherman, D. R., Hichey, M. J., Coulter, S. N., Zhu, Y. Q., Warrener, P., Nguyen, L. Y., Shawar, R. M., Folger, K. R., and Stover, C. K. (1999). Characterization of *Pseudomonas aeruginosa* efflux pump contributing to aminoglycoside impermeability. *Antimicrob. Agents Chemother.* **43**, 2975–2983

47. Ziha-Zafiri, I., Llanes, C., Köhler, T., Pechère, J. C., and Plésiat, P. (1999). In vivo emergence of multidrug-resistant mutants of *Pseudomonas aeruginosa* overexpressing the active efflux system *MexA–MexB–OprM*. *Antimicrob. Agents Chemother.* **43**, 287–291.

48. Saito, K., Yoneyama, H., and Nakae, T. (1999). NalB type mutations causing the overexpression of the MexAB-OprM efflux pump are located in the MexR gene of the *Pseudomonas aeruginosa* chromosome. *FEMS Microbiol. Lett.* **179**, 67–72.

49. Fukuda, H., Hosaka, M., Iyobe, S., Gotoh, N., Nishino, T., and Hirai, K. (1995). *nfxC*-type quinolone resistance in a clinical isolate of *Pseudomonas aeruginosa*. *Antimicrob. Agents Chemother.* **39**, 790–792.

50. Michéa-Hamzehpour, M., Auckenthaler, R., Regamey, P., and Pechère, J. C. (1987). Resistance occurring after fluoroquinolone therapy of experimental *Pseudomonas aeruginosa* peritonitis. *Antimicrob. Agents Chemother.* **31**, 1803–1808.

51. Köhler, T., Michea-Hamzehpour, M., Plésiat, P., Kahr, A. L., and Pechère, J. C. (1997). Differential selection of multidrug efflux system by quinolones in *Pseudomonas aeruginosa.* *Antimicrob. Agent Chemother.* **41**, 2540–2543.

52. Zhanel, G. G., Karlowsky, J. A., Saunders, M. H., Davidson, R. J., Hoban, D. J., Hancock, R. E. W., McLean, I., and Nicolle, L. E. (1995). Development of multiple-antibiotic-resistant (Mar) mutants of *Pseudomonas aeruginosa* after serial exposure to fluoroquinolones. *Antimicrob. Agents Chemother.* **39**, 489–495.

53. Belland, R. J., Morrison, S. G., Ison, C., and Huang, W. M. (1994). *Neisseria gonorrhoeae* acquires mutations in analogous regions of *gyrA* and *parC* in fluoroquinolone-resistant isolates. *Mol. Microbiol.* **14**, 371–380.

54. Tanaka, M., Nakayama, H., Harakoa, M., and Saika, T. (2000). Antimicrobial resistance of *Neisseria gonorrhoeae* and high prevalence of ciprofloxacin-resistant in Japan, 1993 to 1998. *J. Clin. Microbiol.* **38**, 521–525.

55. Hagman, K. E., Lucas, C. E., Balthazar, J. T., Snyder, L., Nilles, M., Judd, R. C., and Shafer, W. M. (1997). The MtrD protein of *Neisseria gonorrhoeae* is a member of the resistance/nodulation/division protein family constituting part of an efflux system. *Microbiology* **143**, 2117–2125.

56. Wang, Y., Huang, W. M., and Taylor, D. E. (1993). Cloning and nucleotide sequence of the *Campylobacter jejuni gyrA* gene and characterization of quinolone-resistance mutations. *Antimicrob. Agents Chemother.* **37**, 457–463.

57. Taylor, D. E., and Chau, A. S. (1997). Cloning and nucleotide sequence of the *gyrA* gene from *Campylobacter fetus* subsp. fetus ATCC 27374 and characterization of ciprofloxacin-resistant laboratory and clinical isolates. *Antimicrob. Agents Chemother.* **41**, 665–671.

58. Zirnstein, G., Li, Y., Swaminathan, B., and Angulo, F. (1999). Ciprofloxacin resistance in *Campylobacter* isolates: Detection of *gyrA* resistance mutations by mismatch amplification mutation assay PCR and DNA sequence analysis. *J. Clin. Microbiol.* **37**, 3276–3280.

59. Gootz, T. D., and Martin, B. A. (1991). Characterization of high-level quinolone resistance in *Campylobacter jejuni. Antimicrob. Agents Chemother.* **35**, 840–845.

60. Charvalos, E., Tselentis, Y., Micheéa-Hamzehpour, M., Köhler, T., and Pechère, J. C. (1995). Evidence for an efflux pump in multidrug-resistant *Campylobacter jejuni. Antimicrob. Agents Chemother.* **39**, 2019–2022.

61. Moore, R. A., Beckthold, B., Wong, S., Kureishi, A., and Bryan, L. E. (1995). Nucleotide sequence of the *gyrA* gene and characterization of ciprofloxacin-resistant mutants of *Helicobacter pylori. Antimicrob. Agents Chemother.* **39**, 107–111.

62. Bina, J. E., Nano, F., and Hancock, R. E. (1997). Utilization of alkaline phosphatase fusions to identify secreted proteins, including potential efflux proteins and virulence factors from *Helicobacter pylori. FEMS Microbiol. Lett.* **148**, 63–68.

63. Musso, D., Drancourt, M., Osscini, S., and Raoult, D. (1996). Sequence of quinolone resistance-determining region of *gyrA* gene for clinical isolates and for an in vitro-selected quinolone-resistant strain of *Coxiella burnetii. Antimicrob. Agents Chemother.* **40**, 870–873.

64. Masecar, B. L., and Robillard, N. J. (1991). Spontaneous quinolone resistance in *Serratia marcescens* due to a mutation in *gyrA. Antimicrob. Agents Chemother.* **35**, 898–902.

65. Power, E. G., Munoz Bellido, J. L., and Phillips, I. (1992). Detection of ciprofloxacin resistance in Gram-negative bacteria due to alterations in *gyrA. J. Antimicrob. Chemother.* **29**, 9–17.

66. Ishii, H., Sato, K., Hoshino, K., Sato, M., Yamaguchi, A., Sawai, T., and Osada, Y. (1991). Active efflux of ofloxacin by a highly quinolone-resistant strain of *Proteus vulgaris. J. Antimicrob. Chemother.* **28**, 827–836.

67. Burns, J. L., Wadsworth, C. D., Barry, J. J., and Goodall, C. P. (1996). Nucleotide sequence analysis of a gene from *Burkholderia* (*Pseudomonas*) *cepacia* encoding an outer membrane lipoprotein involved in multiple antibiotic resistance. *Antimicrob. Agents Chemother.* **40**, 307–313.

68. Morita, Y., Kodama, K., Shiota, S., Mine, T., Kataoka, A., Mizushima, T., and Tsuchiya, T. (1998). NorM, a putative multidrug efflux protein of *Vibrio parahaemolyticus* and its homolog in *Escherichia coli. Antimicrob. Agent Chemother.* **42**, 1778–1782.

69. Sreedharan, S., Oram, M., Jensen, B., Peterson, L. R., and Fisher, L. M. (1990). DNA gyrase *gyrA* mutations in ciprofloxacin-resistant strains of *Staphylococcus aureus*: Close similarity with quinolone-resistance mutations in *Escherichia coli. J. Bacteriol.* **172**, 7260–7262.

70. Ito, H., Yoshida, H., Bogaki-Shonai, M., Niga, T., Hattori, H., and Nakamura, S. (1994). Quinolone-resistance mutations in the DNA gyrase *gyrA* and *gyrB* genes of *Staphylococcus aureus. Antimicrob. Agents Chemother.* **38**, 2014–2023

71. Ferrero, L., Cameron, B., Manse, B., Lagneaux, D., Crouzet, J., Famechon, A., and Blanche, F. (1994). Cloning and primary structure of *Staphylococcus aureus* DNA topoisomerase IV: A primary target of fluoroquinolones. *Mol. Microbiol.* **13**, 641–653.

72. Yamagishi, J., Kojima, T., Oyamada, Y., Fujimoto, K., Hattori, H., Nakamura, S., and Inoue, M. (1996). Alterations in the DNA topoisomerase IV *grlA* gene responsible for quinolone resistance in *Staphylococcus aureus. Antimicrob. Agents Chemother.* **40**, 1157–1163.

73. Yoshida, H., Bogaki, M., Nakamura, S., Ubukata, K., and Konno, M. (1990). Nucleotide sequence and characterization of the *Staphylococcus aureus norA* gene, which confers resistance to quinolones. *J. Bacteriol.* **172**, 6942–6949.

74. Neyfakh, A. A., Borsch, C. M., and Kaatz, G. W. (1993). Fluoroquinolone resistance protein NorA of *Staphylococcus aureus* is a multidrug efflux transporter. *Antimicrob. Agents Chemother.* **37**, 128–129.

75. Beyer, R., Pestova, E., Millichap, J. J., Stosor, V., Noskin, G. A., and Peterson, L. R. (2000). A convenient assay for estimating the possible involvement of efflux of fluoroquinolones by *Streptococcus pneumoniae* and *Staphylococcus aureus*: Evidence for diminished moxifloxacin, sparfloxacin, and trovafloxacin efflux. *Antimicrob. Agents Chemother.* **44**, 798–801.

76. Ferrero, L., Cameron, B., and Crouzet, J. (1995). Analysis of *gyrA* and *grlA* mutations in stepwise-selected ciprofloxacin-resistant mutants of *Staphylococcus aureus. Antimicrob. Agents Chemother.* **39**, 1554–1558.

77. Tanaka, M., Zhang, Y. X., Ishida, H., Akasaka, T., Sato, K., and Hayakawa, I. (1995). Mechanisms of 4-quinolone resistance in quinolone-resistant and methicillin-resistant *Staphylococcus aureus* isolates from Japan and China. *J. Med. Microbiol.* **42**, 214–219.

78. Jones, M. E., Boenink, N. M., Verhoef, J., Kohrer, K., and Schmitz, F. J. (2000). Multiple mutations conferring ciprofloxacin resistance in *Staphylococcus aureus* demonstrate long-term stability in an antibiotic-free environment. *J. Antimicrob. Chemother.* **45**, 353–356.

79. Niga, T., Yoshida, H., Hattori, H., Nakamura, S., and Ito, H. (1997). Cloning and sequencing of a novel gene (*recG*) that affects the quinolone susceptibility of *Staphylococcus aureus. Antimicrob. Agents Chemother.* **41**, 1770–1774.

80. Munoz, R., and De La Campa, A. G. (1996). ParC subunit of DNA topoisomerase IV of *Streptococcus pneumoniae* is a primary target of fluoroquinolones and cooperates with DNA gyrase A subunit in forming resistance phenotype. *Antimicrob. Agents Chemother.* **40**, 2252–2257.

81. Pan, X. S., and Fisher, L. M. (1996). Cloning and characterization of the *parC* and *parE* genes of *Streptococcus pneumoniae* encoding DNA topoisomerase IV: Role in fluoroquinolone resistance. *J. Bacteriol.* **178**, 4060–4069.

82. Tankovic, J., Perichon, B., Duval, J., and Courvalin, P. (1996). Contribution of mutations in *gyrA* and *parC* genes to fluoroquinolone resistance of mutants of *Streptococcus pneumoniae* obtained in vivo and in vitro. *Antimicrob. Agents Chemother.* **40**, 2505–2510.

83. Perichon, B., Tankovic, J., and Courvalin, P. (1997). Characterization of a mutation in the *parE* gene that confers fluoroquinolone resistance in *Streptococcus pneumoniae*. *Antimicrob. Agents Chemother.* **41**, 1166–1167.

84. Gootz, T. D., Zaniewski, R., Haskell, S., Schmieder, B., Tankovic, J., Girard, D., Courvalin, P., and Polzer, R. J. (1996). Activity of the new fluoroquinolone trovafloxacin (CP-99,219) against DNA gyrase and topoisomerase IV mutants of *Streptococcus pneumoniae* selected in vitro. *Antimicrob. Agents Chemother.* **40**, 2691–2697.

85. Janoir, C., Zeller, V., Kitzis, M. D., Moreau, N. J., and Gutmann, L. (1996). High-level fluoroquinolone resistance in *Streptococcus pneumoniae* requires mutations in *parC* and *gyrA*. *Antimicrob. Agents Chemother.* **40**, 2760–2764

86. Alovero, F. L., Pan, X. S., Morris, J. E., Manzo, R. H., and Fisher L. M. (2000). Engineering the specificity of antibacterial fluoroquinolones: Benzenesulfonamide modifications at C-7 of ciprofloxacin changes its primary target in *Streptococcus pneumoniae* from topoisomerase IV to gyrase. *Antimicrob. Agents Chemother.* **44**, 320–325.

87. Gill, M. J., Brenwald, N. P., and Wise, R. (1999). Identification of an efflux pump gene, *pmrA*, associated with fluoroquinolone resistance in *Streptococcus pneumoniae*. *Antimicrob. Agents Chemother.* **43**, 187–189.

88. Nakanishi, N., Yoshida, S., Wakebe, H., Inoue, M., and Mitsuhashi, S. (1991). Mechanisms of clinical resistance to fluoroquinolones in *Enterococcus faecalis*. *Antimicrob. Agents Chemother.* **35**, 1053–1059.

89. Korten, V., Huang, W. M., and Murray, B. E. (1994). Analysis by PCR and direct DNA sequencing of *gyrA* mutations associated with fluoroquinolone resistance in *Enterococcus faecalis*. *Antimicrob. Agents Chemother.* **38**, 2091–2094.

90. Tankovic, J., Mahjoubi, F., Courvalin, P., Duval, J., and Leclerco, R. (1996). Development of fluoroquinolone resistance in *Enterococcus faecalis* and role of mutations in the DNA gyrase *gyrA* gene. *Antimicrob. Agents Chemother.* **40**, 2558–2561.

91. Lynch, C., Courvalin, P., and Nikaido, H. (1997). Active efflux of antimicrobial agents in wild-type strains of *enterococci*. *Antimicrob. Agents Chemother.* **41**, 869–871.

92. Takiff, H. E., Salazar, L., Guerrero, C., Philipp, W., Huang, W. M., Kreiswirth, B., Cole, S. T., Jacobs Jr., W. R., and Telenti, A. (1994). Cloning and nucleotide sequence of *Mycobacterium tuberculosis gyrA* and *gyrB* genes and detection of quinolone-resistance mutations. *Antimicrob. Agents Chemother.* **38**, 773–780.

93. Xu, C., Kreiswirth, B. N., Sreevatsan, S., Musser, J. M., and Drlica, K. (1996). Fluoroquinolone resistance associated with specific gyrase mutations in clinical isolates of multidrug-resistant *Mycobacterium tuberculosis*. *J. Infect. Dis.* **174**, 1127–1130.

94. Kocagoz, T., Hackbarth, C. J., Unsal, I., Rosenberg, E. Y., Nikaido, H., and Chambers, H. F. (1996). Gyrase mutations in laboratory-selected, fluoroquinolone-resistant mutants of *Mycobacterium tuberculosis* H37Ra. *Antimicrob. Agents Chemother.* **40**, 1768–1774.

95. Revel, V., Cambau, E., Jarlier, V., and Sougakoff, W. (1994). Characterization of mutations in *Mycobacterium smegmatis* involved in resistance to fluoroquinolones. *Antimicrob. Agents Chemother.* **38**, 1991–1996.

96. Takiff, H. E., Cimino, M., Musso, M. C., Weisbrod, T., Martinez, R., Delgado, M. B., Salazar, L., Bloom, B. R., and Jacobs Jr., W. R. (1996). Efflux pump of the proton antiporter family confers low-level fluoroquinolone resistance in *Mycobacterium smegmatis*. *Proc. Natl. Acad. Sci. U.S.A.* **93**, 362–366

97. Liu, J., Takiff, H. E., and Nikaido, H. (1996). Active efflux of fluoroquinolones in *Mycobacterium smegmatis* mediated by LfrA, a multidrug efflux pump. *J. Bacteriol.* **178**, 3791–3795.

98. Banerjee, S. K., Bhatt, K., Rana, S., Misra, P., and Chakraborti, P. K. (1996). Involvement of an efflux system in mediating high level of fluoroquinolone resistance in *Mycobacterium smegmatis*. *Biochem. Biophys. Res. Commun.* **226**, 362–368.

99. Daum, T. E., Schaberg, D. R., Terpenning, M. S., Sottile, W. S., and Kauffman, C. A. (1990). Increasing resistance of *Staphylococcus aureus* to ciprofloxacin. *Antimicrob. Agents Chemother.* **34**, 1862–1863.

100. Schaefler, S. (1989). Methicillin-resistant strains of *Staphylococcus aureus* resistant to quinolones. *J. Clin. Microbiol.* **27**, 335–336.

101. Shalit, I., Berger, S. A., Gorea, A., and Frimerman, H. (1989). Widespread quinolone resistance among methicillin-resistant *Staphylococcus aureus* isolates in a general hospital. *Antimicrob. Agents Chemother.* **33**, 593–594.

102 Thornsberry, C. (1994). Susceptibility of clinical bacterial isolates to ciprofloxacin in the United States. *Infection* **22** (Suppl. 2), 80–89.

103. Aldridge, K. E., Gelfand, M. S., Schiro, D. D., and Barg, N. L. (1992). The rapid emergence of fluoroquinolone-methicillin-resistant *Staphylococcus aureus* infections in a community hospital: An in vitro look at alternative antimicrobial agents. *Diag. Microbiol. Infect. Dis.* **15**, 601–608.

104. Fass, R. J., Barnishan, J., and Ayers, L. W. (1995). Emergence of bacterial resistance to imipenem and ciprofloxacin in a university hospital. *J. Antimicrob. Chemother.* **36**, 343–353.

105. George, R. C., Ball, L. C., and Norbury, P. B. (1990). Susceptibility to ciprofloxacin of nosocomial gram-negative bacteria and staphylococci isolated in the UK. *J. Antimicrob. Chemother.* **26** (Suppl. F), 145–156.

106. Scheel, O., Lyon, D. J., Rosdahl, V. T., Adeyemi-Doro, F. A., Ling, T. K., and Cheng, A. F. (1996). In-vitro susceptibility of isolates of methicillin-resistant *Staphylococcus aureus* 1988–1993. *J. Antimicrob. Chemother.* **37**, 243–251.

107. Witte, W., Cuny, C., and Claus, H. (1993). Unrelatedness of multiply resistant *Staphylococcus aureus* with resistance to methicillin and to quinolones (QR-MRSA) as evident from SmaI-digestion patterns of genomic DNA. *Int. J. Med. Microbiol. Virol. Parasitol. Infect. Dis.* **278**, 510–517.

108. Sader, H. S., Pignatari, A. C., Hollis, R. J., Leme, I., and Jones, R. N. (1993). Oxacillin- and quinolone-resistant *Staphylococcus aureus* in Sao Paulo, Brazil: A multicenter molecular epidemiology study. *Infect. Control Hosp. Epidemiol.* **14**, 260–264.

109. Rohner, P., Herter, C., Auckenthaler, R., Pechère, J. C., Waldvogel, F. A., and Lew, D. P. (1989). Synergistic effect of quinolones and oxacillin on methicillin-resistant *Staphylococcus* species. *Antimicrob. Agents Chemother.* **33**, 2037–2041.

110. Schaberg, D. R., Dillon, W. I., Terpenning, M. S., Robinson, K. A., Bradley, S. F., and Kauffman, C. A. (1992). Increasing resistance of enterococci to ciprofloxacin. *Antimicrob. Agents Chemother.* **36**, 2533–2535.

111. Tankovic, J., Mahjoubi, F., Courvalin, P., Duval, J., and Leclerco, R. (1996). Development of fluoroquinolone resistance in *Enterococcus faecalis* and role of mutations in the DNA gyrase *gyrA* gene. *Antimicrob. Agents Chemother.* **40**, 2558–2561.

112. Yee, Y. C., Muder, R. R., Hsieh, M. H., and Lee, T. C. (1992). Molecular epidemiology of endemic ciprofloxacin-susceptible and -resistant Enterobacteriaceae. *Infect. Control Hosp. Epidemiol.* **13**, 706–710.

113. Turnidge, J. (1995). Epidemiology of quinolone resistance: Eastern hemisphere. *Drugs* **49** (Suppl. 2), 43–47.

114. Goldstein, F. W., and Acar, J. F. (1996). Antimicrobial resistance among lower respiratory tract isolates of *Streptococcus pneumoniae*: Results of a 1992-93 Western Europe and USA collaborative surveillance study (The Alexander Project Collaborative Group). *J. Antimicrob. Chemother.* **38** (Suppl. A), 71–84.

115. Spangler, S. K., Jacobs, M. R., Pankuch, G. A., and Appelbaum, P. C. (1993). Susceptibility of 170 penicillin-susceptible and penicillin-resistant pneumococci to six oral cephalosporins, four quinolones, desacetylcefotaxime, Ro 23-9424 and RP 67829. *J. Antimicrob. Chemother.* **31**, 273–280.

116. Chen, D. K., McGeer, A., de Azavedo, J. C., and Low, D. E. (1999). Decreased susceptibility of Streptococcus pneumoniae to fluoroquinolones in Canada. Canadian Bacterial Surveillance network. *New Engl. J. Med.* **22**, 233–239.

117. Suzuki, Y., Koguchi, M., Tanaka, S., Fukayama, S., Ishihara, R., Deguchi, K., Oda, S., Nakane, Y., and Fukumoto, T. (1995). Study of clinically isolated new quinolones-resistant *Haemophilus influenzae*, Part 1. *Jpn. J. Antibiot.* **48**, 1026–1032.

118. Doern, G. V. (1996). Antimicrobial resistance among lower respiratory tract isolates of *Haemophilus influenzae*: Results of a 1992-93 Western Europe and USA collaborative surveillance study (The Alexander Project Collaborative Group). *J. Antimicrob. Chemother.* **38** (Suppl. A), 59–69.

119. Felmingham, D., and Gruneberg, R. N. (1996). A multicentre collaborative study of the antimicrobial susceptibility of community-acquired, lower respiratory tract pathogens 1992-1993: The Alexander Project. *J. Antimicrob. Chemother.* **38** (Suppl. A), 1–57.

120. Berk, S. L., and Kalbfleisch, J. H. (1996). Antibiotic susceptibility patterns of community-acquired respiratory isolates of *Moraxella catarrhalis* in Western Europe and in the USA (The Alexander Project Collaborative Group). *J. Antimicrob. Chemother.* **38** (Suppl. A), 85–96.

121. Arai, S., Gohara, Y., Kuwano, K., and Kawashima, T. (1992). Antimycoplasmal activities of new quinolones, tetracyclines, and macrolides against *Mycoplasma pneumoniae*. *Antimicrob. Agents Chemother.* **36**, 1322–1324.

122. Kenny, G. E., and Cartwright, F. D. (1996). Susceptibilities of *Mycoplasma pneumoniae*, *Mycoplasma hominis*, and *Ureaplasma urealyticum* to a new quinolone, trovafloxacin (CP-99,219). *Antimicrob. Agents Chemother.* **40**, 1048–1049.

123. Renaudin, H., Tully, J. G., and Bebear, C. (1992). In vitro susceptibilities of *Mycoplasma genitalium* to antibiotics. *Antimicrob. Agents Chemother.* **36**, 870–872.

124. Bebear, C. M., Bove, J. M., Bebear, C., and Renaudin, J. (1997). Characterization of *Mycoplasma hominis* mutations involved in resistance to fluoroquinolones. *Antimicrob. Agents Chemother.* **41**, 269–273.

125. Gooding, B. B., Erwin, M. E., Barrett, M. S., Johnson, D. M., and Jones, R. N. (1992). Antimicrobial activities of two investigational fluoroquinolones (CI-960 and E4695) against over 100 *Legionella* spp. isolates. *Antimicrob. Agents Chemother.* **36**, 2049–2050.

126. Miyashita, N., Niki, Y., Kishimoto, T., Nakajima, M., and Matsushima, T. (1997). In vitro and in vivo activities of AM-1155, a new fluoroquinolone, against *Chlamydia* spp. *Antimicrob. Agents Chemother.* **41**, 1331–1334.

127. Kam, K. M., Lo, K. K., Ho, N. K., and Cheung, M. M. (1995). Rapid decline in penicillinase-producing *Neisseria gonorrhoeae* in Hong Kong associated with emerging 4-fluoroquinolone resistance. *Genitourin. Med.* **71**, 141–144.

128. Kam, K. M., Wong, P. W., Cheung, M. M., Ho, N. K. Y., and Lo, K. K. (1996). Quinolone-resistant *Neisseria gonorrhoeae* in Hong Kong. *Sex. Transm. Dis.* **23**, 103–108.

129. Bogaerts, J., Tello, W. M., Akingeneye, J., Mukantabana, V., Van Dyck, E., and Piot, P. (1993). Effectiveness of norfloxacin and ofloxacin for treatment of gonorrhoea and decrease of in vitro susceptibility to quinolones over time in Rwanda. *Genitourin. Med.* **69**, 196–200.

130. Knapp, J. S., Wongba, C., Limpakarnjanarat, K., Young, N. L., Parekh, M. C., Neal, S. W., Buatiang, A., Chitwarakorn, A., and Mastro, T. D. (1997). Antimicrobial susceptibilities of strains of *Neisseria gonorrhoeae* in Bangkok, Thailand: 1994–1995. *Sex. Transm. Dis.* **24**, 142–148.

131. Tapsall, J. W., Shultz, T. R., and Phillips, E. A. (1992). Characteristics of *Neisseria gonorrhoeae* isolated in Australia showing decreased sensitivity to quinolone antibiotics. *Pathology* **24**, 27–31.

132. Bauriaud, R., Seror, C., Lareng, M. B., and Lefevre, J. C. (1992). In vitro sensitivity to antibiotics of genital mycoplasmas isolated in Toulouse: Study of new molecules (macrolides and quinolones). *Pathol. Biol. (Paris)* **40**, 479–482.

133. Schachter, J., and Moncada, J. V. (1989). In vitro activity of ofloxacin against *Chlamydia trachomatis*. *Am. J. Med.* **87**, 14S–16S.

134. Aguiar, J. M., Chacon, J., Canton, R., and Baquero, F. (1992). The emergence of highly fluoroquinolone-resistant *Escherichia coli* in community-acquired urinary tract infections. *J. Antimicrob. Chemother.* **29**, 349–350.

135. Alos, J. I., Gomez-Garces, J. L., Garcia-Bermejo, I., Garcia-Gomez, J. J., Gonzalez-Palacios, R., and Padilla, B. (1993). The prevalence of *Escherichia coli* susceptibility to quinolones and other antibiotics in community-acquired bacteriurias in Madrid. *Med. Clin. (Barcelona)* **101**, 87–90.

136. Akalin, H. E. (1995). Role of quinolones in the treatment of diarrhoeal diseases. *Drugs* **49** (Suppl. 2), 128–131.

137. DuPont, H. L. (1991). Use of quinolones in the treatment of gastrointestinal infections. *Eur. J. Clin. Microbiol. Infect. Dis.* **10**, 325–329.

138. Rao, P. S., Rajashekar, V., Varghese, G. K., and Shivananda, P. G. (1993). Emergence of multidrug-resistant *Salmonella typhi* in rural southern India. *Am. J. Trop. Med. Hyg.* **48**, 108–111.

139. Yague, A., Royo, G., Satorres, J., Gonzalo, N., Martin, C., and Sevillano, A. (1993). Enteric fever caused by multiresistant *Salmonella typhi*: Two autochthonous cases. *Enferm. Infecc. Microbiol. Clin.* **11**, 199–201.

140. Frost, J. A., Kelleher, A., and Rowe, B. (1996). Increasing ciprofloxacin resistance in salmonellas in England and Wales 1991–1994. *J. Antimicrob. Chemother.* **37**, 85–91.

141. David, E., Andronescu, D., Serban, D., and Cocean, S. (1996). The sensitivity of *Salmonella* strains in diarrheal disease to new quinolones compared with other antimicrobial substances. *Bacteriol. Virusol. Parasitol. Epidemiol.* **41**, 43–46.

142. Hoge, C. W., Bodhidatta, L., Tungtaem, C., and Echeverria, P. (1995). Emergence of nalidixic acid resistant *Shigella dysenteriae* type 1 in Thailand: An outbreak associated with consumption of a coconut milk dessert. *Int. J. Epidemiol.* **24**, 1228–1232.

143. Horiuchi, S., Inagaki, Y., Yamamoto, N., Okamura, N., Imagawa, Y., and Nakaya, R. (1993). Reduced susceptibilities of *Shigella sonnei* strains isolated from patients with dysentery to fluoroquinolones. *Antimicrob. Agents Chemother.* **37**, 2486–2489.

144. Engels, D., Madaras, T., Nyandwi, S., and Murray, J. (1995). Epidemic dysentery caused by *Shigella dysenteriae* type 1: A sentinel site surveillance of antimicrobial resistance patterns in Burundi. *Bull. World Health Organ.* **73**, 787–791.

145. Segreti, J., Gootz, T. D., Goodman, L. J., Parkhurst, G. W., Quinn, J. P., Martin, B. A., and Trenholme, G. M. (1992). High-level quinolone resistance in clinical isolates of *Campylobacter jejuni*. *J. Infect. Dis.* **165**, 667–670.

146. Wretlind, B., Stromberg, A., Ostlund, L., Sjogren, E., and Kaijser, B. (1992). Rapid emergence of quinolone resistance in *Campylobacter jejuni* in patients treated with norfloxacin. *Scand. J. Infect. Dis.* **24**, 685–686.

147. Rautelin, H., Renkonen, O. V., and Kosunen, T. U. (1991). Emergence of fluoroquinolone resistance in *Campylobacter jejuni* and *Campylobacter coli* in subjects from Finland. *Antimicrob. Agents Chemother.* **35**, 2065–2069.

148. Takahashi, Y., Masuda, N., Otsuki, M., Miki, M., and Nishino, T. (1997). In vitro activity of HSR-903, a new quinolone. *Antimicrob. Agents Chemother.* **41**, 1326–1330.

149. Megraud, F. (1997). Resistance of *Helicobacter pylori* to antibiotics. *Aliment. Pharmacol. Ther.* **11** (Suppl. 1), 43–53.

150. Westblom, T. U., and Unge, P. (1992). Drug resistance of *Helicobacter pylori*: Memorandum from a meeting at the Sixth International Workshop on *Campylobacter*, *Helicobacter*, and Related Organisms [letter]. *J. Infect. Dis.* **165**, 974–975.

151. Kresken, M., Hafner, D., Mittermayer, H., Verbist, L., Bergogne-Berezin, E., Giamarellou, H., Esposito, S., van Klingeren, B., Kayser, F. H., and Reeves, D. S. (1994). Prevalence of fluoroquinolone resistance in Europe. Study Group "Bacterial Resistance" of the Paul-Ehrlich-Society for Chemotherapy e. V. *Infection* **22** (Suppl. 2), 90–98.

152. Pena, C., Albareda, J. M., Pallares, R., Pujol, M., Tubau, F., and Ariza, J. (1995). Relationship between quinolone use and emergence of ciprofloxacin-resistant *Escherichia coli* in bloodstream infections. *Antimicrob. Agents Chemother.* **39**, 520–524.

153. Weber, P., Plaisance, J. J., and Mancy, C. (1995). Comparative epidemiology of the resistance of enterobacteriaceae, *Staphylococcus* and *Pseudomonas aeruginosa* to fluoroquinolones in an outpatient study. *Presse Med.* **24**, 979–982.

154. Fish, D. N., Piscitelli, S. C., and Danziger, L. H. (1995). Development of resistance during antimicrobial therapy: A review of antibiotic classes and patient characteristics in 173 studies. *Pharmacotherapy* **15**, 279–291.

155. Ball, P. (1994). Bacterial resistance to fluoroquinolones: Lessons to be learned. *Infection* **22** (Suppl. 2), 140–147.

156. Carratala, J., Fernandez-Sevilla, A., Tubau, F., Callis, M., and Gudiol, F. (1995). Emergence of quinolone-resistant *Escherichia coli* bacteremia in neutropenic patients with cancer who have received prophylactic norfloxacin. *Clin. Infect. Dis.* **20**, 557–560 [discussion, 561-563].

157. Guibert, J., and Acar, J. F. (1986). Ofloxacin (RU 43280): Clinical evaluation in urinary and prostatic infections. *Pathol. Biol. (Paris)* **34**, 494–497.

158. Thomas, J. K., Forrest, A., Bhavnani, S. M., Hyatt, J. M., Cheng, A., Ballow, C. H., and Schentag, J. J. (1998). Pharmacodynamic evaluation of factors associated with the development of bacterial resistance in acutely ill patients during therapy. *Antimicrob. Agents Chemother.* **42**, 521–527

159. Baddour, L. M., Hicks, D. V., Tayidi, M. M., Roberts, S. K., Walker, E., Smith, R. J., Sweitzer, D. S., Herrington, J. A., and Painter, B. G. (1995). Risk factor assessment for the acquisition of fluoroquinolone-resistant isolates of *Pseudomonas aeruginosa* in a community-based hospital. *Microb. Drug Resist.* **1**, 219–222.

160. Muder, R. R., Brennen, C., Goetz, A. M., Wagener, M. M., and Rihs, J. D. (1991). Association with prior fluoroquinolone therapy of widespread ciprofloxacin resistance among Gram-negative isolates in a Veterans Affairs medical center. *Antimicrob. Agents Chemother.* **35**, 256–258.

161. Kern, W. V., Andriof, E., Oethinger, M., Kern, P., Hacker, J., and Marre, R. (1994). Emergence of fluoroquinolone-resistant *Escherichia coli* at a cancer center. *Antimicrob. Agents Chemother.* **38**, 681–687.

162. Stratton, C. W., Johnston, P. E., and Haas, D. W. (1994). Lack of correlation between the use of a specific fluoroquinolone and the emergence of fluoroquinolone-resistant isolates of *Pseudomonas aeruginosa*: A tale of two hospitals. *Antimicrob. Infect. Dis. Newsl.* **4**, 25–29.

163. Dalhoff, A. (1994). Quinolone resistance in *Pseudomonas aeruginosa* and *Staphylococcus aureus*: Development during therapy and clinical significance. *Infection* **22** (Suppl. 2), 111–121.

164. Schito, G. C., Acar, and J. F., Bauernfeind, A. (1996). A multinational European survey on the in-vitro activity of rufloxacin and other comparative antibiotics on respiratory and urinary bacterial pathogens. *J. Antimicrob. Chemother.* **38**, 627–639.

165. Gohara, Y., Arai, S., Kuwano, K., Kawashima, T., and Matsu-Ura, I. (1992). In vitro antimicrobial activities of new quinolone antibiotics against *Mycoplasma pneumoniae*. *Nippon Saikingaku Zasshi* **47**, 387–393.

166. Gransden, W. R., Warren, C., and Phillips, I. (1991). 4-Quinolone-resistant *Neisseria gonorrhoeae* in the United Kingdom. *J. Med. Microbiol.* **34**, 23–27.

167. Tauxe, R. V., Puhr, N. D., Wells, J. G., Hargrett-Bean, N., and Blake, P. A. (1990). Antimicrobial resistance of *Shigella* isolates in the USA: The importance of international travelers. *J. Infect. Dis.* **162**, 1107–1111.

CHAPTER 5

Pharmacokinetics and Pharmacodynamics of the Fluoroquinolones

MYO-KYOUNG KIM* and CHARLES H. NIGHTINGALE†

*Department of Pharmacy and Division of Infectious Disease, Hartford Hospital, Hartford, Connecticut 06102-5037, and †Office of Research Administration, Hartford Hospital, Hartford, Connecticut 06102-5037

The Quinolones, Third Edition

INTRODUCTION

The ultimate goal for the usage of fluoroquinolones is to eradicate bacterial pathogens at specific sites of infection, eventually leading to clinical success in the human body without causing adverse reactions. In order to accomplish this, an understanding of pharmacokinetic and pharmacodynamic concepts is crucial. In this chapter, the pharmacokinetic and pharmacodynamic characteristics of commonly utilized fluoroquinolones (ciprofloxacin, levofloxacin, trovafloxacin, moxifloxacin, and gatifloxacin) and gemifloxacin (a fluoroquinolone in clinical phase-development stages in the United States) are reviewed. Reviews for the less frequently used fluoroquinolones such as ofloxacin, sparfloxacin, clinafloxacin, pefloxacin, lomefloxacin, and enoxacin are not incorporated in this chapter. Usage of these fluoroquinolones has declined because of their toxicity profile and their failure to demonstrate expanded microbiological activity compared to other more commonly used fluoroquinolones [1]. (For information on these fluoroquinolones, refer to the second edition of this textbook.)

BASIC CONCEPTS OF PHARMACOKINETICS AND PHARMACODYNAMICS

Fluoroquinolones, like other antibiotics, should be administered to humans in order to reach and affect bacteria residing in the body. Maximal bactericidal effects are achieved when antibiotics, including fluoroquinolones, both arrive at and remain in tissues occupied by the pathogen. This usually results in successful clinical outcomes and is dependent on optimizing concentration and occupancy times of antibiotics in affected tissues without disturbing other noninfected mammalian tissues. Pharmacokinetic methods are commonly employed to illustrate the movement and existence of antibiotics in the body. Pharmacokinetics is defined as the study of the course of antibiotic movement through the body. This includes the processes involving administration of a drug through its elimination from the body.

However, even if an antibiotic reaches and remains in infected tissue, the agent cannot exert its activity against pathogens until it binds to critical sites within pathogens. The field of pharmacodynamics describes the relationship between pharmacokinetics and microbiology. Pharmacodynamics refers to the study of the relationship between drug concentration in the body and the pharmacological effect that the drug exerts on its target. A successful relationship usually culminates in the achievement of clinical efficacy. However, in the context of antibiotics, pharmacodynamics refers to the relationship between an antibiotic concentration in the body and the ability of the antibiotic to adversely affect the life-cycle of a bacterial pathogen.

Once antibiotics reach bacteria in the human body, the goal of therapy should be to kill bacteria completely and thus inhibit selection and stimulation of resistant organisms. To accomplish this goal, antibiotics should be capable of targeting key elements impacting pathogen survival. Specifically, antibiotics should be able to reach the site of infection, target binding sites in the bacteria (e.g., DNA gyrase and/or topoisomerase IV for fluoroquinolones), and inhibit protein synthesis [2,3]. If antibiotics cannot destroy bacteria completely, the surviving bacteria will be either selected and predominate the bacterial population or the surviving bacteria will be stimulated to express various resistance factors. To maximize efficacy and suppress resistance, antibiotics should occupy an adequate number of active sites and stay on the active sites for a sufficient period of time. Since fluoroquinolone interactions with receptors determine their efficacy, prudent utilization of these agents is contingent on characterization of their pharmacodynamic properties.

PHARMACOKINETICS

The pharmacokinetics of antibiotics is the study of antibiotic transit from administration site to specific infection site, and eventually to elimination. This process consists of three steps: absorption, distribution, and elimination. Pharmacokinetic properties are pivotal factors for selecting a judicious antibiotic and choosing an appropriate dosing regimen in order to maximize bacterial eradication and minimize resistance. Since an antibiotic exerts sufficient bactericidal activity only when it reaches and stays at infection sites, clinicians should be familiar not only with the drug's antibacterial activity, but also with its bioavailability, serum concentrations, tissue penetration, mechanism of metabolism and elimination, drug and food interactions, drug-and-drug interactions, drug-and-disease interaction, and other factors that can alter its pharmacokinetics. Moreover, with an understanding that various patient populations can influence half-life or clearance differently, clinicians will be able to select proper doses and dosing schedules needed to optimize antibiotic activity while keeping avoidable side effects and costs to a minimum. This section will address the pharmacokinetic properties of fluoroquinolones.

ABSORPTION

Absorption refers to the passage of drug from the drug's administration site in the body to the general circulation. Bioavailability (F), maximum concentration (C_{max}), and time to achieve maximal concentration (T_{max}) are useful parameters that describe drug absorption.

Bioavailability

The bioavailability (F) of a drug refers to the fraction of the administered dose that is absorbed into the bloodstream. Theoretically speaking, bioavailability is 100% after intravenous administration because the entire dose is infused into the systemic circulation. However, following oral administration of a drug, bioavailability ranges from 0% (no drug absorption) to 100% (complete drug absorption). The most common reason accounting for relatively low bioavailability of oral formulations is the so-called "first-pass effect." It occurs when a portion of an oral dose is biotransformed before it can enter the general circulation. Beermann et al. [4] suggested a possible first-pass effect for ciprofloxacin by demonstrating that the amount of parent compound recovered in the urine after an oral dose (42%) was smaller than that after intravenous administration (62%), while the amounts of metabolites recovered after an oral dose (12%) were larger than that after intravenous administration (9%). However, the first-pass effect for ciprofloxacin is clinically insignificant.

As shown in Table I [5–32], oral formulations of fluoroquinolones exhibit excellent bioavailability. For example, the bioavailability of ciprofloxacin has been reported to be 70–85% [5,18,19]. Because of the bioavailability of ciprofloxacin, a 500-mg capsule is substituted for a 400-mg intravenous dose, thus compensating for the drug's lower bioavailability. The bioavailability of ciprofloxacin has drawn much attention to fluoroquinolones since it was the first oral option for antipseudomonal treatment. Even more impressive bioavailabilities have been observed with other fluoroquinolones, including levofloxacin, moxifloxacin, and gatifloxacin. Their oral administration dose is comparable to their intravenous dose [6–9]. Therefore, the conversion ratio from intravenous dose to oral dose is 1:1. This outstanding feature enables these fluoroquinolones to target a market for treatment of community-acquired pneumonia since they also have good to excellent antimicrobial activity against most typical respiratory tract pathogens, including penicillin-resistant *Streptococcus pneumoniae* [8–10,14–16].

TABLE I Pharmacokinetic Parameters [5–32]

Drug	Dose (mg)	C_{max} (μg/ml)	T_{max} (hr)	Bioavail-ability (%)	V_d (l/kg)	Protein binding (%)	$T_{1/2}$ (hr)	AUC (μg·hr/ml)
Ciprofloxacin	500	2.4	1.2	70–85	2.1–2.5	35	3.0–5.0	11.6
Levofloxacin	500	5.5–6.2	1–2	99	1.09	24–38	7–8	47.7
Trovafloxacin	200	2.2–3.1	1.4	87.6	1.13	70	10–12	26.7
Moxifloxacin	400	3.1–4.5	1–2	86–92	1.84	30–50	12–13	31–48
Gatifloxacin	400	3.4–3.8	1–2	96–98	1.5–2.0	20	7–8	32.4
Gemifloxacin	320	1.0–1.5	0.5–2	~70	3.5	70	6–8	8.0–9.8

C_{max} = maximum drug concentration; T_{max} = time to reach peak concentration; V_d = volume of distribution, $T_{1/2}$ = half-life, AUC = area under the concentration–time curve.

Serum Concentrations

In general, serum concentrations reflect the presence of fluoroquinolones in the human body and generally is considered to be a good surrogate marker for the drug concentration to which the bacteria is exposed. The linearity between escalating doses and serum concentrations (especially C_{max} and AUC) has been well documented for most fluoroquinolones [5–19]. This linear relationship allows for serum concentrations to be predicted as a function of dose. For example, with ciprofloxacin, the C_{max} for each oral dose unit of 100 mg is projected to be about 0.5 μg/ml, and the AUC is approximately 2 μg·hr/ml. Using this rule, the C_{max} and AUC of a 500-mg dose is projected to be about 2.5 μg/ml and 10 μg·hr/ml, respectively [17,18].

Since fluoroquinolones eradicate bacteria through a concentration-dependent eradication relationship within the usual therapeutic dosing range, peak concentration and area under the curve (AUC) are important parameters to be considered. The AUC is used to describe the total amount of drug that reaches and is retained in the blood. In fact, AUC is simply the product of drug concentration and the time of antibiotic duration within the dosing interval (C_p × time). When fluoroquinolones are orally administered, they are rapidly absorbed from the gastrointestinal tract and achieve a C_{max} 1–2 hr following oral administration. Once the C_{max} is attained, the concentration curve of oral administration overlaps with that of intravenous administration. Therefore, for the newer fluoroquinolones, the AUCs of oral and intravenous formulations are similar [6–9,12–16,21].

The specific values for C_{max} and AUC of individual fluoroquinolones are listed in Table I. It is important to remember that these parameters do not necessarily indicate clinical significance. Aside from considering pharmacokinetic parameters such as AUC and C_{max}, clinicians should also examine the intrinsic antibacterial activity (i.e., MICs) of fluoroquinolones in order to evaluate their efficacy. This consideration will be further discussed in the section on "Pharmacodynamics" of this chapter.

DISTRIBUTION

Volume of Distribution

The volume of distribution (V_d) of a drug is defined as the theoretical body space available for its distribution. It is calculated by dividing the amount of drug administered by the peak plasma concentration. High values of V_d (>1 liter/kg) indicate extravascular penetration. As listed in Table I, the V_d values of fluoroquinolones are above 1 liter/kg, suggesting extensive distribution into tissue compartments. Fluoroquinolones are not highly protein bound. As shown in Table I, protein binding of commonly used fluoroquinolones ranges from about 20% for gatifloxacin to 70% for trovafloxacin. Relatively low protein binding may contribute to the high V_d observed in fluoroquinolones. However, since V_d is only a proportionality constant between the dose administered and the observed serum concentration, it is of limited use in predicting fluoroquinolone concentrations in specific tissue or fluid compartments. Therefore, one should consider tissue drug concentrations in determining antibiotic activity in certain tissue infections.

Extravascular Penetration: Fluid, Cellular, and Tissue Penetration

Fluoroquinolones achieve sufficient penetration into body fluids and tissues through passive diffusion across the capillary bed [33]. In the case of kidney penetration, active transport mechanisms also play a role. The extent of passive diffusion depends on lipid solubility, degree of ionization, and serum protein binding of individual antibiotics. High extravascular penetration has been shown for all the fluoroquinolones discussed in this chapter.

Penetration of antibiotics into inflammatory fluid is typically determined by measuring concentrations in skin blisters. The C_{max} and AUC in serum versus the

C_{max} and AUC in blister fluid are listed in Table II. The penetration rates into skin blisters for fluoroquinolones range from about 62% for moxifloxacin (p.o.) to 121% for ciprofloxacin [34–38]. This high penetration value represents good penetration of fluoroquinolones into inflammatory fluid.

Fluoroquinolones have been shown to achieve superior cellular penetration. For example, ciprofloxacin's concentration ratio of human neutrophils to serum concentrations is 4–7 [39,40]. Moxifloxacin's high intracellular concentration was indicated by a concentration ratio of leukocytes to extracellular levels of approximately 5 [41]. Pascual *et al.* [42] demonstrated that the cellular-to-extracellular concentration ratios of trovafloxacin reflected high concentrations of human neutrophils, human peritoneal macrophages, and tissue-cultured epithelial cells; they were 106, 92, and 96% of the serum concentration, respectively.

Fischman *et al.* [43] found that trovafloxacin reached peak concentrations greater than five times the MICs of most Enterobacteriaceae and anaerobes. Tissue concentrations of radiolabeled trovafloxacin were measured by positron emission tomography. In this study, the highest degree of penetration was found in the liver and lung. However, trovafloxacin was also well distributed into many other organs. In general, fluoroquinolones have been documented to penetrate well into various fluids and tissues, including bile, pancreatic juice, peritoneal fluid, pleural exudate, and empyema, aqueous humor, semen, human milk, joint fluid, liver, colon, bone tissue, muscle, fat, skin, and pharyngeal mucosa, cartilage, gall bladder wall, muscle, and skin [5–16,44–52]. Even though the extent of

TABLE II   Peak Concentrations and Areas under the Curve in Serum and Blister Fluid [34–38]

Drug	Dose (mg)	Serum		Blister fluid		Penetration rate (%)
		C_{max} (µg/ml)	AUC (µg·hr/ml)	C_{max} (µg/ml)	AUC (µg·hr/ml)	
Ciprofloxacin	100 i.v.	2.10	2.81	0.58	3.40	121
	500 p.o.	0.46	1.98	0.28	2.32	117
Levofloxacin	NR	NR	NR	NR	NR	94–104
Trovafloxacin	200 p.o.	2.9	24.4	1.2	15.3	63
Moxifloxacin	400 i.v.	3.7	22.9	1.7	16.7	73
	400 p.o.	3.2	19.8	1.6	12.3	62
Gatifloxacin	400 p.o.	4.1	31.4	3.6	36.9	117

NR = not reported.

penetration is different depending on the agent and tissue, favorable tissue penetration is a common feature of fluoroquinolones.

Drug Penetration into Respiratory Tract System

Fluoroquinolones achieve good penetration into respiratory tract tissues. High drug concentrations of bronchial mucosa, alveolar macrophage, and epithelial lining fluid indicate good penetration into the respiratory tract system. The concentrations of these individual agents are listed in Table III [53–59]. As shown in Table III, the ratio of bronchial mucosa to plasma concentration ranges from approximately 1 for trovafloxacin to around 15.6 for ciprofloxacin. In addition,

TABLE III   Penetration of Fluoroquinolones into Respiratory Tract Tissue and Fluid [53–59]

Drug	Sample time (hour)	Plasma concentration (µg/ml)	Lung concentration (mg/kg or mg/l) [mean site/serum ratio]		
			Bronchial mucosa	Alveolar macrophage	Epithelial lining fluid
Ciprofloxacin	2	1.39	21.63 [15.6]	ND	ND
	2.5	2.33	ND	5.4 [2.3]	2.1 [0.9]
	5	1.13	ND	7.6 [6.7]	BDL
	12	0.43	ND	3.8 [8.8]	BDL
Levofloxacin	2	4.9	6.5 [1.3]	41.9 [7.3]	9.0 [1.8]
	6–8	4.0	4.0 [1.0]	38.4 [9.6]	10.1 [2.7]
	12–24	1.2	BDL	13.9 [11.6]	BDL
Trovafloxacin	6	1.41	1.52 [1.07]	19.06 [13.32]	3.01 [2.27]
	12	0.85	1.01 [1.16]	16.22 [16.29]	4.81 [5.53]
	24	0.37	BDL	10.23 [22.55]	0.93 [2.16]
Moxifloxacin	2	3.22	5.36 [1.67]	56.7 [18.59]	20.7 [6.78]
	12	1.14	1.97 [1.74]	54.1 [44.61]	5.9 [5.19]
	24	0.51	1.06 [2.07]	35.9 [70.04]	3.57 [6.95]
Gatifloxacin	2	NR	NR [1.57]	NR [17.51]	NR [1.51]
	4	NR	NR [1.65]	NR [25.25]	NR [1.74]
	12	NR	BDL	NR [36.67]	NR [1.75]
Gemifloxacin	Steady state[a]	1.4	9.52 [7.2]	2.99 [2.6]	0.98 [0.7]

[a]Specific time not published. ND = not determined; BDL = below detection limit; NR = not reported.

the ratio of alveolar macrophage to plasma concentration ranges from about 2.3 (ciprofloxacin) to 70.0 (moxifloxacin). Lastly, the ratio of epithelial lining fluid ranges from around 0.9 (ciprofloxacin) to approximately 7.0 (moxifloxacin). The newer fluoroquinolones, including moxifloxacin, gatifloxacin, and gemifloxacin, achieve bronchial mucosa and epithelial lining fluid concentrations in excess of the MIC values of most common respiratory tract pathogens throughout substantial portions of their dosing intervals [57–59].

Fluoroquinolones have also shown impressive penetration into sputum and nasal tissue. In sputum collected from chronic bronchitis patients, ciprofloxacin concentrations ranged from 1 to 2.3 μg/ml, with corresponding serum concentrations of 2–3 μg/ml [60]. In sputum from cystic fibrosis patients, ciprofloxacin concentrations are similar to or greater than that of serum 2–12 hr after the dose. Also, the sputum AUC of ciprofloxacin is four times that of the serum [61,62]. With ciprofloxacin, serum and nasal secretion AUC and $T_{1/2}$ are comparable [63,64]. In a study that attempted to demonstrate good sinus penetration by moxifloxacin, Gehanno et al. [65] measured sinus concentrations of moxifloxacin in 34 chronic sinusitis patients who received 400-mg q-24 hr for three doses orally. They found that levels in maxillary sinus mucosa, anterior ethmoid mucosa, and nasal polyp tissue were higher than those in plasma. Therefore, the good penetration of fluoroquinolones into various respiratory tract tissues and fluid supports one of several rationales for their utilization in respiratory tract infections.

Drug Penetration into Urinary Tract System and Reproductive System

Good tissue penetration of fluoroquinolones into kidney, prostate tissue, and gynecologic tissue is well documented [5–16,66–77]. This characteristic offers one justification for the use of fluoroquinolones in the treatment of urinary tract or gynecologic infections. After low doses (e.g., oral doses of 100 mg), urine levels of ciprofloxacin have been demonstrated to remain above the required MICs of common urinary pathogens [5,11]. This feature is also characteristic of newer fluoroquinolones, including levofloxacin and moxifloxacin [12–16]. Although only 6–10% of an oral trovafloxacin dose is excreted unchanged in the urine, mean urinary trovafloxacin concentrations 12 and 24 hr after administration of a single 100-mg dose are higher than the MIC_{90} for most urinary pathogens [23,78]. With respect to prostatic tissue, Dan et al. [72] established the mean ratio of tissue to serum concentration to be 0.93. With gynecologic tissue, Martens et al. [79] found that trovafloxacin concentrations in the ovary were approximately 60–100% higher than those in the serum of women undergoing elective hysterectomy. Trovafloxacin tissue concentrations of the myometrium, uterus, fallopian tubes, and cervix were 50–70% of serum levels.

Drug Penetration into Central Nervous System

To date, no fluoroquinolones are FDA approved for the treatment of bacterial meningitis. However, since fluoroquinolones achieve good penetration into cerebrospinal fluid (CSF), there exists a potential for the development of fluoroquinolones for this indication. Currently, acceptable empiric therapy for bacterial meningitis includes the combination of vancomycin and third-generation cephalosporins because of a high prevalence of penicillin-resistant *Streptococcus pneumoniae* [80]. However, effective monotherapy with a long dosing interval is preferred over combination therapy. Also, the penetration rate of vancomycin into the CNS is only 20–30% even with inflamed meninges [81]. For commonly used fluoroquinolones, as shown in Table IV [80,82–90], the fraction of CSF penetration into noninflamed meninges ranges from 5–10% (ciprofloxacin) to 25% (trovafloxacin) of serum concentrations. Moreover, CNS penetration into inflamed meninges is much higher than that of noninflamed meninges. It ranges from 20–40% with gatifloxacin to 50–80% with moxifloxacin. Along with this high degree of CNS penetration, newer fluoroquinolones such as moxifloxacin and gatifloxacin provide sufficient bactericidal activity against most common meningitis pathogens including penicillin-resistant *S. pneumoniae* [14–16]. Lutsar *et al.* [80] employed a rabbit meningitis model to prove that gatifloxacin was effective in the treatment of cephalosporin-resistant pneumococcal meningitis. Interestingly, Iwamoto *et al.* [91] found a drug interaction between fenbufen and some fluoroquinolones, including ciprofloxacin. They demonstrated that fenbufen

TABLE IV   Percentage CSF Penetration [80,82–90]

Drug	Without inflamed meninges	With inflamed meninges
Ciprofloxacin	5–10%	14–26%
Levofloxacin	16%	61%
Trovafloxacin	25%	20–40%
Moxifloxacin	10%	50–80%
Gatifloxacin	ND	20–40%

ND = not determined.

decreased elimination of fluoroquinolones from CSF. However, good CNS penetration is not always advantageous because such drugs may elicit CNS adverse effects in patients with infections outside the CNS. Cutler *et al.* [86] performed a healthy volunteer study in which trovafloxacin, an agent with good CNS penetration, caused a high incidence of CNS side effects, including dizziness (50%), headache (25%), and hypesthesia (17%). All other fluoroquinolones have been associated with CNS toxicity to some extent.

ELIMINATION

Most fluoroquinolones are eliminated primarily by hepatic elimination (metabolism or biotransformation) and renal excretion. Transintestinal elimination is an alternative mode of elimination. As listed in Table V [5–9,44,92–99], approximately half of the doses of ciprofloxacin and trovafloxacin are cleared by this route. However, transintestinal elimination is not an important factor to consider in clinical practice. Instead, renal or hepatic elimination of each agent should be taken into consideration because such information will enable clinicians to tailor the dosage regimen for their patients. The percentages of the dose that are recovered in the urine as parent compound and metabolites for the commonly used fluoroquinolones are listed in Table V.

Ciprofloxacin, levofloxacin, gatifloxacin, and gemifloxacin are highly dependent on renal elimination. Glomerular filtration and active tubular secretion represent major renal excretion pathways. Renal elimination of ciprofloxacin, levofloxacin, and gatifloxacin has been demonstrated to be blocked by probenecid, a competitor for renal secretion [48,100]. In contrast, fluoroquinolones such as moxifloxacin, which are not significantly dependent on renal elimination,

TABLE V   Elimination of Fluoroquinolones (% of dose) [5–9,44,92–99]

Drug	Urine parent compound	Urine metabolites	Feces
Ciprofloxacin			
p.o.	30–45	12–22	~50
i.v.	57–62	9–24	15–20
Levofloxacin	80–90	5	<4
Trovafloxacin	6–7	17	51–63
Moxifloxacin	15–21	10	25
Gatifloxacin	79–88	<0.1	6

do not have significant drug interactions with probenecid. As shown in Table VI [5–10,102–105], with renally eliminated fluoroquinolones, the half-life and AUC in patients with reduced renal function are significantly greater than that in subjects with normal renal functions. Therefore, these agents should be dose adjusted for renal function.

Unlike renally eliminated fluoroquinolones, trovafloxacin primarily relies on hepatic elimination (Table V). Dalvie *et al.* [44] demonstrated that trovafloxacin is metabolized primarily in the liver by glucuronidation, *N*-acetylation, and *N*-sulfoconjugation (phase II hepatic metabolism). They also showed that hepatobiliary excretion is the primary route of elimination. As shown in Table VII [5–10,31,106–108], the half-life and AUC of trovafloxacin in patients with reduced liver function are significantly higher compared to healthy subjects, while the difference in half-life and AUC of other fluoroquinolones between these two populations is not significant (below 25% of difference). Table VIII [11–16,109] lists metabolites of each fluoroquinolone discussed in this chapter. While moxifloxacin is partially eliminated via metabolism, this does not occur via oxidative processes. Therefore, the usual drug interactions with other compounds, most of which occur by competitive inhibition of oxidative metabolism, do not occur with moxifloxacin.

Prolonged half-life is another significant characteristic of the newer-generation fluoroquinolones. As listed in Table I, the half-lives of levofloxacin, trovafloxacin, moxifloxacin, gatifloxacin, and gemifloxacin in healthy subjects are in the range of 8–12 hr [5–16]. Because of their long half-lives, these fluoroquinolones can be administered once daily. However, long half-life is not always beneficial. It would

TABLE VI   Comparison of Half-Life and AUC in Humans with Normal Renal Function and with Reduced Renal Function [5–10,102–105]

Drug	Normal renal function (NRF)		Reduced renal function (RRF)		Dose adjust-ment
	$T_{1/2}$ (hr)	AUC (μg·hr/ml)	$T_{1/2}$ (hr) [RRF-to-NRF ratio]	AUC (μg·hr/ml) [RRF-to-NRF ratio]	
Ciprofloxacin	3.5–4.3	9.8–15.6	7.1–6.3 [1.6–1.8]	20.2–26.8 [1.7–2.1]	Yes
Levofloxacin	7–8	48	9–76 [1.1–10.8]	90–264 [1.8–5.5]	Yes
Trovafloxacin	10–12	NA	12–15 [1.0–1.5]	NA	No
Moxifloxacin	12–13	31–48	15–16 [1.2–1.3]	36–44 [≈1.0]	No
Gatifloxacin	NR	NR	NR	NR [1.2]	Yes
Gemifloxacin	NR	NR	NR [7–10]	NR [1.7–2.4]	Yes

NA = not available; NR = not reported.

TABLE VII   Comparison of Half-Life and AUC in Humans with Normal Hepatic Function and with Reduced Liver Function [5–10,31,106–108]

Quinolones	Normal liver function (NLF)		Reduced liver function (RLF)		Dose adjust-ment
	$T_{1/2}$ (hr)	AUC (μg·hr/ml)	$T_{1/2}$ (hr) [RLF-to-NLF ratio]	AUC (μg·hr/ml) [RLF-to-NLF ratio]	
Ciprofloxacin	3.5–4.2	16–19	3.7 [≈1.0]	18–21 [≈1.0]	No
Levofloxacin	ND (No changes expected due to negligible hepatic elimination)				No
Trovafloxacin	10–12	12.6	18.2 [1.5–1.8]	47.3 [3.8]	Yes
Moxifloxacin	NR	NR	NR [≈1.0]	NR [23]	No
Gatifloxacin	9.3	37.4	8.9 [≈1.0]	46.2 [1.2]	No
Gemifloxacin	8.0	6.9	8.4–9.2 [1.0–1.2]	9.1–10.2 [1.3–1.5]	No

ND = not determined; NR = not reported.

TABLE VIII   Metabolites of Fluoroquinolones [11–16,109]

Metabolites	Ciprofloxacin	Levofloxacin	Trovafloxacin	Maxifloxacin	Gatifloxacin
Oxo	+				Negligible
N-formyl	+				metabolism
N-sulphonyl	+			+	"
N-acetyl			+		"
N-sulfate			+		"
Desethylenyl	+				"
Glucoronide	+	+	+	+	"

be disadvantageous in patients who develop adverse reactions to the drug. Unlike other newer fluoroquinolones, ciprofloxacin should be administered twice daily due to its relatively short half-life (3–5 hr). As shown in Table I, the half-lives of individual fluoroquinolones display considerable within-study and between-study variation.

SPECIAL POPULATION

The pharmacokinetic parameters of the fluoroquinolones do not depend on gender [5–16,110–112]. Studies performed on the geriatric population demonstrated that advanced age is associated with higher C_{max} and AUC values and slightly reduced total, renal, and nonrenal clearance; this difference is clinically negligible [5–16,111–113]. Drugs such as levofloxacin and gatifloxacin, which are primarily eliminated renally, are more affected by patient age because of the natural decrease in renal function as a function of age. In the pediatric population, pharmacokinetic studies are limited due to the concern for its potential toxicity (arthropathy) in this group. However, Kearns *et al.* [114] performed a study with 14 children and 6 infants in which they examined the tolerability and pharmacokinetics of trovafloxacin (4.0 mg/kg). They demonstrated that all subjects tolerated trovafloxacin well, with no changes in vital signs or laboratory values of renal, hematologic, or hepatic function. They also showed that the pharmacokinetic profile of trovafloxacin in pediatric patients is not significantly different from that in healthy adults.

Disease status may exert some influence on the pharmacokinetic profile of an agent. For example, in addition to exhibiting a high degree of variability, the total clearance of ciprofloxacin in burn patients is generally higher than that anticipated on the basis of renal function [115]. At the present time, no clinically significant change caused by disease status has been documented [116–122]. Grasela *et al.* [116] demonstrated that the pharmacokinetic profile of gatifloxacin was similar in healthy subjects and in patients with acute exacerbation of chronic bronchitis. Cystic fibrosis does not affect the pharmacokinetic profile of ciprofloxacin [117–120]. Acquired immunodeficiency syndrome (AIDS) also does not seem to influence the pharmacokinetics of ciprofloxacin or trovafloxacin [121,122].

DRUG INTERACTIONS

Drug–Food Interaction

The oral absorption of some fluoroquinolones is delayed by the presence of food in the gastrointestinal tract. Thus, peak serum concentrations tend to be somewhat lower and the time to achieve peak concentrations is slightly delayed; this effect is clinically insignificant [123,133,141,142,151,158]. None of the fluoroquinolones listed in Table IX [100,123–165] are significantly affected by food. In contrast, the bioavailability and AUC of ciprofloxacin are significantly affected by administration of dairy products; however, with the addition of high-fat food, these parameters are less affected by dairy products [100]. Interestingly, while coadministered dairy products delay the T_{max} of moxifloxacin, the AUC is unaffected. Since absorption of all fluoroquinolones is inhibited by divalent cations (refer to the section on "Drug–Drug Interactions"), coadministration of high-cation-content food products (especially Ca^{2+}- or Fe^{2+}-supplemented food,

TABLE IX   Food Interactions and Drug Interactions [100,123–165]

Food or agents	Cipro-floxacin	Levo-floxacin	Trova-floxacin	Moxi-floxacin	Gati-floxacin	Gami-floxacin
Food	No ($\uparrow$T$_{max}$)	No ($\uparrow$T$_{max}$)	No ($\uparrow$T$_{max}$)	No ($\uparrow$T$_{max}$)	No	No
Dairy prods.	$\downarrow$F, $\downarrow$AUC	–	–	No ($\uparrow$T$_{max}$)	No	–
Antacid	$\downarrow$F, $\downarrow$AUC	$\downarrow$F, $\downarrow$AUC	$\downarrow$F, $\downarrow$AUC	$\downarrow$F, $\downarrow$AUC	$\downarrow$F, $\downarrow$AUC	$\downarrow$F, $\downarrow$AUC
Ca^{2+} suppls.	$\downarrow$F, $\downarrow$AUC	$\downarrow$F, $\downarrow$AUC	No ($\downarrow$F)	$\downarrow$F	–	–
Iron prep.	$\downarrow$F, $\downarrow$AUC	$\downarrow$F, $\downarrow$AUC	$\downarrow$F, $\downarrow$AUC	$\downarrow$F	$\downarrow$AUC	$\downarrow$F, $\downarrow$AUC
Sucralfate	$\downarrow$F, $\downarrow$AUC	$\downarrow$F, $\downarrow$AUC	$\downarrow$AUC	$\downarrow$F	–	$\downarrow$F, $\downarrow$AUC
Cimetidine	No	No ($\uparrow$T$_{1/2}$)	No	–	No	–
Ranitidine	No	No	–	No	–	–
Omeprazole	–	–	No	–	–	No
N-butylsco-polamine	No ($\downarrow$F)	–	–	–	–	–
Metoclo-pramide	No ($\downarrow$T$_{max}$)	–	–	–	–	–
Probenecid	$\uparrow$AUC, $\uparrow$T$_{1/2}$	No ($\uparrow$T$_{1/2}$)	–	No	$\uparrow$AUC, $\uparrow$T$_{1/2}$	–
Digoxin	–	No	No	No	No	No
Warfarin	$\uparrow$INR	No	No	No	No	No
Glyburide	$\uparrow$hypoglycemia	–	–	–	No	–
Midazolam	–	–	–	–	No	–
Oral contr.	–	–	–	No	–	–
Caffeine	$\uparrow$caffeine	–	No	–	–	–
Theophylline	$\uparrow$AUC	No	No	No	No	No
Morphine	–	–	$\downarrow$AUC	–	–	–
NSAIDs	No	–	No	–	–	–
Phenytoin	$\uparrow$/$\downarrow$phenytoin	–	–	–	–	–
Cyclosporine	No	No	No	–	–	–

No = no clinically significant interaction; F = bioavailability; AUC = area under the curve; T$_{1/2}$ = half-life; T$_{max}$ = time to achieve peak concentration; – = information not available.

or enteral tubing formula) with fluoroquinolones should be avoided to promote reliable administration.

Drug–Drug Interactions

As shown in Table IX [100,123–165], the absorption of all oral fluoroquinolones are affected by di- or trivalent-cation- (Mg^{2+}-, Al^{3+}-, or Ca^{2+}-) containing agents such as antacids, calcium, and iron supplements and sucralfate. The mechanism of this interaction probably arises from the formation of poorly absorbed chelated products consisting of fluoroquinolone molecules and metal cations [132,159].

However, bismuth-based antacids such as bismuth subsalicylate have been demonstrated to have no effect on ciprofloxacin absorption [165]. In order to avoid the interaction between these cation-containing agents and fluoroquinolones, the fluoroquinolones should be administered at least 4 hr before or 8 hr after cation-containing agents [5–10,100,164].

In general, no significant interaction between H_2 blockers and proton pump inhibitors and the commonly used fluoroquinolones has been documented [134,140,148,160]. However, as indicated in Table IX, ciprofloxacin, levofloxacin, trovafloxacin, and gatifloxacin have been documented to interact negligibly with cimetidine, which inhibits the cytochrome P450 enzyme system as well as inducing gastric pH changes [5–9,11–16,140]. Ciprofloxacin, levofloxacin, and moxifloxacin do not interact significantly with ranitidine [5,6,9,11,12,14,148]. Moreover, trovafloxacin and gemifloxacin do not interact with omeprazole [134,160].

N-butylscopolamine bromide prolongs stomach emptying time, thus reducing ciprofloxacin absorption. While this reduction achieves statistical significance, in clinical practice this feature is of minimal importance. Metoclopramide accelerates intestinal peristalsis, leading to decreased T_{max} following concomitant ciprofloxacin administration. However, the C_{max}, AUC, and $T_{1/2}$ of ciprofloxacin are not significantly changed by coadministration with metoclopramide [126]. Since opiates decrease gastrointestinal movement, they are postulated to reduce oral fluoroquinolone absorption. The AUC of trovafloxacin was diminished by morphine, while the pharmacokinetic profile of ciprofloxacin was unchanged [100].

Addition of ciprofloxacin to theophylline or caffeine may increase the concentration of the two agents, resulting in CNS toxicity [127,128]. However, newer fluoroquinolones have not been shown to interact with theophylline or caffeine [136,138,146,155,157,162] (Table IX). Aside from interacting with theophylline and caffeine, ciprofloxacin has been reported to interact with warfarin and glyburide [100]. However, levofloxacin, trovafloxacin, moxifloxacin, gatifloxacin, and gemifloxacin have not been shown to interact with digoxin, warfarin, and glyburide [100,137,147,149,152,153,161,163] (Table IX). The addition of such fluoroquinolones as ciprofloxacin, levofloxacin and trovafloxacin to cyclosporine has been reported to exert no effect on the pharmacokinetic profile of cyclosporine [100]. Coadministration of probenecid with an agent, which is cleared by renal secretion, increases the AUC of this agent. For example, the addition of probenecid to ciprofloxacin increases the AUC of ciprofloxacin. However, the addition of probenecid to trovafloxacin did not affect the pharmacokinetic profiles of these agents because the clearance of these agents is not dependent on renal secretion. No significant pharmacokinetic interactions between fluoroquinolones and β-lactam antibiotics or aminoglycosides have been documented [5–16,100]. Other published interactions are listed in Table IX.

PHARMACODYNAMICS

As mentioned earlier, the pharmacodynamics of antibiotics comprises the study of the relationship between the drug's microbiological properties and its pharmacokinetics. Bacterial time–kill curves, the drug's pharmacokinetic properties in various biological fluids and the post-antibiotic effect, usually characterize pharmacodynamics.

BACTERICIDAL ACTIVITY: TIME–KILL CURVES

In order to measure bactericidal activity, the minimum bactericidal concentration (MBC) to the minimum inhibitory concentration (MIC) ratio is utilized. When this ratio is less than or equal to 2, an antibiotic generally exhibits bactericidal activity. However, no definitive information on this correlation has been published. As opposed to the MBC-to-MIC ratio, a time–kill curve provides more specific information on antibiotic activity. As a commonly employed procedure for creating time–kill curves involves adding an antibiotic (0.5–10 times MIC) to a media containing a test pathogen (approximately 5×10^7 colony-forming units/ml). The added antibiotic can be in constant concentration (static) or in changing concentration as a function of time (dynamic), simulating the drug's pharmacokinetics in the human body. Next, the changes in colony-forming units (cfus) versus time are observed [166]. Since bactericidal activity is defined as the killing of 99.9–99.99% of a pathogen's colonies, a $2–3 \log_{10}$ decrease in cfu/ml in a time–kill curve reflects the bactericidal activity of a specific antibiotic against a tested pathogen. In addition, the time–kill curve provides information on the minimal time required for an antibiotic to achieve 99.9–99.99% eradication.

In general, fluoroquinolones have bactericidal activity against most common pathogens. For example, through MBC testing, ciprofloxacin has been demonstrated to have rapid bactericidal activity within two dilutions of the MIC against most Gram-negative and Gram-positive aerobes. However, it does not achieve bactericidal activity against *P. aeruginosa*, *Proteus* spp., and *Staphylococcus* spp. [167,168]. Newer fluoroquinolones such as moxifloxacin and gatifloxacin have also been shown to have bactericidal activity against most Gram-negative and Gram-positive aerobes [169–173]. In contrast to ciprofloxacin, some of the newer agents (moxifloxacin and gatifloxacin) have superior bactericidal activity against Gram-positive pathogens, including *S. aureus* and *S. pneumoniae*. This bactericidal activity has been confirmed by low MBC-to-MIC ratios and also by time–kill studies [8,9,14–16]. In a time–kill study performed by Boswell *et al.* [171], moxifloxacin was shown to kill *S. aureus* and *S. pneumoniae* within 2.5 and 3.5 hr, respectively. Hosaka *et al.* [172] also demonstrated that gatifloxacin killed more than 99% of *S. aureus* within 1 to 2 hr. Moreover, Hoellman *et al.* [173] showed that gatifloxacin achieved a 99.9% bacterial killing effect against *S. pneumoniae* within 24 hr regardless of penicillin-sensitivity for tested isolates.

Pharmacodynamic Surrogate Markers and Clinical Outcome

In the arena of microbiology and antibiotics, pharmacodynamics is the study of the relationship between drug concentrations in the body and bactericidal activity. Drug concentrations in the body are in most studies represented by serum concentrations. Likewise, antibiotic efficacy is usually reported as minimum inhibitory concentrations (MICs). Even though minimum bactericidal concentrations (MBCs) and serum bactericidal titers (SBTs) are also adopted to describe a specific antibiotic killing efficacy, determination of these factors requires more resources, as opposed to determining an antibiotic's MIC against a particular pathogen.

Therefore, a commonly used pharmacodynamic parameter is the drug's serum or plasma concentration indexed to the microbiological properties of the drug against the pathogen. In such a case, the serum or plasma is accepted as a surrogate marker for the drug concentration surrounding the bacteria. When such a surrogate is used, three parameters—peak concentration to MIC ratio (C_{max}/MIC), area under the curve to MIC ratio (AUC/MIC), and time above MIC (T>MIC)—are commonly employed. As shown in Figure 1, T>MIC refers to the duration of time when drug concentrations are above the MIC. In general, a T>MIC greater than or equal to 50–70% is a reliable predictor for the efficacy of time-dependent antibiotics such as penicillins and macrolides in hosts with normal immunological defenses. C_{max}/MIC refers to the ratio of maximum concentration versus MIC and is not reflected by the dwelling time of the antibiotic in the body. C_{max}/MIC is useful for indicating the bactericidal efficacy of concentration-dependent antibiotics such as aminoglycosides and fluoroquinolones. If C_{max}/MIC is greater than 10, there is a high probability of successful antibiotic treatment, and the emergence of resistance bacteria is minimized. Drusano *et al.* [174] performed a study using a neutropenic rat model treated with lomefloxacin, which showed that C_{max}/MIC was significantly correlated to survival, especially with high ratios (10/1 to 20/1).

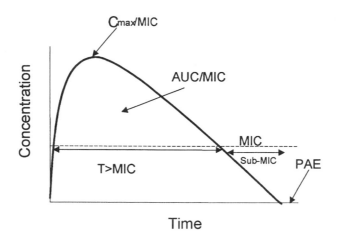

FIGURE 1 Pharmacodynamic surrogate markers.

However, when toxicity prevents acquisition of high C_{max}/MIC values, time factors should be considered as well as peak concentrations. The fluoroquinolone group is a prototype of this scenario. Since AUC incorporates time and concentration factors, the AUC/MIC ratio is the most commonly adopted parameter used to describe fluoroquinolone efficacy. In a pharmacodynamic study of intravenous ciprofloxacin in seriously ill patients, Forrest *et al.* demonstrated that values ranging from 125 to 250 for the AUC/MIC represented significant breakpoints in the time-to-bacterial eradication [175]. This ratio is believed to be of importance for the treatment of infections caused by Gram-negative pathogens. However, AUC/MICs greater than 30 are correlated with antibiotic success for Gram-positive organisms, especially for *Streptococcus pneumoniae*. Lacy *et al.* demonstrated that sustained bactericidal activity against *Streptococcus pneumoniae* occurred when AUC/MIC ranged from 30 to 55 [176].

AUC/MIC also may predict bacterial resistance to fluoroquinolones. Forrest *et al.* [175] demonstrated that resistance to ciprofloxacin developed in patients with nosocomial pneumonia when AUC/MIC were less than 100. Thomas *et al.* [177] supported this by demonstrating an increased probability of resistance during antibiotic therapy with AUC/MICs of <100 in 107 acutely ill patients with nosocomial lower-respiratory tract infection caused by mainly Gram-negative organisms. However, resistance is less likely to occur with AUC/MIC ≥100. Thus, the emergence of resistance with an AUC/MIC <125 validates the likelihood of attaining successful bactericidal activity with AUC/MICs ≥125.

The calculated C_{max}/MIC and AUC/MIC for each fluoroquinolone against *S. pneumoniae* are listed in Table X [5–16,178]. As shown in Table X, C_{max}/MIC ratios for newer fluoroquinolones, including moxifloxacin, gatifloxacin, and gemifloxacin, are higher than those for ciprofloxacin and levofloxacin. In addition, unlike ciprofloxacin, the AUC/MIC ratios of newer fluoroquinolones are substantially greater than 30. For levofloxacin, AUC/MIC varies depending on pathogen MIC. It could be greater than 30 when the MIC of *S. pneumoniae* is 1; the opposite is true when the MIC of *S. pneumoniae* is 2. Finally, it should be kept in mind that these pharmacodynamic surrogate markers are only able to predict the *potential* for bacterial eradication. They usually correlate with clinical cures, but not always. Successful therapy of a patient involves not only drug–bacteria interactions, but other factors such as the pathogenicity of the organism, inoculum size, and the status of the immune system, which is a function of the genetic makeup of the patient, his or her age, and even psychological factors. Clinical outcomes should be confirmed by well-designed clinical studies.

POST-ANTIBIOTIC EFFECTS

The term "post-antibiotic effect" (PAE) refers to persistent suppression of bacterial growth after limited exposure to an antibiotic. The PAE is calculated by the following equation:

$$PAE = T - C,$$

where T is the time required for the cfu count in a test culture to increase $1 \log_{10}$ above the count observed immediately after drug removal, and C is the time needed for the cfu count in an untreated control culture to increase $1 \log_{10}$ above

TABLE X   Calculated Pharmacodynamic Surrogate Markers against *Streptococcus pneumoniae* [5–16,178]

	Dose (mg)	C_{max} (μg/ml)	AUC$_{0-24}$ (μg·hr/ml)	MIC of S. pneu- moniae	C_{max}/ MIC	AUC$_{0-24}$/ MIC
Ciprofloxacin	500	2.4	23.2	2	1.2	11.6
Levofloxacin	500	5.5–6.2	47.7	1–2	2.75–6.2	11.9–47.7
Trovafloxacin	200	2.2–3.1	26.7	0.12–0.25	8.8–25.8	106.8–213.6
Moxifloxacin	400	3.1–4.5	31–48	0.25	12.4–18.0	124–192
Gatifloxacin	400	3.4–3.8	32.4	0.5	6.8–7.6	64.8
Gemifloxacin	320	1.0–1.5	8.0–9.8	0.015–0.03	33.3–100	267–653.3

the count observed immediately after the same procedure used on the test culture for drug removal. Drug removal is performed through dilution, drug inactivation, washing, or filtration. The longer the PAE duration, the less likely that bacterial regrowth will occur during periods of inadequate antibiotic concentrations. The extent of the PAE helps determine the dosing regimen design [179].

The precise mechanism of the PAE for fluoroquinolones is unknown, but it has been attributed to consistent inhibition of DNA replication [181]. Fluoroquinolones have a long-duration PAE, which is a typical characteristic of bactericidal concentration-dependent antibiotics. PAE values of individual fluoroquinolones are listed in Table XI [5–16,182–191]. The PAE of each agent varies greatly depending on the type and MIC of pathogens, inoculum size, drug concentration tested, and other factors, including the growth phase of the organism at the time of exposure, mechanical shaking of the culture, medium type, pH, and medium temperature [166]. The durations of PAE in Table XI were compiled from different studies with different factors influencing PAE duration. Therefore, one cannot make direct comparisons of a number or a range of numbers in each cell. Also, the range of each cell is derived from different drug concentrations or other environmental factors.

Unfortunately, there are drawbacks to measuring PAE duration. One considerable limitation is that bacteria are exposed only once to a fixed concentration of a testing antimicrobial agent for a short period of time. In contrast, in a clinical setting antimicrobial agents are used multiple times. Moreover, the concentrations should remain above the MIC for a relatively longer time than the antibiotic exposure period for PAE testing. Also, the concentration should diminish continuously throughout the dosing interval. These facts suggest that conventional testing may overestimate the PAE as opposed to the PAE in a clinical situation where concentrations are continuously changing.

The other impediment to applying *in vitro* PAE to clinical practice is that host immunity is not considered when the PAE is determined. However, other terminology such as post-antibiotic leukocyte enhancement (PALE) and post-antibiotic sub-MIC effect (PASME) are sometimes utilized to account for host immunity. PALE refers to a phenomenon by which pathogens in the PAE phase are more susceptible to the antibacterial effect of human leukocytes than non-PAE controls. The post-antibiotic sub-MIC effect is reflected by combination of the PAE and the additive effects of exposure to sub-MIC levels [179,180]. In Table XI, the values for sub-MIC effect (SME) and post-antibiotic sub-MIC effect (PASME) of moxifloxacin and gatifloxacin are listed, as well as that for the PAE. The SME is defined as the effect of subinhibitory concentrations of an agent on a strain not previously exposed to the agent. The definition of the PASME is the effect of subinhibitory concentrations of an agent on a strain previously exposed to the agent at concentration greater than MIC. As shown in Table XI, the values

TABLE XI Post-Antibiotic Effects (PAE), Sub-MIC Effects (SME), and Post-Antibiotic Sub-MIC Effects (PASME) [5–16,182–191]

Pathogens	Ciprofloxacin		Levofloxacin		Trovafloxacin	Moxifloxacin			Gatifloxacin			Gemifloxacin
	PAE	PASME	PAE	PASME	PAE	PAE	SME	PASME	PAE	SME	PASME	PAE
S. aureus	0.8–2.5	1.25–12.25	1.8–3.1	5.0–>22.3	–	1.91	11.2	14.1	1.0–2.0	0.0–0.7	1.0–3.8	1.0–1.1
S. pneumoniae	0.5–2.3	0.5–3.3	0.7–2.3	0.63–2.9	3.0–10.6	1.44–3.3	9.0	10.9	1.2–4.0	0.3–7.8	1.6–8.6	0.7–1.5
K. pneumoniae	0.2–0.5	–	–	–	–	1.03	8.0	9.1	–	–	–	0.1–0.2
E. coli	1.2–3.7	–	–	–	3.0	1.01	8.0	10.6	4.8	2.4–>9.6	≥9.6	0.1–0.6
H. influenzae	0.6–2.4	–	2.3–3.0	–	0.8–2.8	2.8–3.5	–	–	–	–	–	2.4–>6
P. aeruginosa	4.5–5.1	–	–	–	0.9	–	–	–	2.2	1.0–1.9	2.8–4.4	2.4–>6
Legionella spp.	1.9–3.6	–	–	–	1.2–2.8	1.2–3.6	–	–	–	–	–	2.3–4.7

– = information not available.

of PASME tend to be higher than that of PAE or the SME because PASME represents the combination effects of PAE and SME.

Despite some of the previously discussed flaws, PAE is generally accepted as a meaningful factor when developing a drug regimen. However, once a drug regimen (especially dosing interval) has been established and demonstrated to be effective in well-designed clinical trials, consideration or discussion of PAE in clinical practice is unimportant. In other words, an established dosage regimen should already incorporate effects of the drug on the bacteria that include the PAE.

CONCLUSION

Fluoroquinolones, especially the newer ones, have considerable and practical pharmacokinetic features, including excellent oral absorption, excellent tissue distribution, significant interstitial fluid levels, substantial phagocytic cellular levels, good lung and urinary concentrations, and long half-lives. In addition, by utilizing pharmacodynamic surrogate markers such as the AUC/MIC ratio, the relationship between pharmacokinetics and antimicrobial activity can be established. Finally, a favorable clinical outcome is expected to result from therapy with the newer fluoroquinolones (moxifloxacin, gatifloxacin, and gemifloxacin) due to their high AUC/MIC ratios.

REFERENCES

1. Ball, P., Mandell, L., Niki, Y., and Tillotson, G. (1999). Comparative tolerability of the newer fluoroquinolone antibiotics. *Drug Saf.* **21**, 407–421.
2. Janoir, C., Zeller, V., Kitzis, M. D., Moreau, N. J., and Gutmann, L. (1996). High-level fluoroquinolone resistance in *Streptococcus pneumoniae* requires mutations in parC and gyrA. *Antimicrob. Agents Chemother.* **40**, 2760–2764.
3. Gootz, T. D., Zaniewski, R., Haskell, S., Schmieder, B., Tankovic, J., Girard, D., Courvalin, P., and Polzer, R. J. (1996). Activity of the new fluoroquinolone trovafloxacin (CP-99,219) against DNA gyrase and topoisomerase IV mutants of *Streptococcus pneumoniae* selected in vitro. *Antimicrob. Agents Chemother.* **40**, 2691–2697.
4. Beermann, D., Scholl, H., Wingender, W., Forster, D., Beubler, E., and Kukovetz, W. R. (1986). In "Proceedings 1st International Ciprofloxacin Workshop, Leverkusen, 1985" (H. C. Neu and H. Weuta, eds.), pp. 141–146. Excerpta Medica, Amsterdam.
5. Product Information (1997). Cipro™, Ciprofloxacin. Bayer Corporation, West Haven, CT.
6. Product Information (1996). Levaquin™, Levofloxacin. Ortho-McNeil Pharmaceutical Corporation, Raritan, NJ.
7. Product Information (1998). Trovan™, Trovafloxacin. Roerig, Division of Pfizer Inc., New York.
8. Product Information (1999). Tequin™, Gatifloxacin. Bristol-Myers Squibb Company, Princeton.
9. Product Information (1999). Avelox™, Moxifloxacin. Bayer Corporation, West Haven, CT.

10. Product Information (1999). Gemifloxacin (microbiological and pharmacokinetic profile). SmithKline Beecham Pharmaceuticals, Philadelphia.

11. Davis, R., Markham, A., and Balfour, J. A. (1996). Ciprofloxacin: An updated review of its pharmacology, therapeutic efficacy and tolerability. *Drugs* **51**, 1019–1074.

12. Davis, R., and Bryson, H. M. (1994). Levofloxacin: A review of its antibacterial activity, pharmacokinetics and therapeutic efficacy. *Drugs* **47**, 677–700.

13. Haria, M., and Lamb, H. M. (1997). Trovafloxacin. *Drugs* **54**, 435–445.

14. Balfour, J. A., and Lamb, H. M. (2000). Moxifloxacin: A review of its clinical potential in the management of community-acquired respiratory tract infections. *Drugs* **59**, 115–139.

15. Nightingale, C. H. (2000). Moxifloxacin, a new antibiotic designed to treat community-acquired respiratory tract infections: A review of microbiologic and pharmacokinetic–pharmacodynamic characteristics. *Pharmacotherapy* **20**, 245–256.

16. Perry, C. M., Barman Balfour, J. A., and Lamb, H. M. (1999). Gatifloxacin. *Drugs* **58**, 683–696.

17. Bergan, T., Thorsteinsson, S. B., Kolstad, I. M., and Johnsen, S. (1986). Pharmacokinetics of ciprofloxacin after intravenous and increasing oral doses. *Eur. J. Clin. Microbiol.* **5**(2), 187–192.

18. Bergan, T., Thorsteinsson, S. B., Solberg, R., Bjornskau, L., Kolstad, I. M., and Johnsen, S. (1987). Pharmacokinetics of ciprofloxacin: Intravenous and increasing oral doses. *Am. J. Med.* **82**(4A), 97–102.

19. Bergan, T., Delin, C., Johansen, S., Kolstad, I. M., Nord, C. E., and Thorsteinsson, S. B. (1986). Pharmacokinetics of ciprofloxacin and effect of repeated dosage on salivary and fecal microflora. *Antimicrob. Agents Chemother.* **29**(2), 298–302.

20. Chien, S. C., Rogge, M. C., Gisclon, L. G., Curtin, C., Wong, F., Natarajan, J., Williams, R. R., Fowler, C. L., Cheung, W. K., and Chow, A. T. (1997). Pharmacokinetic profile of levofloxacin following once-daily 500 mg oral or intravenous doses. *Antimicrob. Agents Chemother.* **41**, 2256–2260.

21. Fish, D., and Chow, A. (1997). The clinical pharmacokinetics of levofloxacin. *Clin. Pharmacokinet.* **32**, 101–119.

22. Teng, R., Dogolo, L. C., Willavize, S., Friedman, H. L., and Vincent, J. (1997). Oral bioavailability of trovafloxacin with and without food in healthy volunteers. *J. Antimicrob. Chemother.* **39**(SB), 87–92.

23. Teng, R., Liston, T. E., and Harris, S. C. (1996). Multiple-dose pharmacokinetics and safety of trovafloxacin in healthy volunteers. *J. Antimicrob. Chemother.* **37**, 955–963.

24. Teng, R., Harris, S. C., Nix, D. E., Schentag, J. J., Foulds, G., and Liston, T. E. (1995). Pharmacokinetics and safety of trovafloxacin (CP-99,219), a new quinolone antibiotic, following administration of single oral doses to healthy male volunteers. *J. Antimicrob. Chemother.* **36**(2), 385–394.

25. Vincent, J., Venitz, J., Teng, R., Baris, B. A., Willavize, S. A., Polzer, R. J., and Friedman, H. L. (1997). Pharmacokinetics and safety of trovafloxacin in healthy male volunteers following administration of single intravenous doses of the prodrug, alatrofloxacin. *J. Antimicrob. Chemother.* **39** (Suppl. B), 75–80.

26. Kubitza, D., Stass, H., Wingender, W., and Kuhlmann, J. (1996). Bay 12-8039 (I), a new 8-methoxy-quinolone: Safety, tolerability, and steady state pharmacokinetics in healthy male volunteers. *Abstr. 36th Intersci. Conf. Antimicrob. Agents Chemother.*, New Orleans. Abstr. #125.

27. Stass, H., Dalhoff, A., Kubitza, D., and Schuhly, U. (1998). Pharmacokinetics, safety, and tolerability of ascending single doses of moxifloxacin, a new-8-methoxyquinolone, administered to healthy subjects. *Antimicrob. Agents Chemother.* **42**, 2060–2065.

28. Nakashima, M., Uematsu, T., Kosuge, K., Kusajima, H., Ooie, T., Masuda, Y., Ishida, R., and Uchida, H. (1995). Single- and multiple-dose pharmacokinetics of AM-1155, a new 6-fluoro-8-methoxy quinolones, in humans. *Antimicrob. Agents Chemother.* **39**, 2635–2640.

29. Allen, A., Bygate, E., Teillol-Foo, M., Oliver, S. D, Johnson, M. R., and Ward, C. (1999). Pharmacokinetics and tolerability of gemifloxacin after administration of single oral doses to healthy volunteers [poster]. *21st Int. Cong. Chemother.*, Birmingham, UK, Abstr. #P440. *J. Antimicrob. Chemother.* **44** (Suppl. A), 137.

30. Allen, A., Bygate, E., Teillol-Foo, M., Oliver, S. D, Johnson, M. R., and Ward, C. (1999). Multiple-dose pharmacokinetics and tolerability of gemifloxacin following oral doses to healthy volunteers [poster]. *21st Int. Cong. Chemother.*, Birmingham, UK, Abstr. #P418. *J. Antimicrob. Chemother.* **44** (Suppl. A), 133.

31. Saliba, F., Isaac, L., Barker, P. J., Bird, N., Allen, A., Montague, T., and Romain, D. (2000). The pharmacokinetics and tolerability of a single oral dose of gemifloxacin in patients with mild or moderate hepatic impairment [poster]. *Abstr. 3rd Eur. Cong. Chemother.*, Madrid.

32. Young, C. L. (2000). Personal communication.

33. Bergan, T., Engeset, A., and Olszewski, W. (1987). Dose serum protein binding inhibit tissue penetration of antibiotics? *Rev. Infect. Dis.* **9**(4), 713–718.

34. Crump, B., Wise, R., and Dent, J. (1983). Pharmacokinetics and tissue penetration of ciprofloxacin. *Antimicrob. Agents Chemother.* **24**(5), 784–786.

35. Wise, R., Lockley, R. M., Webberly, M., and Dent, J. (1984). Pharmacokinetics of intravenously administered ciprofloxacin. *Antimicrob. Agents Chemother.* **26**(2), 208–210.

36. Wise, R., Mortiboy, D., Child, J., and Andrews, J. M. (1996). Pharmacokinetics and penetration into inflammatory fluid of trovafloxacin (CP-99,219). *Antimicrob. Agents Chemother.* **40**, 47–49.

37. Muller, M., Stass, H., Brunner, M., Moller, J. G., Lackner, E., and Eichler, H. G. (1999). Penetration of moxifloxacin into peripheral compartments in humans. *Antimicrob. Agents Chemother.* **43**(10), 2345–2349.

38. Wise, R., Andrews, J. M., Ashby, J. P., and Marshall, J. (1999). A study to determine the pharmacokinetics and inflammatory fluid penetration of gatifloxacin following a single oral dose. *J. Antimicrob. Chemother.* **44**(5), 701–704.

39. Easmon, C. S., and Crane, J. P. (1985). Uptake of ciprofloxacin by human neutrophils. *J. Antimicrob. Chemother.* **16**(1), 67–73.

40. Easmon, C. S., Crane, J. P., and Blowers, A. (1986). Effect of ciprofloxacin on intracellular organisms: In-vitro and in-vivo studies. *J. Antimicrob. Chemother.* **18** (Suppl. D), 43–48.

41. Garcia, I., Pascual, A., and Perea, E. J. (1994). Intracellular penetration and activity of BAY Y 3118 in human polymorphonuclear leukocytes. *Antimicrob. Agents Chemother.* **38**(10), 2426–2429.

42. Pascual, A., Garcia, I., Ballesta, S., and Perea, E. J. (1996). Uptake and intracellular activity of trovafloxacin in human phagocytes and tissue cultured epithelial cells. *Abstr. 36th Intersci. Conf. Antimicrob. Agents Chemother.*, New Orleans. Abstr. #A3.

43. Fischman, A. J., Babich, J. W., Bonab, A. A., Alpert, N. M., Vincent, J., Callahan, R. J., Correia, J. A., and Rubin, R. H. (1998). Pharmacokinetics of [18F]trovafloxacin in healthy human subjects studied with positron emission tomography. *Antimicrob. Agents Chemother.* **42**(8), 2048–2054.

44. Dalvie, D. K., Khosla, N., and Vincent, J. (1997). Excretion and metabolism of trovafloxacin in humans. *Drug Metab. Dispos.* **25**, 423–427.

45. Brogard, J. M., Jehl, F., Arnaud, J. P., Levy, P., Peladan, F., Blickle, J. F., and Monteil, H. (1985). Ciprofloxacin: Evaluation of its biliary elimination in man. *Schweiz. Med. Wochenschr.* **115**(13), 448–453.

46. Pederzoli, P., Falconi, M., Bassi, C., Vesentini, S., Orcalli, F., Scaglione, F., Solbiati, M., Messori, A., and Martini, N. (1987). Ciprofloxacin penetration in pancreatic juice. *Chemotherapy* **33**(6), 397–401.

47. Lockley, M. R., Waldron, R., Wise, R., and Donovan, I. A. (1986). Intraperitoneal penetration of ciprofloxacin. *Eur. J. Clin. Microbiol.* **5**(2), 209–210.

48. Shimada, J., Yamaji, T., Ueda, Y., Uchida, H., Kusajima, H., and Irikura, T. (1983). Mechanism of renal excretion of AM-715, a new quinolone carboxylic acid derivative, in rabbits, dogs, and humans. *Antimicrob. Agents Chemother.* **23**(1), 1–7.

49. Melnik, G., Schwesinger, W. H., Dogolo, L. C., Teng, R., and Vincent, J. (1998). Concentrations of trovafloxacin in colonic tissue and peritoneal fluid after intravenous infusion of the prodrug alatrofloxacin in patients undergoing colorectal surgery. *Am. J. Surg.* **176** (Suppl. 6A), 14S–17S.

50. Fong, I. W., Ledbetter, W. H., Vandenbroucke, A. C., Simbul, M., and Rahm, V. (1986). Ciprofloxacin concentrations in bone and muscle after oral dosing. *Antimicrob. Agents Chemother.* **29**(3), 405–408.

51. Daschner, F. D., Westenfelder, M., and Dalhoff, A. (1986). Penetration of ciprofloxacin into kidney, fat, muscle and skin tissue. *Eur. J. Clin. Microbiol.* **5**(2), 212–213.

52. Wittmann, D. H., and Kotthaus, E. (1986). Further methodological improvement in antibiotic bone concentration measurements: Penetration of ofloxacin into bone and cartilage. *Infection* **14** (Suppl. 4), S270–S273.

53. Schuler, P., Zemper, K., Borner, K., Koeppe, P., Schaberg, T., and Lode, H. (1997). Penetration of sparfloxacin and ciprofloxacin into alveolar macrophages, epithelial lining fluid, and polymorphonuclear leucocytes. *Eur. Respir. J.* **10**(5), 1130–1136.

54. Fabre, D., Bressolle, F., Gomeni, R., Arich, C., Lemesle, F., Beziau, H., and Galtier, M. (1991). Steady-state pharmacokinetics of ciprofloxacin in plasma from patients with nosocomial pneumonia: Penetration of the bronchial mucosa. *Antimicrob. Agents Chemother.* **35**(12), 2521–2525.

55. Andrews, J. M., Honeybourne, D., Jevons, G., Brenwald, N. P., Cunningham, B., and Wise, R. (1997). Concentrations of levofloxacin (HR 355) in the respiratory tract following a single oral dose in patients undergoing fibre-optic bronchoscopy. *J. Antimicrob. Chemother.* **40**(4), 573–577.

56. Andrews, J. M., Honeybourne, D., Brenwald, N. P., Bannerjee, D., Iredale, M., Cunningham, B., and Wise R. (1997). Concentrations of trovafloxacin in bronchial mucosa, epithelial lining fluid, alveolar macrophages and serum after administration of single or multiple oral doses to patients undergoing fiber-optic bronchoscopy. *J. Antimicrob. Chemother.* **39**, 797–802.

57. Soman, A., Honeybourne, D., Andrews, J., Jevons, G., and Wise, R. (1999). Concentrations of moxifloxacin in serum and pulmonary compartments following a single 400 mg oral dose in patients undergoing fibre-optic bronchoscopy. *J. Antimicrob. Chemother.* **44**(6), 835–838.

58. Honeybourne, D., Andrews, J. M., Wise, R., Stahlberg, H. J., and Goehler, K. (in press). Tissue penetration of gatifloxacin into bronchial mucosa, epithelial lining fluid and alveolar macrophages after administration of a single 400 mg oral dose. Manuscript submitted for publication.

59. Bromley, I., and Allen, A. (2000). Penetration of gemifloxacin into bronchial mucosa, epithelial lining fluid and alveolar macrophages in healthy volunteers [poster]. *Abstr. 3rd Eur. Cong. Chemother.*, Madrid.

60. Davies, B. L., Maesen, F. P., and Baur, C. (1986). Ciprofloxacin in the treatment of acute exacerbations of chronic bronchitis. *Eur. J. Clin. Microbiol.* **5**(2), 226–231.

61. Bender, S. W., Dalhoff, A., Shah, P. M., Strehl, R., and Posselt, H. G. (1986). Ciprofloxacin pharmacokinetics in patients with cystic fibrosis. *Infection* **14**(1), 17–21.

62. Smith, M. J., White, L. O., Bowyer, H., Willis, J., Hodson, M. E., and Batten, J. C. (1986). Pharmacokinetics and sputum penetration of ciprofloxacin in patients with cystic fibrosis. *Antimicrob. Agents Chemother.* **30**(4), 614–616.

63. Ullmann, U., Giebel, W., Dalhoff, A., and Koeppe, P. (1986). Single and multiple dose pharmacokinetics of ciprofloxacin. *Eur. J. Clin. Microbiol.* **5**(2), 193–196.

64. Darouiche, R., Perkins, B., Musher, D., Hamill, R., and Tsai, S. (1990). Levels of rifampin and ciprofloxacin in nasal secretions: Correlation with MIC_{90} and eradication of nasopharyngeal carriage of bacteria. *J. Infect. Dis.* **162**(5), 1124–1127.

65. Gehanno, P., Stass, H., and Arvis, P. (1999). Penetration of moxafloxacin into sinus tissues following multiple oral dosing. *9th Eur. Conf. Clin. Microbiol. Infect. Dis.*, Berlin, 21–24 March 1999.

66. Duben, W., Student, A., Jablonski, M., and Malottke, R. (1986). Tissue concentration and effectiveness of ofloxacin in surgical patients. *Infection* **14** (Suppl. 1), S70–S72.

67. Waldron, R., Arkell, D. G., Wise, R., and Andrews, J. M. (1986). The intraprostatic penetration of ciprofloxacin. *J. Antimicrob. Chemother.* **17**(4), 544–545.

68. Boerema, J. B., Debruyne, F. M., and Dalhoff, A. (1984). Intraprostatic concentrations of ciprofloxacin after intravenous administration [letter]. *Lancet* **2**(8404), 695–696.

69. Boerema, J. B., Dalhoff, A., and Debruyne, F. M. (1985). Ciprofloxacin distribution in prostatic tissue and fluid following oral administration. *Chemotherapy* **31**(1), 13–18.

70. Dalhoff, A., and Eickenberg, H. U. (1985). Tissue distribution of ciprofloxacin following oral and intravenous administration. *Infection* **13**(2), 78–81.

71. Dalhoff, A., and Weidner, W. (1984). Diffusion of ciprofloxacin into prostatic fluid. *Eur. J. Clin. Microbiol.* **3**(4), 360–362.

72. Dan, M., Golomb, J., Gorea, A., Braf, Z., and Berger, S. A. (1986). Concentration of ciprofloxacin in human prostatic tissue after oral administration. *Antimicrob. Agents Chemother.* **30**(1), 88–89.

73. Gombert, M. E., du Bouchet, L., Aulicino, T. M., Berkowitz, L. B., and Macchia, R. J. (1987). Intravenous ciprofloxacin versus cefotaxime prophylaxis during transurethral surgery. *Am. J. Med.* **82** (Suppl. 4A), 130–132.

74. Grabe, M., Forsgren, A., and Bjork, T. (1986). Concentrations of ciprofloxacin in serum and prostatic tissue in patients undergoing transurethral resection. *Eur. J. Clin. Microbiol.* **5**(2), 211–212.

75. Hoogkamp-Korstanje, J. A., van Oort, H. J., Schipper, J. J., and van der Wal, T. (1984). Intraprostatic concentration of ciprofloxacin and its activity against urinary pathogens. *J. Antimicrob. Chemother.* **14**(6), 641–645.

76. Dalhoff, A. and Weuta, H. (1987). Penetration of ciprofloxacin into gynecologic tissues. *Am. J. Med.* **82**(4A), 133–138.

77. Segev, S., Rubinstein, E., Shick, J., Rabinovitch, O., and Dolitsky, M. (1986). Penetration of ciprofloxacin into female pelvic tissues. *Eur. J. Clin. Microbiol.* **5**(2), 207–209.

78. Brighty, K. E., and Gootz, T. D. (1997). The chemistry and biological profile of trovafloxacin. *J. Antimicrob. Chemother.* **39** (Suppl. B), 1–14.

79. Martens, M. G., Maccato, M., Van Hook, C., and Vincent, J. (1998). Penetration of trovafloxacin into gynecologic tissues. *Am. J. Surg.* **176** (Suppl. 6A), 18S–22S.

80. Lutsar, I., Friedland, I. R., Wubbel, L., McCoig, C. C., Jafri, H. S., Ng, W., Ghaffar, F., and McCracken Jr., G. H. (1998). Pharmacodynamics of gatifloxacin in cerebrospinal fluid in experimental cephalosporin-resistant pneumococcal meningitis. *Antimicrob. Agents Chemother.* **42**(10), 2650–2655.

81. Charles, F. C., Armstrong, L. L., Ingrim, N. B., and Lance, L. L. (1998–99). "Drug Information Handbook," 6th ed. Lexi-Comp Inc., Hudson, OH. American Pharmaceutical Association.
82. Valainis, G., Thomas, D., and Pankey, G. (1986). Penetration of ciprofloxacin into cerebrospinal fluid. *Eur. J. Clin. Microbiol.* **5**(2), 206–207.
83. Wolff, M., Boutron, L., Singlas, E., Clair, B., Decazes, J. M., and Regnier, B. (1987). Penetration of ciprofloxacin into cerebrospinal fluid of patients with bacterial meningitis. *Antimicrob. Agents Chemother.* **31**(6), 899–902.
84. Fish, D. N., and Chow, A. T. (1997). The clinical pharmacokinetics of levofloxacin. *Clin. Pharmacokin.* **32**(2), 101–109.
85. Nau, R., Schmidt, T., Kaye, K., Froula, J. L., and Tauber, M. G. (1995). Quinolone antibiotics in therapy of experimental pneumococcal meningitis in rabbits. *Antimicrob. Agents Chemother.* **39**(3), 593–597.
86. Cutler, N. R., Vincent, J., Jhee, S. S., Teng, R., Wardle, T., Lucas, G., Dogolo, L. C., and Sramek, J. J. (1997). Penetration of trovafloxacin into cerebrospinal fluid in humans following intravenous infusion of alatrofloxacin. *Antimicrob. Agents Chemother.* **41**, 1298–1300.
87. McCoig, C. C., Wubbel, L., Jafri, H. S., Lutsar, I., Bastero, R., Olsen, K., Shelton, S., Friedland, I. R., and McCracken, G. H. (1999). Pharmacodynamics of trovafloxacin in experimental pneumococcal meningitis: Basis for dosage selection in children with meningitis. *J. Antimicrob. Chemother.* **43**(5), 683–688.
88. Ostergaard, C., Sorensen, T. K., Knudsen, J. D., and Frimodt-Moller, N. (1998). Evaluation of moxifloxacin, a new 8-methoxyquinolone, for treatment of meningitis caused by a penicillin-resistant pneumococcus in rabbits. *Antimicrob. Agents Chemother.* **42**(7), 1706–1712.
89. Ooie, T., Suzuki, H., Terasaki, T., and Sugiyama, Y. (1996). Comparative distribution of quinolone antibiotics in cerebrospinal fluid and brain in rats and dogs. *J. Pharmacol. Exp. Ther.* **278**(2), 590–596.
90. Davey, P. G., Charter, M., Kelly, S., Varma, T. R., Jacobson, I., Freeman, A., Precious, E., and Lambert, J. (1994). Ciprofloxacin and sparfloxacin in penetration into human brain tissue and their activity as antagonists of GABAA receptor of rat vagus nerve. *Antimicrob. Agents Chemother.* **38**(6), 1356–1362.
91. Iwamoto, K., Ichikawa, N., Naora, K., and Hirano, H. (1995). Effect of fenbufen on the penetration of quinolone antibiotics into cerebrospinal fluid: Comparative study with 5 quinolones. *Drugs* **49** (Suppl. 2), 349–351.
92. Hoffken, G., Lode, H., Prinzing, C., Borner, K., and Koeppe, P. (1985). Pharmacokinetics of ciprofloxacin after oral and parenteral administration. *Antimicrob. Agents Chemother.* **27**(3), 375–379.
93. Gonzalez, M. A., Uribe, F., Moisen, S. D., Fuster, A. P., Selen, A., Welling, P. G., and Painter, B. (1984). Multiple-dose pharmacokinetics and safety of ciprofloxacin in normal volunteers. *Antimicrob. Agents Chemother.* **26**(5), 741–744.
94. Dalvie, D. K., Khosla, N., and Vincent, J. (1997). Excretion and metabolism of trovafloxacin in humans. *Drug Metab. Dispos.* **25**(4), 423–427.
95. Stass, H., Dalhoff, A., Kubitza, D., and Schuhly, U. (1998). Pharmacokinetics, safety, and tolerability of ascending single doses of moxifloxacin, a new 8-methoxy quinolone, administered to healthy subjects. *Antimicrob. Agents Chemother.* **42**(8), 2060–2065.
96. Stass, H., Dalhoff, A., and Kubitza, D. (1997). Bay 12-8039: Study on the food effect after oral administration of 200-mg SD to healthy volunteers [poster]. *Abstr. 8th Eur. Cong. Clin. Microbiol. Infect. Dis.*, Lausanne.

97. Kubitza, D., Strass, H. H., Wingender, W., and Kuhlmann, J. (1996). Bay 12-8039 (I), a new 8-methoxy-quinolone: Safety, tolerability, and steady state pharmacokinetics in healthy male volunteers. *Abstr. 36th Intersci. Conf. Antimicrob. Agents Chemother.*, New Orleans. Abstr. #F25.

98. Nakashima, M., Uematsu, T., Kosuge, K., Kusajima, H., Ooie, T., Masuda, Y., Ishida, R., and Uchida, H. (1995). Single- and multiple-dose pharmacokinetics of AM-1155, a new 6-fluoro-8-methoxy quinolone, in humans. *Antimicrob. Agents Chemother.* **39**(12), 2635–2640.

99. Lober, S., Ziege, S., Rau, M., Scheiber, G., Koeppe, P., and Lode, H. (1998). Gatifloxacin:pharmacokinetics and interaction with Maalox. *Abstr. 38th Intersci. Conf. Antimicrob. Agents Chemother.*, San Diego. Abstr. #A23.

100. Product information reference in Micromedex, Vol. 104. (1975–2000). Micromedex Inc.

101. Stass, H., Dietrich, H., and Sachse, R. (1997). Influence of a four-times dosing of 500-mg probenecid on kinetics of Bay 12-8039 after administration of a single 400-mg dose in healthy male volunteers. *Abstr. 37th Intersci. Conf. Antimicrob. Agents Chemother.*, Toronto. Abstr. #F-154.

102. Gasser, T. C., Ebert, S. C., Graversen, P. H., and Madsen, P. O. (1987). Ciprofloxacin pharmacokinetics in patients with normal and impaired renal function. *Antimicrob. Agents Chemother.* **31**(5), 709–712.

103. Stass, H., Halabi, A., and Delesen, H. (1998). No dose adjustment needed for patients with renal impairment receiving oral BAY 12-8039(M). *Abstr. 38th Intersci. Conf. Antimicrob. Agents Chemother.*, San Diego. Abstr. #A14.

104. Kawada, Y., Kanimoto, Y., and Takahashi, Y. (1998). Pharmacokinetics of gatifloxacin in patients with impaired renal function. *Antiinfect. Drugs Chemother.* **16** (Suppl. 1), 69.

105. Allen, A., Walls, C. M., McDonnell, D., Bird, N., and Lewis, A. (2000). Pharmacokinetics of the novel fluoroquinolone gemifloxacin administered to patients with severe renal impairment and patients on dialysis [poster]. *Abstr. 3rd Eur. Cong. Chemother.*, Madrid.

106. Anderson, K. E., Egger, N. G., Goeger, D. E., Teng, R., Dogolo, L. C., Willavize, S., and Vincent, J. (1997). The safety, toleration and pharmacokinetics of trovafloxacin in patients with hepatic impairment. *Abstr. 37th Intersci. Conf. Antimicrob. Agents Chemother.*, Toronto. Abstr. #A65.

107. Stass, H., Kubitza, D., and Von Bergmann, K. (1999). No dose adjustment is needed for moxifloxacin in subjects suffering from hepatic impairment. *Clin. Microbiol. Infect.* **5** (Suppl. 3), 291.

108. Grasela, D., Christofalo, B., and Lacreta, F. (1998). Single-dose safety and pharmacokinetics of oral gatifloxacin in subjects with hepatic impairment. *Abstr. 38th Intersci. Conf. Antimicrob. Agents Chemother.*, San Diego. Abstr. #A30.

109. Stass, H., and Kubitza, D. (1999). Pharmacokinetics and elimination of moxifloxacin after oral and intravenous administration in man. *J. Antimicrob. Chemother.* **43** (Suppl. B), 83–90.

110. Hoffler, D., Dalhoff, A., Gau, W., Beermann, D., and Michl, A. (1984). Dose- and sex-independent disposition of ciprofloxacin. *Eur. J. Clin. Microbiol.* **3**(4), 363–366.

111. Teng, R., Dogolo, L. C., Willavize, S. A., and Vincent, J. (1995). Effect of age and gender on the pharmacokinetics of CP-99,219, a new quinolone antibiotic, in healthy volunteers. *Abstr. 35th Intersci. Conf. Antimicrob. Agents Chemother.*, San Francisco. Abstr. #F238.

112. Vincent, J., Teng, R., Dogolo, L. C., Schumacher, D., Willavize, S. A., and Friedman, H. L. (1996). Trovafloxacin and ofloxacin profiles in ambulatory subjects matched for age and gender. *Abstr. 36th Intersci. Conf. Antimicrob. Agents Chemother.*, New Orleans. Abstr. #A6.

113. von Rosenstiel, N., and Adam, D. (1994). Quinolone antibacterials. An update of their pharmacology and therapeutic use. *Drugs* **47**(6), 872–901.

114. Kearns, G. L., Bradley, J. S., Reed, J. S., and Vincent, J. (1997). Trovafloxacin pharmacokinetics in infants and children. *Abstr. 37th Intersci. Conf. Antimicrob. Agents Chemother.*, Toronto. Abstr. #A104.

115. Garrelts, J. C., Jost, G., Kowalsky, S. F., Krol, G. J., and Lettieri, J. T. (1996). Ciprofloxacin pharmacokinetics in burn patients. *Antimicrob. Agents Chemother.* **40**(5), 1153–1159.

116. Grasela, T., Cirincione, B., Christofalo, B., Pierce, P., Hiles, C., and Grasela, D. (1998). Population pharmacokinetics of gatifloxacin in adults with acute bacterial exacerbation of chronic bronchitis. *Abstr. 38th Intersci. Conf. Antimicrob. Agents Chemother.*, San Diego. Abstr. #A28.

117. LeBel, M., Bergeron, M. G., Vallee, F., Fiset, C., Chasse, G., Bigonesse, P., and Rivard, G. (1986). Pharmacokinetics and pharmacodynamics of ciprofloxacin in cystic fibrosis patients. *Antimicrob. Agents Chemother.* **30**(2), 260–266.

118. Pedersen, S. S., Jensen, T., and Hvidberg, E. F. (1987). Department of Clinical Microbiology, Rigshospitalet, Copenhagen, Denmark: Comparative pharmacokinetics of ciprofloxacin and ofloxacin in cystic fibrosis patients. *J. Antimicrob. Chemother.* **20**(4), 575–583.

119. Smith, M. J., White, L. O., Bowyer, H., Willis, J., Hodson, M. E., and Batten, J. C. (1986). Pharmacokinetics and sputum penetration of ciprofloxacin in patients with cystic fibrosis. *Antimicrob. Agents Chemother.* **30**(4), 614–616.

120. Bender, S. W., Dalhoff, A., Shah, P. M., Strehl, P., and Posselt, H. G. (1986). Ciprofloxacin pharmacokinetics in patients with cystic fibrosis. *Infection* **14**(1), 17–21.

121. Owens Jr., R. C., Patel, K. B., Banevicius, M. A., Quintiliani, R., Nightingale, C. H., and Nicolau, D. P. (1997). Oral bioavailability and pharmacokinetics of ciprofloxacin in patients with AIDS. *Antimicrob. Agents Chemother.* **41**(7), 1508–1511.

122. Lacy, M., Nicolau, D., Nightingale, C., Geffken, A., Teng, R., Vincent, J., and Quintiliani, R. (1997). The pharmacokinetics of trovafloxacin in patients with AIDS. *Abstr. 37th Intersci. Conf. Antimicrob. Agents Chemother.*, Toronto. Abstr. #A64.

123. Ledergerber, B., Bettex, J. D., Joos, B., Flepp, M., and Luthy, R. (1985). Effect of standard breakfast on drug absorption and multiple-dose pharmacokinetics of ciprofloxacin. *Antimicrob. Agents Chemother.* **27**(3), 350–352.

124. Hoffken, G., Lode, H., Prinzing, C., Borner, K., and Koeppe, P. (1985). Pharmacokinetics of ciprofloxacin after oral and parenteral administration. *Antimicrob. Agents Chemother.* **27**(3), 375–379.

125. Hoffken, G., Borner, K., Glatzel, P. D., Koeppe, P., and Lode, H. (1985). Reduced enteral absorption of ciprofloxacin in the presence of antacids. *Eur. J. Clin. Microbiol.* **4**(3), 345.

126. Bergan, T. (1998). Pharmacokinetics of the fluoroquinolones. In "The Quinolones," 2nd ed. (V. T. Andriole, ed.), pp. 143–182. Academic Press, San Diego.

127. Wijnands, W. J. E., Vree, T. B., and van Herwaarden, C. L. (1986). The influence of quinolone derivatives on theophylline clearance. *Br. J. Clin. Pharmacol.* **22**, 677–683.

128. Raoof, S., Wallschlager, C., and Khan, F. (1987). Ciprofloxacin increases serum levels of theophylline. *Am. J. Med.* **82** (Suppl. 4A), 115–118.

129a Kamada, A. K. (1990). Possible interaction between ciprofloxacin and warfarin. *Ann. Pharmacother.* **24**, 27–28.

129b Dillard, M. L., Fink, R. M., and Parkerson, R. (1992). Ciprofloxacin–phenytoin interaction. *Ann. Pharmacother.* **26**, 262–263.

130. Brouwers, P. J., De Boer, L. E., Guchelaar, H. J. (1997). Ciprofloxacin–phenytoin interaction. *Ann. Pharmacother.* **31**, 498.

131. Job, M. L., Arn, S. K., Strom, J. G., Jacobs, N. F., and D'Souza, M. J. (1994). Effect of ciprofloxacin on the pharmacokinetics of multiple-dose phenytoin serum concentrations. *Ther. Drug Monit.* **16**, 427–431.

132. Shiba, K., Sakamoto, M., Nakazawa, Y., and Sakai, O. (1995). Effects of antacid on absorption and excretion on new quinolones. *Drugs* **49** (Suppl. 2), 360–361.

133. Teng, R., Dogolo, L. C., Willavize, S. A., Friedman, H. L., and Vincent, J. (1997). Oral bioavailability of trovafloxacin with and without food in healthy volunteers. *J. Antimicrob. Chemother.* **39** (Suppl. B), 87–92.

134. Teng, R., Dogolo, L. C., Willavize, S. A., Friedman, H. L., and Vincent, J. (1997). Effect of Maalox and omeprazole on the bioavailability of trovafloxacin. *J. Antimicrob. Chemother.* **39** (Suppl. B), 93–97.

135. LeBel, M., Dogolo, L., Teng, R., and Vincent, J. (1997). Contrasting effects of divalent and trivalent cation-containing antacids on the bioavailability of trovafloxacin. *Abstr. 20th Int. Cong. Chemother.*, Sydney. Abstr. #2257.

136. LeBel, M., Teng, R., Dogolo, L. C., Willavize, S., Friedman, H. L., and Vincent, J. (1996). The effect of steady-state trovafloxacin on the steady-state pharmacokinetics of caffeine in healthy subjects. *Abstr. 36th Intersci. Conf. Antimicrob. Agents Chemother.*, New Orleans. Abstr. #A1.

137. Purkins, L., Kleinermans, D., Brown, S., and Willavize, S. (1997). Effects of orally administered trovafloxacin on the steady-state pharmacokinetics of digoxin: Results of double-blind, placebo-controlled, parallel-group study. *Abstr. 20th Int. Cong. Chemother.*, Sydney. Abstr. #2261.

138. Vincent, J., Teng, R., Dogolo, L. C., Willavize, S. A., and Friedman, H. L. (1997). Effect of trovafloxacin, a new fluoroquinolone antibiotic, on the steady-state pharmacokinetics of theophylline in healthy volunteers. *J. Antimicrob. Chemother.* **39** (Suppl. B), 81–86.

139. Teng, R., Dogolo, L. C., Willavize, S. A., Friedman, H. L., and Vincent, J. (1997). Effect of Maalox and omeprazole on the bioavailability of trovafloxacin. *J. Antimicrob. Chemother.* **39** (Suppl. B), 93–97.

140. Purkins, L., Oliver, S., and Willavize, S. (1997). An open, placebo-controlled, two-way crossover study to investigate the effects of cimetidine on the steady-state pharmacokinetics of trovafloxacin. *Abstr. 20th Int. Cong. Chemother.*, Sydney. Abstr. #2260.

141. Lettieri, J., Agarwal, V., and Lui, P. (in press). Effect of food on a single 400-mg moxifloxacin in healthy male subjects. *Clin. Pharmacol.*

142. Stass, H., and Kubitza, D. (1998). Study to assess the interaction between moxifloxacin and diary products in healthy volunteers. *Antiinfect. Drugs Chemother.* **16** (Suppl. 1), 74.

143. Stass, H. H., Schuhly, U., Wandel, C., Moller, J. G., and Delesen, H. (1999). Study to evaluate the interaction between oral moxifloxacin and sucralfate in healthy volunteers. *Abstr. 39th Intersci. Conf. Antimicrob. Agents Chemother.*, San Francisco. Abstr. #7.

144. Stass, H., and Kubitza, D. (1998). Study to evaluate the interaction between moxifloxacin and iron supplements. *Abstr. 2nd Eur. Cong. Chemother., 7th Biennial Conf. Antiinfect. Agents Chemother.*, Hamburg. Abstr. #T154.

145. Stass, H., and Wandel, C. (1999). No significant interaction between oral moxifloxacin and calcium supplements in healthy volunteers. *J. Antimicrob. Chemother.* **44** (Suppl. A), 132.

146. Stass, H., Kubitza, D., and Schwietert, R. (1997). Bay 12-8039 does not interact with theophylline [poster]. *Abstr. 20th Int. Cong. Chemother.*, Sydney.

147. Horstmann, R., Delesen, H., and Dietrich, D. (1998). No drug–drug interaction between moxifloxacin and β-acetyldigoxin. *J. Clin. Pharmacol.* **38**, 879.

148. Stass, H., and Ochmann, K. (1997). Study to evaluate the interaction between Bay 12-8039 and ranitidine [poster]. *Abstr. 20th Int. Cong. Chemother.*, Sydney.

149. Muller, F. O., Hundt, H. K. L., Muir, A. R., Potgieter, M. A., Terblanche, J., Toerien, C. J., and Stass, H. (1998). Study to investigate the influence of 400-mg BAY 12-8039 given once daily to healthy volunteers on PK and PD of warfarin. *Abstr. 38th Intersci. Conf. Antimicrob. Agents Chemother.*, San Diego. Abstr. #A13.

150. Sachse, R., Stass, H., and Delesen, H. (1999). Lack of interaction between moxifloxacin and combined oral contraceptive steroids. *Clin. Microbiol. Infect.* **5** (Suppl. 3), 141.

151. Shiba, K., Sakamoto, M., Saito, A., Sakai, O., Ueda, Y., Kusajima, H., and Ishida, R. (1995). Effect of ferrous sulfate, tea and milk on absorption of AM-1155, a 6-fluoro-8-methoxy quinolone in humans. *Abstr. 35th Intersci. Conf. Antimicrob. Agents Chemother.*, San Francisco. Abstr. #A43.

152. Olsen, S. J., Udermann, H. D., Kaul, S., Kollia, G. D., Birkhofer, M. J., and Grasela, D. M. (1999). Pharmacokinetic of concomitantly administered gatifloxacin and digoxin. *Abstr. 39th Intersci. Conf. Antimicrob. Agents Chemother.*, San Francisco. Abstr. #199.

153. Grasela, D., Lacreta, F., Kollia, G., Randall, D., Stoltz, R., and Berger, S. (1999). Lack of effect of multiple dose gatifloxacin on oral glucose tolerance glucose and insulin homeostasis, and glyburide pharmacokinetics in patients with type II non-insulin-dependent diabetes mellitus. *Abstr. 39th Intersci. Conf. Antimicrob. Agents Chemother.*, San Francisco. Abstr. #196.

154. Gajjar, D. A., Lacreta, F. P., Kollia, G. D., Uderman, H. D., Swingle, M., Randall, D. M., and Grasela, D. M. (1999). Lack of effect of gatifloxacin on the pharmacokinetics of midazolam, a model substrate for cytochrome P4503A activity, in healthy adult volunteers. *Abstr. 39th Intersci. Conf. Antimicrob. Agents Chemother.*, San Francisco. Abstr. #197.

155. Niki, Y., Hashiguchi, K., Miyashita, N., Nakajima, M., and Matsushima, T., and Soejima, R. (1996). Effect of AM-1155 on serum concentration of theophylline. *Abstr. 36th Intersci. Conf. Antimicrob. Agents Chemother.*, New Orleans. Abstr. #F73.

156. Stahlberg, H. J., Gohler, K., and Guillame, M. (1999). Effects of gatifloxacin on the pharmacokinetics of theophylline in healthy young volunteers. *J. Antimicrob. Chemother.* **44** (Suppl. A), 136.

157. Manita, S., Toriumi, C., Kusajima, H., and Momo, K. (1998). The influence of gatifloxacin on pharmacokinetics and metabolism of theophylline in rats and humans. *Abstr. 38th Intersci. Conf. Antimicrob. Agents Chemother.*, San Diego. Abstr. #A16a.

158. Allen, A., Bygate, E., Clark, D., Lewis, A., and Pay, V. (2000). The effect of food on the bioavailability of oral gemifloxacin in healthy volunteers [poster]. *Abstr. 3rd Eur. Cong. Chemother.*, Madrid.

159. Allen, A., Vousden, M., Porter, A., Lewis, A., and Teillol-Foo, M. (1999). Effect of Maalox on the bioavailability of gemifloxacin in healthy volunteers [poster]. *Abstr. 21st Int. Cong. Chemother.*, Birmingham, UK, Abstr. #P421. *J. Antimicrob. Chemother.* **44** (Suppl. A), 133.

160. Allen, A., Vousden, M., Lewis, A., and Teillol-Foo, M. (1999). Effect of omeprazole on the pharmacokinetics of oral gemifloxacin in healthy volunteers [poster]. *Abstr. 21st Int. Cong. Chemother.*, Birmingham, UK, Abstr. #P423. *J. Antimicrob. Chemother.* **44** (Suppl. A), 134.

161. Davy, M., Bird, N., Rost, K. L., and Fuder, H. (1999). Lack of effect of gemifloxacin on the steady-state pharmacodynamics of warfarin in healthy volunteers [poster]. *Abstr. 21st Int. Cong. Chemother.*, Birmingham, UK, Abstr. #P417. *J. Antimicrob. Chemother.* **44** (Suppl. A), 132.

162. Davy, M., Allen, A., Bird, N., Rost, K. L., and Fuder, H. (1999). Lack of effect of gemifloxacin on the steady-state pharmacodynamics of theophylline in healthy volunteers [poster]. *Abstr. 21st Int. Cong. Chemother.*, Birmingham, UK, Abstr. #P419. *J. Antimicrob. Chemother.* **44** (Suppl. A), 133.

163. Vousden, M., Allen, A., Lewis, A., and Ehren, N. (1999). Lack of pharmacokinetic interaction between gemifloxacin and digoxin in healthy elderly volunteers. *Chemotherapy* **45**(6), 485–490.

164. Allen, A., Bygate, E., and Faessel, H. (2000). The effect of ferrous sulphate and sucralfate on the bioavailability of oral gemifloxacin in healthy volunteers [poster]. *Abstr. 3rd Eur. Cong. Chemother.*, Madrid.

165. Lomaestro, B. M., and Bailie, G. R. (1995). Absorption interactions with fluoroquinolones. 1995 update. *Drug Saf.* **12**(5), 314–333.

166. Amsterdam, D. (1996). Susceptibility testing of antimicrobials in liquid media. In "Antibiotics in Laboratory Medicine" (V. Lorian, ed.), 4th ed., pp. 52–111. Williams & Wilkins, Baltimore.

167. Auckenthaler, R., Michea-Hamzehpour, M., and Pechere, J. C. (1986). In-vitro activity of newer quinolones against aerobic bacteria. *J. Antimicrob. Chemother.* **17** (Suppl. B), 29–39.

168. Lagast, H., Husson, M., and Klastersky, J. (1985). Bactericidal activity of ciprofloxacin in serum and urine against *Escherichia coli, Pseudomonas aeruginosa, Klebsiella pneumoniae, Staphylococcus aureus* and *Streptococcus faecalis*. *J. Antimicrob. Chemother.* **16**(3), 341–347.

169. Bauernfeind, A., Eberlein, E., Schneider, I. (1998). Comparative bactericidal kinetics of gatifloxacin (AM1155) at varous dosages in a pharmacodynamic model. *J. Antimicrob. Chemother.* **16** (Suppl. 1), 69.

170a. Boswell, F. J., Andrews, J. M., and Wise, R. (1997). Pharmacodynamic properties of BAY 12-8039 on Gram-positive and Gram-negative organisms as demonstrated by studies of time–kill kinetics and postantibiotic effect. *Antimicrob. Agents Chemother.* **41**(6), 1377–9.

170b. Visalli, M. A., Jacobs, M. R., and Appelbaum, P. C. (1997). Antipneumococcal activity of BAY 12-8039, a new quinolone, compared with activities of three other quinolones and four oral beta-lactams. *Antimicrob. Agents Chemother.* **41**(12), 2786–2789.

171. Boswell, F. J., Andrews, J. M., Wise, R., and Dalhoff, A. (1999). Bactericidal properties of moxifloxacin and post-antibiotic effect. *J. Antimicrob. Chemother.* **43** (Suppl. B), 43–49.

172. Hosaka, M., Yasue, T., Fukuda, H., Tomizawa, H., Aoyama, H., and Hirai, K. (1992). In vitro and in vivo antibacterial activities of AM-1155, a new 6-fluoro-8-methoxy quinolone. *Antimicrob. Agents Chemother.* **36**(10), 2108–2117.

173. Hoellman, D. B., Lin, G., Jacobs, M. R., and Appelbaum, P. C. (1999). Anti-pneumococcal activity of gatifloxacin compared with other quinolone and non-quinolone agents. *J. Antimicrob. Chemother.* **43**(5), 645–649.

174. Drusano, G. L., Johnson, D. E., Rosen, M., and Standiford, H. C. (1993). Pharmacodynamics of a fluoroquinolone antimicrobial agent in a neutropenic rat model of pseudomonas sepsis. *Antimicrob. Agents Chemother.* **37**(3), 483–490.

175. Forrest, A., Nix, D. E., Ballow, C. H, Goss, T. F., Birmingham, M. C., and Schentag, J. J. (1993). Pharmacodynamics of intravenous ciprofloxacin in seriously ill patients. *Antimicrob. Agents Chemother.* **37**(5), 1073–1081.

176. Lacy, M. K., Lu, W., Xu, X., Tessier, P. R., Nicolau, D. P., Quintiliani, R., and Nightingale, C. H. (1999). Pharmacodynamic comparisions of levofloxacin, ciprofloxacin, and ampicillin against *Streptococcus pneumoniae* in an *in vitro* model infection. *Antimicrob. Agents Chemother.* **43**, 672–677.

177. Thomas, J. K., Forrest, A., Bhavnani, S. M., Hyatt, J. M., Cheng, A., Ballow, C. H., and Schentag, J. J. (1998). Pharmacodynamic evaluation of factors associated with the development of bacteria resistance in acutely ill patients during therapy. *Antimicrob. Agents Chemother.* **42**, 521–527.

178. Doern, G. V., Pfaller, M. A., Erwin, M. E., Brueggemann, A. B., and Jones, R. N. (1998). The prevalence of fluoroquinolone resistance among clinically significant respiratory tract isolates of *Streptococcus pneumoniae* in the United States and Canada—1997 results from the SENTRY Antimicrobial Surveillance Program. *Diag. Microbiol. Infect. Dis.* **32**(4), 313–316.

179. Craig, W. A., and Gunmundsson, S. (1996). Postantibiotic effect. In "Antibiotics in Laboratory Medicine." (V. Lorian, ed.), 4th ed., pp. 296–329. Williams & Wilkins, Baltimore, Maryland.

180. Cars, O., and Odenholt-Tornqvist, I. (1993). The postantibiotic sub-MIC effect in vitro and in vivo. *J. Antimicrob. Chemother.* **31**, 159–166.

181. Guan, L., Blumenthal, R. M., and Burnham, J. C. (1992). Analysis of macromolecular biosynthesis to define the quinolone-induced postantibiotic effect in *Escherichia coli. Antimicrob. Agents Chemother.* **36**(10), 2118–2124.

182. Maggiolo, F., Capra, R., Bartoli, A., Silanos, M. A., Tellarini, M., and Suter, F. (1997). Subinhibitory concentrations of Bay 128039: Pharmacodynamics effect in vitro. *Abstr. 37th Intersci. Conf. Antimicrob. Agents Chemother.*, Toronto. Abstr. #F147.

183. Davidson, R. J., Fuller, J., and Low, D. E. (1998). Pharmacodynamic properties of moxifloxacin, levofloxacin, and clarithromycin in *Streptococcus pneumoniae* and *Haemophilus influenzae*. *Abstr. 38th Intersci. Conf. Antimicrob. Agents Chemother.*, San Diego. Abstr. #E200.

184. Odenholt, E., Lowdins, E., and Cars, O. (1998). In vitro pharmacodynamic studies of grepafloxacin and trovafloxacin. *Abstr. 38th Intersci. Conf. Antimicrob. Agents Chemother.*, San Diego. Abstr. #A107.

185. Moore, T., Kershner, K., Donald, B., Rittenhouse, S., and Coleman, K. (1999). PAE of gemifloxacin and ciprofloxacin against Gram-positive and Gram-negative organisms. *Abstr. 39th Intersci. Conf. Antimicrob. Agents Chemother.*, San Francisco. Abstr. #2298.

186. Licata, L., Smith, C. E., Goldschmidt, R. M., Barrett, J. F., and Frosco, M. (1997). Comparison of the postantibiotic and postantibiotic sub-MIC effects of levofloxacin and ciprofloxacin on *Staphylococcus aureus* and *Streptococcus pneumoniae*. *Antimicrob. Agents Chemother.* **41**(5), 950–955.

187. Spangler, S. K., Lin, G., Jacobs, M. R., and Appelbaum, P. C. (1998). Postantibiotic effect and postantibiotic sub-MIC effect of levofloxacin compared to those of ofloxacin, ciprofloxacin, erythromycin, azithromycin, and clarithromycin against 20 pneumococci. *Antimicrob. Agents Chemother.* **42**(5), 1253–1255.

188. Pankuch, G. A., Jacobs, M. R., and Appelbaum, P. C. (1999). Post-antibiotic and post-antibiotic sub-MIC effect of gatifloxacin against Gram-positive and -negative bacteria. *Abstr. 39th Intersci. Conf. Antimicrob. Agents Chemother.*, San Francisco. Abstr. #538.

189. Clark, C. L., Credito, K. L., Appelbaum, P. C., and Jacobs, M. R. (2000). PAE of gemifloxacin, a novel broad-spectrum quinolone, compared with 11 other drugs against *Haemophilus influenzae* [poster]. *Abstr. 3rd Eur. Cong. Chemother.*, Madrid.

190. Dubois, J., and St.-Pierre, C. (1999). Comparative in vitro activity and PAE of gemifloxacin against *Legionella* spp. [poster]. *Abstr. 21st Int. Cong. Chemother.*, Birmingham, UK. Abstr. #434.

191. Clark, C. L., Credito, K. L., Jacobs, M. R., and Appelbaum, P. C. (2000). PAE of gemifloxacin compared with five other quinolones against pneumococcus [poster]. *Abstr. 3rd Eur. Cong. Chemother.*, Madrid.

CHAPTER 6

Use of Quinolones in Urinary Tract Infection and Prostatitis

LINDSAY E. NICOLLE

Department of Internal Medicine, University of Manitoba, Health Sciences Centre, and St. Boniface Hospital, Winnipeg, Manitoba R3A 1R9

INTRODUCTION

The first fluoroquinolone antimicrobials introduced, including norfloxacin, ciprofloxacin, and ofloxacin, were excreted primarily into the urine, and had an antimicrobial spectrum effective for all important uropathogens. The unique ability to offer oral therapy effective for *Pseudomonas aeruginosa* infection was an important contribution to the management of urinary infection. Thus, the quinolones have been extensively evaluated for use in the treatment of urinary tract infection. All quinolone antimicrobials are effective in the treatment of acute uncomplicated urinary tract infection, with 3 days of therapy the optimal duration. They are also effective as oral or parenteral therapy in the treatment of infections with susceptible organisms of complicated urinary tract infection and acute uncomplicated pyelonephritis. The use of these agents in recurrent complicated infection may, however, be limited by recurrence with resistant organisms. The quinolones offer a theoretical advantage in treatment of prostatitis because of good diffusion into the prostate relative to other antimicrobials. However, a high frequency of relapse of prostatic infection is the norm, even with quinolone therapy. The newer quinolone antimicrobials have an expanded anaerobic and Gram-positive spectrum, but these organisms are less important as uropathogens. Some of these newer agents also have decreased urinary excretion, but studies suggest they are as effective in the treatment of complicated urinary infection and pyelonephritis as the early quinolones.

The quinolone antimicrobials are an important therapeutic option in the management of urinary infection. They are indicated for the treatment of acute uncomplicated urinary infection, acute uncomplicated pyelonephritis, complicated urinary infection, and prostatitis. There is now widespread clinical experience with these agents that documents their importance in antimicrobial therapy of urinary infections.

URINARY TRACT INFECTION

Urinary infection is the most common bacterial infection in adults. As many as 20% of women experience recurrent urinary infection [1], and acute urinary infection is a common reason for hospitalization, especially in older populations [2]. Management of this problem generates considerable costs in physician visits, investigations, hospitalization, and antimicrobial therapy. The diverse clinical presentations of urinary infection include acute uncomplicated urinary tract infection, acute nonobstructive pyelonephritis, complicated urinary tract infection and, in men, prostatitis. In addition, asymptomatic bacteriuria is common [3].

Acute uncomplicated urinary infection is symptomatic lower tract (bladder) infection, or acute cystitis [3]. This syndrome occurs primarily in women with normal genitourinary tracts. The classic clinical presentation includes lower tract symptoms of frequency, urgency, dysuria, and suprapubic discomfort. For some women, frequent recurrent infection is common. The determinants of acute uncomplicated urinary infection are both genetic and behavioral. Sexual intercourse is the most frequent precipitating factor, and the use of spermicides or a diaphragm for birth control increases the frequency of infection. Women with acute uncomplicated urinary infection are effectively treated with a short course of antibiotics, and long-term low-dose or post-intercourse antimicrobial prophylactic therapy may prevent recurrent infection.

Acute nonobstructive pyelonephritis is infection of the kidney, following ascension of organisms from the bladder. It occurs primarily in women who also experience acute uncomplicated urinary infection [3]. The classic clinical manifestations include fever, flank pain, and tenderness with or without associated lower tract symptoms. *E. coli* is isolated in 90% of infections, and strains are characterized by a unique virulence determinant, the P pilus (gal–gal receptor) [4]. Diabetics may be more likely to develop pyelonephritis [2], and diabetics and the elderly are more likely to be bacteremic with pyelonephritis.

Complicated urinary infection occurs in the setting of functional or structural abnormalities of the genitourinary tract [3]. Infections may be asymptomatic or symptomatic. Genitourinary abnormalities lead to recurrent infection by preventing complete voiding, which is the major defense against urinary infection. In addition, some bacteria may establish a nidus in protected environments within the genitourinary tract where antimicrobial therapy cannot eradicate the organism, leading to recurrent infection. Examples include struvite (infection) stones and foreign bodies, such as stents or indwelling catheters, that become coated with bacterial biofilm. Individuals with complicated urinary infection will usually experience frequent recurrent infection if the underlying abnormality cannot be corrected.

Bacterial prostatitis is bacterial infection of the prostate gland [5]. It occurs in men at any age but is more frequent with increasing age. Acute bacterial prostatitis generally occurs in younger men and is associated with high fever, urinary retention, and, occasionally, abscess formation in the prostate. Chronic bacterial prostatitis is more common. It may be asymptomatic. Symptoms are variable, including lower perineal pain and dysuria. Bacteria in the prostate may be a source for recurrent episodes of cystitis in men. Antimicrobial therapy will usually ameliorate acute symptoms but is seldom successful in permanent eradication of bacteria from the prostate [6].

Asymptomatic bacteriuria is common. It increases with increasing age for both men and women but is uncommon in healthy men under 60 years of age [7]. Among elderly institutionalized individuals with multiple comorbidities, the prevalence is 25–50%. Pregnant women with untreated asymptomatic bacteriuria are at increased risk of acute pyelonephritis later in pregnancy, which may precipitate premature labor [8]. Asymptomatic bacteriuria is associated with a high frequency of bacteremia and sepsis following invasive genitourinary procedures [9]. Treatment of asymptomatic bacteriuria in these two clinical situations—pregnancy and invasive genitourinary interventions—prevents adverse outcomes. In other situations, treatment of asymptomatic bacteriuria has not been shown to be effective in improving clinical outcomes, and therapy is not indicated.

The microbiologic diagnosis of urinary infection requires a urine specimen cultured quantitatively that has been collected in a manner to limit contamination [3]. For acute uncomplicated urinary infection, $\geq 10^2$ cfu/ml of any uropathogen, together with pyuria, is sufficient for diagnosis. For acute nonobstructive pyelonephritis, a quantitative count of $\geq 10^4$ cfu/ml of organisms is sufficient for diagnosis. In complicated urinary tract infection $\geq 10^5$ cfu/ml is diagnostic, and asymptomatic bacteriuria is diagnosed if two consecutive specimens with $\geq 10^5$ cfu/ml of the same organism(s) are isolated. The standard diagnostic test for bacterial prostatitis is the triple glass test, which compares quantitative culture and pyuria on urethral, midstream, prostatic massage, and postprostatic massage specimens. This test, however, is of questionable clinical utility, and is infrequently used in clinical practice [10].

The IDSA/FDA guidelines [3] provide specific criteria for assessing efficacy of antimicrobials in clinical trials of urinary tract infection (Table I). Outcome should be determined at both short-term (5–9 days posttherapy) and long-term (4–6 weeks posttherapy) follow-up. Recurrent infection, either relapse with the pretherapy-infecting organism or reinfection with a new organism, is common for many individuals with urinary infection. Anticipated cures are higher for acute uncomplicated urinary infection and acute nonobstructive pyelonephritis than for complicated urinary infection or bacterial prostatitis.

TABLE I   Proposed IDSA/FDA Guidelines for Clinical Trials in Urinary Infection [3]

	Expected cure	
	5–9 days[a]	4–6 weeks[a]
Acute uncomplicated UTI	>85%	60%
Acute pyelonephritis	>80%	>60%
Complicated UTI	>65%	>40%
UTI in men	>75%	>50%
Asymptomatic bacteriuria	>75%	>50%

[a]Posttherapy.

PHARMACOLOGY

The successful treatment of urinary infection requires adequate antimicrobial levels in the urine [11]. Thus, effective antimicrobials are generally excreted into the urine by glomerular filtration or tubular secretion, with limited tubular reabsorption. It has been suggested that tissue rather than urine levels are the determinants of effective therapy of pyelonephritis. Published reports, however, are consistent in suggesting that urinary rather than serum levels predict cure, and antimicrobials such as nitrofurantoin and norfloxacin, which do not achieve therapeutic tissue levels, are effective treatment for pyelonephritis. Back-diffusion of antimicrobials from the concentrated tubular solution into the renal interstitium and infected medullary tissues may contribute to cure in this situation. Treatment of prostatitis is particularly difficult [5]. Most antibiotics diffuse poorly into the prostate, as only lipid-soluble drugs cross the lipid membrane of the prostatic epithelium. The inflammation associated with acute infection increases antimicrobial penetration. Prostatic stones are also common in older men and serve as a nidus from which bacteria cannot be eradicated, leading to recurrent infection.

As a group, the initial quinolone antimicrobials generally achieved high urinary antibiotic levels (Table II). Urinary excretion varied from <50% for pefloxacin to almost 100% for ofloxacin or levofloxacin. Norfloxacin achieves therapeutic levels only in the urine and feces. Several of the quinolones also excrete active metabolites of the parent compound into the urine. Some more recent quinolones with expanded Gram-positive and anaerobic coverage, such as sparfloxacin, trovafloxacin, and grepafloxacin, have low urinary excretion (<10% of active drug), while moxifloxacin and gemifloxacin have somewhat higher excretion. Urinary levels of all these agents, however, still remains above the MICs of most infecting organisms for extended periods.

The reported penetration of quinolones into the prostate is variable [12,19]. Quinolone levels in prostatic fluid are usually <1 mg/liter, but are higher in seminal fluid and prostatic tissue. Concentrations in seminal fluid vary from 2 to 5 mg/liter, and in prostatic adenoma tissue from 1 to 4 µg/g. Prostatic fluid levels are consistently 20–50% of serum levels, while seminal fluid levels are usually about twice serum levels. There is some variability among quinolones in penetration [19]. Ciprofloxacin, enoxacin, and lomefloxacin all produce higher prostatic concentrations than norfloxacin, ofloxacin and fleroxacin.

MICROBIOLOGY

Acute uncomplicated urinary infection and acute nonobstructive pyelonephritis are diseases primarily caused by *Escherichia coli* [3]. This organism is responsible

TABLE II Excretion of Active Antimicrobial into the Urine, and Representative Urinary Levels for Quinolone Antimicrobials [11–18]

Antimicrobial	Urinary excretion[a]	Urinary levels; dose
Ciprofloxacin	65%[a]	>2 µg/ml 12–24 hr; 500 mg
Clinafloxacin	50–72%	14.7–147 mg/l; 25–200 mg
Enoxacin	50–75%[a]	>8 at 24–48 hr; 600 mg
Fleroxacin	44–61%	200–800 mg for 8 hr; 100–200 mg
Gatifloxacin	82–88%	221–953 µg/ml 2–6 hr post; 100–600 mg
Gemifloxacin	20–30%	–
Grepafloxacin	8% in 24 hr	15 µg/ml at 8–12 hr; 400 mg
Lomefloxacin	76% in 24 hr	100–250 µ/ml for 12 hr; 200 mg
Moxifloxacin	18–20% in 48 hr	1.4–137.6 mg/l in first 24 hr; 50–800 mg
Norfloxacin	45–60%[a]	168–417 at 0–3 hr; 400 mg
Ofloxacin/ Levofloxacin	77-95%	126–438 µ/ml 0–3 hr; 100 mg
Pefloxacin	15% parent drug 24–50% metabolities; major norfloxacin	42 µ/ml for 0–24 hr; 800 mg
Sparfloxacin	9–10%	13.7 mg/l over 6 hr; 400 mg
Trovofloxacin	7%	–

[a]Includes active metabolites.

for 75–80% of episodes of acute uncomplicated urinary infection and 90% of episodes of acute nonobstructive pyelonephritis. *Klebsiella pneumoniae*, *Proteus mirabilis*, and *Staphylococcus saprophyticus* are isolated in most non-*E. coli* infections. The bacteriology of complicated urinary infection is more varied [20]. *E. coli* is still frequently isolated, particularly in initial episodes. Recurrent infection is common, and repeated courses of antimicrobial therapy lead to isolation of organisms of increased antimicrobial resistance. *Klebsiella pneumoniae*, *Citrobacter* species, *Enterobacter* species, *Morganella morganii*, *Proteus mirabilis*, *Providencia stuartii*, and *Pseudomonas aeruginosa* are frequently isolated. Gram-positive organisms isolated include *Enterococcus* species, group B streptococci, and coagulase-negative staphylococci. The etiology of bacterial prostatitis is not as well characterized. Generally, organisms isolated in chronic prostatitis are similar to those of complicated urinary infection [5]. For acute bacterial prostatitis, *Staphylococcus aureus* is also a common pathogen.

The Gram-negative uropathogens are included in the bacterial spectrum of the quinolones. For some organisms, particularly *P. aeruginosa*, a quinolone offers a unique advantage, as it may be the only effective oral therapy. *Enterococcus* spp. is an important Gram-positive organism isolated, usually, in complicated urinary infection. Some quinolones, such as ofloxacin and ciprofloxacin, have enterococcal activity, but these agents are not as effective for enterococci as for Gram-negative uropathogens. The expanded spectrum of the new quinolones with improved anaerobic and Gram-positive activity provides little, if any, additional microbiologic benefit in therapy of urinary infection. The improved Gram-positive coverage may, however, provide improved enterococcal coverage.

The microbiologic spectrum of the quinolones is restricted by development of quinolone resistance in some clinical settings. Repeated courses of quinolone therapy for complicated urinary infection, particularly *P. aeruginosa* infection, results in emergence of quinolone-resistant organisms [21]. This may particularly be a problem in the institutional setting, where the prevalence of quinolone resistance may be high due to intense antimicrobial use [22].

CLINICAL STUDIES

LIMITATIONS OF AVAILABLE STUDIES

The pharmacokinetic and susceptibility profiles of the quinolone antimicrobials led these agents to be identified early in clinical development as an important therapeutic advance in the treatment of urinary infection. Many clinical trials have assessed the efficacy of the quinolones in management of urinary infection. Unfortunately, methodological problems make some studies difficult to interpret and compromise a critical assessment of the clinical role for these agents. Problems in trials include lack of blinding, small subject numbers, enrollment of different clinical presentations of urinary infection, failure to provide both short- and long-term outcomes, and lack of relevant antimicrobial comparators. In addition, many clinical trials have been published only in abstract form. In the following discussion, we review a number of published studies that help define the role of quinolone therapy in urinary infection, but we do not summarize all the reported clinical trials.

ACUTE UNCOMPLICATED URINARY INFECTION

Early studies with the quinolones for acute uncomplicated urinary infection evaluated minimal therapeutic courses. Single-dose therapy was studied with

norfloxacin, ciprofloxacin, ofloxacin, enoxacin, fleroxacin, pefloxacin, and rufloxacin (Table III). Generally, single-dose treatment was effective. A consistent
observation in virtually all these studies, however, is failure of single-dose
quinolone therapy for *S. saprophyticus* infection. As this organism is usually the
second most frequently isolated in acute cystitis, quinolone therapy as a single
dose cannot be recommended.

TABLE III   Single-Dose (SD) Therapy for Treatment of Acute Uncomplicated Urinary Infection

		Outcome (% cure)			
		5-9 days		4-6 weeks	
Regimen	Comparator[a]	R[c]	C[d]	R	C
Norfloxacin 800 mg [23]	400 mg b.i.d., 3d	81	94	78[a]	88
Norfloxacin 1200 mg [24]	400 mg b.i.d., 7d	84	98	63[a]	83
Ciprofloxacin 100 mg [25]	250 mg, SD	84	89	74	79
Ciprofloxacin 250 mg [26]	750 mg, SD	81	83	64	74
Ciprofloxacin 250 mg [27]	500 mg, SD	81	93	62	79
Ciprofloxacin 500 mg [28]	250 b.i.d., 7d	89[a]	98	82	93
Enoxacin 600 mg [29]	200 mg b.i.d., 3d	76	89	67	82
Enoxacin 400 mg [30]	Trimethoprim 600 mg, SD	69	85	–	–
Ofloxacin 100 mg [31]	TMP/SMX 160/800, 3–7d	73[a]	93	–	–
Ofloxacin 100 mg [32]	–	94	–	80	–
Ofloxacin 200 mg [33]	TMP/SMX 320/1600	85	71	81	79
	Fosfomycin trometamol 3 g		69		82
Ofloxacin 200 mg [34]	200 mg o.d., 3 d		95		98[a]
	TMP/SMX 160/800 mg 7d	93	92	81	89
Norfloxacin 800 mg [35]	–	88	–	–	–
Ciprofloxacin 500 mg	–	97	–	–	–
Ofloxacin 400 mg	–	97	–	–	–
Fleroxacin 400 mg [36]	Amoxicillin 3g, SD	97	56	–	–
Fleroxacin 400 mg [37]	200 mg o.d., 7d	88	96	91	89
	Ciprofloxacin 250 mg b.i.d., 7d	–	96	–	93
Pefloxacin 800 mg [38]	Norfloxacin 400 mg b.i.d. 5d	88	87	79	72
Peflexacin 800 mg [39]	Rufloxacin 400 mg SD	84	88	85	91
Rufloxacin 400 mg [40]	Norfloxacin 400 b.i.d., 3d	94	99	–	–

[a]Same agent as single-dose (SD) regimen unless other stated.

[b]Significant difference compared to comparator.

[c]R = regimen.

[d]C = comparator.

Three days of therapy for acute uncomplicated urinary infection has been studied for many quinolone antimicrobials (Table IV). Studies consistently show short-term cure rates of ≥85% and 3-day therapy equivalent in outcome to longer courses of 5 or 7 days. Three-day therapy has been effective for *S. saprophyticus* infection in most reports, although one study with lomefloxacin reported relatively poorer cure rates with this organism with 3- compared to 7-day therapy [51]. These clinical trials suggest that 3 days is the optimal duration of therapy

TABLE IV   Studies of 3-Day Therapy for Treatment of Acute Uncomplicated Urinary Infection

| Regimen (3 days) | Comparator[a] | Bacteriologic cure (%) | | | |
| | | 5–9 days | | 4–6 weeks | |
		R	C	R	C
Norfloxacin 400 mg b.i.d. [41]	Naladixic acid 660 mg daily	96	96	89	89
Norfloxacin 400 mg b.i.d. [42]	Naladixic acid 660 mg daily	92[b]	80	–	–
Norfloxacin 400 mg b.i.d. [43]	TMP-SMX DS b.i.d., 10d	96	100	91	95
Norfloxacin 400 mg b.i.d. [44]	400 mg b.i.d., 7d	94	97	81[b]	92
Norfloxacin 400 mg b.i.d. [45]	400 mg b.i.d., 7d	92	95	82	88
Ofloxacin 200 mg b.i.d. [46]	200 mg b.i.d., 7d	96	91	88	86
	Ofloxacin 300 mg b.i.d., 7d		96		100
	TMP/SMX DS b.i.d., 7d		93		88
Ofloxacin 200 mg o.d. [47]	TMP/SMX DS b.i.d., 7d	85	82	–	–
Ofloxacin 200 mg b.i.d. [48]	Cefixime 400 mg o.d., 3d	86	83	80	77
Ofloxacin 100 mg b.i.d. [49]	Cefuroxime axetil 125/b.i.d., 3d	89	80	–	–
Enoxacin 200 mg b.i.d. [50]	Cefuroxime axetil 125 b.i.d., 7d	86	71	75	50
Ciprofloxacin 100 mg b.i.d. [27]	250 b.i.d., 7d	93	92	87	85
Ciprofloxacin 250 mg b.i.d.		90	–	76	–
Ciprofloxacin 500 mg o.d.	500 o.d., 5d	92	90	80	71
	Norfloxacin 400 mg b.i.d., 7d		94		84
Lomefloxacin 400 mg o.d. [51]	400 mg o.d., 7d	88	93	81	82
	Norfloxacin 400 mg b.i.d., 7d		93		85
Lomefloxacin 400 mg o.d. [52]	Norfloxacin 400 mg b.i.d., 3d	91	95	87	89
Temafloxacin 400 mg o.d. [53]	Ciprofloxacin 400 mg b.i.d., 7 d	97	96	–	–
Gemifloxacin 320 mg o.d.[c]	Ciprofloxacin 250 mg b.i.d.	95	94	–	–
Levofloxacin 250 mg o.d.[d]	Ofloxacin 200 mg b.i.d.	98	97	–	–

[a]Same antimicrobial as 3-day agent unless stated.

[b]Significant difference between regimens.

[c]*Abstr. 3rd Eur. Cong. Chemother.*, Madrid, 2000.

[d]*Abstr. 38th Intersci. Conf. Antimicrob. Agents Chemother.*, San Diego.

with quinolones for acute uncomplicated urinary infection. Whether 3-day therapy is the optimal duration for postmenopausal women has not been adequately evaluated. Comparative studies with antimicrobials of other classes are limited, and it is difficult to comment on the relative effectiveness of quinolones. The different quinolone antimicrobials, however, are likely equivalent for treatment of acute uncomplicated urinary infection. The quinolones have also been evaluated for longer courses of therapy of 5–10 days [12,54] (Tables III and IV), and, while effective, these longer courses do not seem to offer an advantage over 3-day therapy. The Infectious Diseases Society of America (IDSA) guidelines suggest that 3 days is the optimal duration, and that evidence supports the use of norfloxacin, ciprofloxacin, ofloxacin, or fleroxacin [55].

Acute uncomplicated urinary infection is characterized by recurrence, sometimes at a high frequency. Recurrent infection is usually reinfection with bacterial flora colonizing the gut, vagina, and periurethral area. Early recurrent infection may be less likely to occur if antimicrobial therapy for treatment of the acute episode is effective in eradicating uropathogens from the gut and vaginal reservoirs. Ofloxacin given for 3 or 7 days was as effective as TMP/SMX treatment in suppressing rectal and vaginal *E. coli* colonization [44]. Norfloxacin was more effective than trimethoprim–sulfamethoxazole in eradicating the infecting organism from fecal flora after 7-day therapy, with TMP/SMX associated with more frequent emergence of resistance and reinfections [56]. In another study, however, TMP/SMX had equivalent efficacy to norfloxacin in eradicating colonizing bacteria [57]. Thus, quinolone therapy has been shown to be effective in decreasing colonization when used in treatment of acute uncomplicated urinary infection.

Recurrent infection may be prevented by prophylactic low-dose antimicrobial therapy, given either post-intercourse or daily, or thrice weekly for several months. Norfloxacin given as 200 mg daily is effective as prophylaxis for at least 12 months [58], and was significantly more effective than nitrofurantoin in preventing symptomatic recurrences in one study [59]. In a second study, norfloxacin was equivalent to nitrofurantoin in preventing symptomatic episodes, but significantly more effective in suppressing potential uropathogens in fecal flora [60]. Ciprofloxacin prophylaxis was effective as either 125 mg daily or post-intercourse and significantly decreased symptomatic episodes compared to the period prior to prophylactic therapy [61]. The post-intercourse prophylactic regimen, however, required use of only one-third the amount of drug. Ofloxacin 100 mg, norfloxacin 200 mg, or ciprofloxacin 125 mg were equally effective as single-dose post-intercourse prophylaxis [62]. Other quinolone antimicrobials are also likely effective for prophylaxis of acute uncomplicated urinary infection, but clinical trials to support efficacy have not been reported.

ACUTE NONOBSTRUCTIVE PYELONEPHRITIS

There are relatively few reported studies that have restricted subject enrollment to patients with the clinical syndrome of acute nonobstructive pyelonephritis (Table V). These patients have, however, often been included in trials of complicated urinary infection. In studies restricted to pyelonephritis, two comparative studies of norfloxacin with TMP/SMX enrolled small study numbers, but reported equivalence of these regimens [63,64]. Norfloxacin had significantly better cure rates than cefadroxil [65] and loracarbef [66], consistent with previous studies suggesting lower efficacy of β-lactam antibiotics in treatment of pyelonephritis [71]. Two studies evaluating ciprofloxacin [67,68] are difficult to assess as a 5-day course of therapy was used rather than the 10–14 days recommended

TABLE V   Studies of Quinolone Therapy in the Treatment of Acute Uncomplicated Pyelonephritis

| Regimen | Comparator | Bacteriologic outcome (% cure) | | | |
| | | 5–9 days | | 4–6 weeks | |
		R	C	R	C
Norfloxacin 400 b.i.d., 10d [63]	TMP/SMX DS b.i.d. 10d	100	100	86	90
Norfloxacin 400 b.i.d., 7d [64]	TMP/SMX DS b.i.d. 10d	67	92	–	–
Norfloxacin 400 b.i.d., 14d [65]	Cefadroxil 1g b.i.d., 14d	91	59%[a]	82	44%[a]
Norfloxacin 400 mg b.i.d. [66]	loracarbef 400 mg b.i.d.	81	88	83	64%[a]
Ciprofloxacin 100 mg IV → 250 po b.i.d.; 5d [67]	Netilmicin 2 mg/kg q.12 hr, 5d	88	88	65	82
Ciprofloxacin 250 b.i.d. 5d after gentamicin 10 mg/kg/dose [68]	Ciprofloxacin 250 b.i.d., to 5 days after stable on gentamicin	94	92	–	–
Ciprofloxacin 500 mg b.i.d. [69]	Rufloxacin 200 mg o.d.	83	64	72	78
Lomefloxacin 400 mg b.i.d. [70]	TMP/SMX DS b.i.d.	100	89%[a]	80	67
Gemifloxacin 320 mg o.d.[b]	Levofloxacin 250 mg o.d.	100	87	–	–

[a]Significant difference.

[b]Abstr. 3rd Eur. Cong. Chemother., Madrid, 2000.

as standard duration [3]. These two studies do suggest equivalence of oral quinolone therapy with parenteral therapy of aminoglycosides, which was also given for only 5 days. Lomefloxacin was superior in outcome to TMP/SMX at short-term follow-up in one trial [70], but the two regimens were equivalent at long-term follow-up. In a study available in abstract only, gemifloxacin was superior to levofloxacin at short-term follow-up for treatment of pyelonephritis.

In aggregate, these studies suggest that oral quinolone therapy with norflox-acin, ciprofloxacin, or lomefloxacin is effective for treatment of acute pyelo-nephritis, with short- and long-term outcomes meeting the standards of the FDA/IDSA guidelines [3]. Quinolone therapy is likely superior to β-lactam therapy, and of equal efficacy with TMP/SMX for susceptible organisms [55]. Ofloxacin, levofloxacin, enoxacin, fleroxacin, pefloxacin, and gemifloxacin are also likely effective for treatment of acute pyelonephritis. Quinolones with very low renal clearance require further clinical evaluation for treatment of this syndrome to determine their efficacy.

COMPLICATED URINARY INFECTION

Quinolones are effective for treatment of complicated urinary infection caused by susceptible organisms (Table VI). Treatment duration varies from 7 to 14 days. Relapse and reinfection rates remain high, approaching 50% by 6 weeks. This is the anticipated outcome when the underlying genitourinary abnormalities that promote infection have not been reversed [3]. Comparative studies between two quinolones, or with antibiotics of other classes, have usually reported equivalence, although occasional studies report significantly improved outcomes for qui-nolones at short- or long-term follow-up, but not both [75,78,82,90,98]. In one comparative trial, ciprofloxacin was superior to sparfloxacin at short-term follow-up, raising the possibility that the newer quinolones with decreased renal clearance are not as effective in treatment of complicated urinary infection as the earlier agents [98]. Thus, the newer, expanded-spectrum quinolones require further evaluation in the treatment of this syndrome.

P. aeruginosa is frequently isolated in recurrent complicated urinary infection. This organism warrants special consideration, as quinolones are usually the only oral therapy effective for *P. aeruginosa* infection, and resistance frequently develops during antimicrobial therapy. Some studies have specifically addressed treatment of *P. aeruginosa* infection [83,84]. Emergence of resistance of *P. aeruginosa* to a quinolone while on therapy has been repeatedly reported, with rates up to 18% observed [99]. This is most likely to occur in the face of persistent genitourinary abnormalities, including foreign bodies such as catheters or stents.

Infrequently, suppressive therapy is indicated for the management of compli-cated urinary infection when underlying abnormalities cannot be corrected.

Quinolones have been evaluated for prolonged, suppressive therapy for subjects with recurrent relapsing infection. Therapy of 3 months or longer with norfloxacin maintained sterility of urine more effectively than 1 month of norfloxacin followed by placebo [100]. In another study, norfloxacin 400 mg b.i.d. for 3 months was compared with 400 mg daily for the final 2 months [99]. This study reported surprisingly high cure rates of 75 and 83% at 2 months posttherapy, but longer follow-up is necessary. Finally, ciprofloxacin, 100 mg at bedtime for 6 months decreased the frequency of symptomatic infection in subjects with spinal cord injury and was not associated with recurrent infection with resistant organisms [101]. Thus, norfloxacin and ciprofloxacin are effective in the limited situations when prolonged therapy is appropriate for management of recurrent complicated urinary infection.

BACTERIAL PROSTATITIS

Bacterial prostatitis is a difficult entity to diagnose clinically and microbiologically, and difficult to treat. There are few studies that specifically evaluate treatment of prostatic infection, although studies of recurrent urinary infection in elderly men will frequently include a high proportion with associated prostatic infection. Norfloxacin [102], ciprofloxacin [103,104], ofloxacin [82], pefloxacin [105], temafloxacin [106,107], and rufloxacin [108] have been evaluated for the treatment of prostatitis. Schaeffer and Darras [102] treated 15 men with prostatitis who had failed prior regimens of TMP/SMX or indanyl carbenicillin with 28 days of norfloxacin 400 mg b.i.d. Five (36%) of 14 with follow-up relapsed less than 2 months posttherapy, and 3 (21%) had reinfections at 1 week to 3 years posttherapy. Thus, only 43% had long-term cures. In a comparative study of norfloxacin with trimethoprim–sulfamethoxazole, each given for 4–6 weeks, Sabbaj et al. [75] reported cure rates of 92% for norfloxacin and 67% for TMP/SMX at 1 to 3 weeks posttherapy in 40 men with positive expressed prostatic secretions. A longer follow-up, however, is needed for adequate evaluation of efficacy. Weidner and Schiefer reported 9 (60%) of 15 men with chronic bacterial prostatitis who had previously failed treatment with TMP/SMX or TMP had eradication after 2 weeks therapy with ciprofloxacin, but the duration of follow-up was not stated [103]. In a second study [104], their group reported 10 (63%) men who had failed previous therapy but remained cured at 21- to 36-month follow-up after treatment with ciprofloxacin 500 mg b.i.d. for 4 weeks. Cox [87] reported that ofloxacin and indanyl carbenicillin had similar bacteriologic outcomes (100%) in 23 patients, but the follow-up (5–9 days) was too short to be relevant. Guibert et al. [105] reported that 23 (74%) of 31 patients treated with pefloxacin 400 mg b.i.d. for 3 to 105 days (median 28 days) were cured, but follow-up was only 4 weeks. Cox [106] reported cure rates of 86% at 4 weeks

TABLE VI Studies of Quinolone Therapy for the Treatment of Complicated Urinary Tract Infection

| Comparator | Special features | Bacteriologic cure (%) | | | |
| | | 5–9 days | | 4–6 weeks | |
		Quin.	Comp.	Quin.	Comp.
Norfloxacin 400 mg b.i.d.					
Amoxicillin 500 mg t.i.d. [72]	Geriatric, symptomatic and asymptomatic	95	75	–	–
TMP/SMX 160/800 b.i.d. [73]	Combined; 3 comparative, one open study	75	62	33	25
None [74]	Men only	75	N/A	–	N/A
TMP/SMX 160/800 mg b.i.d. [75]	Recurrent UTI, men; 4-6 weeks therapy	–	–	93	80*
None [76]	Spinal cord injured	50	–	16	–
Standard parenteral regimens [77]	Hospital-acquired	96	88	–	–
Standard parenteral regimens [78]	Hospital-acquired	100	88	–	–
Ciprofloxacin 250-500 mg b.i.d.					
TMP/SMX 160/800 mg b.i.d. [79]	Ambulatory urology patients	88	86	68	67
TMP/SMX 160/800 mg b.i.d. [80]	Hospital inpatient	–	–	88; 94	87
TMP 100 b.i.d. [81]	Geriatric patients, some asymptomatic	94	75	75	56
Parenteral aminoglycoside [82]	Catheterized subjects	63	15*	21	23
None [83]	P. aeruginosa only	89	NA	64	NA
None [84]	P. aeruginosa only	–	NA	44	NA
Norfloxacin 400 mg b.i.d. [85]		79	72	–	–
Ofloxacin 300 mg b.i.d.					
Rufloxacin 200 mg o.d. [86]		81	90	–	–
Carbenicillin 765 mg q6h [87]		100	75	–	–
TMP/SMX [87]		92	95	–	–

Regimen	Comments				
Enoxacin 200, 400 mg b.i.d.					
None [88]	Elderly	90	NA	69	NA
Lomefloxacin 400 mg o.d.					
Norfloxacin 400 b.i.d. [89]		86	74	74	48
TMP/SMX 160/800 mg b.i.d. [90]		88	52*	64	47
Ciprofloxacin 500 mg b.i.d. [91]		97	96	–	–
Fleroxacin 400 mg o.d. po or i.v.					
Ofloxacin 200 mg b.i.d. [92]	Hospitalized	80	91	–	–
Ceftazidime 1.5–6 g daily [93]	Includes pyelonephritis	94	95	82	85
None [94]	Sequential i.v.–p.o.	81	NA	–	–
None [95]	Sequential i.v.–p.o.	–	NA	65	NA
Pefloxacin 400 mg b.i.d.					
Cefotaxime 1 g t.i.d. [96]		92	82	68	80
Temafloxacin 400 mg b.i.d.					
Norfloxacin 400 mg b.i.d. [97]		95	96	–	–
Sparfloxacin 100 mg o.d.					
Ciprofloxacin 500 mg b.i.d. [98]		73	81*	63	67
Gatifloxacin 400 mg o.d.**					
Ciprofloxacn 500 mg o.d.	Includes pyelonephritis	88	83	77	72
Gemifloxacin 320 mg o.d.†					
Levofloxacin 250 mg o.d.		87	86	–	–

*Significant difference between regimens.

**Abstr. 39th Intersci. Conf. Antimicrob. Agents Chemother., San Francisco.

†Abstr. 3rd Eur. Cong. Chemother., Madrid, 2000.

posttreatment with temafloxacin 400 mg b.i.d. for 28 days in 112 men with chronic bacterial prostatitis, but Naber *et al.* [107] reported cure of only 68% at a similar time in 61 men treated with the same regimen. Finally, Boerema *et al.* [108] reported cure rates of 79% at 4 weeks posttherapy in 27 men treated with rufloxacin 200 mg daily for 4 weeks for chronic bacterial prostatitis.

There are too few studies to allow an assessment of the comparative effectiveness of quinolones with other agents in the treatment of bacterial prostatitis. The limited information suggests that, despite an apparent advantage of diffusion into the prostate, the overall efficacy of treatment with quinolones is not substantially different from other antimicrobials, particularly TMP/SMX. This reflects the difficulties inherent in diagnosing and managing this clinical problem. It is anticipated that at least 50% of individuals will relapse within 3 months of discontinuation of therapy, even when therapy is extended as long as 4 to 12 weeks. Even with the availability of the quinolone antimicrobials, chronic bacterial prostatitis remains a frustrating clinical challenge.

CONCLUSION

The pharmacokinetic properties and microbiologic spectrum of the quinolones make these agents important in the management of urinary tract infection. Studies of different clinical presentations of urinary infection have consistently documented the efficacy of quinolone antimicrobials in the management of urinary tract infection. They offer a unique advantage in treating urinary infection in cases where the infecting organism is resistant to other available oral antimicrobials. Where the underlying organism is susceptible, outcomes with quinolone therapy are generally equivalent to other agents, particularly trimethoprim–sulfamethoxazole. The effectiveness of quinolones is, however, limited by resistance emergence in some particularly complicated infections, and by the inherent limitations of any antimicrobial therapy when persistent genitourinary abnormalities promote infection, or with bacterial prostatitis. This class of drugs is, however, an important addition to the antimicrobial options available for treatment of urinary infection and prostatitis, and is widely used for these indications.

REFERENCES

1. Johnson, J. R., and Stamm, W. E. (1989). Urinary tract infections in women: Diagnosis and treatment. *Ann. Intern. Med.* **111**, 906–917.

2. Nicolle, L. E., Friesen, D., Harding, G. K. M., and Roos, L. L. (1996). Hospitalization for acute pyelonephritis in Manitoba, Canada, during the period from 1989–1992: Impact of diabetes, pregnancy, and aboriginal origin. *Clin. Infect. Dis.* **22**, 1051–1056.

3. Rubin, R. H., Shapiro, E. D., Andriole, V. T., Davis, R. J., and Stamm, W. E. (1992). Evaluation of new anti-infective drugs for the treatment of urinary tract infection. *Clin. Infect. Dis.* **15** (Suppl. 1), S216–S227.

4. Johnson, J. R. (1991). Virulence factors in *Escherichia coli* urinary tract infection. *Clin. Microbiol. Rev.* **4**, 80–128.

5. Nickel, J. C. (1996). Prostatitis. In "Antibiotic Therapy in Urology" (S. G. Mulholland, ed.), pp. 57–69. Lippincott-Raven, Philadelphia.

6. Leigh, D. A. (1993). Prostatitis: An increasing problem for diagnosis and management. *J. Antimicrob. Chemother.* **32** (Suppl. A), 1–9.

7. Nicolle, L. E. (in press). Asymptomatic bacteriuria in the elderly. *Infect. Dis. Clin. N. Amer.*

8. Nicolle, L. E. (1994). Screening for asymptomatic bacteriuria in pregnancy. In "The Canadian Guide to Clinical Preventive Health Care" (The Canadian Task Force on the Periodic Health Exam), pp. 100–107. Health Canada, Canada Communication Group.

9. Cafferkey, M. T., Falkener, F. R., Gillespie, W. A., *et al.* (1982). Antibiotics for the prevention of septicaemia in urology. *J. Antimicrob. Chemother.* **9**, 471–476.

10. Lipsky, B. A. (1989). Urinary tract infections in men: Epidemiology, pathophysiology, diagnosis, and treatment. *Ann. Intern. Med.* **110**, 138–150.

11. Nicolle, L. E. (1996). Measurement and significance of antibiotic activity in the urine. In "Antibiotics in Laboratory Medicine," 4th ed. (V. Lorian, ed.), pp. 793–812. Williams & Wilkins, Baltimore.

12. Naber, K. G. (1989). Use of quinolones in urinary tract infections and prostatitis. *Rev. Infect. Dis.* **11** (Suppl. 5), S1321–S1337.

13. Child, J., Andrews, J. M., and Wise, R. (1995). Pharmacokinetics and tissue penetration of the new fluoroquinolone grepafloxacin. *Antimicrob. Agents Chemother.* **39**, 513–515.

14. Montay, G. (1996). Pharmacokinetics of sparfloxacin in healthy volunteers and patients: A review. *J. Antimicrob. Chemother.* **37** (Suppl. A), 27–40.

15. Nakashima, M., Uematsu, T., Kosuge, K., Kusajima, H., Ooie, T., Masuda, Y., Ishida, R., and Uchida, H. (1995). Single and multiple dose pharmacokinetics of AM-1155, a new 6-fluoro-8-methoxy quinolone, in humans. *Antimicrob. Agents Chemother.* **39**, 2635–2640.

16. Allen, A., Vousden, M., Porter, A., and Lewis, A. (1999). Effect of Maalox on the bioavailability of oral gemifloxacin in healthy volunteers. *Chemotherapy* **45**, 504–511.

17. Stass, H., Dalhoff, A., Kubitza, D., and Schuhly, U. (1998). Pharmacokinetics, safety, and tolerability of ascending single doses of moxifloxacin, a new 8-methoxy quinolone, administered to healthy subjects. *Antimicrob. Agents Chemother.* **42**, 2060–2065.

18. Bron, N. J., Dorr, M. B., Mant, T. G., Webb, C. L., and Vassos, A. B. (1996). The tolerance and pharmacokinetics of clinafloxacin in healthy subjects. *J. Antimicrob. Chemother.* **38**, 1023–1029.

19. Andriole, V. T. (1991). Use of quinolones in treatment of prostatitis and lower urinary tract infections. *Eur. J. Clin. Microbiol. Infect. Dis.* **10**, 342–350.

20. Nicolle, L. E. (1997). A practical guide to the management of complicated urinary tract infections. *Drugs* **53**, 583–592.

21. Ena, J., Amador, C., Martinez, C., and Oritz de la Table, V. (1995). Risk factors for acquisition of urinary tract infections caused by ciprofloxacin resistant *Escherichia coli*. *J. Urol.* **153**, 117–120.

22. Flournoy, D. J. (1994). Antimicrobial susceptibilities from nursing home residents in Oklahoma. *Gerontology* **40**, 53–56.

23. Saginur, R., Nicolle, L. E., and the Canadian Infectious Diseases Society Clinical Trials Study Group (1992). Single-dose compared with 3-day norfloxacin treatment of uncomplicated urinary tract infection in women. *Arch. Intern. Med.* **152**, 1233–1237.

24. Arau-Boger, R., Leibovici, L., and Danon, Y. L. (1994). Urinary tract infections with low and high colony counts in young women. *Arch. Intern. Med.* **154**, 300–304.

25. Garlando, F., Rietiker, S., Tauber, M. G., Flepp, M., Meier, B., and Luthy, R. (1987). Single-dose ciprofloxacin at 100 versus 250 mg for treatment of uncomplicated urinary tract infections in women. *Antimicrob. Agents Chemother.* **31**, 354–356.

26. Raz, R., Rottensterich, E., Hefter, H., Kennes, Y., and Potasman, I. (1989). Single-dose ciprofloxacin in the treatment of uncomplicated urinary tract infection in women. *Eur. J. Clin. Microbiol. Infect. Dis.* **8**, 1040–1042.

27. Karachalios, G. N., Georgiopoulos, A. N., Nasopoulou-Papadimitriou, D. D., and Adracta, D. J. (1991). Value of single-dose ciprofloxacin in the treatment of acute uncomplicated urinary tract infection in women. *Drugs Exp. Clin. Res.* **17**, 521–524.

28. Iravani, A., Tice, A. D., McCarty, J., Sikes, D. H., Nolen, T., Gallis, H. A., Whalen, E. P., Tosiello, R. L., Heyd, A., Kowalsky, S. F., Echols, R. M., and the Urinary Tract Infection Study Group (1995). Short courses of ciprofloxacin treatment for acute uncomplicated urinary tract infection in women: The minimum effective dose. *Arch. Intern. Med.* **155**, 485–494.

29. Backhouse, C. I., and Matthews, J. A. (1989). Single-dose enoxacin compared with 3-day treatment for urinary tract infection. *Antimicrob. Agents Chemother.* **33**, 877–880.

30. Bailey, R. R., Gorrie, S. I., Peddie, B. A., and Davies, P. R. (1987). Double-blind, randomized trial comparing single dose enoxacin and trimethoprim for treatment of bacterial cystitis. *N.Z. Med. J.* **100**, 618–619.

31. o.d.e, B., Walder, M., and Forsgren, A. (1987). Failure of a single dose of 100 mg ofloxacin in lower urinary tract infections in females. *Scand. J. Infect. Dis.* **19**, 677–679.

32. Raz, R., Genesin, J., Gonen, E., Shmilovitz, M., Hefter, H., and Potasman, I. (1988). Single low-dose ofloxacin for the treatment of uncomplicated urinary tract infection in young women. *J. Antimicrob. Chemother.* **22**, 945–949.

33. Naber, K. G., and Thyroff-Friesinger, U. (1990). Fosfomycin trometamol versus ofloxacin/cotrimoxazole as single-dose therapy of acute uncomplicated urinary tract infection in females: A multicentre study. *Infection* **18** (Suppl. 2), S70–S76.

34. Hooton, T. M., Johnson, C., Winter, C., Kuwamura, L., Rogers, M. E., Roberts, P. L., and Stamm, W. E. (1991). Single-dose and three-day regimens of ofloxacin versus trimethoprim–sulfamethoxazole for acute cystitis in women. *Antimicrob. Agents Chemother.* **35**, 1479–1483.

35. Pfau, A., and Sacks, T. G. (1993). Single-dose quinolone treatment in acute uncomplicated urinary tract infection in women. *J. Urol.* **149**, 532–534.

36. Whitby, M., Brown, P., Silagy, C., and Rana, C. (1993). Comparison of fleroxacin and amoxicillin in the treatment of uncomplicated urinary tract infections in women. *Am. J. Med.* **94** (Suppl. 3A), 97S–100S.

37. Iravani, A. (1993). Multicenter study of single-dose and multiple-dose fleroxacin versus ciprofloxacin in the treatment of uncomplicated urinary tract infections. *Am. J. Med.* **94** (Suppl. 3A), 89S–96S.

38. Van Balen, F. A. M., Touw-Otten, F. W. M. M., and deMelker, R. A. (1990). Single-dose pefloxacin versus five-day treatment with norfloxacin in uncomplicated cystitis in women. *J. Antimicrob. Chemother.* **26** (Suppl. B), 153–160.

39. Jardin, A., and Cesana, M. (1995). French Multicenter Urinary Tract Infection Rufloxacin group: Randomized, double-blind comparison of single-dose regimens of rufloxacin and pefloxacin for acute, uncomplicated cystitis in women. *Antimicrob. Agents Chemother.* **39**, 215–220.

40. Del Rio, G., Dalet, F., Aguilar, L., Caffaratti, J., and Dal-Rem, R. (1996). Single-dose rufloxacin versus 3-day norfloxacin treatment of uncomplicated cystitis: Clinical evaluation and pharmacodynamic considerations. *Antimicrob. Agents Chemother.* **40**, 408–412.

41. Reeves, D. S., Lacey, R. W., Mummey, R. V., Mahemdra, M., Bint, A. J., and Nervsom, S. W. B. (1984). Treatment of acute urinary infection by norfloxacin or nalidixic acid/citrate: A multi-centre comparative study. *J. Antimicrob. Chemother.* **13** (Suppl. B), 99–105.

42. Vogel, R., Deaney, N. B., Round, E. M., Vanden Burg, M. J., and Currie, W. J. C. (1984). Norfloxacin, amoxycillin, cotrimoxazole and nalidixic acid: A summary of 3-day and 7-day therapy studies in the treatment of urinary tract infections. *J. Antimicrob. Chemother.* **13** (Suppl. B), 113–120.

43. Stein, G. E., Mummaur, N., Goldstein, E. J. C., *et al.* (1987). A multicenter comparative trial of three-day norfloxacin vs. ten-day sulfamethoxazole and trimethoprim for the treatment of uncomplicated urinary tract infections. *Arch. Intern. Med.* **147**, 1760–1762.

44. The Inter-Nordic Urinary Tract Infection Study Group (1988). Double-blind comparison of 3-day versus 7-day treatment with norfloxacin in symptomatic urinary tract infections. *Scand. J. Infect. Dis.* **20**, 619–624.

45. Trienekens, T. A. M., London, N. H. H. J., Houben, A. W., de Jong, R. A. M., and Stobberingh, E. E. (1993). Treating acute urinary tract infections: An RCT of 3-day versus 7-day norfloxacin. *Can. Fam. Phys.* **39**, 514–518.

46. Hooton, T. M., Latham, R. H., Wong, E. S., Johnson, C., Roberts, P. L., and Stamm, W. E. (1989). Ofloxacin versus trimethoprim–sulfamethoxazole for treatment of acute cystitis. *Antimicrob. Agents Chemother.* **33**, 1308–1312.

47. Basista, M. P. (1991). Randomized study to evaluate efficacy and safety of ofloxacin vs. trimethoprim and sulfamethoxazole in treatment of uncomplicated urinary tract infection. *Urology* **37** (Suppl.), 21–27.

48. Raz, R., Rottensterich, E., Leshem, Y., and Tabenkin, H. (1994). Double-blind study comparing 3-day regimens of cefixime and ofloxacin in treatment of uncomplicated urinary tract infections in women. *Antimicrob. Agents Chemother.* **38**, 1176–1177.

49. Naber, K. G., and Koch, E. M. W. (1993). Cefuroxime axetil vs. ofloxacin for short-term therapy of acute uncomplicated lower urinary tract infections in women. *Infection* **21**, 34–45.

50. Brumfitt, W., Hamilton-Miller, M. T., and Walker, S. (1993). Enoxacin relieves symptoms of recurrent urinary infections more rapidly than cefuroxime axetil. *Antimicrob. Agents Chemother.* **37**, 1558–1559.

51. Neringer, R., Forsgren, A., Hansson, C., o.d.c, B., and the South Swedish Lolex Study Group (1992). Lomefloxacin versus norfloxacin in the treatment of uncomplicated urinary tract infections: Three day versus seven day treatment. *Scand. J. Infect. Dis.* **24**, 773–780.

52. Nicolle, L. E., Dubois, J., Martel, A. Y., Harding, G. K. M., Shafran, S. D., and Conly, J. M. (1993). Treatment of acute uncomplicated urinary tract infections with 3 days of lomefloxacin compared with treatment with 3 days of norfloxacin. *Antimicrob. Agents Chemother.* **37**, 574–579.

53. Stein, G. E., and Philip, E. (1992). Comparison of three-day temafloxacin with seven-day ciprofloxacin treatment of urinary tract infections in women. *J. Fam. Pract.* **34**, 180–185.

54. Malenverni, R., and Glauser, M. P. (1988). Comparative studies of fluoroquinolones in the treatment of urinary tract infections. *Rev. Infect. Dis.* **10**, S153–S163.

55. Warren, J. W., Abrutyn, E., Hebel, J. R., Johnson, J. R., Schaeffer, A. J., and Stamm, W. E. (1999). Guidelines for antimicrobial treatment of uncomplicated acute bacterial cystitis and acute pyelonephritis in women. *Clin. Infect. Dis.* **29**, 745–758.

56. Haase, D. A., Harding, G. K. M., Thomson, M. J., Kennedy, J. K., Urias, B. A., and Ronald, A. R. (1984). Comparative trial of norfloxacin and trimethoprim–sulfamethoxazole in the treatment of women with localized acute, symptomatic urinary tract infections and antimicrobial effect on periurethral and fecal microflora. *Antimicrob. Agents Chemother.* **26**, 481–484.

57. Schaeffer, A. J., and Sisney, G. A. (1985). Efficacy of norfloxacin in urinary tract infections: Biological effects on vaginal and fecal flora. *J. Urol.* **133**, 628–630.

58. Nicolle, L. E., Harding, G. K. M., Thomson, M., Kennedy, J., Urias, B., and Ronald, A. R. (1989). Prospective randomized, placebo-controlled trial of norfloxacin for the prophylaxis of recurrent urinary tract infection in women. *Antimicrob. Agents Chemother.* **33**, 1032–1035.

59. Raz, R., and Boger, S. (1991). Long-term prophylaxis with norfloxacin versus nitrofurantoin in women with recurrent urinary tract infection. *Antimicrob. Agents Chemother.* **35**, 1241–1242.

60. Brumfitt, W., Hamilton-Miller, J. M. T., Smith, G. W., and Al-Wali, W. (1991). Comparative trial of norfloxacin and macrocrystalline nitrofurantoin in the prophylaxis of recurrent urinary tract infection in women. *Quart. J. Med. New Series* **81**, 811–820.

61. Melebos, M. D., Asbach, H. W., Gerbarz, E., Zarakovitis, I. E., Weingaertner, K., and Naber, K. G. (1997). Post-intercourse versus daily ciprofloxacin prophylaxis for recurrent urinary tract infections in pre-menopausal women. *J. Urol.* **157**, 935–939.

62. Pfau, A., and Sacks, T. G. (1994). Effective postcoital quinolone prophylaxis of recurrent urinary tract infections in women. *J. Urol.* **152**, 136–138.

63. Guerra, J. G., Falconi, E., Balomino, J. C., Benaviali, L., and Antunez de Mayolo, E. (1983). Clinical evaluation of norfloxacin versus co-trimoxazole in urinary tract infections. *Eur. J. Clin. Microbiol. Infect. Dis.* **2**, 260–265.

64. Sabbaj, J., Hougland, J. L., and Shih, W. J. (1985). Multiclinic comparative study of norfloxacin and trimethoprim–sulfamethoxazole for treatment of urinary tract infections. *Antimicrob. Agents Chemother.* **27**, 297–301.

65. Sandberg, T., Englund, G., Lincoln, K., and Nilsson, L.-G. (1990). Randomized double-blind study of norfloxacin and cefadroxil in the treatment of acute pyelonephritis. *Eur. J. Clin. Microbiol. Infect. Dis.* **9**, 317–323.

66. Hyslop, D. L., and Bischoff, W. (1992). Loracarbef versus cefaclor and norfloxacin in the treatment of uncomplicated pyelonephritis. *Am. J. Med.* **92** (Suppl. 6A), 86S–94S.

67. Bailey, R. R., Lynn, K. L., Robson, R. A., Peddie, B. A., and Smith, A. (1992). Comparison of ciprofloxacin with netilmicin for the treatment of acute pyelonephritis. *N.Z. Med. J.* **115**, 102–103.

68. Bailey, R. R., Begg, E. J., Smith, A. H., Robson, R. A., Lynn, K. L., Chambers, S. T., Barday, M. L., and Hornibrook, J. (1996). Prospective, randomized, controlled study comparing two dosing regimens of gentamicin/oral ciprofloxacin switch therapy for acute pyelonephritis. *Clin. Nephrol.* **46**, 183–186.

69. Bach, D., Berg-Segers, A., Hubner, A., Breukeler, G., Cesana, M., and Pletan, Y. (1995). Rufloxacin once daily versus ciprofloxacin twice daily in the treatment of patients with acute uncomplicated pyelonephritis. *J. Urol.* **154**, 19–24.

70. Mouton, Y., Ajana, F., Chidiac, C., Capron, M. H., Home, P., and Masquelier, A.-M. (1992). A multicenter study of lomefloxacin and trimethoprim–sulfamethoxazole in the treatment of uncomplicated acute pyelonephritis. *Am. J. Med.* **92** (Suppl. 4A), 87S–90S.

71. Penson, A. G., Philbrick, J. T., Lindbeck, G. H., and Schorling, J. B. (1992). Oral antibiotic therapy for acute pyelonephritis. A methodologic review of the literature. *J. Gen. Intern. Med.* **7**, 544–553.

72. Leigh, D. A., Smith, E. C., and Marriner, J. (1984). Comparative study using norfloxacin and amoxycillin in the treatment of complicated urinary tract infections in geriatric patients. *J. Antimicrob. Chemother.* **13** (Suppl. B), 79–83.

73. Goldstein, E. J. C., Alpert, M. L., Najem, A., Eng, R. H. K, Ginsburg, B. P., Kahn, R. M., and Cherubin, C. E. (1987). Norfloxacin in the treatment of complicated and uncomplicated urinary tract infections. *Am. J. Med.* **82** (Suppl. 6B), 65–69.

74. Corrado, M. L., Grad, C., and Sabbaj, J. (1987). Norfloxacin in the treatment of urinary tract infections in men with and without identifiable urologic complications. *Am. J. Med.* **82** (Suppl. 6B), 70–74.

75. Sabbaj, J., Hoagland, V. L., and Cook, T. (1986). Norfloxacin versus co-trimoxazole in the treatment of recurring urinary tract infections in men. *Scand. J. Infect. Dis.* **48** (Suppl.), 48–53.

76. Waites, K. B., Canupp, K. C., and DeVivo, M. J. (1991). Efficacy and tolerance of norfloxacin in treatment of complicated urinary tract infection in outpatients with neurogenic bladder secondary to spinal cord injury. *Urology* **38**, 589–596.

77. Cox, C. E., McCabe, R. E., and Grad, C. (1987). Oral norfloxacin versus parenteral treatment of nosocomial urinary tract infection. *Am. J. Med.* **82** (Suppl. 6B), 59–64.

78. Cherubin, C., and Stilwell, S. (1986). Norfloxacin versus parenteral therapy in the treatment of complicated urinary tract infections and resistant organisms. *Scand. J. Infect. Dis.* **48** (Suppl.), 32–37.

79. Boerema, J. B. J., Willems, F. T. C., and Veheggen, W. J. H. M. (1989). Ciprofloxacin versus cotrimoxazole in the treatment of patients with complicated urinary tract infections. *Drug Invest.* **1**, 18–23.

80. Williams, A. H., and Grüneberg, R. N. (1986). Ciprofloxacin and co-trimoxazole in urinary tract infection. *J. Antimicrob. Chemother.* **18** (Suppl. D), 107–110.

81. Newsom, S. W. B., Murphy, P., and Matthews, J. (1986). A comparative study of ciprofloxacin and trimethoprim in the treatment of urinary tract infections in geriatric patients. *J. Antimicrob. Chemother.* **18** (Suppl. D), 111–115.

82. Fang, G., Brennen, C., Wagener, M., Swanson, D., Hilf, M., Zadecky, L., DeVine, J., and Yu, V. L. (1991). Use of ciprofloxacin versus use of aminoglycosides for therapy of complicated urinary tract infection: Prospective, randomized clinical and pharmacokinetic study. *Antimicrob. Agents Chemother.* **35**, 1849–1855.

83. Leigh, D. A., Emmanuel, F. X. S., and Petch, J. J. (1986). Ciprofloxacin therapy in complicated urinary tract infections caused by *Pseudomonas aeruginosa* and other resistant bacteria. *J. Antimicrob. Chemother.* **18** (Suppl. D), 117–121.

84. Brown, E. M., Morris, R., and Stephenson, T. P. (1986). The efficacy and safety of ciprofloxacin in the treatment of chronic *Pseudomonas aeruginosa* urinary tract infection. *J. Antimicrob. Chemother.* **18** (Suppl. D), 123–127.

85. Schaeffer, A. J., and Anderson, R. U. (1992). Efficacy and tolerability of norfloxacin vs. ciprofloxacin in complicated urinary tract infection. *Urology* **40**, 446–449.

86. Mattina, R., Cocuzza, C. E., Cesana, M., and the Italian Multicentre UTI Rufloxacin Group (1993). Rufloxacin once daily versus ofloxacin twice daily for treatment of complicated cystitis and upper urinary tract infections. *Infection* **21**, 106–111.

87. Cox, C. E. (1989). Ofloxacin in the management of complicated urinary tract infections, including prostatitis. *Am. J. Med.* **87** (Suppl. 6C), 61S–68S.

88. Huttunen, M., Kunnas, K., and Saloranta, P. (1988). Enoxacin treatment of urinary tract infections in elderly patients. *J. Antimicrob. Chemother.* **21** (Suppl. B), 105–111.

89. Hoepelman, I. M., Havinga, W. H., Bemi, R. A., Zwinkelo, M., de Wit, M. A. M., de Hond, H. A. P. M., Boon, T. A., Visser, M. R., van Asbeck, F. W. A., and Verhoef, J. (1993). Safety and efficacy of lomefloxacin versus norfloxacin in the treatment of complicated urinary tract infections. *Eur. J. Clin. Microbiol. Infect. Dis.* **12**, 343–347.

90. Nicolle, L. E., Louie, T. J., Dubois, J., Martel, A., Harding, G. K. M., and Sinave, C. P. (1994). Treatment of complicated urinary tract infections with lomefloxacin compared with trimethoprim–sulfamethoxazole. *Antimicrob. Agents Chemother.* **38**, 1368–1373.

91. Cox, C. E. (1992). A comparison of the safety and efficacy of lomefloxacin and ciprofloxacin in the treatment of complicated or recurrent urinary tract infections. *Am. J. Med.* **92** (Suppl. 4A), 82S–86S.

92. Naber, K. G., and Sigl, G. (1993). Fleroxacin versus ofloxacin in patients with complicated urinary tract infections: A controlled clinical study. *Am. J. Med.* **94** (Suppl. 3A), 114S–117S.

93. Cox, C. E. (1993). Comparison of intravenous fleroxacin with ceftazidime for treatment of complicated urinary tract infections. *Am. J. Med.* **94** (Suppl. 3A), 118S–125S.

94. Gelfand, M. S., Simmons, B. P., Craft, R. B., Grogan, J., and Amarshi, N. (1993). A sequential study of intravenous and oral fleroxacin in the treatment of complicated urinary tract infection. *Am. J. Med.* **94** (Suppl. 3A), 126S–130S.

95. de Gier, R., Karperien, A., Bouter, K., Zqinkels, M., Verhoef, J., Knol, W., Boon, T., and Hoepelman, I. M. (1995). A sequential study of intravenous and oral fleroxacin for 7 or 14 days in the treatment of complicated urinary tract infections. *Int. J. Antimicrob. Agents* **6**, 27–30.

96. Timmerman, C., Hoepelman, I., de Hond, J., Boon, T., Schreinemachers, L., Mensink, H., and Verhoef, J. (1992). Open, randomized comparison of pefloxacin and cefotaxime in the treatment of complicated urinary tract infections. *Infection* **20**, 34–37.

97. Cox, C. E. (1991). Oral temafloxacin compared to norfloxacin for the treatment of complicated urinary tract infections. *Am. J. Med.* **91** (Suppl. 6A), 129S–133S.

98. Naber, K. G., DiSilverio, F., Geddes, A., and Guibert, J. (1996). Comparative efficacy of sparfloxacin versus ciprofloxacin in the treatment of complicated urinary tract infection. *J. Antimicrob. Chemother.* **37** (Suppl. A), 135–144.

99. Boerema, J. B. J., and van Saene, H. K. F. (1986). Norfloxacin treatment in complicated urinary tract infection. *Scand. J. Infect. Dis.* **48** (Suppl.), 20–26.

100. Sheehan, G. J., Harding, G. K. M., Haase, D. A., Thomson, M. J., Urias, B., Kennedy, J. K., Hoban, D. J., and Ronald, A. R. (1988). Double-blind randomized comparison of 24 weeks of norfloxacin and 12 weeks of norfloxacin followed by 12 weeks of placebo in the therapy of complicated urinary tract infection. *Antimicrob. Agents Chemother.* **32**, 1292–1293.

101. Biering-Sorensen, F., Hoiby, N., Nordbenbo, A., Ravnborg, M., Bruun, B., and Rahm, V. (1994). Ciprofloxacin as prophylaxis for urinary tract infection: Prospective, randomized, cross-over, placebo controlled study in patients with spinal cord lesion. *J. Urol.* **151**, 105–108.

102. Schaeffer, A. J., and Darras, F. S. (1990). The efficacy of norfloxacin in the treatment of chronic bacterial prostatitis refractory to trimethoprim–sulfamethoxazole and/or carbenicillin. *J. Urol.* **144**, 690–693.

103. Weidner, W., and Schiefer, H. G. (1991). Chronic bacterial prostatitis: Therapeutic experience with ciprofloxacin. *Infection* **19** (Suppl. 3), S165–S166.

104. Weidner, W., Schiefer, H. G., and Brahler, E. (1991). Refractory chronic bacterial prostatitis: A re-evaluation of ciprofloxacin treatment after a median follow-up of 30 months. *J. Urol.* **146**, 350–352.

105. Guibert, J., Boutelier, R., and Guyot, A. (1990). A clinical trial of pefloxacin in prostatitis. *J. Antimicrob. Chemother.* **26** (Suppl. B), 161–166.

106. Cox, C. E. (1991). Treatment of chronic bacterial prostatitis with temafloxacin. *Am. J. Med.* **91** (Suppl. 6A), 134S–139S.

107. Naber, K. G., Boerema, J. B. J., Bischoff, W., Blenk, H., Focht, J., Carpentier, P., and Sylvester, J. (1991). An assessment of temafloxacin in the treatment of chronic bacterial prostatitis. *J. Antimicrob. Chemother.* **28** (Suppl. C), 97–96.

108. Boerema, J. B. J., Bischoff, W., Foeht, J., and Naber, K. G. (1991). An open multicentre study on the efficacy and safety of rufloxacin in patients with chronic bacterial prostatitis. *J. Antimicrob. Chemother.* **28**, 587–597.

CHAPTER 7

Use of the Quinolones in Sexually Transmitted Diseases

RICHARD P. DICARLO and DAVID H. MARTIN

Department of Medicine, Louisiana State University School of Medicine, New Orleans, Louisiana 70112

The Quinolones, Third Edition

INTRODUCTION

There are more than 25 infectious organisms that can be sexually transmitted and cause disease [1]. However, sexually transmitted diseases (STDs) are often categorized by clinical syndrome for purposes of empiric management. Aside from HIV infection, the major syndromes (and their most commonly associated pathogens) are male urethritis (*Neisseria gonorrhoeae, Chlamydia trachomatis, Ureaplasma urealyticum*, and herpes simplex virus), mucopurulent cervicitis (same organisms as male urethritis, with the exception of *U. urealyticum*), pelvic inflammatory disease (*N. gonorrhoeae, C. trachomatis, Mycoplasma hominis*, and vaginal anaerobes), vaginitis/vaginosis (*Candida albicans, Trichomonas vaginalis, Gardnerella vaginalis, Mobiluncus* spp., and other anaerobes), and genital ulcer disease (herpes simplex virus, *Treponema pallidum, Haemophilus ducreyi, C. trachomatis*, and *Calymmatobacterium granulomatis*).

Over the past 10 years, the quinolones have become increasingly important in the therapy of many STDs. Several factors have contributed to this. First, quinolones have excellent *in-vitro* activity against many of the above pathogens. Second, the prevalence of penicillin- and tetracycline-resistant strains of *N. gonorrhoeae* and sulfonamide-resistant strains of *H. ducreyi* have increased, requiring newer agents to treat these organisms. Third, quinolones may play a role in the empiric approach to treatment when there is an advantage to using a single agent that is active against the multiple pathogens that can cause a particular STD syndrome. Fourth, quinolones can be used as a single oral dose for some STDs. This is desirable because of improved compliance, and also because of the ease and safety of administering an oral antibiotic as opposed to an intramuscular injection. Finally, most quinolones achieve high concentrations in gynecologic and urogenital tract tissues [2–5]. Penetration into gynecologic tissues has been most frequently studied with ciprofloxacin, where concentrations have generally exceeded serum levels by two- to fivefold [5]. Concentrations in the fallopian tubes, ovaries, fundus myometrium, and cervix ranged from 0.62 to 3.3 mg/kg 2 hours after either a single dose or multiple preoperative doses (while serum levels ranged from 0.6 to 1.3 mg/liter) [4].

The efficacy of quinolones for many STDs has been established through multiple clinical trials. *N. gonorrhoeae* has been most extensively studied, and many agents have proved efficacious. Ofloxacin has proven an effective therapy for *C. trachomatis*, and the early data on sparfloxacin for this infection looks promising as well. Ofloxacin also has been shown to be effective in the treatment of pelvic inflammatory disease. Ciprofloxacin, norfloxacin, rosoxacin, and fler-oxacin are all effective as single agents for chancroid. Additionally, there are preliminary data that quinolones may be effective for donovanosis. Thus far, quinolones have not been highly effective for the treatment of bacterial vaginosis.

However, some of the newer agents with improved anaerobic activity may be promising for this disease. Unfortunately, quinolones have not demonstrated good activity against *T. pallidum*, and there is currently no role for these drugs in the treatment of syphilis. Details of the role of quinolones in the treatment of infections caused by the above organisms are provided in the following sections.

GONOCOCCAL INFECTIONS

BACKGROUND

Neisseria gonorrhoeae is a Gram-negative coccus that can infect a variety of columnar and cuboidal epithelial membranes. Included are the urethral mucosa, endocervical mucosa, rectal mucosa, Bartholin's glands, fallopian tubes, epididymis, pharynx, and conjunctiva. The organism attaches to these surfaces by means of pili and outer-membrane proteins, then penetrates into the submucosal tissues, where it usually stimulates the formation of microabscesses. Subsequently, there is disruption of the mucosal membrane and exudate formation, resulting in the characteristic purulent discharge.

The incidence of *N. gonorrhoeae* infection in the United States has decreased steadily since the late 1970s, but in 1998 the rate was still approximately 133 cases per 100,000, which represents an 8.9% increase from the rate in 1997 [6]. The vast majority of clinical infections caused by *N. gonorrhoeae* are urethritis in men and endocervicitis in women. However, other sites may be involved. Up to 44% of women with gonorrhea have positive rectal cultures for *N. gonorrhoeae*, although there are usually no rectal symptoms [7–9]. A review from the 1970s found that 45% of men who have sex with men (MSM) with gonorrhea had rectal involvement [9]. This percentage decreased during the 1980s [10], as sexual habits among MSM changed, but more recent studies have reported an increasing incidence of infection at this site [11,12]. Pharyngeal infection may be present in 10–20% of heterosexual women and MSM with gonorrhea but is much less frequent in heterosexual men [8,13]. Inoculation of the conjunctiva in adults is uncommon but can result in severe conjunctivitis. *N. gonorrhoeae* can ascend the genital tract and cause epididymitis in men and pelvic inflammatory disease in women. Finally, disseminated gonococcal infection (DGI) occurs with a frequency of 1% or less in those with local disease. This syndrome most frequently results in bacteremia, arthralgias, septic arthritis, and skin lesions, rarely resulting in endocarditis or meningitis.

Penicillinase-producing *N. gonorrhoeae* (PPNG) was first documented in the mid-1970s, and became increasingly prevalent during the 1980s. A 3.2- or 4.4-mD plasmid is most commonly responsible for this type of resistance. In 1998, 3.0%

of gonococcal isolates tested under the Centers for Disease Control (CDC) Gonococcal Isolate Surveillance Project (GISP) produced penicillinase [14]. Reported rates of PPNG have been much higher in certain U.S. cities and in other parts of the world [15,16]. Plasmid-mediated tetracycline resistance (TRNG) in the United States was first documented in 1985 [17], and 6.6% of 1998 GISP isolates exhibited this type of resistance. Chromosomal resistance to penicillin and tetracycline has also become increasingly prevalent. In 1998, 5.1% of GISP isolates had chromosomal resistance to penicillin, 6.8% had chromosomal resistance to tetracycline, and another 7.2% had chromosomal resistance to both [14]. The development of widespread resistance to penicillin and tetracycline has resulted in the use of quinolones and third-generation cephalosporins as first-line treatment for gonococcal infections in much of the world.

IN-VITRO ACTIVITY OF QUINOLONES AGAINST NEISSERIA GONORRHOEAE

Most quinolone antibiotics have good *in-vitro* activity against *N. gonorrhoeae*. Table I summarizes the activity against strains obtained at the University College Hospital, London, in the 1980s [18]. Strains with known resistance were excluded from this analysis; the MIC_{90} ranged from 0.002 mg/liter with clinafloxacin to 0.12 mg/liter with pefloxacin. More recent studies of new quinolones such as gatifloxacin, gemifloxacin, and sitafloxacin have yielded similar results, and these are also summarized in Table I [19–26]. The presence of plasmid-mediated or chromosomal resistance to penicillin has little effect on the susceptibility of *N. gonorrhoeae* to the quinolones [27].

CLINICAL STUDIES

Many quinolones have proven effective for uncomplicated gonococcal infection in clinical trials [28–56]. Table II summarizes the single-dose regimens that have had better than 95% cure rates. A single 100-mg dose of ciprofloxacin is the lowest single dose that has been effective [39]. Several regimens have been associated with a high failure rate. A single 100-mg dose of acrosoxacin had a success rate of only 28% [57]. A single 1200-mg dose of flumequine had a success rate of only 74% [58], but multidose regimens with this compound have been successful. Trovafloxacin has been effective [59], but newly discovered problems with toxicity have restricted the use of this drug to serious infections in hospitalized patients. Of the newer fluoroquinolones, gatifloxacin has most recently demonstrated efficacy for uncomplicated gonococcal infections [56].

TABLE I   *In-Vitro* Activity of Quinolone Antibiotics
against *N. Gonnorhea* [18–26]

Drug	MIC_{90} (mg/liter)
Clinafloxacin	0.002
Ciprofloxacin	0.008
Levofloxacin	0.015
Ofloxacin	0.03
Sparfloxacin	0.06
Fleroxacin	0.06
Enoxacin	0.06
Norfloxacin	0.06
Rosoxacin	0.06
Pefloxacin	0.12
Gemifloxacin	0.006–2
Gatifloxacin	0.004–0.06
Sitafloxacin	0.002–0.004

TABLE II   Single Doses of Quinolones with Proven
Efficacy in the Treatment of Gonorrhea

Drug	Effective dosage (in mg)
Ciprofloxacin	100, 250, 500, 2000
Ofloxacin	200, 400, 600, 800
Norfloxacin	400, 600, 800
Pefloxacin	400, 800
Enoxacin	200, 400, 600
Fleroxacin	400
Rosoxacin	200, 300, 400
Sparfloxacin	200
Temofloxacin	200, 400
Difloxacin	200
Gatifloxacin	400, 600

Not only do quinolones have a high efficacy rate, but it also appears that they rapidly eliminate *N. gonorrhoeae* from the lower urinary tract in men. Quantitative urine cultures were negative 2 hours after a single 500-mg dose of ciprofloxacin in five men with gonococcal urethritis who were tested; urethral swab cultures 24 hours after a single dose were also negative in a small number of men [60]. The majority of clinical-trial experience has been in men with gonococcal urethritis. However, there is ample evidence that single-dose quinolones are equally effective in women with gonococcal cervicitis [29,56].

Clinical trials of quinolones for gonococcal urethritis and cervicitis have established that these drugs can also eliminate *N. gonorrhoeae* from the rectum and pharynx. Effective single-dose regimens have included ciprofloxacin 250 and 500 mg, ofloxacin 400 mg, fleroxacin 400 mg, norfloxacin 800 mg, and gatifloxacin 400 or 600 mg [29,32,39,40,48,56,61].

Gonococcal keratoconjunctivitis in adults is uncommon. Current recommendations for treatment of this condition from the CDC are saline lavage plus a single 1-g dose of intramuscular ceftriaxone [62]. In a study carried out in Rwanda, a single 1200-mg dose of oral norfloxacin effectively cured eight patients with gonococcal keratoconjunctivitis [63]. Gonococcal conjunctivitis is more common among neonates, but quinolones are contraindicated for this age group. There have been no more recent studies of treatment for DGI in the published literature. Current CDC recommendations for treatment of this condition are hospitalization, an intravenous or intramuscular third-generation cephalosporin until there has been clear clinical improvement, followed by oral cefixime or ciprofloxacin to complete 7 days of therapy. Intravenous ciprofloxacin or ofloxacin are recommended for initial treatment in patients allergic to β-lactam antibiotics [62].

Quinolones have been used for the treatment of gonorrhea outside of clinical trials since the mid-1980s. In various parts of Southeast Asia, norfloxacin was introduced in 1985. Ofloxacin, ciprofloxacin, and pefloxacin have also been used extensively in this region [16]. In the United States, ciprofloxacin has been used as first-line therapy for uncomplicated gonorrhea in certain public health clinics since 1989 [64]. The CDC currently recommends a 500-mg dose of ciprofloxacin or a 400-mg dose of ofloxacin as first-line agents [62]. Lower doses have proven effective, but these recommendations stem in part from concern about the development of isolates with quinolone resistance and the potential for treatment failures [65].

It should be noted that quinolones have no activity against *T. pallidum* and, therefore, would not be effective in aborting an incubating syphilis infection transmitted concomitantly with *N. gonorrhoeae*. This is a theoretical concern that is of little consequence in populations with a low incidence of syphilis, but may be a significant consideration in those with a high incidence.

RESISTANCE OF *N. GONORRHOEAE* TO THE QUINOLONES

Quinolone resistance in *N. gonorrhoeae* is conferred by mutations that alter the molecular structure of the A and B subunits of DNA gyrase (GyrA and GyrB respectively) or mutations that alter the parC subunit structure of topoisomerase. Strains with mutations in the GyrB subunit usually have low-level resistance, whereas mutations in GyrA are associated with higher-level resistance [66]. In addition, strains with mutations at both the GyrA and parC subunits may have higher MICs than those with a mutation in GyrA alone [67]. Transfer of these mutations between strains of *N. gonorrhoeae* has been demonstrated *in vitro* [68]. Reduced uptake of quinolones has also been demonstrated among gonococcal isolates [69,70], and this may be an additional clinically important resistance mechanism, although the genetic basis is unknown.

Criteria for determining resistance, intermediate susceptibility, and susceptibility of *N. gonorrhoeae* to various quinolones have been proposed [71] and are shown in Table III. Treatment failure with a quinolone is usually due to a strain that has an MIC to ciprofloxacin of 1.0–2.0 mg/liter or greater. Strains that show intermediate susceptibility usually can be effectively treated with high doses of quinolones. A 500-mg dose of ciprofloxacin results in a peak serum level of 2.5 mg/liter [72], which should be more than adequate to treat an isolate with an MIC <0.5 mg/liter. However, treatment failure does not always correlate completely with *in-vitro* activity. A 1998 study from Singapore found that there was an 8% ciprofloxacin failure rate among gonococcal infections with organisms showing intermediate sensitivity to the quinolones [73]. Furthermore, use of quinolones in this setting may result in additional mutations conferring higher-level resistance.

TABLE III   Proposed Criteria for Gonococcal Susceptibility to Various Quinolones[a]

Drug	Resistant MIC (mg/l)	Intermediate sensitivity MIC (mg/l)	Susceptible MIC (mg/l)
Ciprofloxacin	≥1.0	0.125–0.5	≤0.06
Ofloxacin	≥2.0	0.5–1.0	≤0.25
Enoxacin	≥1.0	0.5	≤0.25
Lomefloxacin	≥2.0	0.25–1.0	≤0.125
Norfloxacin	≥1.0	0.5	≤0.25

[a]Adapted from Knapp *et al.* (1995) [71].

Therefore, quinolone treatment of infections caused by strains with intermediate sensitivity should be avoided.

As quinolone use for the treatment of gonorrhea has increased, resistance to these agents has become more widespread. Resistant strains have been isolated in Australia, Canada, Hong Kong, Japan, Republic of the Philippines, India, Bangladesh, China, Thailand, Rwanda, Spain, Finland, Russia, the United Kingdom, and the United States. Strains with intermediate susceptibility have been reported from the above countries as well as Greece [74], The Netherlands [75], the Canary Islands, and the West Indies [76]. Treatment failure with enoxacin was first reported in 1986 [77]. Treatment failures with the 250-mg dose of ciprofloxacin were first reported in the United Kingdom in 1990 [78]. Since then, there have been reports of treatment failures with the 500-mg dose of ciprofloxacin [79–81], the 400-mg dose of ofloxacin [50,82], the 600-mg dose of norfloxacin [50], levofloxacin 100 mg t.i.d. for 7 days [83], and with sparfloxacin 100 mg t.i.d. for 5 days [84].

Surveillance reports indicate that the prevalence of quinolone resistance in some geographic areas is increasing. In Hong Kong, 0.5% of strains exhibited quinolone resistance in 1992 [85], and this increased to 24% of strains in 1996 [86]. The Republic of the Philippines, Australia, and other Pacific Rim countries have also had an increase in percentage of resistant isolates [76,87–89], as have selected cities in India [90], China [91], and Bangladesh [92]. Additionally, the level of resistance may be increasing in these areas. In the late 1990s, strains with MICs ≥ 8.0 mg/liter to ciprofloxacin have been reported [80,93,94]. Resistance is still uncommon in the United States, where only 0.1% of GISP isolates had an MIC to ciprofloxacin ≥ 1.0 mg/liter. However, GISP data also indicate that the percentage of isolates with decreased susceptibility to ciprofloxacin has increased from 0.4% in 1990 to 0.9% in 1998 [14]. Furthermore, a high percentage of these isolates are clustered in relatively few geographic regions. A study of one such cluster in Ohio and western Pennsylvania found that 80% of the organisms were indistinguishable by pulsed-field gel electrophoresis [95]. This suggests the spread of a single clone rather than selection due to antibiotic pressure. Nonetheless, areas with a high prevalence of these strains are fertile ground for the emergence of high-level resistance. Therefore, quinolones probably should not be used in this setting.

In-vitro data with gatifloxacin suggest that it may have reasonable activity even in the face of GyrA and ParC mutations that confer high levels of resistance to other quinolones [19, 96]. Whether this drug will be clinically useful against these isolates, however, remains unproven.

CHLAMYDIA TRACHOMATIS

BACKGROUND

Chlamydia trachomatis is considered to be the most common STD pathogen in the United States. Most infections are asymptomatic, but the organism is an important cause of the following diseases: urethritis in men and women, endocervicitis, epididymitis, pelvic inflammatory disease, conjunctivitis in adults and infants, pneumonia in infants, and lymphogranuloma venereum. Additionally, this organism is recognized as a "trigger" of Reiter's syndrome in genetically susceptible individuals. As a consequence of clinically inapparent fallopian tube infections, *C. trachomatis* is probably the major cause of obstructive infertility and ectopic pregnancy today. Reviews of the epidemiology, microbiology, and clinical aspects of chlamydial infections are available elsewhere [97–99].

IN-VITRO ACTIVITY OF QUINOLONES
AGAINST *C. TRACHOMATIS*

Many of the quinolones have been studied *in vitro* for activity against *C. trachomatis*. The results of a number of these studies are summarized in Table IV. Only the MIC_{90} data are presented, as in most studies MICs and MBCs for *C. trachomatis* are identical or no more than twofold different. Furthermore, there is some controversy over the true definition of what constitutes an MBC for this obligate intracellular pathogen [100]. The range of MICs varies from 16–32 mg/liter for norfloxacin and 16 for enoxacin to 0.06–0.125 and 0.016–0.25 for the newer quinolones grepafloxacin and trovafloxacin, respectively. Based on achievable serum and tissue levels, one would predict that the drugs on the high end of the MIC range—including pefloxacin, enoxacin, and norfloxacin—would not be effective for chlamydial infections. As discussed below, this appears to be true for norfloxacin at least. Drugs with MICs in the range of 1–4 mg/liter might be effective, while those with MICs ≤0.5 mg/liter would be quite likely to have clinical activity.

CLINICAL STUDIES

In fact, the *in-vitro* susceptibility data summarized in Table IV appear to correlate well with the clinical efficacy of these drugs in humans with chlamydial infections. Norfloxacin was the first of the modern generation of quinolones to be studied for chlamydial infections, and it was found to be ineffective [101]. As

TABLE IV *In-Vitro* Activity of Quinolone Antibiotics against
C. trachomatis

Drug	MIC_{90} (mg/l)	Reference
Sparfloxacin	0.6	[163]
Grepafloxacin	0.06–0.125	[164,165]
Trovafloxacin	0.25	[166]
Temafloxacin	0.25	[167]
Tosufloxacin	0.25	[168]
Gatifloxacin	0.25	[169]
Lomefloxacin	0.25	[168]
Ofloxacin	0.5–1	[170,171]
Ciprofloxacin	1–2	[172,173]
Rufloxacin	4	[174]
Fleroxacin	2–4	[175,176]
Pefloxacin	8	[175]
Enoxacin	16	[173]
Norfloxacin	16–32	[172,173,175]

can be seen in Table IV, the *C. trachomatis* MIC_{90} of norfloxacin is high, and, given the achievable serum and tissue levels as described in the pharmacokinetics chapter of this book (Chapter 5), the failure of this drug to eradicate *C. trachomatis in vivo* is not surprising. Ciprofloxacin is much more active *in vitro* against *C. trachomatis* than is norfloxacin, and the early clinical experience with this drug suggested that it might be effective [102], but several later studies showed that the bacteriologic failure rates were unacceptably high [103–106]. Hooton *et al.* studied doses as high as 1 g twice daily and observed a 38% failure rate. Furthermore, 52% of men taking 750 mg twice daily were bacteriological failures [106]. In the study by Fong *et al.*, 12 of 20 (60%) of chlamydia-infected men with nongonococcal urethritis (NGU) treated with 750 mg of ciprofloxacin b.i.d. failed or relapsed [103].

In contrast to the results with ciprofloxacin, ofloxacin in doses of 300 mg twice daily or 400 mg once daily for a total of 7 days has been shown to be very effective for chlamydial infections, even though the *in-vitro* activity of this drug against *C. trachomatis* is only approximately twofold better than ciprofloxacin. In five randomized trials involving both men and women, ofloxacin was equally effective as the standard doxycycline treatment regimen [107–111].

Given the fact that fleroxacin is less active *in vitro* against *C. trachomatis* than ciprofloxacin, it is of interest that this drug also appears to be effective clinically for chlamydial infections. Among 15 males treated with 600 mg once daily, there were no failures, and among 11 women similarly treated there was only 1 [112]. Zeigler *et al.* reported a similar experience from Europe [113]. Among drugs with $MIC_{90}s$ in the range of 1 to 4 mg/liter, pharmacokinetics probably play a critical role in determining activity. The area under the curve per 100-mg dose unit for fleroxacin, ofloxacin, and ciprofloxacin are 19.5, 9.6, and 2.0 mg·hr/liter, respectively [114]. Dividing the AUC by the upper end of the *C. trachomatis* MIC range for each of the drugs results in ratios of approximately 5 for both fleroxacin and ofloxacin, but only 1 for ciprofloxacin. Dividing the AUC by the MIC may be a useful way of predicting quinolone activity against *C. trachomatis*. Forrest *et al.* have demonstrated the effectiveness of this approach in predicting the clinical outcome of other bacterial infections treated with ciprofloxacin [115].

Several drugs with $MIC_{90}s$ less than 0.5 mg/liter have been studied in patients with chlamydial infections, and all appear to be effective. Temafloxacin, one of the first of these, was actually licensed for the treatment of chlamydial infections in the United States but was withdrawn from the market because of toxicity. Two other drugs, grepafloxacin and trovafloxacin, which are highly active against chlamydia both *in vitro* and *in vivo*, also were withdrawn from the market. Tosufloxacin in doses of 150 mg three times daily for 14 days cured 13 men with *C. trachomatis* and NGU [116]. More extensive data are available for grepafloxacin, trovafloxacin, and sparfloxacin, all of which have $MIC_{90}s$ ranging from 0.016 to 0.25 mg/liter for chlamydia. McCormack *et al.* observed *C. trachomatis* eradication rates of 96.3% (78/81) in women and 100% (36/36) in men treated with 400 mg of grepafloxacin daily for 7 days. Outcomes were similar in the doxycycline-treated comparison group [117].

In a dose-ranging study of trovafloxacin conducted in New Orleans and Indianapolis, we found that doses ranging from 200 mg once daily for 7 and 5 days to as little as 50 mg given daily for 7 days appeared to be effective in both men and women [118]. A large multicenter randomized trial has demonstrated the clinical efficacy of trovafloxacin for human chlamydial infections [119].

In a large multicenter European study, doxycycline 200 mg twice daily for 7 days was compared to two different doses of sparfloxacin: 200 mg once followed by 100 mg daily for 2 days and 200 mg once followed by 100 mg daily for 6 days. The 7-day regimen was clearly equal to the doxycycline regimen (3 of 74 failures/relapses versus 2 failures/relapses in the doxycycline group), but the 3-day regimen did not appear to be as effective (10/70 failures/relapses) [120].

Lymphogranuloma venereum (LGV) is caused by biologically more virulent *C. trachomatis* immunotypes. These organisms have the same antibiotic susceptibility patterns as the more common immunotypes that cause urethritis in men and endocervicitis in women. Generally, this syndrome is treated for a period of 3 weeks instead of the 1-week course recommended for uncomplicated chlamydial infections. Based on this experience, a 3-week course of any of the quinolones clinically effective for the common chlamydial syndromes as discussed above should also be effective for LGV, though there are no published data.

In summary, there appear to be five quinolones that have been adequately studied and have been found to be effective consistently for uncomplicated *C. trachomatis* infection: ofloxacin, grepafloxacin, trovafloxacin, sparfloxacin, and fleroxacin. The advantage of the latter four drugs over ofloxacin is that they are effective when given once a day, reflecting the *in-vitro* studies cited above. However, since all of these drugs are proprietary and therefore the cost is relatively high, none have an advantage over the macrolide azithromycin given as a single 1-g dose for the treatment of chlamydial infections [121]. Additionally, all four quinolones with enhanced chlamydial activity *in vitro* are relatively toxic. Grepafloxacin was taken off the U.S. market because of rare but life-threatening cardiotoxicity, and the use of trovafloxacin has been limited to severe infections in hospitalized patients because of hepatic toxicity. Though still available in the United States, sparfloxacin has significant phototoxicity problems, as does fleroxacin, which is marketed only outside the United States. Therefore, ofloxacin remains the only quinolone indicated for chlamydial infections in this country.

PELVIC INFLAMMATORY DISEASE

Pelvic inflammatory disease (PID) is a syndrome that appears to be caused by a variety of organisms. Studies in which laparoscopically obtained specimens for culture were obtained have demonstrated *C. trachomatis*, *N. gonorrhoeae*, *M. hominis*, and a variety of vaginal aerobic and anaerobic bacteria in the fallopian tubes and the pelvis itself [122]. Based on these observations, current treatment recommendations include a number of different combination regimens designed to provide coverage for all of these organisms. Unfortunately, there are few comparative studies available to tell us which of the recommended regimens might be the best or, in fact, whether such broad-spectrum coverage, particularly for anaerobes, is even necessary in all cases.

Since some of the older quinolones do not have significant activity against anaerobic bacteria, the experience with these drugs in the treatment of PID is of particular interest. Ofloxacin as a single agent has been compared to the combination of single-dose cefoxitin plus multidose doxycycline in two well-designed clinical trials for outpatient treatment of PID [123,124]. In these studies, ofloxacin was equally effective as the standard regimen both clinically and microbiologically. A possible explanation for these observations is that anaerobes play a small role, if any, in the pathogenesis of early or mild PID. This hypothesis is supported by laparoscopic studies suggesting that anaerobes are more likely to be present in patients with severe disease, including tuboovarian abscesses than in those with mild infections [125,126]. However, in view of the fact that long-term follow-up studies using endpoints such as ectopic pregnancy, infertility, or tubal scarring as determined by second-look laparoscopy have not been done, it is not possible to be certain that better anti-anaerobic coverage does not provide some additional benefit. For this reason, the Centers for Disease Control and Prevention's STD Treatment Guidelines continue to recommend the addition of metronidazole to ofloxacin for the treatment of PID [62]. This issue may become less important as the results of ongoing PID treatment studies of new quinolones with better *in-vitro* anaerobic activity become available. At this point, it appears likely that at least some of these drugs will be recommended in the future for single-drug therapy of PID.

CHANCROID

BACKGROUND

Chancroid is a common cause of genital ulcer disease in developing nations. It has been an uncommon disease in North America since the advent of the antibiotic era, although it has caused sporadic localized outbreaks. The etiologic agent is *Haemophilus ducreyi*, a Gram-negative bacillus. Rapid diagnostic tests for this organism are not commercially available nor is premade culture media. Therefore, most cases of chancroid are diagnosed clinically and treated empirically. *H. ducreyi* is resistant to penicillin, and most strains are resistant to tetracycline. Resistance to trimethoprim and to trimethoprim–sulfamethoxazole has been reported with increasing frequency [127]. *H. ducreyi* is sensitive to ceftriaxone, which can be used effectively in a single dose [128]. Of the macrolide antibiotics, azithromycin appears to have the greatest activity [129], and it can also be used effectively in a single dose [130]. Quinolone antibiotics have good *in-vitro* activity against *H. ducreyi*, although they may be less effective than ceftriaxone or azithromycin when used in a single dose [128].

IN-VITRO ACTIVITY OF QUINOLONES AGAINST *HAEMOPHILUS DUCREYI*

The results of many studies of the *in-vitro* activity of quinolones against *H. ducreyi* are summarized in Table V. The MIC_{90} has ranged from 16 mg/liter for nalidixic acid [131] to 0.008 mg/liter for ciprofloxacin [132,133]. Most comparative studies have found that ciprofloxacin has the greatest activity against this

TABLE V   *In-Vitro* Activity of Quinolone Antibiotics against *H. ducreyi*

Drug	MIC_{90} (mg/l)	Reference
Ciprofloxacin	0.008–0.5	[129,131–134,177]
Ofloxacin	0.03–2	[134,177]
Fleroxacin	0.06	[132–137]
Sparfloxacin	0.02	[136]
Difloxacin	0.03–0.12	[135,177]
Norfloxacin	0.06–1	[131,134,177]
Pefloxacin	<0.06–0.12	[131,134]
Enoxacin	0.12	[134]
Rosoxacin	0.06–0.12	[134,135]
Nalidixic acid	16	[131]

pathogen [129,131,132,134,135]. However, one isolate with an MIC of 2.0 has been reported from Thailand [133]. Sparfloxacin [136], fleroxacin [132,137], ofloxacin [133,134], difloxacin [135], rosoxacin [134,135], and norfloxacin [129,131] have also shown good activity. It should be noted that *H. ducreyi* is difficult to culture and that surveillance data about antibiotic sensitivity are limited. Whether or not quinolone resistance has begun to emerge to a significant degree worldwide is currently unknown [86].

CLINICAL STUDIES

Quinolone regimens that have been effective for the treatment of chancroid are shown in Table VI. Most of these studies used clinical healing as the measure of efficacy. In single-dose trials, efficacy has ranged from 63% with a single 300-mg dose of rosoxacin [138] to 100% with a single 500-mg dose of ciprofloxacin [139,140]. Pooling the data from a number of studies, the overall efficacy of single-dose quinolone regimens for chancroid was 88% (307/348) [138–146]. While the number of published studies is limited, it appears that the quinolones may be most effective for chancroid when used in multidose regimens. Several investigators have reported efficacy rates of 98 to 100% for multidose ciprofloxacin regimens [139,141,147]. Pooling the data from studies of multidose regimens, the overall efficacy was 94% (186/197) [138,139,141,148]. The improved results with multidose regimens may be due to the theoretical need to maintain tissue levels above the MIC_{95} for 48 hours in order to treat chancroid effectively [149]. Currently, ciprofloxacin 500 mg b.i.d. for 3 days is the only quinolone regimen recommended for chancroid in the CDC STD treatment guidelines [62].

TABLE VI   Quinolone Regimens Effective for the Treatment of Chancroid

Regimen	Efficacy (clinical response)	Reference
Ciprofloxacin 500 mg once	76–100%	[139–142,147]
Ciprofloxacin 500 mg q. 12 hr (2 doses)	98%	[139]
Ciprofloxacin 500 mg q. 12 hr for 3 days	100%	[141]
Ciprofloxacin 250 mg q. day for 3 days	100%	[147]
Fleroxacin 200 mg once	88%	[143]
Fleroxacin 400 mg once	78–94%	[143,145,146]
Norfloxacin 800 mg single dose	94%	[144]
Rosoxacin 300 mg single dose	63%	[138]
Rosoxacin 150 mg q. 12 hr for 3 days	95%	[138]
Enoxacin 400 mg q. 12 hr (3 doses)	89%	[148]

DONOVANOSIS

Calymmatobacterium granulomatis is the etiologic agent of donovanosis, a major cause of genital ulcer disease in Asia, Africa, and some parts of the Caribbean [150]. The causative organism is difficult to propagate, so nothing is known about its *in-vitro* susceptibility to antibiotics. Clinically, many different antibiotics have been effective, including tetracycline, macrolides, aminoglycosides, trimethoprim/sulfamethoxazole, chloramphenicol, and, to a lesser degree, the β-lactams. However, treatment failures are common with all of these drugs, necessitating repeated therapeutic courses, and/or combination therapy. Two reports of individual cases and a small case series have suggested that both ciprofloxacin and norfloxacin may be effective for this disease [151,152].

BACTERIAL VAGINOSIS

Bacterial vaginosis is a polymicrobic condition that usually results in a mild to moderate amount of vaginal discharge and a pungent odor. This condition may be an important risk factor for preterm low-birth-weight delivery [153] as well as for PID [154]. The responsible organisms include *Gardnerella vaginalis*, a facultative anaerobe, as well as various strict anaerobes such as nonfragilis *Bacteroides*, *Prevotella*, and *Mobiluncus* species [155]. Currently available quinolones do not have good activity against these organisms. Based on a review by Ridgway, enoxacin, norfloxacin, fleroxacin, and pefloxacin have $MIC_{90}s$ against *Gardnerella* that range from 8 to 32 mg/liter [27]. Ciprofloxacin, ofloxacin, and levofloxacin have better activity, with $MIC_{90}s$ ranging from 1.0 to 2.0 mg/liter.

Newer quinolones have anaerobic activity that may make them effective against bacterial vaginosis. *In-vitro* analysis has demonstrated that gemifloxacin has good activity against *Bacteroides* and *Prevotella* species [156]. Sparfloxacin also has activity against these species that is better than ofloxacin and levofloxacin [157]. Clinafloxacin and sitafloxacin have even better activity against these organisms [157,158]. Sitafloxacin also has good *in-vitro* activity against *Gardnerella vaginalis* and *Mobiluncus* [158]. However, there are no published clinical trials using these newer agents for the treatment of this condition.

A few clinical trials using ciprofloxacin and ofloxacin have been reported. Two studies comparing 7-day courses of ofloxacin to 7-day courses of metronidazole have demonstrated that ofloxacin failed to cure bacterial vaginosis in a majority of patients [159,160]. One study of 22 women with nonspecific vaginosis who took ciprofloxacin 500 mg b.i.d. for 7 days reported that 73% had both clinical and bacteriological cures, and that 91% had a clinical cure or improvement [161]. Another trial found that only 8 of 14 women who took ciprofloxacin 250 mg b.i.d. for 7 days had cure or clinical improvement [162]. Both were noncomparative trials, and further evidence of clinical success with ciprofloxacin is not available in the published literature.

SPECIAL TOXICITY CONSIDERATIONS WHEN QUINOLONES ARE USED FOR TREATING SEXUALLY TRANSMITTED DISEASES

There are a few special considerations concerning the contraindications for quinolones that deserve special attention in the context of STD treatment. Quinolones are contraindicated in pregnancy, having been rated as pregnancy class C drugs by the Food and Drug Administration. Since early pregnancy is also a possibility in young women who have acquired an STD secondary to unprotected sex, quinolones must be used with caution in this setting. Therefore, a cephalosporin should be available as alternative treatment for uncomplicated gonococcal infections in clinics that use quinolones as first-line therapy for this disease. Alternatively, rapid urine pregnancy tests must be performed before a quinolone is administered to a potentially pregnant woman. Regardless of the approach, the treatment algorithm is complicated by the special precautions that must be taken with quinolones in potentially pregnant women.

Another consideration is that quinolones are not indicated for the treatment of children under 17 years of age (see Chapters 11, 14, and 15). This limits the use of quinolones in clinics that treat large numbers of adolescents. While it is very unlikely that any adolescent would be harmed by a single dose of a quinolone given to treat gonorrhea, especially given the lack of problems with quinolone therapy in children with cystic fibrosis, nonetheless, alternative drugs should be available for treating STDs in adolescents for medicolegal reasons.

CONCLUSION

The quinolones as a class of antibiotics are very useful in the treatment of gonorrhea as they are quite effective in single doses and are relatively inexpensive. A significant problem is the emergence of quinolone-resistant *N. gonorrhoeae* in many developing countries throughout the world. Whenever quinolones are used for treating gonorrhea, the maximum recommended dose should be used in order to slow the emergence of resistance. While the use of some newer quinolones for treatment of chlamydia has been limited by toxicity considerations, ofloxacin remains effective for these infections. The drawback of quinolones for this organism is that multidose therapy is necessary, which increases the cost. Currently, however, quinolones are the only drugs that are well tolerated and effective against both *N. gonorrhoeae* and *C. trachomatis*. Ofloxacin appears to be effective for pelvic inflammatory disease as a single agent, despite its relatively poor activity against anaerobes. Better anaerobic coverage by several of the newer quinolones suggests that these drugs may have a role in treating this condition in the future. The presently available quinolones are not effective for bacterial vaginosis, but, again, newer generations of the drugs with better anaerobic coverage may prove to be effective. Many of the quinolones are active against the causative agent of chancroid, *H. ducreyi*. Multidose therapy is currently recommended, as the failure rates may be somewhat higher with single-dose therapy. Finally, early work suggests that the quinolones may be effective in the treatment of donovanosis.

REFERENCES

1. Eng, T. R., and Butler, W. T. (1997). "The Hidden Epidemic: Confronting Sexually Transmitted Diseases." National Academy Press, Washington, DC.
2. Walker, R. C., and Wright, A. J. (1987). Symposium on antimicrobial agents: The quinolones. *Mayo Clin. Proc.* **62**, 1007–1012.
3. Andriole, V. T. (1988). Clinical overview of the newer 4-quinolone antibacterial agents. In "The Quinolones" (V. T. Andriole, ed.), pp. 173–177. Academic Press, San Diego.

4. Gerstner, G. J., Dalhoff, A., and Weuta, H. (1988). Single and multiple dose pharmacokinetics of ciprofloxacin in gynecologic tissues. *Infection* **16**, S24–S28.

5. Dalhoff, A., and Weuta, H. (1987). Penetration of ciprofloxacin into gynecologic tissues. *Am. J. Med.* **27**, 133–138.

6. Division of STD Prevention (1999). "Sexually Transmitted Diseases Surveillance, 1998." U.S. Department of Health and Human Services, Public Health Service, Atlanta.

7. McCormack, W. M., Stumacher, R. J., Johnson, K., and Donner, A. (1977). Clinical spectrum of gonococcal infection in women. *Lancet* **1**, 1182–1185.

8. Handsfield, H. H., Knapp, J. S., Diehr, P. K., and Holmes, K. K. (1980). Correlation of auxotype and penicillin susceptibility of *Neisseria gonorrhoeae* with sexual preference and clinical manifestations of gonorrhea. *Sex. Transm. Dis.* **7**, 1–5.

9. Klein, E. J., Fisher, L. S., Chow, A. W., and Guze, L. B. (1977). Anorectal gonococcal infection. *Ann. Intern. Med.* **83**, 340–346.

10. Centers for Disease Control and Prevention (1984). Declining rate of rectal and pharyngeal gonorrhea among males—New York City. *MMWR* **33**, 295–297.

11. Evans, B. G., Catchpole, M. A., Heptonstall, J., Mortimer, J. Y., McCarrigle, C. A., Nicoll, A. G., Waight, P., Gill, O. N., and Swan, A. V. (1993). Sexually transmitted diseases and HIV-1 infection among homosexual men in England and Wales. *Br. Med. J.* **306**, 426–428.

12. Ross, J. D., McMillan, A., and Young, H. (1991). Changing trends of gonococcal infection in homosexual men in Edinburgh. *Epidemiol. Infect.* **107**, 585–590.

13. Wiesner, P. J., Tronca, E., Bonin, P., Pedersen, A. H., and Holmes, K. K. (1973). Clinical spectrum of pharyngeal gonococcal infection. *New Engl. J. Med.* **25**, 181–185.

14. Division of STD Prevention (1999). "Sexually Transmitted Diseases Surveillance, 1998—GISP Report." U.S. Department of Health and Human Services, Public Health Service, Atlanta.

15. Division of STD Prevention (1996). "Sexually Transmitted Diseases Surveillance, 1995." U.S. Department of Health and Human Services, Public Health Service, Atlanta.

16. Sivayathorn, A. (1995). The use of fluoroquinolones in sexually transmitted diseases in Southeast Asia. *Drugs* **49**, 123–127.

17. Centers for Disease Control and Prevention (1985). Tetracycline resistant *Neisseria gonorrhoeae*—Georgia, Pennsylvania, New Hampshire. *MMWR* **34**, 563–570.

18. Ridgway, G. L. (1993). Quinolones in sexually transmitted diseases. *Drugs* **45**, 134–138.

19. Biedenbach, D. J., Beach, M. L., and Jones, R. N. (1998). Antimicrobial activity of gatifloxacin tested against *Neisseria gonorrhoeae* using three methods and a collection of fluoroquinolone-resistant strains. *Diag. Microbiol. Infect. Dis.* **32**, 307–311.

20. Makino, M., Miyazaki, Y., Ohno, A., Matsumoto, T., Fuyuya, N., and Yamaguchi, K. (1999). In vitro antibacterial activity of gemifloxacin against common respiratory tract pathogens and urinary tract pathogens isolated in Japan. *39th Intersci. Conf. Antimicrob. Agents Chemother.*, San Francisco.

21. Vazquez, J. A., de la Fuente, L., Gimenez, M. J., and Aguilar, L. (2000). In vitro activity of gemifloxacin and 12 other antimicrobials against 400 isolates of *Neisseria gonorrhoeae*. *Abstr. 3rd Eur. Cong. Chemother.*, Madrid.

22. Huczko, E, Valera, L., Conetta, B, Stickle, T., Macko, A., and Fung-Tome, J. (2000). Susceptibility of bacterial isolates to gatifloxacin and ciprofloxacin from clinical trials during the 1997–98 period. *39th Intersci. Conf. Antimicrob. Agents Chemother.*, San Francisco.

23. Deshpande, I. M., Erwin, M. E, Beach, M. L., and Jones, R. N. (2000). Anti-gonococcal activity of gemifloxacin using fluoroquinolone-resistant strains and developing in-vitro susceptibility test methods and quality control guidelines. *39th Intersci. Conf. Antimicrob. Agents Chemother.*, San Francisco.

24. Zenilman, J. M., Neumann, T. M., Patton, M., and Reichart, C. (1993). Antibacterial activities of OPC-17116, ofloxacin, and ciprofloxacin against 200 isolates of *Neisseria gonorrhoeae*. *Antimicrob. Agents Chemother.* **37**, 2244–2246.

25. Deguchi, T., Yasuda, M., Nakano, M., Kanematsu, E., Ozeki, S., Ishihara, S., Saito, I., and Kawada, Y. (1997). Antimicrobial activity of a new fluoroquinolone, DU-6859a, against quinolone-resistant clinical isolates of *Neisseria gonorrhoeae* with genetic alterations in the GyrA subunit of DNA gyrase and the ParC subunit of topoisomerase IV. *J. Antimicrob. Chemother.* **39**, 247–249.

26. Carlyn, C. J., Doyle, L. J., Knapp, C. C., Ludwig, M. D., and Washington, J. A. (1995). Activities of three investigational fluoroquinolones (BAY y 3118, DU-6859a, and clinafloxacin) against *Neisseria gonorrhoeae* isolates with diminished susceptibilities to ciprofloxacin and ofloxacin. *Antimicrob. Agents Chemother.* **39**, 1606–1608.

27. Ridgway, G. L. (1995). Quinolones in sexually transmitted diseases: Global experience. *Drugs* **49**, 115–122.

28. Echols, R. M., Heyd, A., O'Keefee, B. J., and Schacht, P. (1994). Single-dose ciprofloxacin for the treatment of uncomplicated gonorrhea: A worldwide summary. *Sex. Transm. Dis.* **21**, 345–352.

29. Hook III, E. W., Jones, R. B., Martin, D. H., Bolan, G. A., Mroczkowski, T. F., Neumann, T. M., Haag, J. J., and Echols, R. (1993). Comparison of ciprofloxacin and ceftriaxone as single-dose therapy for uncomplicated gonorrhea in women *Antimicrob. Agents Chemother.* **37**, 1670–1673.

30. Roddy, R. E., Handsfield, H. H., and Hook III, E. W. (1986). Comparative trial of single-dose ciprofloxacin and ampicillin plus probenecid for treatment of gonococcal urethritis in men. *Antimicrob. Agents Chemother.* **20**, 267–269.

31. Bryan, J. P., Hira, S. K., Brady, W., Luo, N., Mwale, C., Mpoko, G., Krieg, R., Siwiwaliondo, E., Reichart, C., Waters, C., *et al.* (1990). Oral ciprofloxacin versus ceftriaxone for the treatment of urethritis from resistant *Neisseria gonorrhoeae* in Zambia. *Antimicrob. Agents Chemother.* **34**, 819–822.

32. Scott, G. R., McMillan, A., and Young, H. (1987). Ciprofloxacin versus ampicillin and probenecid in the treatment of uncomplicated gonorrhoea in men. *J. Antimicrob. Chemother.* **21**, 117–121.

33. Lassus, A., Karppinen, L., Ingervo, L., Jeskanen, L., Reitamo, S., Happonen, H. P., and Karkulahti, R. (1989). Ciprofloxacin versus amoxycillin and probenecid in the treatment of uncomplicated gonorrhoea. *Scand. J. Infect. Dis.* **60**, 58–61.

34. Balachandran, T., Roberts, A. P., Evans, B. A., and Azadian, B. S. (1992). Single-dose therapy of anogenital and pharyngeal gonorrhoea with ciprofloxacin. *Int. J. AIDS STD* **3**, 49–51.

35. Loo, P. S., Ridgway, G. L., and Oriel, J. D. (1985). Single dose ciprofloxacin for treating gonococcal infections in men. *Genitourin. Med.* **61**, 302–305.

36. Shahmanesh, M., Shukla, S. R., Phillips, I., Westwood, A., and Thin, R. N. (1986). Ciprofloxacin for treating urethral gonorrhoea in men. *Genitourin. Med.* **62**, 86–87.

37. Avonts, D., Fransen, L., Vielfont, J., Stevens, A., Hendrickx, K., and Piot, P. (1988). Treating uncomplicated gonococcal infection with 250 mg or 100 mg ciprofloxacin in a single oral dose. *Genitourin. Med.* **64**, 134–134.

38. Aznar, J., Prados, R., Rodriguez-Pichardo, A., Hernandez, I., de Miguel, C., and Perea, E. J. (1986). Comparative clinical efficacy of two different single-dose ciprofloxacin treatments for uncomplicated gonorrhea. *Sex. Transm. Dis.* **13**, 169–171.

39. Thorpe, E. M., Schwebke, J. R., Hook III, E. W., Rompalo, A., McCormack, W. M., Mussari, K. L., Giguere, G. C., and Collins, J. J. (1996). Comparison of single-dose cefuroxime axetil with ciprofloxacin in treatment of uncomplicated gonorrhea caused by penicillinase-producing

and non-penicillinase-producing *Neisseria gonorrhoeae* strains *Antimicrob. Agents Chemother.* **40**, 2775–2780.

40. Smith, B. L., Mogabgab, W. J., Dalu, A. Z., Jones, R. B., Douglas, J. M., Handsfield, H. H., Hook III, E. W., Viner, B. L., Shands, J. W. J., and McCormack, W. M. (1993). Multicenter trial of fleroxacin versus ceftriaxone in the treatment of uncomplicated gonorrhea. *Am. J. Med.* **22**, 81S–84S.

41. Lassus, A., Abath Filho, L., Santos Jr., M. F., and Belli, L. (1992). Comparison of fleroxacin and penicillin G plus probenecid in the treatment of acute uncomplicated gonococcal infections *Genitourin. Med.* **68**, 317–320.

42. Lassus, A., Renkonen, O. V., and Ellmen, J. (1988). Fleroxacin versus standard therapy in gonococcal urethritis. *J. Antimicrob. Chemother.* **22**, 223–225.

43. Bogaerts, J., Tello, W. M., Akingeneye, J., Mukantabana, V., Van Dyck, E., and Piot, P. (1993). Effectiveness of norfloxacin and ofloxacin for treatment of gonorrhoea and decrease of in vitro susceptibility to quinolones over time in Rwanda. *Genitourin. Med.* **63**, 196–200.

44. Bogaerts, J., Martinez Tello, W., Verbist, L., Piot, P., and Vandepitte, J. (1987). Norfloxacin versus thiamphenicol for treatment of uncomplicated gonorrhea in Rwanda. *Antimicrob. Agents Chemother.* **31**, 434–437.

45. Panikabutra, K., Lee, C. T., Ho, B., and Bamberg, P. (1988). Single dose oral norfloxacin or intramuscular spectinomycin to treat gonorrhoea (PPNG and non-PPNG infections): Analysis of efficacy and patient preference. *Genitourin. Med.* **64**, 235–240.

46. Mitsuya, H., Asaka, H., Segawa, A., Fukatsu, H., Otani, S., Yoshida, K., Okamura, K., Murase, T., Asano, H., Obata, K., *et al.* (1989). Treatment of gonococcal urethritis with norfloxacin [Japanese]. *Hinyokika Kiyo, Acta Urologica Japonica* **35**, 705–709.

47. Cristiano, P. (1989). Clinical trial of norfloxacin in the treatment of uncomplicated gonococcal urethritis: Preliminary report. *Drugs Exp. Clin. Res.* **15**, 33–35.

48. Romanowski, B., Wood, H., Draker, J., and Tsianco, M. C. (1986). Norfloxacin in the therapy of uncomplicated gonorrhea. *Antimicrob. Agents Chemother.* **30**, 514–515.

49. Mogabgab, W. J. (1991). Single-dose oral temafloxacin versus parenteral ceftriaxone in the treatment of gonococcal urethritis/cervicitis. *Am. J. Med.* **91**, 145S–149S.

50. Vagaskar, S. R., Fernandez, R. J., Wagle, U. D., and Rajani, N. D. (1990). Rosoxacin in the treatment of uncomplicated acute gonococcal urethritis. *J. Postgrad. Med.* **36**, 191–193.

51. Leow, Y. H., Chan, R. K., Cheong, L. L., Goh, C. L., and Nadarajah, M. (1995). Comparing the efficacy of pefloxacin and ciprofloxacin in the treatment of acute uncomplicated gonococcal urethritis in males. *Ann. Acad. Med., Singapore* **2**, 515–518.

52. Cheong, L. L., Chan, R. K., and Nadarajah, M. (1992). Pefloxacin and ciprofloxacin in the treatment of uncomplicated gonococcal urethritis in males. *Genitourin. Med.* **58**, 260–262.

53. Stolz, E., Wagenvoort, J. H., and van der Willigen, A. H. (1987). Quinolones in the treatment of gonorrhoea and *Chlamydia trachomatis* infections. *Pharmaceut. Weekbl., Scient. Ed.* **11**, S82–S86.

54. Smith, B. L., Cummings, M., Benes, S., Draft, K., and McCormack, W. M. (1989). Evaluation of difloxacin in the treatment of uncomplicated urethral gonorrhea in men. *Antimicrob. Agents Chemother.* **33**, 1721–1723.

55. Moi, H., Morel, P., Gianotti, B., Barlow, D., Phillips, I., and Jean, C. (1996). Comparative efficacy and safety of single oral doses of sparfloxacin versus ciprofloxacin in the treatment of acute gonococcal urethritis in men. *J. Antimicrob. Chemother.* **37**, 115–122.

56. Stoner, B. P., Douglas, J. M., Martin, D. H., Hook III, E. W., Leone, P., McCormack, W. M., Mroczkowski, T. F., Jones, R., Yang, J., and Baumgartner, T. (1999). Randomized, double-blind,

multicenter trial of single-dose gatifloxacin compared with ofloxacin for the treatment of uncomplicated gonorrhea. *39th Intersci. Conf. Antimicrob. Agents Chemother.*, San Francisco.

57. Handsfield, H. H., Judson, F. N., and Holmes, K. K. (1981). Treatment of uncomplicated gonorrhea with rosoxacin. *Antimicrob. Agents Chemother.* **20**, 625–629.

58. Svindland, H. B., Svarva, P. L., and Maeland, J. A. (1982). Quinolone derivative, flumequine, as short-term treatment for gonorrhoea. *Br. J. Vener. Dis.* **58**, 317–320.

59. Hook III, E. W., Pinson, G. B., Blalock, C. J., and Johnson, R. B. (1995). Dose-ranging study of CP-99,219 (trovafloxacin) for treatment of uncomplicated gonorrhea. *Antimicrob. Agents Chemother.* **40**, 1720–1721.

60. Haizlip, J., Isbey, S. F., Hamilton, H. A., Jerse, A. E., Leone, P. A., Davis, R. H., and Cohen, M. S. (1995). Time required for elimination of *Neisseria gonorrhoeae* from the urogenital tract in men with symptomatic urethritis: Comparison of oral and intramuscular single-dose therapy. *Sex. Transm. Dis.* **22**, 145–148.

61. Coker, D. M., Ahmed-Jushuf, I., Arya, O. P., Chessbrough, J. S., and Pratt, B. C. (1989). Evaluation of single-dose ciprofloxacin in the treatment of rectal and pharyngeal gonorrhoea. *J. Antimicrob. Chemother.* **24**, 271–272.

62. Centers for Disease Control and Prevention (1998). 1998 Guidelines for Treatment of Sexually Transmitted Diseases. *MMWR*.

63. Kestelyn, P., Bogaerts, J., Stevens, A. M., Piot, P., and Meheus, A. (1989). Treatment of adult gonococcal keratoconjunctivitis with oral norfloxacin. *Am. J. Ophthalmol.* **108**, 516–523.

64. Zenilman, J. M. (1996). Gonococcal susceptibility to antimicrobials in Baltimore, 1988–1994. What was the impact of ciprofloxacin as first-line therapy for gonorrhea? *Sex. Transm. Dis.* **23**, 213–218.

65. Moran, J. S. (1996). Ciprofloxacin for gonorrhea—250 mg or 500 mg? *Sex. Transm. Dis.* **23**, 165–167.

66. Deguchi, T., Yasuda, M., Nakano, M., Ozeki, S., Kanematsu, E., Kawada, Y., Ezaki, T., and Saito, I. (1996). Uncommon occurrence of mutations in the gyrB gene associated with quinolone resistance in clinical isolates of *Neisseria gonorrhoeae*. *Antimicrob. Agents Chemother.* **40**, 2437–2438.

67. Deguchi, T., Yasuda, M., Nakano, M., Ozeki, S., Ezaki, T., Saito, I., and Kawada, Y. (1996). Quinolone-resistant *Neisseria gonorrhoeae*: Correlation of alterations in the GyrA subunit of DNA gyrase and the ParC subunit of topoisomerase IV with antimicrobial susceptibility profiles *Antimicrob. Agents Chemother.* **40**, 1020–1023.

68. Belland, R. J., Morrison, S. G., Ison, C., and Huang, W. M. (1994). *Neisseria gonorrhoeae* acquires mutations in analogous regions of gyrA and parC in fluoroquinolone-resistant isolates *Mol. Microbiol.* **14**, 371–380.

69. Corkill, J. E., Percival, A., and Lind, M. (1991). Reduced uptake of ciprofloxacin in a resistant strain of *Neisseria gonorrhoeae* and transformation of resistance to other strains. *J. Antimicrob. Chemother.* **28**, 601–604.

70. Deguchi, T., Saito, I., Tanaka, M., Sato, K.-I., Deguchi, K.-I., Yasuda, M., Nakano, M., Nishino, Y., Kanematsu, E., Ozeki, S., and Kawada, Y. (1997). Fluoroquinolone treatment failure in gonorrhea: Emergence of a *Neisseria gonorrhoeae* strain with enhanced resistance to fluoroquinolones. *Sex. Transm. Dis.* **24**, 247–250.

71. Knapp, J. S., Hale, J. A., Neal, S. W., Wintersheid, K., Rice, R. J., and Whittington, W. L. (1995). Proposed criteria for interpretation of susceptibilities of strains of *Neisseria gonorrhoeae* to ciprofloxacin, ofloxacin, enoxacin, lomefloxacin, and norfloxacin. *Antimicrob. Agents Chemother.* **39**, 2442–2445.

72. Vance-Bryan, K., Guay, D. R., and Rotschafer, J. C. (1990). Clinical pharmacokinetics of ciprofloxacin. *Clin. Pharmacokin.* **19**, 434–461.

73. Ng, P. P., Chan, R. K., and Linnanmäki, E. (1998). Gonorrhea treatment failure and ciprofloxacin resistance. *Int. J. STD AIDS* **9**, 323–325.

74. Tzelepi, E., Avgerinou, H., Kyriakis, K. P., Tzouvelekis, L. S., Flemetakis, A., Kalogeropoulou, A., and Frangouli, E. (1997). Antimicrobial susceptibility and types of *Neisseria gonorrhoeae* in Greece: Data for the period 1990 to 1993. *Sex. Transm. Dis.* **24**, 378–385.

75. Van de Laar, M. J., van Duynhoven, Y. T., Dessens, M., van Santen, M., and van Klingeren, B. (1997). Surveillance of antibiotic resistance in *Neisseria gonorrhoeae* in The Netherlands, 1977-1995. *Genitourin. Med.* **73**, 510–517.

76. Knapp, J. S., Fox, K. K., Trees, D. L., and Whittington, W. L. (1997). Fluoroquinolone resistance in Neisseria gonorrhoeae. *Emerg. Infect. Dis.* **3**, 33–39.

77. Wagenvoort, J. H., van der Willigen, A. H., and van Noort, J. A. (1986). Decreased sensitivity of *Neisseria gonorrhoeae* to quinolone compounds. *Eur. J. Clin. Microbiol.* **5**, 685–685.

78. Jephcott, A. E., and Turner, A. (1990). Ciprofloxacin resistance in gonococci. *Lancet* **335**, 165–165.

79. Tapsall, J. W., Shultz, T. R., Lovett, R., and Munro, R. (1992). Failure of 500-mg ciprofloxacin therapy in male urethral gonorrhoea. *Med. J. Aust.* **156**, 143–143.

80. Tapsall, J. W., Limnios, E. A., Thacker, C., Donovan, B., Lynch, S. D., Kirby, L. J., Wise, K. A., and Carmody, C. J. (1995). High-level quinolone resistance in *Neisseria gonorrhoeae*: A report of two cases. *Sex. Transm. Dis.* **22**, 310–311.

81. Centers for Disease Control and Prevention (1995). Fluoroquinolone resistant *Neisseria gonorrhoeae*: Colorado and Washington. *MMWR* **20**, 761–764.

82. Kam, K. M., Wong, P. W., Cheung, M. M., Ho, N. K. Y., and Lo, K. K. (1996). Quinolone-resistant *Neisseria gonorrhoeae* in Hong Kong. *Sex. Transm. Dis.* **23**, 103–108.

83. Tanaka, M., Sagiyama, K., Haraoka, M., Saika, T., Kobayashi, I., and Naito, S. (1999). Genotypic evolution in a quinolone-resistant *Neisseria gonorrhoeae* isolate from a patient with clinical failure of levofloxacin treatment. *Urologica Internationalis* **62**, 64–68.

84. Tanaka, M., Nakayama, H., Haraoka, M., Nagafuji, T., Saika, T., and Kobayashi, I. (1998). Analysis of quinolone resistance mechanisms in a sparfloxacin-resistant clinical isolate of *Neisseria gonorrhoeae*. *Sex. Transm. Dis.* **25**, 489–493.

85. Kam, K. M., Lo, K. K., Lai, C. F., Lee, Y. S., and Chan, C. B. (1993). Ofloxacin susceptibilities of 5,667 *Neisseria gonorrhoeae* strains isolated in Hong Kong. *Antimicrob. Agents Chemother.* **37**, 2007–2008.

86. Ison, C., Dillon, J. R., and Tapsall, J. W. (1998). The epidemiology of global antibiotic resistance among *Neisseria gonorrhoeae* and *Haemophilus ducreyi*. *Lancet* **351**, 8–11.

87. Klausner, J. D., Aplasca, M. R., Mesola, V. P., Bolan, G., Whittington, W. L., and Holmes, K. K. (1999). Correlates of gonococcal infection and of antimicrobial resistant *Neisseria gonorrhoeae* among female sex workers, Republic of the Phillipines, 1996–1997. *J. Infect. Dis.* **179**, 729–733.

88. Tapsall, J. W., Limnios, E. A., and Shultz, T. R. (1998). Continuing evolution of the pattern of quinolone resistance in *Neisseria gonorrhoeae* isolated in Sydney, Australia. *Sex. Transm. Dis.* **25**, 415–417.

89. Aplasca, M. R., Pato-Mesola, V., Klausner, J., Tuazon, C., Whittington, W. L., and Holmes, K. K. (1997). High rates of failure after treatment with ciprofloxacin: Are fluoroquinolones no longer useful for gonorrhea treatment? *Abstr. 4th Int. Cong. AIDS in Asia and the Pacific*, Manila.

90. Divekar, A. A., Grogate, A. S., and Shivkar, L. K. (2000). Association between auxotypes, serogroups, and antibiotic susceptibilities of *Neisseria gonorrhoeae* isolated from women in Mumbai, India. *Sex. Transm. Dis.* **26**, 358–363.

91. Guoming, L., Chen, Q., and Shengchun, W. (2000). Resistance to *Neisseria gonorrhoeae* epidemic strains to antibiotics. *Sex. Transm. Dis.* **27**, 115–118.

92. Bhuiyan, B. U., Rahman, M., Miah, M. R., Nahar, S., Islam, N., Ahmed, M., Rahman, K. M., and Albert, M. J. (1999). Antimicrobial susceptibilities and plasmid contents of *Neisseria gonorrhoeae* isolates from commercial sex workers in Dhaka, Bangladesh: Emergence of high level resistance to ciprofloxacin. *J. Clin. Microbiol.* **37**, 1130–1136.

93. Turner, A., Gough, K. R., Jephcott, A. E., and McClean, A. N. (1995). Importation into the UK of a strain of *Neisseria gonorrhoeae* resistant to penicillin, ciprofloxacin and tetracycline. *Genitourin. Med.* **71**, 331–332.

94. Birley, H., McDonald, P., Carey, P., and Fletcher, J. (1994). High level ciprofloxacin resistance in *Neisseria gonorrhoeae*. *Genitourin. Med.* **14**, 292–293.

95. Kilmarx, P. H., Knapp, J. S., Xia, M., St. Louis, M. E., Neal, S. W., Sayers, D., Doyle, L. J., Roberts, M. C., and Whittington, W. L. (1998). Intercity spread of gonococci with decreased susceptibility to fluoroquinolones: A unique focus in the United States. *J. Infect. Dis.* **177**, 677–682.

96. Deguchi, T., Yasuda, M., Nakano, M., Ozeki, S., Kanematsu, E., Fukuda, H., Maeda, S., Saito, I., and Kawada, Y. (1997). Comparison of in vitro antimicrobial activity of AM-1155 with those of tosufloxacin and fleroxacin against clinical isolates of *Neisseria gonorrhoeae* harboring quinolone resistance alterations in GyrA and Parc. *Chemotherapy* **43**, 239–244.

97. Peterson, H. B., Walker, C. K., Kahn, J. G., Washington, A. E., Eschenbach, D. A., and Faro, S. (1991). Pelvic inflammatory disease. Key treatment issues and options. *JAMA* **266**(18), 2605–2611.

98. Martin, D. H. (1994). *Chlamydia trachomatis* infections. In "Obstetrical and Gynecological Infectious Diseases" (J. G. Pastorek, ed.), pp. 491–505. Raven, New York.

99. Black, C. M. (1997). Current methods of laboratory diagnosis of *Chlamydia trachomatis* infections. *Clin. Microbiol. Rev.* **10**, 160–184.

100. Bowie, W. R., Lee, C. K., and Alexander, E. R. (1978). Prediction of the efficacy of antimicrobial agents in treatment of infections due to *Chlamydia trachomatis*. *J. Infect. Dis.* **138**, 655–659.

101. Bowie, W. R., Willets, V., and Siegel, N. (1986). Failure of norfloxacin to eradicate *Chlamydia trachomatis* in nongonococcal urethritis. *Antimicrob. Agents Chemother.* 30, 594.

102. Oriel, J. D. (1986). Ciprofloxacin in the treatment of gonorrhoea and non-gonococcal urethritis. *J. Antimicrob. Chemother.* **18**, 129–132.

103. Fong, I. W., Linton, W., Simbul, M., Thorup, R., McLaughlin, B., Rahm, V., and Quinn, P. A. (1987). Treatment of nongonococcal urethritis with ciprofloxacin. *Am. J. Med.* **82**, 311–316.

104. Perea, E. J., Aznar, J., Herrera, A., Mazuecos, J., and Rodriguez-Pichardo, A. (1989). Clinical efficacy of new quinolones for therapy of nongonococcal urethritis. *Sex. Transm. Dis.* **16**, 7–10.

105. Jeskanen, L., Karppinen, L., Ingervo, L., Reitamo, S., Happonen, H. P., and Lassus, F. (1989). Ciprofloxacin versus doxycycline in the treatment of uncomplicated urogenital *Chlamydia trachomatis* infections. A double-blind comparative study. *Scand. J. Infect. Dis.* **60**, 62–65.

106. Hooton, T. M., Rogers, E., Medina, T. G., Kuwamura, L. E., Ewers, C., Roberts, P. L., and Stamm, W. E. (1990). Ciprofloxacin compared with doxycycline for nongonococcal urethritis. Ineffectiveness against *Chlamydia trachomatis* due to relapsing infection. *JAMA* **264**, 1418–1421.

107. Judson, F. N., Beals, B. S., and Tack, K. J. (1986). Clinical experience with ofloxacin in sexually transmitted diseases. *Infection* **14**, 309–310.

108. Ibsen, H. H. W., Moller, B. R., Halkier-Sorensen, L., and From, E. (1989). Treatment of nongonococcal urethritis: Comparison of ofloxacin and erythromycin. *Sex. Transm. Dis.* **16**, 32–35.

109. Mogabgab, W. J., Holmes, B., Murray, M., Beville, R., Lutz, F. B., and Tack, K. J. (1990). Randomized comparison of ofloxacin and doxycycline for chlamydia and ureaplasma urethritis and cervicitis. *Chemotherapy* **36**, 70–76.

110. Kitchen, V. S., Donegan, C., Ward, H., Thomas, B., Harris, J. R. W., and Taylor-Robinson, D. (1990). Comparison of ofloxacin with doxycycline in the treatment of non-gonococcal urethritis and cervical chlamydial infection. *J. Antimicrob. Chemother.* **26**, 99–105.

111. Hooton, T. M., Batteiger, B. E., Judson, F. N., Spruance, S. L., and Stamm, W. E. (1992). Ofloxacin versus doxycycline for treatment of cervical infection with *Chlamydia trachomatis*. *Antimicrob. Agents Chemother.* **36**, 1144–1146.

112. Martin, D. H., Mroczkowski, T. F., Richelo, B. N., St. Clair, P. J., and Pizzuti, D. J. (1990). Randomized double blind study of fleroxacin (F) and doxycycline (D) for the treatment of *Chlamydia trachomatis* (Ct) genital tract infections. *3rd Int. Symp. New Quinolones*, Vancouver.

113. Ziegler, C., Stary, A., Mailer, H., Kopp, W., Gebhart, W., and Soltz-Szots, J. (1992). Quinolones as an alternative treatment of chlamydial, mycoplasma, and gonococcal urogenital infections. *Dermatology* **185**, 128–131.

114. Bergan, T. (1988). Pharmacokinetics of fluorinated quinolones. In "The Quinolones" (V. T. Andriole, ed.), pp. 119–145. Academic Press, San Diego.

115. Forrest, A., Nix, D. E., Ballow, C. H., Goss, T. F., Birmingham, M. C., and Schentag, J. J. (1993). Pharmacodynamics of intravenous ciprofloxacin in seriously ill patients. *Antimicrob. Agents Chemother.* **37**, 1073–1081.

116. Tanaka, M., Matsumoto, T., Kumazawa, J., Nakayama, H., Urabe, H., Miyazaki, Y., Kano, M., and Nanri, K. (1994). Tosufloxacin in the treatment of nongonococcal urethritis, including *Chlamydia trachomatis*. *Clin. Therap.* **16**, 819–823.

117. McCormack, W. M., Martin, D. H., Hook III, E. W., and Jones, R. B. (1998). Daily oral grepafloxacin vs. twice daily oral doxycycline in the treatment of *Chlamydia trachomatis* endocervical infection. *Infect. Dis. Obstet. Gynecol.* **6**, 109–115.

118. Martin, D. H., Jones, R. B., and Johnson, R. B. (1999). A phase-II study of trovafloxacin for the treatment of *Chlamydia trachomatis* infections. *Sex. Transm. Dis.* **26**, 369–373.

119. McCormack, W. M., Dalu, Z. A., Martin, D. H., Hook III, E. W., Laisi, R., Kell, P., Pluck, N. D., and Johnson, R. B. (1999). Double-blind comparison of trovafloxacin and doxycycline in the treatment of uncomplicated chlamydial urethritis and cervicitis: Trovafloxacin Chlamydial Urethritis/Cervicitis Study Group *Sex. Transm. Dis.* **26**, 531–536.

120. Phillips, I., Dimian, C., Barlow, D., Moi, H., Stolz, E., Weidner, W., and Perea, E. (1996). A comparative study of two different regimens of sparfloxacin versus doxycycline in the treatment of nongonococcal urethritis in men. *J. Antimicrob. Chemother.* **37**, 123–134.

121. Martin, D. H., Mroczkowski, T. F., Dalu, A. Z., McCarty, J., Jones, R. B., Hopkins, S. J., and Johnson, R. B. (1992). A controlled trial of a single dose of azithromycin for the treatment of chlamydial urethritis and cervicitis. *New Engl. J. Med.* **327**, 921–925.

122. Westrom, L., and Mardh, P.-A. (1990). Acute pelvic inflammatory disease (PID). In "Sexually Transmitted Diseases" (K. K. Holmes, P. A. Mardh, P. F. Sparling, P. J. Wiesner, W. Cates, S. M. Lemon, and W. E. Stamm, eds.), pp. 593–613. McGraw-Hill, New York.

123. Wendel Jr., G. D., Cox, S. M., Bawdon, R. E., Theriot, S. K., Heard, M. C., and Nobles, B. J. (1991). A randomized study of ofloxacin versus cefoxitin and doxycycline in the outpatient treatment of acute salpingitis. *Am. J. Obstet. Gynecol.* **164**, 1390–1396.

124. Martens, M. G., Gordon, S., Yarborough, D. R., Faro, S., Binder, D., and Berkeley, A. (1993). Multicenter randomized trial of ofloxacin versus cefoxitin and doxycycline in outpatient treatment of pelvic inflammatory disease: Ambulatory PID Research Group. *South. Med. J.* **86**, 604–610.

125. Mardh, P.-A. (1980). An overview of infectious agents of salpingitis, their biology, and recent advances in methods of detection. *Am. J. Obstet. Gynecol.* **138**, 933–951.

126. Gjonnaess, H., Dalaker, K., Anestad, G., Mardh, P.-A., Kvile, G., and Bergan, T. (1982). Pelvic inflammatory disease: Etiologic studies with emphasis on chlamydial infection. *Obstet. Gynecol.* **59**, 550–555.

127. Van Dyck, E., Bogaerts, J., Smet, H., Tello, W. M., Mukantabana, V., and Piot, P. (1994). Emergence of *Haemophilus ducreyi* resistance to trimethoprim–sulfamethoxazole in Rwanda. *Antimicrob. Agents Chemother.* **38**, 1647–1648.

128. Schulte, J. M., and Schmid, G. P. (1995). Recommendations for treatment of chancroid, 1993. *Clin. Infect. Dis.* **20**, S39–S46.

129. Slaney, L., Plummer, F., Ronald, A. R., Degagne, P., Hoban, D., and Brunham, R. C. (1990). *In vitro* activity of azithromycin, erythromycin, ciprofloxacin and norfloxacin against *Neisseria gonorrhoeae*, *Haemophilus ducreyi* and *Chlamydia trachomatis*. *J. Antimicrob. Chemother.* **25** (Suppl. A), 1–5.

130. Martin, D. H., Sargent, S. J., Wendel Jr., G. D., McCormack, W. M., Spier, N. A., and Johnson, R. B. (1995). Comparison of azithromycin and ceftriaxone for the treatment of chancroid. *Clin. Infect. Dis.* **21**, 409–414.

131. Jones, B. M., Geary, I., Lee, M. E., and Duerden, B. I. (1985). Activity of pefloxacin and thirteen other antimicrobial agents in vitro against isolates from hospital and genitourinary infections. *J. Antimicrob. Chemother.* **17**, 739–746.

132. Abeck, D., Johnson, A. P., Dangor, Y., and Ballard, R. C. (1988). Antibiotic susceptibilities and plasmid profiles of *Haemophilus ducreyi* isolates from southern Africa. *J. Antimicrob. Chemother.* **22**, 437–444.

133. Knapp, J. S., Back, A. F., Babst, A. F., Taylor, D., and Rice, R. J. (1993). In vitro susceptibilities of isolates of *Haemophilus ducreyi* from Thailand and the United States to currently recommended and newer agents for treatment of chancroid. *Antimicrob. Agents Chemother.* **37**, 1552–1555.

134. Wall, R. A., Mabey, D. C., Bello, C. S., and Felmingham, D. (1985). The comparative in-vitro activity of twelve 4-quinolone antimicrobials against *Haemophilus ducreyi*. *J. Antimicrob. Chemother.* **16**, 165–168.

135. Dangor, Y., Miller, S. D., Exposto, F. d.L., and Koornhof, H. J. (1988). Antimicrobial susceptibilities of southern African isolates of *Haemophilus ducreyi*. *Antimicrob. Agents Chemother.* **32**, 1458–1460.

136. Aldridge, K. E., Cammarata, C. L., and Martin, D. H. (1993). Comparison of in vitro activities of various parenteral and oral antimicrobial agents against endemic *Haemophilus ducreyi*. *Antimicrob. Agents Chemother.* **37**, 1986–1988.

137. Le Saux, N. M., Slaney, L. A., Plummer, F. A., Ronald, A. R., and Brunham, R. C. (1987). In vitro activity of ceftriaxone, cefetamet (Ro 15-8074), ceftetrame (Ro 19-5247; T-2588), and fleroxacin (Ro 23-6240; AM-833) versus *Neisseria gonorrhoeae* and *Haemophilus ducreyi*. *Antimicrob. Agents Chemother.* **31**, 1153–1154.

138. Haase, D. A., Ndinya-Achola, J. O., Nash, R. A., D'Costa, L. J., Hazlett, D., Lubwama, S., Nsanze, H., and Ronald, A. R. (1986). Clinical evaluation of rosoxacin for the treatment of chancroid. *Antimicrob. Agents Chemother.* **30**, 39–41.

139. Bodhidatta, L., Taylor, D. N., Chitwarakorn, A., Kuvanont, K., and Echeverria, P. (1988). Evaluation of 500- and 1000-mg doses of ciprofloxacin for the treatment of chancroid. *Antimicrob. Agents Chemother.* **32**, 723–725.

140. Traisupa, A., Wongba, C., and Tesavibul, P. (1988). Efficacy and safety of a single dose therapy of a 500-mg ciprofloxacin tablet in chancroid patients. *Infection* **16**, S44–S45.

141. Naamara, W., Plummer, F. A., Greenblatt, R. M., D'Costa, L. J., Ndinya-Achola, J. O., and Ronald, A. R. (1987). Treatment of chancroid with ciprofloxacin: A prospective, randomized clinical trial. *Am. J. Med.* **82**, 317–320.

142. Bogaerts, J., Kestens, L., Martinez Tello, W., Akingeneye, J., Mukantabana, V., Verhaegen, J., Van Dyke, E., and Piot, P. (1995). Failure of treatment for chancroid in Rwanda is not related to human immunodeficiency virus infection: In vitro resistance of *Haemophilus ducreyi* to trimethoprim–sulfamethoxazole. *Clin. Infect. Dis.* **20**, 924–930.

143. MacDonald, K. S., Cameron, D. W., D'Costa, L., Ndinya-Achola, J. O., Plummer, F. A., and Ronald, A. R. (1989). Evaluation of fleroxacin (RO 23-6240) as single-oral-dose therapy of culture-proven chancroid in Nairobi, Kenya. *Antimicrob. Agents Chemother.* **33**, 612–614.

144. Ariyarit, C., Mokamukkul, B., Chitwarakorn, A., Wongba, C., Buatiang, A., Singharaj, P., and Kuvanont, K. (1988). Clinical and microbiological efficacy of a single dose of norfloxacin in the treatment of chancroid. *Scand. J. Infect. Dis.* **56**, 55–58.

145. Tyndall, M. W., Plourde, P. J., Agoki, E., Malisa, W., Ndinya-Achola, J. O., Plummer, F. A., and Ronald, A. R. (1993). Fleroxacin in the treatment of chancroid: An open study in men seropositive or seronegative for the human immunodeficiency virus type 1. *Am. J. Med.* **94**, 85S–88S.

146. Plourde, P. J., D'Costa, L. J., Agoki, E., Ombetti, J., Ndinya-Achola, J. O., Slaney, L. A., Ronald, A. R., and Plummer, F. A. (1992). A randomized, double-blind study of the efficacy of fleroxacin versus trimethoprim–sulfamethoxazole in men with culture-proven chancroid. *J. Infect. Dis.* **165**, 949–952.

147. Behets, F. M., Liomba, G., Lule, G., Dallabetta, G., Hoffman, I. F., Hamilton, H. A., Moeng, S., and Cohen, M. S. (1995). Sexually transmitted diseases and human immunodeficiency virus control in Malawi: A field study of genital ulcer disease. *J. Infect. Dis.* **171**, 451–455.

148. Naamara, W., Kunimoto, D. Y., D'Costa, L., Ndinya-Achola, J. O., Nsanze, H., Ronald, A. R., and Plummer, F. A. (1988). Treating chancroid with enoxacin. *Genitourin. Med.* **64**, 189–192.

149. Ronald, A. R., Corey, L., McCutchan, J. A., and Handsfield, H. H. (1992). Evaluation of new anti-infective drugs for the treatment of chancroid: Infectious Diseases Society of America and the Food and Drug Administration. *Clin. Infect. Dis.* **15**, S108–S114.

150. Hart, G. (1990). Donavanosis. In "Sexually Transmitted Diseases" (K. K. Holmes, P. A. Mardh, P. F. Sparling, P. J. Wiesner, W. Cates, S. M. Lemon, and W. E. Stamm, eds.), pp. 273–277. McGraw-Hill, New York.

151. Ramanan, C., Sarma, P. S., Ghorpade, A., and Das, M. (1990). Treatment of donovanosis with norfloxacin. *Int. J. Derm.* **29**, 298–299.

152. Ahmed, B. A., and Tang, A. (1996). Successful treatment of donovanosis with ciprofloxacin. *Genitourin. Med.* **72**, 73–74.

153. Hillier, S. L., Nugent, R. P., Eschenbach, D. A., Krohn, M. A., Gibbs, R. S., Martin, D. H., Cotch, M. F., Edelman, R., Pastorek Jr., J. G., Rao, A. V., *et al.* (1995). Association between bacterial vaginosis and preterm delivery of a low-birth-weight infant: The Vaginal Infections and Prematurity Study Group. *New Engl. J. Med.* **333**, 1737–1742.

154. Eschenbach, D. A. (1993). Bacterial vaginosis and anaerobes in obstetric–gynecologic infection. *Clin. Infect. Dis.* **16**, S282–S287.

155. Rein, M. F. (1993). Vulvovaginitis and cervicitis. In "Principles and Practice of Infectious Diseases" (G. L. Mandell, J. E. Bennett, and R. Dolin, eds.), pp. 1074–1090. Churchill Livingstone, New York.

156. Tanaka, K., Kato, N., and Watanabe, K. (1999). Comparative in vitro antibacterial activity of gemifloxacin against anaerobic bacteria. *39th Intersci. Conf. Antimicrob. Agents Chemother.*, San Francisco.

157. Hecht, D. W., and Wexler, H. M. (1996). In vitro susceptibility of anaerobes to quinolones in the United States. *Clin. Infect. Dis.* **23**, S2–S8.

158. Kato, N., Kato, H., Tanaka-Bando, K., Watanabe, K., and Ueno, K. (1996). Comparison of in vitro activities of DU-6859a and other fluoroquinolones against Japanese isolates of anaerobic bacteria. *Clin. Infect. Dis.* **1**, S31–S35.

159. Nayagam, A. T., Smith, M. D., Ridgway, G. L., Allason-Jones, E., Robinson, A. J., and Stock, J. (1992). Comparison of ofloxacin and metronidazole for the treatment of bacterial vaginosis. *Int. J. AIDS STD* **3**, 204–207.

160. Covino, J. M., Black, J. R., Cummings, M., Zwickl, B., and McCormack, W. M. (1993). Comparative evaluation of ofloxacin and metronidazole in the treatment of bacterial vaginosis. *Sex. Transm. Dis.* **20**, 262–264.

161. Carmond, O., Hernandez-Gonzalez, S., and Kobelt, R. (1987). Ciprofloxacin in the treatment of nonspecific vaginitis. *Am. J. Med.* **82**, 321–323.

162. Fredricsson, B., Englund, K., Nord, C. E., and Weintraub, L. (1992). Could bacterial vaginosis be due to the competitive suppression of lactobacilli by aerobic microorganisms? *Gynecol. Obstet. Invest.* **33**, 119–123.

163. Perea, E. J., Aznar, J., Garcia-Iglesias, M. C., and Pascual, A. (1996). Comparative in-vitro activity of sparfloxacin against genital pathogens. *J. Antimicrob. Chemother.* **37**, 19–25.

164. Martin, D. H., Mroczkowski, T. F., and Paliaro, C. (1994). In vitro activity of OPC-17116, ofloxacin and doxycycline versus recent clinical isolates of *C. trachomatis*. *34th Intersci. Conf. Antimicrob. Agents Chemother.*, Orlando.

165. Kimura, M., Kishimoto, T., Niki, T., and Soejima, R. (1993). In vitro and in vivo antichlamydial activities of newly developed quinolone antimicrobial agents. *Antimicrob. Agents Chemother.* **37**, 801–803.

166. Jones, R. B., Van Der Pol, B., and Johnson, R. B. (1997). Susceptibility of *Chlamydia trachomatis* to trovafloxacin. *J. Antimicrob. Chemother.* **39** (Suppl. B), 63–65.

167. Segreti, J. (1991). In vitro activity of temafloxacin against pathogens causing sexually transmitted diseases. *Am. J. Med.* **91**, 24S–26S.

168. Segreti, J., Hirsch, D. J., Harris, A. A., Kapell, K. S., Orbach, H., and Kessler, H. A. (1990). In vitro activity of tosufloxacin (A-61827; T-3262) against selected pathogens. *Antimicrob. Agents Chemother.* **34**, 971–973.

169. Roblin, P. M., and Hammerschlag, M. R. (1999). In vitro activity of gatifloxacin against *Chlamydia trachomatis* and *Chlamydia pneumoniae*. *J. Antimicrob. Chemother.* **44**, 549–551.

170. Gruneberg, R. N., Felmingham, D., O'Hare, M. D., Robbins, M. J., Perry, K., Wall, R. A., *et al.* (1988). The comparative in-vitro activity of ofloxacin. *J. Antimicrob. Chemother.* **22**, 9–19.

171. Sambri, V., Rumpianesi, F., Xerri, L., and Cevenini, R. (1989). In-vitro activity of ofloxacin against *Chlamydia trachomatis*. *J. Chemother.* **1**, 231–232.

172. Ridgway, G. L., Mumtaz, G., Gabriel, F. G., and Oriel, J. D. (1984). The activity of ciprofloxacin and other 4-quinolones against *Chlamydia trachomatis* and *Mycoplasmas* in vitro. *Eur. J. Clin. Microbiol.* **3**, 344–346.

173. Anzar, J., Cabellero, M. C., Lozano, M. C., de Miguel, C., Palomares, J. C., and Perea, E. J. (1985). Activities of new quinolone derivatives against genital pathogens. *Antimicrob. Agents Chemother.* **27**, 76–78.

174. Furneri, P. M., Bazzano, M., Campo, L., Cesana, M., and Tempera, G. (1994). In vitro activity of rufloxacin against *Listeria monocytogenes*, *Legionella pneumophila* and *Chlamydia trachomatis*. *Chemotherapy* **40**, 104–108.

175. Martin, D. H. (1988). In vitro activity of RO23-6240, a new fluoroquinolone, against *Chlamydia trachomatis* [abstract]. *Ann. Mtg. Am. Feder. Clin. Res. (Southern Section)*, New Orleans, p. 59.

176. Maeda, H., Fujii, A., Nakata, K., Arakawa, S., and Kamidono, S. (1988). In vitro activities of T-3262, NY-198, fleroxacin (AM-833; RO 23-6240), and other new quinolone agents against clinically isolated *Chlamydia trachomatis* strains. *Antimicrob. Agents Chemother.* **32**, 1080–1081.

177. Liebowitz, L. D., Saunders, J., Fehler, G., Ballard, R. C., and Koornhof, H. J. (1986). In vitro activity of A-56619 (difloxacin), A-56620, and other new quinolone antimicrobial agents against genital pathogens. *Antimicrob. Agents Chemother.* **30**, 948–950.

CHAPTER 8

Treatment of Respiratory Infections with Quinolones

PAUL B. IANNINI,* MICHAEL S. NIEDERMAN,† and VINCENT T. ANDRIOLE‡

*Department of Medicine, Danbury Hospital, Danbury, Connecticut 06810, and Yale University School of Medicine, New Haven, Connecticut 06520, †Division of Pulmonary and Critical Care Medicine, Winthrop-University Hospital, Mineola, New York 11501, and Department of Medicine, State University of New York at Stony Brook, Stony Brook, New York, 11794, and ‡Yale University School of Medicine, New Haven, Connecticut 06520-8022

INTRODUCTION

Respiratory infections are a common source of morbidity and mortality, with pneumonia being the leading cause of death from infectious diseases in the United

States [1]. Community-acquired pneumonia (CAP) occurs in more than 4 million people annually and has a mortality rate that varies in relation to the severity of illness, as reflected by the site of therapy. Ambulatory patients with CAP have a mortality rate well below 5%, whereas those who enter the hospital (20–25% of all patients with CAP) have a mortality rate of 12–25%, with a further increase in mortality rate for those requiring admission to an intensive care unit and mechanical ventilation [2]. Nosocomial pneumonia is the second or third most common hospital-acquired infection but is the leading cause of mortality from all nosocomial infections. More than half of all patients who die as a result of nosocomial infection have pneumonia, and the crude mortality rate for ventilator-associated pneumonia (VAP) may exceed 50% [3–5]. Although hospital-acquired pneumonia (HAP) occurs in patients with severe illness, the infection itself, rather than the concomitant comorbid conditions, is responsible for up to one-half of all deaths that occur in patients with this illness [5], reflecting a high "attributable mortality," particularly in medical (rather than trauma) patients.

Acute bronchitis is a common illness that is generally of viral etiology and runs a self-limited course, rarely requiring therapy. However, acute exacerbation of chronic bronchitis (AECB) is frequently the result of bacterial infection, and is an often-underestimated source of morbidity and mortality. Approximately 15 million Americans have chronic obstructive pulmonary disease, and up to 12 million of them also have chronic bronchitis, defined as chronic productive cough with sputum production for at least 3 months of the year during two consecutive years [6]. Patients with this illness are prone to frequent exacerbation, and up to one-third of patients have <3 exacerbation per year, one-third have 3–4 exacerbations per year, and the remaining third have >4 exacerbations per year. Although AECB is often regarded as a minor illness, as many as 20–60% of patients admitted to an intensive care unit (ICU) with this diagnosis will require mechanical ventilation, with an associated mortality rate of 10–30% [7].

Guidelines for the therapy of these common respiratory infections have been developed that consider the likely bacterial pathogens and the need for prompt empiric therapy [1,9]. The ability to define an exact etiologic pathogen for many patients with respiratory infection remains an elusive goal, achieved in no more than half of all patients with acute lung infection [1,8]. *S. pneumoniae* was the leading cause of CAP, accounting for 25% of all cases and a third of cases with no confirmed etiology by routine diagnostic testing in a recent report that utilized cultures of blood, sputum, and transthoracic needle aspiration as well as serology [10]. Antibiotic therapy can provide definite benefits for patients with CAP, HAP, and AECB, but it must be selected based on knowledge of the clinical spectrum of the disease, the antibiotic susceptibility of likely pathogens in the geographic region, and the principals of pharmacology. Although there are many choices available to achieve an effective antibiotic regimen, the increasing rate of resistance to antibiotics of the common typical bacterial pathogens and the evolving role of atypical pathogens have prompted an increased use of antibiotic combinations. The newer quinolones have excellent activity against both typical and atypical pathogens, including those that have become resistant to a variety of antibiotic classes, and suggest new approaches to effective therapy.

CLINICAL ISSUES IN THE THERAPY OF RESPIRATORY INFECTION

COMMUNITY-ACQUIRED PNEUMONIA

Initial antibiotic therapy of CAP is most often empiric and should be directed at the pathogens that are most likely to be present. The pathogen-specific associated mortality rate is highest for *Streptococcus pneumoniae* and *Legionella* [11]. At a minimum, these two pathogens should be reliably treated by the therapy selected. Most studies of this illness have shown that even with extensive diagnostic testing a specific etiologic diagnosis is established in less than half of patients, and the responsible pathogen is often not identified for days (by culture) to weeks (by serology) after the patient is clinically diagnosed with CAP [1]. This low yield has led the American Thoracic Society (ATS) to recommend limited diagnostic testing in patients with CAP, reserving serologic testing for epidemiological purposes and for nonresponding patients, and sputum cultures for situations of suspected resistant or unusual pathogens [1]. This approach, if extensively used, may introduce bias into the reporting of antibiotic susceptibility for respiratory isolates because only those patients requiring hospitalization would be cultured. The reliability of a sputum Gram stain to guide initial empiric therapy has remained controversial. This test can be either sensitive or specific, depending on the criteria employed, but it cannot be both. Thus, if a Gram stain of expectorated sputum is used, many patients with the finding of any Gram-positive diplococci, a sensitive criterion for a "positive" result, may not grow *S. pneumoniae*. However, if the criterion used is a predominance of Gram-positive diplococci, then most sputum samples with a "positive" result will yield *S. pneumoniae* on culture, but many patients infected with this organism will have a negative result [12]. A Gram stain can be used to guide and focus initial therapy when a highly specific criterion is used. However, it is common to overinterpret the presence of *S. pneumoniae*, and to fail to recognize less apparent organisms such as *Haemophilus influenzae* [13].

The Infectious Disease Society of America (IDSA) guidelines recommend the use of Gram stain as a guide to selection of antibiotic therapy, and cultures of blood and expectorated sputum in patients who are to be hospitalized, as well as testing for *Legionella* for seriously ill patients who do not have an alternative diagnosis, especially if they are greater than age 40, immunocompromised, or not responding to β-lactam antibiotics [9]. Fluoroquinolones are recommended by the IDSA guidelines as first-line choices of therapy for both ambulatory and hospitalized patients with CAP [9].

The ATS has recommended that initial empiric therapy be based on an assessment of three factors: age 60 or greater with or without comorbid illness; the severity of illness (mild, moderate, or severe); and the locus of therapy (outpatient or inpatient). Application of these factors separates patients into four groups, each with its own rank order of likely pathogens and suggested therapy [1]. The first group is outpatients with mild to moderate pneumonia younger than age 60 without comorbid illness. The second group is outpatients with mild to moderate pneumonia who are either older than age 60 or who have comorbid illness or both. The third group is inpatients with moderate pneumonia of all ages. The last is inpatients of any age with severe pneumonia, usually treated in the ICU. Guidelines are of necessity dynamic recommendations that must be adjusted periodically for changes in bacterial resistance patterns, the recognition of new pathogens, or the availability of new antibiotics. New guidelines are currently under development by the ATS, IDSA, and CDC (Centers for Disease Control) for the treatment of CAP. The guideline employed is less important than rapid institution of antibiotic therapy within 8 hours of hospitalization and collection of blood cultures within 24 hours, both of which are associated with improved survival [14].

Several studies have suggested that empiric therapy directed at the likely etiologic pathogens leads to an improved outcome for patients with CAP, and establishing a specific etiologic diagnosis has not been shown to be useful from a survival viewpoint [15,16]. In the setting of severe CAP, if initial empiric therapy is successful and the patient is clinically improving within 72 hours, mortality is low; this is not the case if initial empiric therapy is ineffective [15]. In one study of severe CAP, the mortality of patients who received effective empiric therapy was 11%, whereas those who received initially ineffective therapy (usually with a therapeutic agent with an inadequate spectrum of activity) had a mortality rate of 60% [15]. Patients without severe illness are also effectively treated by empiric regimens directed at the most likely pathogens. A study of nearly 4500 hospitalized non-ICU patients reported that patients treated with a β-lactam antibiotic (second- or third-generation cephalosporin, or ampicillin–sulbactam), with or without a macrolide, in accordance with the ATS guidelines, had a significantly lower mortality rate than patients who were treated with a nonrecommended regimen [17]. Interestingly, when a macrolide was added along with the β-lactam, mortality was lower. Gleason et al. [18] reviewed 12,945 patients aged 65 or greater hospitalized with CAP and reported on the association between antibiotic therapy and 30-day mortality. The use of a β-lactam/β-lactamase inhibitor plus a macrolide and of an aminoglycoside plus any other antibiotic lead to increased 30-day mortality rates with HRs (hazard reductions) of 1.77 and 1.21, respectively, while initial treatment with a second-generation cephalosporin plus a macrolide (HR = 0.71), a nonpseudomonal third generation cephalosporin plus a macrolide (HR = 0.74), or a fluoroquinolone alone (HR = 0.64) were independently associated with reduced 30-day mortality [18]. These data fit well with more recent findings that atypical pathogens may be found in more than half of all patients with CAP whether hospitalized or not, although these organisms often coexist with bacterial pathogens [19,20]. Thus, in CAP it may be necessary to treat broadly with antibiotics that are effective for organisms that include *S. pneumoniae*, *H. influenzae*, atypical pathogens, and possibly enteric Gram-negatives. The effectiveness of a β-lactam–macrolide combination or a quinolone may reflect the importance of using a regimen directed against this spectrum of organisms. Studies comparing the newer quinolones to combinations of a β-lactam and a macrolide or of an azalide suggest that some of the newer quinolone antibiotics are at least equally, and perhaps more, effective [21,22]. Patients with bacteremic pneumococcal pneumonia caused by penicillin-resistant strains have also been shown to have increased risk of adverse outcome and may benefit from therapy with quinolones that are active against penicillin-resistant strains [23].

The availability of quinolone antibiotics with a spectrum of antimicrobial activity that is effective for patients with CAP may be advantageous for the management of two other issues. The first is in deciding which patients should be admitted to the hospital. Several studies have better-defined criteria for admission, making it clear that certain "low-risk" patients can be identified, and these individuals can be treated at home [24]. With the availability of oral antibiotics that achieve high concentrations in lung tissue and serum, it may be possible to treat certain patients who are "borderline" for admission in an outpatient setting. The quinolone class of antibiotics is particularly well suited for this application. The second management issue in CAP that was the focus of a 1995 study is the early switch from intravenous to oral therapy, a goal that can often be achieved by day 3 or 4 of hospitalization and facilitates early discharge [25]. Criteria for early oral therapy have been defined, but the quinolones are well suited to this purpose because many agents are available in both intravenous and oral forms (e.g., ciprofloxacin, ofloxacin, levofloxacin, trovafloxacin, and gatifloxacin), and the serum levels achieved with either route of administration are similar, facilitating an early switch to oral therapy. The highly bioavailable agents levofloxacin, gatifloxacin, and moxifloxacin provide serum levels after oral administration that are equivalent to those achieved with parenteral administration. The use of intravenous lines could potentially be avoided for the nearly 80% of patients who are hospitalized but are capable of taking oral medications.

HOSPITAL-ACQUIRED PNEUMONIA

Empiric therapy also becomes a consideration for patients with suspected HAP because of diagnostic difficulties not only in establishing the identity of the etiologic pathogen but also in defining whether a patient actually has pneumonia or a noninfectious cause of lung infiltrates and fever. Nosocomial pneumonia is defined clinically as the presence of a new or progressive lung infiltrate in the presence of at least two of the following: fever, purulent sputum, and leukocytosis [8]. This definition is sensitive but not specific, and not all patients who satisfy these clinical criteria are subsequently confirmed as having had pneumonia. This lack of specificity is particularly true in mechanically ventilated patients. In addition, hospitalized patients are frequently colonized by potentially pathogenic microorganisms, and it is sometimes difficult to determine which of the multiple organisms present in a sputum culture are colonizing organisms and which, if any, are causing infection. A variety of quantitative culture methods, generally utilizing sampling techniques through a bronchoscope, have been developed to define the presence of pneumonia and establish the identity of the etiologic pathogen. At the time of this writing, these techniques remain of unproven value as a guide to therapy that can influence the outcome of patients with HAP [26,27]. There is a benefit to selecting timely and appropriate empiric therapy for patients with suspected ventilator-associated pneumonia. In one study, mortality rate was significantly reduced if initial empiric therapy was active against the pathogens that were subsequently isolated from sampling secretions through a bronchoscope. However, if initial therapy was inactive against the subsequently confirmed pathogens, mortality remained high despite being later modified on the basis of cultures obtained via a bronchoscope [27].

The bacteriology of HAP differs from CAP, but appropriate empiric therapy can be selected by stratifying patients based on the time of onset of pneumonia (<day 5 of hospitalization vs. ≥day 5), the severity of illness (mild to moderate vs. severe), and the presence of risk factors for specific organisms. The ATS guidelines for HAP classify patients, based on these factors, into one of three groups: patients with no risk factors for specific organisms who have either mild to moderate pneumonia beginning any time or severe pneumonia of early onset; those with risk factors for specific organisms with mild to moderate pneumonia beginning any time; and those with severe pneumonia with either risk factors for specific pathogens or beginning at or after day 5 of hospitalization [8].

In the therapy of HAP, the ATS guidelines recommend single-agent antibiotic therapy for the majority of patients, except those with severe pneumonia who are at risk for infection with *P. aeruginosa*. In patients with nosocomial pneumonia, monotherapy with agents from a number of antibiotic classes, including the quinolones, has proven effective, even for those with severe illness [28]. If *P.*

aeruginosa is suspected, combination therapy leads to improved survival, when compared to monotherapy, in the presence of bacteremia [29]. The emergence of resistance during monotherapy, even with the most potent quinolones or β-lactams, has been a problem that might be reduced by the use of combinations of antipseudomonal antibiotics from different classes [28]. The use of combination therapy for HAP to achieve antibacterial synergy is not an important consideration in the absence of neutropenia. One other advantage of combination therapy is that it can provide coverage for a large number of potential pathogens, but the advent of new antimicrobial agents, including the quinolones, provides the opportunity for similar coverage with a single agent.

Combination therapy for patients with HAP has traditionally been an antipseudomonal β-lactam with an aminoglycoside. However, in one study of severe HAP [30], the addition of an aminoglycoside to imipenem did not enhance the efficacy of imipenem alone and did not prevent the emergence of resistance during therapy. This lack of synergy may be related to poor penetration of aminoglycosides into pulmonary secretions and the inactivity of this class of agents at acid pH that commonly exists in the lungs of patients with pneumonia. In addition, whether they are dosed once daily or by more traditional regimens, aminoglycosides have a predictable incidence of nephrotoxicity [31]. The ATS guidelines for HAP suggest ciprofloxacin as an alternative to an aminoglycoside in combination therapy regimens because of its spectrum of antimicrobial activity and excellent penetration into lung tissue, without a substantial risk of nephrotoxicity. Other antipseudomonal quinolones could also be used in this setting, but among the agents that are currently available or in development, only trovafloxacin and, possibly, gemifloxacin have adequate activity against this pathogen. There has been a marked increase in the rate of resistance of *P. aeruginosa* to both ciprofloxacin and levofloxacin in the late 1990s [32].

ACUTE EXACERBATIONS OF CHRONIC BRONCHITIS

The use of antibiotics for acute exacerbation of chronic bronchitis (AECB) has been controversial, with some investigators suggesting that there is no rationale for their use. However, a metaanalysis [33] of nine large placebo-controlled trials of antibiotics for AECB found a clear benefit to therapy, particularly if it was used in patients with at least two of the three cardinal symptoms of exacerbation: increased dyspnea, increased sputum volume, and increased sputum purulence. Patients with at least two of these symptoms who received antibiotics, rather than placebo, had a significantly higher rate of resolution of symptoms, a lower rate of relapse, and often a more rapid return to baseline of peak flow rates. In addition to leading to an overall improved outcome, the use of certain antibiotics can lead to a prolonged time between exacerbations. In a summary of a number of clinical trials, Chodosh [34] observed that quinolones are not only effective for AECB but also may be associated with longer disease-free intervals than when other agents are used.

In most studies of AECB, investigators have assumed that all antibiotics are equivalent. The Canadian Bronchitis Guidelines [6] have emphasized that there may be differences among patients with AECB and that a classification scheme should be used to guide antibiotic therapy. The necessity for this approach arises from the appearance of organisms that are likely to be antibiotic resistant and that may be common in certain populations, particularly the more severely ill patients with frequent exacerbations and multiple courses of antibiotic therapy. Resistant organisms in AECB include penicillin-resistant *S. pneumoniae* and β-lactamase-producing *H. influenzae* and *M. catarrhalis*. Stratification schemes take into account concerns about antibiotic resistance and the realization that exacerbation can be a potentially serious event, and that certain high-risk patients may benefit from a more aggressive approach to antibiotic therapy because the "cost of failure" of initial therapy may be great.

Based on these considerations, patients with AECB can be classified into three groups: patients with simple bronchitis who are younger than age 65, have fewer than three episodes of exacerbation per year, and an FEV_1 >50% of predicted; complicated patients with bronchitis over the age of 65 or have more than three episodes of exacerbation per year or an FEV_1 <50% of predicted; and patients with complicated bronchitis (as defined previously) who also have comorbid illness [6]. Following this classification, simple bronchitis can be treated with any of a group of first-line antibiotics, whereas the complicated patients are initially treated with second-line agents, which include among them the quinolones. The increasing rate of resistance of *S. pneumoniae* to earlier quinolones such as ciprofloxacin and levofloxacin as well as penicillin, macrolides, and sulfamethoxazole–trimethoprim, may necessitate the use of the newer quinolones with enhanced activity for these resistant strains.

PHARMACOLOGICAL ADVANTAGES FOR THE USE OF QUINOLONES IN RESPIRATORY INFECTION

PENETRATION INTO LUNG TISSUE

A number of studies have documented the finding that quinolones penetrate well into respiratory sites of infection, but the relevance of this property to the clinical efficacy of these agents has remained uncertain. The quinolones, as a class, are poorly protein bound, and have a low molecular weight and a zwitterionic structure, which favors their penetration into tissue where the levels of concentrations achieved may exceed those achieved in serum. One way of expressing the relative concentration of these agents in sputum is to report the ratio of the sputum concentration to the MIC for certain common organisms. Ciprofloxacin, for example, has a sputum/MIC ratio greater than 10, after standard doses, for *H. influenzae*, *M. catarrhalis*, and a number of enteric Gram-negatives [35–37]. Similar ratios can also be achieved against other organisms if the dose is increased to the upper range of tolerability (1500 mg orally per day with ciprofloxacin). A second method to express the relative activity of the quinolones is a calculation that employs the numerical value of the measured area under the serum concentration–time curve for 24 hr (AUC) and dividing by the MIC of the target organism. The resulting value, the AUIC, is the area under the curve that remains above the MIC. Clinical studies have shown that the AUIC ratio should be greater than 125 to achieve rapid bacterial eradication during therapy and also to prevent regrowth with resistant organisms [38]. A study [38] of acutely ill patients reported that, when the AUIC for ciprofloxacin exceeded 125 for the target organism, the likelihood of clinical and microbiologic cure was 80 and 82%, respectively. The cure rates were only 42 and 26% when the AUIC was below 125. Concentrations of various quinolones in sputum, bronchial mucosa, lung tissue, neutrophils, and alveolar macrophages have been measured, but it has been hard to correlate these findings with specific clinical outcomes. However, the ability to achieve high concentrations at sites of infection could have clinical advantages. High concentrations in pulmonary tissues can be achieved with either intravenous or oral therapy. Therefore, it is possible to use oral quinolone therapy for "borderline" patients and still achieve high serum and lung tissue concentrations, thereby potentially avoiding the need for admission in certain circumstances (mild to moderate nursing-home-acquired pneumonia). A study [39] of healthy subjects showed that the serum AUC for ciprofloxacin given orally at 750 mg two times per day was comparable to the AUC for the same drug given intravenously at 400 mg three times per day. In addition, reliable entry of quinolones into lung tissue might be an advantage for helping to rapidly switch inpatient antibiotic therapy of pneumonia from intravenous to oral formulations, facilitating earlier discharge from the hospital. Most of the available quinolones achieve concentrations in lung tissue that exceed serum concentrations. For example, after 500 mg of ciprofloxacin orally, peak serum concentration (in µg/ml) is 2.5, the concentration in bronchial secretions is 1.0 µg/ml, in lung tissue (after 750 mg) 4.9 µg/g, and the concentration in neutrophils and macrophages is four- to eightfold higher than in the extracellular fluid surrounding these cells [37]. Ofloxacin 400 mg p.o. achieves a peak concentration in serum of 4.0 µg/ml), in bronchial secretions (after 200 mg) of 4.5 µg/ml, and in lung tissue (after 200 mg) of 2.2 µg/g. Four newer quinolones—grepafloxacin, levofloxacin, sparfloxacin, and trovafloxacin—have their peak serum levels after standard doses summarized in Table I, along with their known concentrations at respiratory sites [36,40]. In reviewing these data, it is clear that all of these newer agents concentrate at a variety of respiratory sites, achieving higher levels than in the serum. These observations

TABLE I Concentrations of Quinolones in Serum and Respiratory Sites (after oral dosing)

	Cipro-floxacin, 500 mg	Grepa-floxacin, 400 mg	Levo-floxacin, 500 mg	Spar-floxacin, 400 mg	Trova-floxacin, 200 mg	Moxi-floxacin, 400 mg	Gati-floxacin, 400 mg	Gemi-floxacin, 320 mg
Serum (max)[a] (µg/ml)	2.5	1.7	6.6	1.6	2.9	3.4	3.3	1.48
Lung biopsy (µg/g)	4.9[b]	4.9[c]		1.3[c]	1.5[c]	1.5–2.0 x serum		
Bronchial sec.[d] (µg/ml)	1.0							
BAL[e] (µg/ml)					6.1			
ELF[f] (µg/ml)		17.8		5.6	3.0–10.0 x serum			
Phagocytes	4–8 x ECF[g]	5–9 x serum		5–9 x serum	10.0–34.0	19–32		

[a]Maximal serum concentration after oral dose.
[b]After 750-mg dose.
[c]Concentration in bronchial mucosa.
[d]Bronchial secretions.
[e]Bronchoalveolar lavage fluid.
[f]Epithelial lining fluid.
[g]Extracellular fluid surrounding phagocytic cells.

TABLE II   Serum Concentrations in Relation to Antimicrobial Activity of New Quinolones against Common Respiratory Pathogens

	C_{max} serum (μg/ml)	S. pneumoniae (C_{max}/MIC)	H. influenzae (C_{max}/MIC)
Clinafloxacin, 200 mg	1.5	12	187
Grepafloxacin, 400 mg	1.5	6.0	25
Levofloxacin, 500 mg	6.6	6.6	220
Sparfloxacin, 400 mg	1.6	6.4	80
Trovafloxacin, 200 mg	2.9	12	240
Gatifloxacin, 400 mg	3.3	6.7	112
Moxifloxacin, 400 mg	3.0	12.0	50
Gemifloxacin, 320 mg	1.5	48	370

suggest that, if the serum levels of a quinolone exceed the MIC of a target organism (see what follows and Table II), then the concentrations at relevant respiratory sites are even higher, and the antibacterial action in the lung is likely higher as well.

MECHANISM OF KILLING

Quinolones act by inhibiting bacterial topoisomerase enzymes that are crucial for DNA physiology. DNA gyrase is the commonly employed name for topoisomerase II, and this enzyme is the primary target for quinolones in Gram-negative organisms and is composed of two dimers of *gyrA* and *gyrB*. The primary function of DNA gyrase is to induce negative supercoils in double-stranded bacterial DNA to facilitate replication, repair, and transcription. Quinolones inhibit this enzyme and prevent its cellular functions [41,42]. The exact mechanism of action is not fully understood but appears to involve trapping or stabilizing of the gyrase–DNA complex after strand breakage and before resealing, creating a lethal injury to the organism. Topoisomerase IV is the primary target for most quinolones in Gram-positive organisms and is composed of two dimers of *parC* and *parE*. The primary function of this enzyme is to separate the two circular, interlinked copies of the parent bacterial DNA that result from replication so that each can take its place in the two new daughter cells. This reaction is called catenation/decatenation, and when topoisomerase IV is bound by quinolones separation cannot take place and leads to rapid cell death. DNA gyrase is the primary target for norfloxacin, ofloxacin, ciprofloxacin, and levofloxacin, and topoisomerase IV is the secondary less-affected target. The affinity of these quinolones to different bacterial target enzymes explains the superb activity of these drugs against Gram-negative organisms and their lesser activity against Gram-positive organisms. Trovafloxacin, gatifloxacin, moxifloxacin, and gemifloxacin have increased affinity for topoisomerase IV as well as DNA gyrase and are therefore much more active against *S. pneumoniae* [43]. The organism must develop mutations at both these target sites for resistance to develop [43]. First-step bacterial mutations of DNA gyrase result in a four- to eightfold increase in the MIC_{90} to ofloxacin, ciprofloxacin, and levofloxacin. These first-step mutants may not be killed by the maximum serum concentrations achieved by these quinolones and can go on to further mutation and an additional four- to eightfold increase in the MIC. Thus, an isolate with an MIC of 1.0 µg/ml will result in a first-step mutant with an MIC of 4.0-8.0 µg/ml. These first-step mutants would not be killed by a maximum serum concentration of 3.5 µg/ml and second-step mutation would result in a new MIC of 16–64 µg/ml and would be highly resistant. The newer quinolones—such as moxifloxacin, gatifloxacin, and gemifloxacin—would still be very active against these first-step mutants because the topoisomerase IV target is unaltered, and the MIC unchanged, resulting in cell death at the usual maximal serum concentration achieved and no opportunity for second-step mutation. Similarly, first-step mutation of the topoisomerase IV target would not affect the MIC because the DNA gyrase target would remain sensitive and the organism killed. Resistance should develop only when two simultaneous mutations occurred in the two different genes that encode for DNA gyrase (usually *gyrA*) and topoisomerase IV (usually *parC*). The mutation frequency for each of these mutations is low, and simultaneous mutations of two different genes would likely be a rare event [44]. The rank order of activity for mutant *S. pneumoniae* is from least to most active, ciprofloxacin, levofloxacin, followed by gatifloxacin, moxifloxacin, sparfloxacin, trovafloxacin [45]. Chen and colleagues [47] have reported that gemifloxacin is the most active against ciprofloxacin-resistant strains.

The quinolones are bactericidal antibiotics that kill in a concentration-dependent fashion, rather than in relation to time above the MIC of the target organism. This means that optimal antibacterial activity can be achieved with infrequent dosing, and with high peak concentrations and high AUCs. In addition, because quinolones have a post-antibiotic effect (PAE) against both Gram-positive and Gram-negative organisms, they can continue to kill even after local concentrations fall below the MIC of the target organism [41,46]. These properties make the quinolones well suited to infrequent dosing, with the ideal being once-daily dosing, particularly given the relatively long half-life of the newer compounds. The only factor limiting a switch to once-daily dosing for all quinolones is the toxicity associated with high doses, particularly concerns related to neurotoxicity and possible seizures.

MICROBIOLOGIC ADVANTAGES OF QUINOLONES FOR RESPIRATORY INFECTION

As discussed above, the therapy of respiratory infections is often empiric, necessitating employment of agents with a broad range of antimicrobial activity. The quinolones fit this description, having activity against common Gram-positive and Gram-negative organisms as well as a number of common atypical pathogens. Large microbiological surveys of common respiratory pathogens have reported a continued increase in penicillin resistance of *S. pneumoniae*, with overall resistance approaching 50% and high-level resistance (2.0μg/ml) approaching 15%–19% [48,49]. Macrolide resistance is present in nearly half the penicillin-resistant strains of *S. pneumoniae* and in 20–24% of strains overall [50,51]. Macrolide resistance in *S. pneumoniae* can be caused by methylation of a single amino acid at the ribosomal binding site, leading to high-level resistance of >16.0 μg/ml to erythromycin, clarithromycin, azithromycin, clindamycin, and streptogramin B, and is designated as the MLSв phenotype. The second mechanism of macrolide resistance is through a membrane efflux pump system that keeps the intracellular level of these drugs very low. There is no cross-resistance to lincosamines or streptogramins, and this pure macrolide resistance is termed the M phenotype. The resistance level of these efflux strains is generally 16 μg/ml or less, but can be substantially higher. The high intracellular levels that macrolides and azalides achieve in pulmonary macrophages and the high pulmonary epithelial lining fluid concentrations were considered high enough to prove effective against efflux-resistant strains of *S. pneumoniae*. However, a more recent report of patients who developed macrolide-resistant (MLSв and M phenotypes) *S. pneumoniae* bacteremia while on macrolide or azalide therapy has cast some doubt on the ability of tissue levels without effective serum levels to prevent bacteremia even in the presence of low-level resistance [52]. The development of gatifloxacin, gemifloxacin, moxifloxacin, and sparfloxacin represents a true advance over older agents because of enhanced activity against Gram-positive organisms, particularly *S. pneumoniae* (both penicillin-sensitive and penicillin-resistant [53–63]. *S. pneumoniae* resistant to 4.0 μg/ml of ciprofloxacin have been reported in 2.9% of isolates from Canada [47], and 5.5% in Hong Kong [64], and in Canada to correlate with an increased use of quinolones [47]. This is not a class-wide resistance, as these isolates were susceptible to levofloxacin 63%, trovafloxacin 77%, gatifloxacin 75%, moxifloxacin 88%, and gemifloxacin 100% [47]. In addition, agents such as trovafloxacin, moxifloxacin, gatifloxacin, and gemifloxacin have the added appeal of activity against respiratory anaerobes, a potential advantage in the therapy of both CAP and HAP if aspiration is suspected [65,66]. *H. influenzae* and *M. catarrhalis* that are β-lactamase positive now account for close to 40 and 90% of strains, respectively [48,49,51]. These commonly encountered Gram-negative organisms have MIC values of less than 0.07 μg/ml to the quinolones regardless of their ability to produce β-lactamase [63].

ACTIVITY AGAINST COMMON RESPIRATORY PATHOGENS

Streptococcus pneumoniae

With the earlier quinolones ciprofloxacin and ofloxacin, concern about widespread use for respiratory infection focused on the borderline activity of these agents against *S. pneumoniae* when compared to their activity against Gram-negative organisms. Considering the serum and tissue concentrations achieved by these drugs (Table I and text above), it is clear that adequate activity against *S. pneumoniae* is best achieved when dosing is maximized. In a study of severe pneumonia, *S. pneumoniae* was always eradicated by ciprofloxacin when a dosage of 400 mg i.v. every 8 hr was used [28]. The MIC_{90} of ciprofloxacin against *S. pneumoniae* has been reported at between 0.5 and 8.0 μg/ml, typically falling around 2.0 μg/ml. Similarly, the MIC_{90} for ofloxacin against this organism has varied from 2 to 8 μg/ml, with a typical value being 2.0 μg/ml. Levofloxacin, which is the L-isomer of ofloxacin, is twice as active on a weight basis and thus has an MIC_{90} of 2.0 μ/ml [46,55,67,68]. New quinolones have been developed that have markedly enhanced Gram-positive activity, particularly against *S. pneumoniae*, compared to older agents. These quinolones include sparfloxacin, moxifloxacin, and gatifloxacin, and they are approved for usage as well as gemifloxacin, which is currently under clinical evaluation. Grepafloxacin has been withdrawn from usage, and trovafloxacin usage has been restricted because of safety concerns. The development of clinafloxacin is currently on hold. On an MIC basis, they are highly active against *S. pneumoniae*, with MIC_{90} values <0.25 μg/ml for gemifloxacin, 0.25 μg/ml for moxifloxacin, and 0.5 μg/ml for gatifloxacin [36,40,53–55,63,67,69]. With standard doses, their rank order of activity can be expressed as the ratio of maximal serum concentration (C_{max}) to MIC_{90} for common organisms; these data appear in Table II for *S. pneumoniae* and *H. influenzae*. This method of comparing the activity of these agents may be particularly well suited to quinolones because their bactericidal activity is dependent on the height of the concentration achieved and its ratio to the MIC. This is a way of expressing how many multiples of the MIC can be achieved by a single dose. All the newer quinolones have pharmacokinetic and pharmacodynamic properties that allow once-daily dosing [36,70–73].

Penicillin-resistant *S. pneumoniae* generally have minor cross-resistance to quinolones, and thus an agent that is active against penicillin-sensitive organisms is equally active against penicillin-resistant organism [47,53–57,60,61]. Baquero [53] has reported similar activity with sparfloxacin and has speculated that the C_{max}/MIC ratios for the new quinolones (Table II) are high enough to predict that resistance is less likely to develop than with the previous generation of quinolones.

Atypical Pathogens

With data from both inpatients and outpatients showing that as many as half of all CAP patients have serologic evidence of atypical pathogen infection, activity against these organisms may be an important attribute of an antibiotic used for lower respiratory tract infections [19,20]. Ciprofloxacin and ofloxacin have documented *in-vitro* activity against *Legionella* spp. and *Chlamydia pneumoniae*; and sparfloxacin, levofloxacin, trovafloxacin, moxifloxacin, gatifloxacin, and gemifloxacin are also active against these pathogens [40,67,69,74–83]. In general, sparfloxacin, trovafloxacin, levofloxacin, moxifloxacin, gatifloxacin, and gemifloxacin appear more active against *C. pneumoniae* than ofloxacin and ciprofloxacin [40,67,74–83], and are also more active against *Mycoplasma pneumoniae*. The newer agents may also be more active against *Legionella* spp., with MIC values equal to 0.05 µg/ml, but ciprofloxacin and sparfloxacin retain excellent activity against these organisms.

Haemophilus influenzae

The major concern with *H. influenzae* is the production of β-lactamase by 40% of clinical isolates, which has rendered ampicillin and amoxicillin unreliable as empiric antibiotic choices for lower respiratory tract infections. Quinolones are not susceptible to destruction by these bacterial enzymes; and, as shown in Table II, the serum concentrations of the new quinolones, as well as those of the older quinolones, far exceed the MIC of *H. influenzae*, making the quinolones a highly active class of antibiotics against these organisms.

Anaerobes

The role of anaerobes in routine respiratory infections is controversial. Although anaerobes are important sources of infection in patients with aspiration pneumonia and lung abscess, their role as copathogens for patients with CAP and HAP is uncertain. Dore and colleagues [84] have studied 130 patients with VAP and found that 30 had anaerobes isolated on a protected specimen brush, but in only 4 patients were anaerobes isolated in the absence of aerobes, and the need for specific therapy was not defined. The presence of anaerobes was more likely in patients with an altered level of consciousness and with early-onset pneumonia. In another study [90] of patients with nosocomial aspiration evaluated by protected-specimen brush cultures, the bacteriology was complex, involving both Gram-positive and Gram-negative organisms, implying that treatment with a narrow-spectrum agent, such as penicillin, would not be effective against all of the organisms isolated. This spectrum of pathogens identified could be adequately treated by the newer quinolones that have activity against anaerobic bacteria as well as Gram-positive and Gram-negative organisms.

Ciprofloxacin and ofloxacin have limited activity against important respiratory tract anaerobes such as *Bacteroides fragilis* [65,66]; and the newer agents sparfloxacin and levofloxacin are only slightly more active on an MIC basis [40]. The most active agents against anaerobes are clinafloxacin, trovafloxacin, moxifloxacin, and gatifloxacin. Clinical trials in patients with aspiration pneumonia and lung abscess have not yet been conducted.

Enteric Gram-Negatives, Including *Pseudomonas aeruginosa*

Gram-negative rods are potential pathogens in CAP patients of advanced age, with comorbid illness, or severe disease. These organisms are also a concern in patients with HAP, but *P. aeruginosa* is the most commonly identified Gram-negative in patients who are treated with long-term mechanical ventilation (>5 days). In treating patients with suspected Gram-negative infection, a distinction must be made as to whether *P. aeruginosa* is suspected, because the number of antibiotics active against this organism is limited and they must be specifically chosen. A number of studies [37] have shown that monotherapy with a variety of agents, including the quinolone ciprofloxacin, is associated with a high rate (>30%) of selection of resistance during the therapy of initially sensitive organisms. Therefore, therapy should involve a combination of agents, and the quinolones can be used for this purpose, in place of an aminoglycoside, when combined with a β-lactam agent. Among the quinolones, the most active against a broad range of Gram-negatives including *P. aeruginosa* is ciprofloxacin, but following the introduction of levofloxacin as a respiratory quinolone (MIC$_{90}$ of 2.0), there has been an increase in the rate of resistance of *P. aeruginosa* to both agents that may approach 25% [88]. Ciprofloxacin also has excellent activity against other Gram-negatives including the Enterobacteriaceae, which have developed high-level resistance to third-generation cephalosporins [28], as do the newer quinolones such as levofloxacin, gatifloxacin, moxifloxacin, and gemifloxacin. The increasing rate of resistance of nosocomial Gram-negative rods that produce extended spectrum β-lactamases or are of the AMP C type provides another important potential role for the quinolones [88].

The newer quinolones are not as active against *P. aeruginosa* as ciprofloxacin, but trovafloxacin does have excellent activity against this organism and may exhibit synergy with β-lactam agents such as ceftazidime [89]. This study [89], which employed checkerboard titration to evaluate synergy, found trovafloxacin to be synergistic with ceftazadime for two of nine strains of *P. aeruginosa*, but found no synergy between amikacin and trovafloxacin. These data support the logic of using an antipseudomonal β-lactam–quinolone combination rather than a quinolone–aminoglycoside combination and suggest that quinolones may have some of the same synergistic properties that have been observed for the aminoglycosides when they are used with β-lactam agents. Some clinical microbiology laboratories assume that all quinolones have relatively similar susceptibility patterns and interpret evidence of activity of one agent against a specific organism to extend to the entire class of quinolones. *P. aeruginosa* susceptibility to one quinolone does not reliably equate to susceptibility to all quinolones. Chidiac *et al.* [90] have studied a strain of *P. aeruginosa* susceptible to ciprofloxacin but resistant to ofloxacin and have shown that this difference in susceptibility patterns correlated with differences in clearance of the organism in an animal model of pneumonia in response to therapy with the different quinolones. When infected animals were treated with ciprofloxacin, all survived, but only half survived with ofloxacin treatment. These data suggest that differences in susceptibility of *P. aeruginosa* to different quinolones can relate to *in-vivo* differences in efficacy.

CLINICAL EFFICACY OF QUINOLONES FOR THE THERAPY OF RESPIRATORY TRACT INFECTIONS

COMMUNITY-ACQUIRED PNEUMONIA

A number of clinical trials [59,91–95] have shown the efficacy of ciprofloxacin and ofloxacin for community-acquired pneumonia in comparison to a variety of standard agents. In a metaanalysis [85,95] of ciprofloxacin vs. other comparators, equivalent or better efficacy was found, even for patients infected with *S. pneumoniae*. Although failures of ciprofloxacin have been reported in CAP patients infected with *S. pneumoniae*, many of these patients were treated with relatively low-dose therapy. When ciprofloxacin is used in high doses (400 mg t.i.d. intravenously or 750 mg b.i.d. orally), efficacy against *S. pneumoniae* is comparable to that of other antibiotics [28,35,58]. Patients who have been reported to develop *S. pneumoniae* meningitis during ciprofloxacin therapy for CAP usually received a dose of less than 1000 mg a day.

Ciprofloxacin has been effective for the therapy of both moderate and severe CAP, and has allowed for the use of sequential intravenous/oral therapy. A study of 122 hospitalized CAP patients treated intravenously with ciprofloxacin 200 mg b.i.d. followed by oral therapy with 500 mg b.i.d. [97] showed equal efficacy when compared to intravenous ceftazidime. This study established the basis for an early switch from intravenous to oral therapy when using a quinolone antibiotic, and demonstrated efficacy that was comparable to prolonged intravenous therapy with a widely used and effective agent. In patients with more severe illness, intravenous ciprofloxacin at doses of 400 mg t.i.d. was comparable to intravenous imipenem at doses of 1 g t.i.d., but patients were treated with parenteral agents for the entire course of therapy [28]. However, in another study [93] of 217 patients with severe forms of CAP, the efficacy of intravenous followed by oral therapy was shown to be comparable to the efficacy of parenteral ceftriaxone followed by oral antibiotic therapy. Another population that has been treated with sequential parenteral/oral therapy using ciprofloxacin is the elderly, and efficacy comparable to ceftazidime has also been demonstrated for this group [94]. This study suggests the possibility of using single-agent oral therapy in the "borderline" patient with moderate illness in a nursing-home setting, thereby avoiding hospitalization in carefully selected circumstances.

Ofloxacin has also been used effectively for patients with CAP and HAP, facilitating a rapid switch from parenteral to oral therapy in those who respond rapidly to initial therapy [96]. In one study [68] of 212 patients with CAP, 76 had documented *S. pneumoniae* infection, and ofloxacin at a dose of 200 mg b.i.d. achieved a clinical cure rate of 97%.

Clinical trials [53,59,97–105] in CAP have also shown efficacy for the new quinolones, including levofloxacin, sparfloxacin, trovafloxacin, moxifloxacin, and gatifloxacin. Levofloxacin is approved for the therapy of pneumonia caused by highly resistant strains of *S. pneumoniae*. In studies of sparfloxacin compared to amoxicillin (e.g., [58]), equivalent overall efficacy was observed between the two therapies, with eradication of *S. pneumoniae* in 88.8% of 1137 patients who received either sparfloxacin or amoxicillin. In trials with sparfloxacin, adverse events have been reported with comparable frequency for both the quinolone and the comparator arms; however, phototoxicity was more frequent with sparfloxacin, and use of this agent necessitates avoidance of exposure to direct and indirect sunlight whenever possible. Therapy of CAP with sparfloxacin at doses of 400 mg initially followed by 200 mg daily had a higher incidence of side effects than in therapy trials of AECB that used lower doses [97].

Another clinical trial of CAP [22] compared trovafloxacin to ceftriaxone and erythromycin in 443 patients randomized to therapy with either intravenous alatrofloxacin followed by oral trovafloxacin, both at a dose of 200 mg daily, or intravenous ceftriaxone, with or without erythromycin, followed by oral cefpodoxime. Both arms of the study showed equivalent efficacy, with a clinical success rate of 90% with the use of trovafloxacin. Interestingly, all-cause mortality was 3.6% with trovafloxacin vs. 7.0% with ceftriaxone, and all subjects with penicillin-resistant *S. pneumoniae* were clinically cured by trovafloxacin. Clinical success was achieved in patients with *S. pneumoniae* bacteremia in 13 of 14 patients treated with trovafloxacin as compared to 8 of 9 patients treated with ceftriaxone.

A clinical trial comparing the efficacy of 10 days of therapy with moxifloxacin 400 mg p.o., q.d. vs. clarithromycin 500 mg p.o., b.i.d. in 382 patients reported equal rates of clinical resolution (95%) and bacteriologic resolution (96%) [100]. An open nonblinded study of moxifloxacin 400 mg p.o., q.d. in 196 patients with CAP treated for 10 days reported a 93% overall clinical resolution rate (95% CI = 88.1%, 95.9%) and a 91% bacteriologic response rate (95% CI = 84%, 96%) [101].

Gatifloxacin, 400 mg p.o., q.d. was compared to clarithromycin 500 mg p.o., b.i.d. in 372 patients with CAP treated for 7–14 days, and comparable rates of clinical cure of 95 and 93%, respectively (95% CI = –4.2%, 9.1%), were achieved as well as comparable rates of bacteriologic eradication, 98 and 93%, respectively [102]. Thirty-five pretreatment isolates in this study were resistant to clarithromycin and excluded from evaluation for efficacy. Gatifloxacin, 400 mg p.o., q.d. was also compared to levofloxacin 500 mg p.o., q.d. in a second study of patients with CAP and was reported to be both clinically, 96 vs. 94%, and bacteriologically, 98 vs. 93%, equivalent [103]. Eradication of *S. pneumoniae* in this study was reported in 100% (12/12) of patients treated with gatifloxacin but in only 78% (14/18) treated with levofloxacin. Another study compared gatifloxacin 400 mg i.v. and p.o., q.d. to the combination of ceftriaxone 1.0–2.0 g i.v., q.d. ± erythromycin 500 mg i.v., q.i.d., followed by clarithromycin 500 mg p.o., b.i.d. in 283 patients with CAP, and reported equal efficacy clinically, 97 vs. 91% (95% CI = –2.5%, 17.6%), and microbiologically, 95 and 95% [104]. Niederman *et al.* [105] have reported on an analysis of data from four multinational CAP trials of patients treated with moxifloxacin 400 mg p.o., q.d. vs. either clarithromycin 500 mg p.o., b.i.d. or amoxicillin 500 or 1000 mg p.o., t.i.d. that has a statistically significant reduction in mortality ($p = 0.045$) for the 701 moxifloxacin-treated patients of 0.57% as compared to 1.70% of the 705 patients treated with the comparators. A trend toward improved survival with the use of quinolones for patients with CAP may be evolving when the results of this study are interpreted in the light of previously discussed studies [98,104,105].

HOSPITAL-ACQUIRED PNEUMONIA

Ciprofloxacin has been a useful drug for the treatment of HAP, and it, along with other quinolones, is recommended as initial empiric therapy in the ATS hospital-acquired pneumonia guidelines. However, if *P. aeruginosa* is suspected, as is the case with late-onset HAP or severe HAP in the presence of risk factors (such as prior antibiotic therapy or corticosteroid therapy), then ciprofloxacin is the only currently recommended quinolone, and it should be used as part of a combination regimen [8]. In one study [68] of HAP involving 109 patients treated with ofloxacin, 94 had clinical success, but 15 patients required addition of other antibiotics because of poor clinical response. Most patients did not have severe pneumonia, and *P. aeruginosa* was not a frequent pathogen.

One of the largest studies [28] of HAP using quinolone therapy was a comparative study of ciprofloxacin and imipenem that was limited to patients with severe pneumonia. A total of 405 patients were studied, and 78% had nosocomial pneumonia (the remainder had severe CAP), and a total of 79% were mechanically ventilated. Patients received monotherapy with either ciprofloxacin 400 mg every 8 hr or imipenem 1 g every 8 hr, although additional therapy for suspected anaerobic or staphylococcal infection was permitted. The patients who received ciprofloxacin had a significantly higher clinical response rate than the imipenem-treated patients (69 vs. 56%) and also had a significantly higher eradication rate for the Enterobacteriaceae group of organisms (93 vs. 66%) [28]. Neither monotherapy was highly effective for the 23% of patients with *P. aeruginosa* infection, because resistance commonly developed during monotherapy, although it took at least 72 hr to develop. Thus, monotherapy can be effective for nonpseudomonal infection in the setting of severe nosocomial pneumonia. With these data in mind, an effective strategy for severe HAP would be to start with a combination regimen involving ciprofloxacin and an antipseudomonal β-lactam. Once the results of tracheal aspiration and blood cultures are available, therapy can be reassessed, and if *P. aeruginosa* is present, then combination therapy should continue. However, if *P. aeruginosa* is absent (as was the case nearly 75% of the time in the severe pneumonia study cited previously), then therapy can be finished using ciprofloxacin alone.

The data reviewed have established ciprofloxacin as an accepted standard for the therapy of severe HAP. Trovafloxacin has also been studied [99] for nosocomial pneumonia. Using intravenous alatrofloxacin, followed by oral trovafloxacin, 300 mg daily, 267 patients were studied in comparison to ciprofloxacin with optional metronidazole. A second antipseudomonal agent could be added for patients in either arm, if indicated by culture data. Both arms of the study had comparable clinical success (77%) and comparable mortality. *Pseudo-*

monas aeruginosa was isolated from 26 patients and was eradicated 67% of the time with trovafloxacin, compared to 55% of the time with ciprofloxacin.

As discussed previously, if quinolones are used in seriously ill patients with potentially resistant pathogens such as *P. aeruginosa*, it is necessary to use an optimal dose, as reflected by an AUIC above 125. The higher the AUIC, the greater the clinical success and the more rapid the bacteriologic eradication [38]. Thus, the appropriate dose of ciprofloxacin for this indication is 400 mg three times a day and of trovafloxacin 300 mg daily. The efficacy of the other new quinolones in severe HAP is not yet established, but only levofloxacin, gatifloxacin, and clinafloxacin have intravenous formulations available, and it is unlikely that the other agents, with only oral formulations, will be considered for this indication.

ACUTE EXACERBATIONS OF CHRONIC BRONCHITIS

On the basis of the bacteriologic considerations in chronic bronchitis and the antimicrobial spectrum of the quinolones, these agents represent an excellent choice for the more complicated patient with AECB. These patients are defined as having either advanced age, FEV_1 <50% of predicted, serious comorbidity, or exacerbation more than three times per year. They are particularly prone to infection with more complex and potentially drug-resistant organisms than are patients without these clinical risk factors. Chodosh [34, 109] has shown that quinolones are particularly useful for patients with AECB because they lead to long disease-free intervals, exceeding 200 days, making them comparable to the most effective antibiotics yet studied. Clinical trials with ciprofloxacin have shown efficacy similar to comparator agents when doses of 750 mg b.i.d. are used [34]. Ofloxacin has also been effective for this indication in doses varying from 400 mg daily to 400 mg b.i.d. [34]. The newer quinolones sparfloxacin and trovafloxacin have also been studied and found to be as effective as comparator agents. Sparfloxacin has been as effective as amoxicillin or ofloxacin [99].

Moxifloxacin and gatifloxacin have both proven to be effective in the therapy of AECB. Gatifloxacin, 400 mg q.d. was compared to cefuroxime axetil 250 mg q.d. in 211 patients, treated for 7–10 days, the majority of whom had type I exacerbation [106]. Clinical cure was achieved in 89% of the gatifloxacin-treated patients as compared to 77% treated with cefuroxime axetil, and bacteriologic eradication of *S. pneumoniae* in 7 out of 7 and of *H. influenzae* in 10 out of 10 patients receiving gatifloxacin vs. 3 of 8 and 9 of 12 in patients receiving cefuroxime axetil [106]. A second study reported the results of combined data from 697 patients enrolled in a double-blinded, randomized multicenter study, with 210 patients treated using an open protocol who received either gatifloxacin

400 mg q.d., cefuroxime axetil 250 mg b.i.d. or levofloxacin 500 mg q.d., all for 7–10 days [107]. Overall bacteriologic eradication was achieved in 93% of gatifloxacin-treated patients as compared to 88% in those treated with the comparators, and *S. pneumoniae* by 100% with gatifloxacin, 88% with levofloxacin, and 56% with cefuroxime axetil [107].

Moxifloxacin 400 mg p.o., q.d. for 5 days has been compared with clarithromycin 500 mg p.o., b.i.d. for 7 days in 750 patients. Clinical cure assessed at 7 days after the end of therapy was equivalent to 89% for moxifloxacin vs. 88% for clarithromycin, but the bacteriologic response rate was superior for moxifloxacin, 77 vs. 62%, as compared to clarithromycin (95% CI = 3.6%, 26.9%) [108]. A second study, employing the same dosages and routes of administration but with a length of therapy of either 5 or 10 days for moxifloxacin vs. 10 days for clarithromycin in 936 patients, 491 of whom had positive sputum cultures pretherapy, reported equivalent efficacy and valid response rates of 89 and 91% for moxifloxacin for 5 and 10 days vs. 91% for clarithromycin for 10 days and equivalent bacteriologic responses [109]. The availability of reliable therapy with only 5 days of therapy with moxifloxacin has appeal in terms of the aspects of patient compliance and convenience. Similar studies with gatifloxacin for 5 days are currently in progress.

The measurement of outcomes, such as the relapse-free time interval and the rate of hospitalization, in patients with AECB is gaining acceptance as an acceptable indicator of differences in efficacy. Pooled data from four multinational trials comparing moxifloxacin 400 mg p.o., q.d. with either clarithromycin 500 mg p.o., b.i.d., cefixime 400 mg p.o., q.d., or cefuroxime axetil 500 mg p.o., b.i.d. in the treatment of patients with AECB reported a statistical significance in the rate of hospitalization ($p = 0.020$) for the 192 moxifloxacin-treated patients at 0.94% compared to patients treated with the comparators at 1.84% [105].

CONCLUSION

The quinolone antibiotic class is extremely useful for the therapy of common respiratory infections, including community-acquired pneumonia, hospital-acquired pneumonia, and acute exacerbation of chronic bronchitis. The appeal of these agents relates to their antimicrobial spectrum of activity combined with pharmacokinetic advantages that include excellent penetration into respiratory tissue and high bioavailability with oral therapy. The newest members of the quinolone class, moxifloxacin and gatifloxacin, have the added advantages of superb activity against multidrug-resistant *S. pneumoniae*, two bacterial targets that impede resistance development, improved activity against anaerobes, metabolism that does not rely on the cytochrome P450 system, and dosage that need not be altered in the setting of renal or hepatic impairment (moxifloxacin) or hepatic impairment alone (gatifloxacin). Gemifloxacin, while still under investigation, shares many of these properties. Current clinical practice has several important opportunities for quinolone use, including the therapy of difficult-to-treat infections (AECB in complicated patients and patients with severe nosocomial pneumonia), the early switch from intravenous to oral therapy in patients with either CAP or HAP, and the possibility of using oral therapy for patients who would otherwise require admission for parenteral therapy with other antimicrobials (i.e., nursing-home-acquired pneumonia). The newer quinolones—moxifloxacin, gatifloxacin, levofloxacin, sparfloxacin, trovafloxacin, and gemifloxacin—have major advantages over their predecessors ciprofloxacin and ofloxacin. Most notably, the newest agents—moxifloxacin, gatifloxacin, and gemifloxacin—are highly active against *S. pneumoniae*, including penicillin-sensitive, penicillin-resistant, and macrolide-resistant strains, as well as other Gram-positives, Gram-negatives, and atypical pathogens. Trovafloxacin has activity against both *P. aeruginosa* and respiratory tract anaerobes, but the use of this agent has been greatly restricted because of hepatic toxicity. The place of these agents in the future management of respiratory infection is still being defined, but the new quinolones are likely to become the drugs of choice for many patient groups.

REFERENCES

1. Niederman, M. S., Bass, J. B., Campbell, G. D., Fein, A. M., Grossman, R. F., Mandell, L. A., Marrie, T. J., Sarosi, G. A., Torres, A., and Yu, V. L. (1993). Guidelines for the initial management of adults with community-acquired pneumonia: Diagnosis, assessment of severity, and initial antimicrobial therapy. *Am. Rev. Respir. Dis.* **148**, 1418–1426.
2. Fine, M. J., Smith, M. S., Carson, C. A., Mutha, S. S., Sankey, S. S., Weissfeld, L. A., and Kapoor, W. N. (1996). Prognosis and outcomes of patients with community-acquired pneumonia: A meta-analysis. *JAMA* **275**, 134–141.
3. Gross, P. A., Neu, H. C., Aswapokee, P., *et al.* (1980). Deaths from nosocomial infection: Experience in a university hospital and a community hospital. *Am. J. Med.* **68**, 219.
4. Gross, P. A., and Van Antwerpen, C. (1983). Nosocomial infections and hospital deaths: A case control study. *Am. J. Med.* **75**, 658.
5. Fagon, J. Y., Chastre, J., Vaugnat, A., Trouillet, J. L., Novara, A., and Gibert, C. (1996). Nosocomial pneumonia and mortality among patients in intensive care units. *JAMA* **275**, 866–869.
6. Baiter, M. S., Hyland, R. H., Low, D. E., *et al.* (1994). Recommendations on the management of chronic bronchitis: A practical guide for Canadian physicians. *Can. Med. Assoc. J.* **151**(10) (Suppl.), 5–23.

7. Seneff, M. G., Wagner, D. P., Wagner, R. P., Zimmerman, J. W., and Knaus, W. A. (1995). Hospital and 1-year survival of patients admitted to intensive care units with acute exacerbation of chronic obstructive pulmonary disease. *JAMA* **274**, 1852–1857.

8. Campbell, G. D., Niederman, M. S., Broughton, W. A., *et al.* (1996). Hospital-acquired pneumonia in adults: Diagnosis, assessment of severity, initial antimicrobial therapy, and preventative strategies: A consensus statement. *Am. J. Respir. Crit. Care. Med.* **153**, 1711–1725.

9. Bartlett, J., Breiman, R., Mandell, L., and File, T. (1998). Community-acquired pneumonia in adults: Guidelines for management (Infectious Disease Society of America). *Clin. Infect. Dis.* **26**, 811–838.

10. Ruiz-Gonzalez, A., Falquera, M., Nogues, A., and Rubio-Caballero, A. (1999). Is *Streptococcus pneumoniae* the leading cause of pneumonia of unknown etiology? A microbiologic study of lung aspirates in consecutive patients with community-acquired pneumonia. *Am. J. Med.* **106**, 385–390.

11. Fine, M., Smith, M., Carson, C., Mutha, S., Sankey, S., Weissfeld, L., and Kapoor, W. (1996). Prognosis and outcomes of patients with community-acquired pneumonia: A meta-analysis. *JAMA* **275**, 134–141.

12. Rein, M. F., Gwaltney Jr., J. M., O'Brien, W. M., Jennings, R. H., and Mandell, G. L. (1978). Accuracy of Gram's stain in identifying pneumococci in sputum. *JAMA* **239**, 2671–2673.

13. Fine, M. J., Orloff, J. J., Rihs, J. D., Vickers, R. M., Kominos, S., Kapoor, W. N., Arena, V. C., and Yu V. L. (1991). Evaluation of housestaff physicians' preparation and interpretation of sputum Gram stains for community-acquired pneumonia. *J. Gen. Intern. Med.* **6**, 189–198.

14. Meehan, T., Fine, M., Krumholtz, H., Scinto, J., Galusha, D., Mockalis, J., Weber, G., Petrillo, M., Houch, P., and Fine, J. (1997). Quality of care, process and outcomes in elderly patients with pneumonia. *JAMA* **278**, 2080–2084.

15. Leroy, O., Santré, C., Beuscart, C., *et al.* (1995). A five-year study of severe community-acquired pneumonia with emphasis on prognosis in patients admitted to an intensive care unit. *Intensive Care Med.* **21**, 24–31.

16. Pachon, J., Pradosm, M. D., Capote, F., Cuello, J. A., Garnacho, J., and Verano, A. (1990). Severe community-acquired pneumonia: Etiology, prognosis, and treatment. *Am. Rev. Respir. Dis.* **142**, 369–373.

17. Gordon, G. S., Throop, D., Berberian, L., Niederman, M., Bass, J., Alemayehu, D., and Mellis, S. (1996). Validation of the therapeutic recommendations of the American Thoracic Society (ATS) guidelines for community-acquired pneumonia in hospitalized patients. *Chest* **110**, 55S.

18. Gleason, P., Meehan, T., Fine, J., Galusha, D., and Fine, M. (1999). Association between initial antimicrobial therapy and medical outcomes for hospitalized elderly patients with pneumonia. *Arch. Int. Med.* **159**, 2511–2512.

19. Lieberman, D., Schlaeffer, F., Boldur, I., *et al.* (1996). Multiple pathogens in adult patients admitted with community-acquired pneumonia: A one-year prospective study of 346 consecutive patients. *Thorax* **51**, 179–184.

20. Marrie, T. J., Peeling, R. W., Fine, M. J., Singer, D. E., Coley, C. M., and Kapoor, W. N. (1996). Ambulatory patients with community-acquired pneumonia: The frequency of atypical agents and clinical course. *Am. J. Med.* **101**, 509–515.

21. File, T. M., Segreti, J., Dunbar, L., *et al.* (1997). A multicenter, randomized study comparing the efficacy and safety of intravenous and/or oral levofloxacin versus ceftriaxone and/or cefuroxime axetil in treatment of adults with community-acquired pneumonia. *Antimicrob. Agents Chemother.* **41**, 1965–1972.

22. Niederman, M., Traub, S., Ellison, W., and Williams, D. (1997). A double-blind, randomized, multicenter, global study in hospitalized community-acquired pneumonia (CAP) comparing

trovafloxacin with ceftriaxone and erythromycin. *Abstr. 37th Intersci. Conf. Antimicrob. Agents Chemother.*, Toronto. Abstr. #LM-72.

23. Metlay, J., Hofman, J., Cetron, M., Fine, M., Farley, M., Whitney, C., and Breiman, R. (2000). Impact of penicillin on medical outcomes for adult patients with bacteremic pneumococcal pneumonia. *Clin. Infect. Dis.* **30**, 520–528.

24. Fine, M. J., Auble, T. E., Yearly, D. M., Hanusa, B. H., Weissfeld, L. A., Singer, D. E., Coley, C. M, Marrie, T. J., and Kapoor, W. N. (1997). A prediction rule to identify low-risk patients with community-acquired pneumonia. *New Engl. J. Med.* **366**, 243–250.

25. Ramirez, J. A. (1995). Switch therapy in adult patients with pneumonia. *Clin. Pulm. Med.* **2**, 327–333.

26. Niederman, M. S., Torres, A., and Summer, W. (1994). Invasive diagnostic testing is not needed routinely to manage suspected ventilator-associated pneumonia. *Am. J. Respir. Crit. Care. Med.* **150**, 565–569.

27. Luna, C. M., Vujacich, P., Niederman, M. S., *et al.* (1997). Impact of BAL data on the therapy and outcome of ventilator-associated pneumonia. *Chest* **111**, 676–685.

28. Fink, M. P., Snydman, D. R., Niederman, M. S., *et al.* (1994). Treatment of severe pneumonia in hospitalized patients: Results of a multicenter, randomized, double-blind trial comparing intravenous ciprofloxacin with imipenem–cilastatin. *Antimicrob. Agents Chemother.* **38**, 547–557.

29. Hilf, M., Yu, V. L., Sharp, J., Zuravleff, J. J., Korvick, J. A., and Muder, R. R. (1989). Antibiotic therapy for *Pseudomonas aeruginosa* bacteremia: Outcome correlations in a prospective study of 200 patients. *Am. J. Med.* **87**, 540–546.

30. Cometta, A., Baumgartner, J. D., Lew, D., *et al.* (1994). Prospective randomized comparison of imipenem monotherapy with imipenem plus netilmicin for treatment of severe infections in nonneutropenic patients. *Antimicrob. Agents Chemother.* **38**, 1309–1313.

31. Hatala, R., Dinh, T., and Cook, D. J. (1996). Once-daily aminoglycoside dosing in immunocompetent adults: A meta-analysis. *Ann. Intern. Med.* **124**, 717–725.

32. Diekema, D., Pfaller, M., Jones, R., Doern, G., Winokur, P., Gales, A., Sader, H., Kugler, K., and Beach, M. (1999). Survey of bloodstream infections due to Gram-negative bacilli: Frequency of occurrence and antimicrobial susceptibility of isolates collected in the United States, Canada, and Latin America for the SENTRY antimicrobial surveillance program, 1997. *Clin. Infect. Dis.* **29**, 595–607.

33. Saint, S., Bent, S., Vittinghoff, E., and Grady, D. (1995). Antibiotics in chronic obstructive pulmonary disease exacerbations: A meta-analysis. *JAMA* **273**, 957–960.

34. Chodosh, S. (1996). Use of quinolones for the treatment of acute exacerbations of chronic bronchitis. *Am. J. Med.* **96** (Suppl. 56A), S93–S100.

35. Andriole, V. (1988). Clinical review of the newer 4-quinolone antibacterial agents. In "The Quinolones" (V. T. Andriole, ed.), pp. 155–200. Academic Press, San Diego.

36. Stein, G. (1996). Pharmacokinetics and pharmacodynamics of newer fluoroquinolones. *Clin. Infect. Dis.* **23** (Suppl.), S19–S24.

37. Sonnesyn, S., and Gerding, D. (1994). Antimicrobials for the treatment of respiratory infection. In "Respiratory Infections: A Scientific Basis for Management" (M. Niederman, G. Sarosi, and J. Glassroth, eds.), pp. 511–537. Saunders, Philadelphia.

38. Forrest, A., Nix, D., Ballow, C., Goss, T., Birmingham, M., and Schentag, J. (1993). Pharmacodynamics of intravenous ciprofloxacin in seriously ill patients. *Antimicrob. Agents Chemother.* **37**, 1073–1081.

39. Shah, A., Lettieri, J., Kaiser, L., Echols, R., and Heller, A. H. (1994). Comparative pharmacokinetics and safety of ciprofloxacin 400 mg iv thrice daily versus 750 mg po twice daily. *J. Antimicrob. Chemother.* **33**, 795–801.

40. Stein, G. E. (1997). Fluoroquinolones: The next generation. In "Proceedings of a Meeting on 'Issues in Pharmacology,'" 1–6 March." Carnes Communications, Valley Forge.

41. Hendershot, E. (1995). Fluoroquinolones. *Infect. Dis. Clin. N. Amer.* **9**, 715–730.

42. Gootz, T., Zaniewski, R., Haskell, S., *et al.* (1996). Activity of the new fluoroquinolone trovafloxacin (CP-99,219) against DNA gyrase and topoisomerase IV mutants of *Streptococcus pneumoniae* selected in vitro. *Antimicrob. Agents Chemother.* **40**, 2691–2697.

43. Zhao, X., Xu, C., and Domagala, J. (1997). DNA topoisomerase targets of the fluoroquinolones: A strategy for avoiding resistance. *Proc. Natl. Acad. Sci. U.S.A.* **94**, 13991–13996.

44. Fukuda, H., and Hiramatsu, K. (1999). Primary targets of fluoroquinolones in *Streptococcus pneumoniae*. *Antimicrob. Agents Chemother.* **43**, 410–412.

45. Jones, M., Sahm, D., Martin, N., Scheuring, S., Heisig, P., Thornsbury, C., Kohrer, K., and Schmitz, F. (2000). Prevalence of *gyrA, gyrB, parC,* and *parE* mutations in clinical isolates of *Streptococcus pneumoniae* with decreased susceptibilities to different fluoroquinolones and originating from worldwide surveillance studies during the 1997–98 respiratory season. *Antimicrob. Agents Chemother.* **44**, 462–466.

46. Child, J., Mortiboy, D., Andrews, J., Chow, A., and Wise, R. (1995). Open-label crossover study to determine pharmacokinetics and penetration of two dose regimens of levofloxacin into inflammatory fluid. *Antimicrob. Agents Chemother.* **39**, 2749–2751.

47. Chen, D., McGeer, A., De Azavedo, J., and Low, D. (1999). Decreased susceptibility of *Streptococcus pneumoniae* to fluoroquinolones in Canada. *New Engl. J. Med.* **341**, 233–239.

48. Thornsbury, C., Jones, M., and Hickey, M. (1999). Resistance surveillance of *Streptococcus pneumoniae, Haemophilus influenzae* and *Moraxella catarrhalis* isolated in the United States, 1997–1998. *J. Antimicrob. Chemother.* **44**, 749–759.

49. Thornsbury, C., Oglive, P., and Holley, H. (1999). Survey of susceptibilities of *Streptococcus pneumoniae, Haemophilus influenzae,* and *Moraxella catarrhalis* isolates to 26 antimicrobial agents: A prospective U.S. study. *Antimicrob. Agents Chemother.* **43**, 2612–2623.

50. Iannini, P., Ovittore, L., and Ross, L. (2000). Characterization of erythromycin resistance in *Streptococcus pneumoniae* in a defined suburban area. *Respir. Med.* **94**(14), A11.

51. Doern, G., Pfaller, M., Kugler, K., Freeman, J., and Jones, R. (1998). Prevalence of antimicrobial resistance among respiratory tract isolates of *Streptococcus pneumoniae* in North America: 1997 results from the SENTRY antimicrobial surveillance program. *Clin. Infect. Dis.* **27**, 764–770.

52. Garau, H., Lonks, J., Gomez, L., Xercavins, M., and Medeiros, A. (2000). Failure of macrolide therapy in patients with bacteremia due to macrolide resistant *Streptococcus pneumoniae*. *Proc. ICMASKO-5*, Seville. Abstr. #7.09.

53. Baquero, F., and Canton, R. (1996). In-vitro activity of sparfloxacin in comparison with currently available antimicrobials against respiratory tract pathogens. *J. Antimicrob. Chemother.* **37**, 1–18.

54. Sefton, A., Maskel, J., Seymour, A., Minassian, M., and Williams, J. (1996). Comparative in-vitro activity of CP-99219, a new quinolone, against respiratory pathogens. *J. Antimicrob. Chemother.* **37**, 803–808.

55. Crokaert, F., Aoun, M., Duchateau, V., Grenier, P., Vandermies, A., and Klastersky, M. (1996). In vitro activity of trovafloxacin (CP-99,219), sparfloxacin, ciprofloxacin, and fleroxacin against respiratory pathogens. *Eur. J. Clin. Microbiol. Infect. Dis.* **15**, 696–698.

56. Niki, Y., Tamada, S., Nakabayashi, M., and Soejima, R. (1995). Sparfloxacin, a new generation fluoroquinolone against *S. pneumoniae* respiratory infections. *Drugs* **49** (Suppl.), 420–422.

57. Girard, A., Girard, D., Gootz, T., Falella, J., and Cimochowski, C. (1995). In vivo efficacy of trovafloxacin (CP-99,219), a new quinolone with extended activities against gram-positive pathogens, *Streptococcus pneumoniae* and *Bacteroides fragilis. Antimicrob. Agents Chemother.* **39**, 2210–2216.

58. Giamarellou, H. (1995). Activity of quinolones against Gram-positive cocci: Clinical features. *Drugs* **49** (Suppl.), 58–66.

59. Cruciani, M., and Basetti, D. (1994). The fluoroquinolones as treatment for infection caused by Gram-positive bacteria. *J. Antimicrob. Chemother.* **33**, 403–417.

60. Klugman, K., and Gootz, T. (1997). In-vitro and in-vivo activity of trovafloxacin against *Streptococcus pneumoniae. J. Antimicrob. Chemother.* **39** (Suppl. B), 51–55.

61. Olsson-Liljequist, B., Hoffman, B., and Hedlund, J. (1996). Activity of trovafloxacin against blood isolates of *Streptococcus pneumoniae* in Sweden. *Eur. J. Clin. Microbiol. Infect. Dis.* **15**, 671–675.

62. Verbist, L., and Verhaegen, J. (1996). In vitro activity of trovafloxacin versus ciprofloxacin against clinical isolates. *Eur. J. Clin. Microbiol. Infect. Dis.* **15**, 683–685.

63. Baurernfeind, A. (1997). Comparison of the antibacterial activities of the quinolones Bay 12-8039, gatifloxacin (AM 1155), trovafloxacin, clinafloxacin, levofloxacin and ciprofloxacin. *J. Antimicrob. Chemother.* **40**, 639–651.

64. Ho, P., Que, T., Tsang, D., Ng, T., Chow, K., and Steo, W. (1999). Emergence of fluoroquinolone resistance among multiple resistant strains of *Streptococcus pneumoniae* in Hong Kong. *Antimicrob. Agents Chemother.* **43**, 1310–1313.

65. Hecht, D., and Wexler, H. (1996). In vitro susceptibility of anaerobes to quinolones in the United States. *Clin. Infect. Dis.* **23** (Suppl.), S2–S8.

66. Goldstein, E. (1996). Possible role for the new fluoroquinolone (levofloxacin, grepafloxacin, trovafloxacin, clinafloxacin, sparfloxacin, and DU-6859a) in the treatment of anaerobic infections: Review of current information on efficacy and safety. *Clin. Infect. Dis.* **23** (Suppl.), S25–S30.

67. Finch, R. (1995). The role of new quinolones in the treatment of respiratory tract infections. *Drugs* **49** (Suppl.), 144–151.

68. Petermann, W. (1991). Ofloxacin in lower respiratory tract infections. *Infection* **19** (Suppl.), S372–S377.

69. Marklein, G. (1996). Quinolones in everyday clinical practice: Respiratory tract infections and nosocomial pneumonia. *Chemotherapy* **42** (Suppl.), 33–42

70. Grasela, D., Lacreta, F., and Uderman, H. (1999). A dose-escalation study of the safety, tolerance and pharmacokinetics (PK) of intravenous (IV) gatifloxacin in healthy adult subjects. *Abstr. 39th Intersci. Conf. Antimicrob. Agents Chemother.*, 17–20 September, San Francisco.

71. Hiemer-Bau, M., Beyer, G., and Stass, H. (1999). Multiple-dose pharmacokinetics (PK) of moxifloxacin (MOX) in serum, urine and saliva [abstract #P769]. *Clin. Microbiol. Infect.* **5** (Suppl. C), 291.

72. Kubitza, D., Stass, H., and Windgender, W. (1996). Bay 12-8039(I), a new 8-methoxy-quinolone: Safety, tolerability (T) and steady-state pharmacokinetics (PK) in healthy male volunteers. *Abstr. 36th Intersci. Conf. Antimicrob. Agents Chemother.*, New Orleans. Abstr. #F25.

73. Allen, A., Bygate, E., Teillool-Foo, M., Johnson, S., and Ward, C. (1999). Pharmacokinetics and tolerability of gemifloxacin after administration of single oral doses to healthy volunteers. *J. Antimicrob. Chemother.* **44** (Suppl. A), 137.

74. Robin, P., and Hammerschlag, M. (1998). In vitro activity of a new 8-methoxyquinolone, BAY 12-8039, against *Chlamydia pneumoniae*. *Antimicrob. Agents Chemother.* **42**, 951–952.

75. Roblin, P., Kutlin, A., and Reznik, T. (1999). Activity of grepafloxacin and other fluoroquinolones and newer macrolides against recent clinical isolates of *Chlamydia pneumoniae*. *Int. J. Antimicrob. Agents.* **12**, 181–184.

76. Bebar, C., Renaudin, H., and Boudjadja, A. (1998). In vitro activity of BAY 132-8039, a new fluoroquinolone against mycoplasmas. *Antimicrob. Agents Chemother.* **42**, 703–704.

77. Duffy, L., Kempf, M., and Crabb, D. (1999). In vitro activity of moxifloxacin and six other new antimicrobials against *Mycoplasma pneumoniae*. *Abstr. 39th Intersci. Conf. Antimicrob. Agents Chemother.*, San Francisco. Abstr. #0367.

78. Dubois, J., and St.-Pierre, C. (1999). In vitro susceptibility study of gatifloxacin against *Legionella* spp. [poster]. *Diag. Microbiol. Infect. Dis.* **33**, 261–266.

79. Miyashiya, N., and Kishimoto, T. (1997). In vitro and in vivo activities of AM-1155, a new fluoroquinolone, against *Chlamydia* spp. *Antimicrob. Agents Chemother.* **41**, 1331–1334.

80. Ishida, K., Kaku, M., and Irifune, K. (1994). In vitro and in vivo activity of AM 1155 against *Mycoplasma pneumoniae*. *J. Antimicrob. Chemother.* **34**, 875–883.

81. Dubois, J., and St.-Pierre, C. (1999). Comparative in vitro activity and postantibiotic effect of gemifloxacin against *Legionella* spp. *J. Antimicrob. Chemother.* **44** (Suppl. A), 136.

82. Duffy, L., Crabb, D., and Searcy, K. (1999). Comparative activity of gemifloxacin and new quinolones, macrolides, tetracycline, and clindamycin against *Mycoplasma* spp. *Abstr. 39th Intersci. Conf. Antimicrob. Agents Chemother.*, San Francisco. Abstr. #1500.

83. Felmingham, D., Robbins, M., Dencer, M., Salman, H., Mathias, I., and Ridgway, G. (1999). In vitro activity of gemifloxacin against *S. pneumoniae*, *H. influenzae*, *M. catarrhalis*, *L. pneumophila* and *Chlamydia* spp. *J. Antimicrob. Chemother.* **44** (Suppl. A), 131.

84. Dore, P., Robert, R., Grollier, G., *et al.* (1996). Incidence of anaerobes in ventilator-associated pneumonia with use of a protected specimen brush. *Am. J. Respir. Crit. Care. Med.* **153**, 1292–1298.

85. Mier, L., Dreyfuss, D., Darchy, B., *et al.* (1993). Is penicillin G an adequate initial treatment for aspiration pneumonia? A prospective evaluation using a protected specimen brush and quantitative cultures. *Intensive Care Med.* **19**, 279–284.

86. Schauman, R., Claros, M., and Pleb, B. (1998). In vitro activity of gatifloxacin against anaerobic bacteria compared with other quinolones and non-quinolones [poster]. *38th Intersci. Conf. Antimicrob. Agents Chemother.*, 24–27 September, San Diego.

87. Ednie, L., Jacobs, M., and Appelbaum, P. (1998). Activities of gatifloxacin compared to seven other agents against anaerobic organisms. *Antimicrob. Agents Chemother.* **42**, 2459–2462.

88. Diekema, D., Pfaller, M., Jones, R., Doern, G., Winokur, P., Galse, C., Sader, H., Kugler, K., and Beach, M. (1999). Survey of bloodstream infections due to Gram-negative bacilli: Frequency of occurrence and antimicrobial susceptibility of isolates collected in the United States, Canada, and Latin America for the SENTRY antimicrobial surveillance program, 1997. *Clin. Infect. Dis.* **29**, 595–607.

89. Miltavic, D., and Wallrauch, C. (1996). In vitro activity of trovafloxacin in combination with ceftazidime, meropenem, and amikacin. *Eur. J. Clin. Microbiol. Infect. Dis.* **15**, 688–693

90. Chidiac, C., Roussel-Delvallez, M., Guery, B., and Beaucaire, G. (1995). Should *Pseudomonas aeruginosa* isolates resistant to one of the fluorinated quinolones be tested for the others? Studies with an experimental model of pneumonia. *Antimicrob. Agents Chemother.* **39**, 677–679.

91. Ball, A. P. (1992). Clinical evidence for the efficacy of ciprofloxacin in lower respiratory tract infections. *Rev. Contemp. Pharmacother.* **3**, 133–142.

92. Khan, F. A, and Basir, R. (1989). Sequential intravenous-oral administration of ciprofloxacin vs. ceftazadime in serious bacterial respiratory tract infections. *Chest* **96**, 528–537.

93. Johnson, R. H., Levine, S., Traub, S. L., *et al.* (1996). Sequential intravenous/oral ciprofloxacin compared to parenteral ceftriaxone in the treatment of hospitalized patients with community-acquired pneumonia. *Infect. Dis. Clin. Pract.* **5**, 265–272.

94. Trenholme, G. M., Schmitt, B. A., Spear, J., Gvazdinskas, L. C., and Levin, S. (1989). Randomized study of intravenous/oral ciprofloxacin versus ceftazadime in the treatment of hospital and nursing home patients with lower respiratory tract infections. *Am. J. Med.* **87** (Suppl. 5A), 116–118.

95. Byl, B., Kaufman, L., Jacobs, F., Derde, M. P., and Thys, J. P. (1993). Ciprofloxacin versus comparative antibiotics in LRTI: A meta-analysis. *Drugs* **45** (Suppl.), 50–51.

96. Gentry, L. O., Rodriguez-Gomez, G., Kohler, R. B., Khan, F. A., and Rytel, M. W. (1992). Parenteral followed by oral ofloxacin for nosocomial and community-acquired pneumonia requiring hospitalization. *Am. Rev. Respir. Dis.* **145**, 31–35.

97. Rubinstein, E. (1996). Safety profile of sparfloxacin in the treatment of respiratory tract infections. *J. Antimicrob. Chemother.* **37** (Suppl.), 145–160.

98. Vincent, J., Venitz, J., Teng, R., *et al.* (1997). Pharmacokinetics and safety of trovafloxacin in healthy male volunteers following administration of single intravenous doses of the prodrug, alatrofloxacin. *J. Antimicrob. Chemother.* **39** (Suppl. B), 75–80.

99. Graham, D, Klein, T., Marti., A., Niederman, M. S., and the Trovan Nosocomial Pneumonia Study Group (1997). A double-blind, randomized, multicenter study in nosocomial pneumonia (NOS) comparing trovafloxacin with ciprofloxacin ± clindamycin/metronidazole. *Abstr. 37th Intersci. Conf. Antimicrob. Agents Chemother.*, Toronto. Abstr. #LM-74.

100. Fogarty, C., Grossman, C., Williams, J., Haverstock, D., and Church, D., for the Community-Acquired Pneumonia Study Group (1999). Efficacy and safety of moxifloxacin vs. Clarithromycin for community-acquired pneumonia. *Infect. Med.* **16**, 748–763.

101. Patel, T., Pearl, J., Williams, J., Haverstock, M., and Church, D., for the Community-Acquired Pneumonia Study Group (2000). Efficacy and safety of 10-days of moxifloxacin 400 mg once daily in the treatment of patients with community-acquired pneumonia. *Respir. Med.* **94**.

102. Ramirez, J., Nguyen, T., Tellier, G., Coppola, G., Bettis, R., Dolmann, A., St.-Pierre, C., and Mayer, H. (1999). Treating community-acquired pneumonia with once-daily gatifloxacin vs. twice-daily clarithromycin. *J. Respir. Infect.* **20** (Suppl.), 541–548.

103. Sullivan, J., McElroy, A., Honsinger, R., McAdoo, M., Harrison, B., Plouffe, J., Gotfried, M., and Mayer, H. (1999). Treating community-acquired pneumonia with once-daily gatifloxacin vs. once-daily levofloxacin. *J. Respir. Infect.* **20** (Suppl.), 549–559.

104. Fogarty, C., Dowell, M., Ellison, T., Vrooman, P., White, B., and Mayer, H. (1999). Treating community-acquired pneumonia in hospitalized patients: Gatifloxacin vs. ceftriaxone/clarithromycin. *J. Respir. Infect.* **20** (Suppl.), 560–569.

105. Niederman, M., Church, D., Haverstock, M., and Springsklee, M. (2000). Does appropriate antibiotic therapy influence outcome in community-acquired pneumonia (CAP) and acute exacerbations of chronic bronchitis (AECB) [abstract #A14]? *Respir. Med.* **94** (Suppl. A), p. E23.

106. DeAbate, A., McIvor, R., McElvaine, P., Skuba, K., and Pierce, P. (1999). Gatifloxacin vs. cefuroxime axetil in patients with acute exacerbations of chronic bronchitis. *J. Respir. Dis.* **20** (Suppl.), S23–S29.

107. Ramirez, A., Molina, J., Dolmann, A., Fogarty, C., DeAbate, A., Breen, J., and Skuba, K. (1999). Gatifloxacin treatment in patients with acute exacerbations of chronic bronchitis: Clinical trial results. *J. Respir. Dis.* **20** (Suppl.), S30–S39.

108. Wilson, R., Kubin, R., Ballin, I., Depperman, K., Bassaris, H., Leophonte, P., Schreurs, A., Torres, A., and Sommerauer, B. (1999). Five-day moxifloxacin therapy compared with 7-day clarithromycin therapy for the treatment of acute exacerbations of chronic bronchitis. *J. Antimicrob. Chemother.* **44**, 501–513.

109. Chodosh, S., DeAbate, C., Haverstock, D., Aneiro, L., Church, D., and the Bronchitis Study Group (2000). Short-course moxifloxacin therapy for treatment of acute bacterial exacerbations of chronic bronchitis. *Respir. Med.* **94**, 18–27.

CHAPTER 9

Use of Quinolones in Surgery and Obstetrics and Gynecology

JOHN WEIGELT,* KAREN BRASEL,* and SEBASTIAN FARO[†]

*Department of Surgery, Medical College of Wisconsin, Milwaukee, Wisconsin 53226,
[†]Department of Obstetrics and Gynecology, Rush Medical College, Rush Presbyterian
and St. Luke's Medical Center, Rush University, Chicago, Illinois 60612

Introduction
Surgical Wound Prophylaxis
Soft Tissue Infection
Intraabdominal Infection
Gynecologic Infections
Postoperative Pelvic Infections
Pelvic Inflammatory Disease
Upper Genital Tract Infection
Pregnancy
Conclusion
References

INTRODUCTION

A number of characteristics make the quinolones attractive in the practice of surgery, obstetrics, and gynecology. These include broad aerobic, facultative, and obligate anaerobic bacterial spectrum of activity, unique mechanism of action, bactericidal capability, acceptable safety profile, intravenous and oral-dose availability, and excellent tissue penetration [1]. In surgery, quinolones are commonly used to treat soft-tissue and intraabdominal infections. Quinolones have also been used for surgical wound prophylaxis. The present quinolones are primarily noted for their activity against aerobic and facultative anaerobic bacteria. In those instances where obligate anaerobic antibacterial activity is indicated, the quinolones currently available must be used in combination with clindamycin or metronidazole. New quinolones offer the promise of antibacterial activity against both aerobic and facultative anaerobic bacteria, as well as against obligate anaerobic bacteria [2,3]. Therefore, the use of these newer quinolones offers the possibility of using single-agent therapy in place of combination therapy for treating complex intraabdominal and pelvic infections. Unfortunately, trovafloxacin, one of the newer quinolones with an expanded spectrum, has been implicated in 14 cases of liver failure, and its use for all approved indications has been severely curtailed by the FDA.

This chapter reviews the current use of fluoroquinolones in surgery and obstetrics and gynecology. Surgical uses include surgical wound prophylaxis and treatment of soft-tissue and intraabdominal infections. Obstetric uses are limited to treatment of postpartum endometritis and wound infection. The fluoroquinolones are suitable for use as a prophylactic agent in women undergoing hysterectomy, treatment of cervical infection by *N. gonorrhoeae* and *C. trachomatis*, pelvic inflammatory disease (PID), postoperative pelvic cellulitis, postpartum endometritis, and wound infection.

SURGICAL WOUND PROPHYLAXIS

Surgical wound prophylaxis decreases surgical wound infection [4]. General principles include an antibiotic that is effective against the expected bacterial challenge, is administered before the surgical incision, has adequate tissue penetration, and is used for a short duration [5]. The quinolones are effective against common pathogens causing surgical wound infections and have excellent penetration into skin and subcutaneous tissues [6,7]. The cost of a prophylactic antibiotic is always a consideration, as well as the concern that excessive use of an antibiotic will result in increased resistance to the agent. Although not used routinely for surgical prophylaxis, the quinolones may offer some advantages as prophylactic agents [8].

Most surgical wound infections are still caused by aerobic Gram-positive and Gram-negative organisms. The quinolones are effective against these pathogens, and a number of studies have been done using quinolones for prophylaxis. Clinical trials in clean wounds include patients having hip or knee replacements, and vascular and cardiac surgery [9,10]. Intravenous and oral administration were used, and surgical infection rates were no different from comparison drugs, which included cefazolin and ceftazidime. Clean contaminated abdominal procedures involving the biliary tract, colon, and urinary tract have been studied [10]. Biliary tract studies commonly used cefazolin as the comparator. All colon studies used metronidazole with the quinolone. Cefuroxime or cefotaxime were the common comparison agents in urinary tract procedures. All these studies revealed that the quinolones were as effective in preventing surgical wound infections as the reference prophylactic agent.

The aerobic and anaerobic spectrum of trovafloxacin made it an ideal prophylactic antibiotic to consider for colon surgery [11]. Trovafloxacin was compared with cefotetan in a multiinstitutional study [12] of patients having colon resections. All patients had a mechanical bowel preparation and parenteral antibiotics. Clinical success was defined as the absence of surgery-related infections. Clinical success was achieved in 79% of patients receiving trovaflox-acin and 82% of patients receiving cefotetan.

Unfortunately, many of the currently available prophylactic quinolone studies involved small patient numbers, used inadequate methods, and reported poorly defined outcomes. In addition, the use of a quinolone for clean wound prophylaxis is controversial. Before widespread use of quinolone prophylaxis can be adopted, better studies of appropriate patient populations must be available. The questions of bacterial resistance and cost must also be addressed.

A concern with any prophylactic antibiotic use is the development of resistance. This is especially true if the same drug is being used for therapeutic purposes. In animal models, successful Gram-positive prophylaxis without developing resistance is documented [13]. Unfortunately, resistance does appear to be associated with misuse of antibiotics [14,15]. Inappropriate use and overuse are commonly suggested as causes of resistance. It is doubtful that proper antimicrobial prophylaxis speeds the of bacterial resistance to any antibiotic.

The cost of prophylaxis is another consideration. The use of quinolone prophylaxis in clean wounds must be questioned considering the low rates of infection and availability of effective agents that are less costly. Before this substitution takes place, a cost-effective analysis should occur. If better bacterial coverage, better patient tolerance, or a better delivery system can be documented, then quinolone prophylaxis should be considered more frequently. However, it is highly unlikely that a parenteral quinolone will be a cost-effective prophylactic agent for the majority of clean and clean contaminated surgical cases.

One potential advantage of the quinolones as perioperative agents is their oral dosage form. Most mistakes in perioperative antibiotic use are associated with administration time [16,17]. Oral administration of perioperative antibiotics is effective and could improve proper use [18]. Oral quinolones have been used preoperatively for prophylaxis in cardiac and biliary tract surgery [19,20]. An oral quinolone should be effective prophylaxis, although whether this method would be cost-effective over short use of older parenteral agents remains to be studied. It does offer the opportunity to avoid missing preoperative parenteral doses, which makes any prophylactic regimen less effective. A quinolone with a longer half-life would also not need to be redosed [21].

In summary, quinolones must be considered to have a rather limited role as a parenteral prophylactic agent. There are simply too many other less costly alternatives. The oral route may offer a new and unique way to provide prophylaxis with these agents for a wide variety of surgical procedures.

SOFT TISSUE INFECTION

The quinolones have no use in uncomplicated skin infections commonly caused by Gram-positive organisms. However, quinolones are useful in complicated skin infections that are caused by multiple organisms, including Gram-negative bacteria [8,22]. If anaerobic bacteria are suspected, two alternatives using quinolones are possible: either combination therapy with an anaerobic agent plus a second-generation quinolone, or monotherapy with a third- or fourth-generation quinolone.

The pharmacokinetics of the quinolones make them ideal for use in patients with soft tissue infections. Inflamed tissues have drug concentrations 1.8 times the serum level [7]. Skin blister quinolone concentration is between 110 and 125% of the serum AUCs. These levels can be achieved with either the intravenous or the oral dosage form [23].

The diabetic patient with a foot infection is always a clinical challenge. Diabetic foot ulcers are usually not a primary infection but are caused by the diabetic neuropathy and subsequent mechanical stresses to the feet of the diabetic patient [24]. Poor vascular supply further complicates these ulcers and may potentiate the risk of infection. Infection can involve soft tissue as well as joints and bone. Treatment is directed at proper diabetic control, foot care, debridement of necrotic tissue, improvement in blood supply, and antibiotics [25].

The bacteriology of diabetic foot lesions is polymicrobial and includes anaerobes, especially when necrotic tissue is present. The number of bacterial isolates is usually greater than two [26–28]. Common Gram-positive isolates include *Staphylococcus aureus* and *Streptococcus* spp. Enterobacteriaceae, including *Escherichia coli*, are common Gram-negative isolates. Other aerobic bacteria include enterococcus, *Proteus* spp., and *Pseudomonas* spp. Anaerobic bacteria commonly include *Peptostreptococcus* spp. and *Bacteroides* spp. Antibiotics remain an important component in treating these infections.

Monotherapy is attractive, but combination therapy is commonly recommended [26]. Unfortunately, the superiority of one regimen over another has not been shown [25,26]. The quinolones have been used to treat lower-extremity infection [29]. Ciprofloxacin at either 1500 or 2000 mg per day orally recorded a 60% success rate at 1 year. This success was better than historical controls treated with cefoxitin or ceftizoxime. The ciprofloxacin patients also had a shorter hospital stay. Another study [30] found no difference between oral ciprofloxacin and parenteral antibiotics. Oral levofloxacin has been compared to oral ciprofloxacin for uncomplicated skin and skin-structure infections. Clinical success was 98% for levofloxacin and 94% for ciprofloxacin [31]. One concern about monotherapy with the quinolones is promotion of methicillin-resistant *Staphylococcus aureus* [32].

Trovafloxacin is effective for soft tissue infection, including diabetic foot infection. The success rates for uncomplicated skin infections are greater than 90%. Trovafloxacin was compared [12] to piperacillin–tazobactam in the treatment of patients with diabetic foot infections. The results were similar, with response rates of 88% for trovafloxacin and 89% for the comparator. Oral trovafloxacin was also compared to amoxicillin–clavulinic acid, with similar results.

Oral antibiotics can be as effective and less costly than parenteral antibiotics for diabetic foot infections [33]. This analysis used oral ciprofloxacin for 10 weeks as one of the treatment choices. Ten days of oral sparfloxacin (400 mg loading dose followed by 200 mg/day) has also been used to treat complicated skin and skin-structure infections in a phase III clinical trial. Unfortunately, photosensitivity reactions occur in 7.4% of patients taking sparfloxacin in contrast to 0.5% on comparator agents [34]. The combination of photosensitivity and prolongation of the Q–T interval has significantly limited the use of this drug.

INTRAABDOMINAL INFECTION

The quinolones have not been routinely used for intraabdominal infections. Quinolones are not mentioned in a policy statement by the Surgical Infection Society regarding treatment of intraabdominal infections [35]. Intraabdominal infections are most commonly mixed infections, with both aerobes and anaerobes. Recommendations promulgated in the early 1990s emphasize single drugs effective against aerobic and anaerobic bacteria as being equivalent to double- or triple-drug therapy for intraabdominal infections [36,37]. Improper empiric selection of antibiotics when treating peritonitis is associated with a significantly higher complication rate and mortality [36].

However, the quinolones do have excellent abdominal tissue penetration. This is especially true for ciprofloxacin. Concentrations of 95% of serum levels are found in peritoneal fluid after ciprofloxacin administration [7]. Ciprofloxacin is observed to be concentrated in pancreatic tissue as well as hepatic tissue [7]. These pharmacokinetic characteristics are attractive and enhance the role quinolones might serve in treatment of intraabdominal infections.

It has been appropriate for quinolones to be excluded as a choice for empiric coverage of intraabdominal infections simply because their spectrum is not appropriate. However, two developments suggest that the use of quinolones in patients with intraabdominal infections may become more common. These are the emphasis on oral therapy and the newer quinolones that have an anaerobic spectrum.

The oral route is being explored as a way to provide effective treatment with and without intravenous therapy. These methods offer the patient and health care market an option for outpatient therapy [38]. Although not completely proven, this approach is suggested as being cost-effective [1]. Patients receive initial doses of intravenous antibiotic and then, when appropriate, are switched to oral forms. An advantage of the quinolones is their availability in both intravenous and oral form. A randomized double-blind multicenter trial [39] compared ciprofloxacin and metronidazole with imipenem–cilastatin for intraabdominal infection. This study compared i.v. therapy with ciprofloxacin–metronidazole, i.v./p.o. therapy with ciprofloxacin–metronidazole, and i.v. therapy with imipenem–cilastatin. The outcomes were equivalent, with all combinations having an overall success rate of at least 80%. The duration of intravenous treatment before switching to oral treatment was 5.2 ± 1.7 days followed by 3.8 ± 3.2 days of oral therapy. The use of other quinolones with similar spectra to ciprofloxacin in this manner may prove to be cost-effective.

The i.v./oral switch method of treatment still requires study. The timing of the switch needs to be better defined. The absorption characteristics of the drug in a patient with acute peritoneal inflammation need to be evaluated. It was recommended that tube feedings and drugs be withheld for 2 hr before the drug is given [39]. Finally, which patients actually need further oral therapy after i.v. therapy and how long oral therapy should continue remain unknown.

The second development making quinolones a more appropriate choice for treating intraabdominal infections is their broader antimicrobial spectrum. Only two quinolones have a broad enough spectrum to be considered for monotherapy of intraabdominal infections. Trovafloxacin and clinafloxacin have aerobic and anaerobic bacterial efficacy [40]. Studies [12,41] in patients with intraabdominal infections demonstrate that trovafloxacin or clinafloxacin alone is as effective as imipenem–cilastatin. The clinical success rate for trovafloxacin was 80%, compared to 83% for imipenem–cilastatin [12]. The clinical success rate for clinafloxacin was 81%, compared to 76% for imipenem–cilastatin [41]. One of the studies comparing trovafloxacin to imipenem–cilastatin used i.v./oral switch therapy.

Clinafloxacin has been removed from further development secondary to photo-toxicity and drug-induced hypoglycemia.

GYNECOLOGIC INFECTIONS

The quinolones appear to be well suited for intraabdominal and pelvic infections because both tend to be polymicrobial. The bacteria involved in these infections typically involve a wide range of Gram-positive and Gram-negative facultative, as well as obligate, anaerobic bacteria. One difference between infections involved in the abdomen and those occurring in the pelvis is that the former are more likely to involve *Bacteroides fragilis*, as well as other members of the *B. fragilis* group. *Prevotella bivia* tends to be frequently involved in mixed pelvic infections. However, *B. fragilis* is frequently found as a coinfecting organism in pelvic abscesses. Although obstetric infection (i.e., postpartum endometritis) tends to be polymicrobial, quinolones are contraindicated in pregnant and breast-feeding women. Thus far, whether quinolones cause teratogenic or developmental abnormalities is not known. Thus, the quinolones appear to have a role in the treatment of intraabdominal and pelvic infections.

Gynecologic infections can be divided into two groups. One group of infections, caused by the patient's endogenous vaginal microflora, are responsible for the majority (probably 95%) of posthysterectomy pelvic infections (Table I) [42]. The remainder of infections are due to exogenous bacteria, primarily sexually transmitted organisms. The patient's endogenous vaginal microflora, in a healthy state or ecosystem, are dominated by *Lactobacillus acidophilus* and other bacteria of low virulence. Although there are many other Gram-positive and Gram-negative bacteria, they are present in low numbers or of inadequate inoculum size and, therefore, are not a threat to cause infection (Table II). If the patient's vaginal ecosystem becomes altered or is disrupted and the pH rises above 5, the growth of *L. acidophilus* is inhibited, whereas the growth of the facultative and obligate anaerobes dominates.

This condition, referred to as bacterial vaginosis (BV), is characterized by a pH above 4.5 (normal is 3.8 to 4.2), the absence of *L. acidophilus* dominance, the absence of white blood cells (WBCs), and the presence of clue cells [43,44]. An understanding of the status of the vaginal ecosystem is important because, if antibiotic prophylaxis is to be successful, the patient must not be infected or have a vaginal microflora that consists of extremely large numbers of bacteria ($>10^6$ bacteria/ml of vaginal fluid) that are potentially virulent. When BV becomes established, the number of bacteria within a genus exceeds 10^6 bacteria/ml of vaginal fluid.

TABLE I   Postoperative Pelvic Infections

Vaginal cuff cellulitis	Pelvic abscess
Pelvic cellulitis	Tuboovarian abscess
Vaginal cuff infected hematoma	Ligneous cellulitis

TABLE II   Bacterial Make-Up of the Vaginal Ecosystem

Lactobacillus acidophilus	*Staphylococcus aureus*
Nondescriptive streptococci	*Staphylococcus epidermidis*
Corynebacterium	*Streptococcus agalactiae*
Diphtheroid	*Enterococcus faecalis*
Escherichia coli	Obligate anaerobes
Enterobacter aerogenes	*Bacteroides fragilis*
Enterobacter cloacae	*Fusobacterium necrophorum*
Gardnerella vaginalis	*Fusobacterium nucleatum*
Klebsiella pneumoniae	*Peptostreptococcus anaerobius*
Morganella morganii	*Prevotella bivia*
Proteus mirabilis	*Prevotella melaninogenica*

Prevention of posthysterectomy pelvic infection and postpartum endometritis is based on the use of both meticulous surgical techniques and prophylactic antibiotics. Many published studies [45,46] demonstrate that the administration of a single dose of an antibiotic prior to commencement of surgery has successfully reduced the incidence of postoperative pelvic infection. Antibiotics used prophylactically in gynecologic and obstetric surgery are usually administered intravenously 30 to 60 minutes prior to the onset of surgery. Quinolones have been studied sparingly as prophylactic agents in gynecologic surgery. A study [47] comparing metronidazole–cefuroxime vs. ciprofloxacin found the two regimens to be comparable. In the metronidazole–cefuroxime group, none of the 58 patients developed a postoperative infection. In the group that received ciprofloxacin, 3 of 54 patients developed a postoperative infection. A multicenter study [47a] was performed comparing orally administered trovafloxacin to cefoxitin given intravenously. Trovafloxacin was found to be as efficacious as cefoxitin in preventing postoperative pelvic infections in patients undergoing hysterectomy. However, at one center patients administered trovafloxacin also received bictria. Patients who received bictria and trovafloxacin were found to have a higher incidence of postoperative pelvic infection. The bictria bound the trovafloxacin and prevented its absorption. In the absence of bictria, trovafloxacin administered orally was as efficacious as cefoxitin as a prophylactic agent in preventing postoperative pelvic infections.

POSTOPERATIVE PELVIC INFECTIONS

Postoperative pelvic infections (e.g., postpartum endometritis and posthysterectomy pelvic cellulitis) are typically polymicrobial, involving aerobic, facultative, and obligate anaerobic bacteria. Antibiotics are administered empirically and, therefore, must provide a broad spectrum of activity against a variety of bacteria. The standard antibiotic regimen of choice is clindamycin and gentamicin. However, the β-lactam antibiotics also provide a broad spectrum of antibacterial activity (Table III). In general, when administered alone the quinolones do not have the necessary spectrum of activity and, therefore, are not suitable for treatment of postpartum endometritis or posthysterectomy pelvic infection [48]. In one study comparing ciprofloxacin to clindamycin–gentamicin, ciprofloxacin was found to be effective in only 71% of the cases. This is compared to the combination of clindamycin–gentamicin, which cured 85% of patients with postpartum endometritis. If either ciprofloxacin or ofloxacin is used to treat postoperative pelvic infections, it should be combined with an anaerobic agent such as clindamycin or metronidazole. The newer quinolones levofloxacin and trovafloxacin are considered to be active against the obligate anaerobic bacteria and, therefore, suitable for treatment of postoperative pelvic infection. However, levofloxacin has only moderate activity against obligate anaerobic bacteria [49]. Trovafloxacin appears to have a broader spectrum of activity against obligate anaerobic bacteria and can be used as a single agent in the treatment of these infections. Initial studies comparing trovafloxacin to clindamycin–gentamicin have shown that the former has efficacy equal to that of the latter antibiotic regimen.

TABLE III β-Lactam Antibiotics for Use in Treating Pelvic Infections

Penicillins	Cephalosporins
Ampicillin-sulbactam (Unasyn)	Cefotetan
Piperacillin-tazobactam (Zosyn)	Cefoxitin
Ticarcillin-clavulanic acid (Timentin)	Ceftizoxime

PELVIC INFLAMMATORY DISEASE

Pelvic inflammatory disease (PID) is a spectrum of disease that begins with cervicitis and may progress to endometritis and, eventually, salpingitis. The most common cause of this spectrum of disease is *Neisseria gonorrhoeae* and/or *Chlamydia trachomatis*. The standard for treating a patient with either chlamydial or gonococcal cervicitis is to treat for the presence of both. Treatment for gonococcal cervicitis requires administration of one of the following in a single dose:

1. Ceftriaxone 125 mg intramuscularly
2. Cefixime 400 mg orally
3. Ciprofloxacin 500 mg orally
4. Ofloxacin 400 mg orally
5. Cefuroxime axetil 1 g orally
6. Cefpodoxime proxetil 200 mg orally
7. Enoxacin 400 mg orally
8. Lomefloxacin 400 mg orally
9. Norfloxacin 800 mg orally
10. Spectinomycin 2 g intramuscularly
11. Ceftizoxime 500 mg intramuscularly
12. Cefotaxime 500 mg intramuscularly
13. Cefotetan 1 g intramuscularly
14. Cefoxitin 2 g intramuscularly

All patients treated for gonococcal cervicitis should be treated for the presence of *C. trachomatis*. Patients treated for chlamydial cervicitis should also be treated for the presence of *N. gonorrhoeae*, because approximately 40 to 60% of patients will be simultaneously infected with both organisms. All the agents listed above, with the exception of ciprofloxacin, enoxacin, ofloxacin, and trovafloxacin, must be used in conjunction with an agent effective against *C. trachomatis*. Quinolones such as ciprofloxacin, enoxacin, ofloxacin, and trovafloxacin are effective against *C. trachomatis*, although not in a single dose [50–53].

Interestingly, in one study [54] investigators found that neither ciprofloxacin nor doxycycline was efficacious in treating chlamydial urogenital infection in a population that included 157 male patients and 43 female patients. There were a total of 32 failures in the ciprofloxacin group and 20 in the doxycycline group. The failure to achieve higher eradication rates was caused by treating female patients with cervical infection and not actually knowing the stage of infection (i.e., whether the patient had endometritis or salpingitis). Failure to eradicate the organism may place the patient at risk for infertility or ectopic pregnancy. This study raises a significant concern with regard to the reliability of doxycycline, which is the gold standard for treating chlamydial cervical infection. In a study [55] comparing ofloxacin and doxycycline, 40 patients were randomized to receive either drug. Two patients in the ofloxacin group and four in the doxycycline group failed treatment.

Thus far, the only quinolone with proven efficacy approved for the treatment of both *C. trachomatis* and *N. gonorrhoeae* is ofloxacin [56]. Trovafloxacin has been shown in several studies to be as effective as doxycycline in treating chlamydial cervical infection. Sparfloxacin is also very active against common genital pathogens [57]. The difference between ofloxacin and trovafloxacin is that the former is administered twice daily, while the latter is administered once per day.

UPPER GENITAL TRACT INFECTION

Involvement of the upper genital tract can be divided artificially into endometritis and salpingitis. However, the two probably cannot be separated clinically, and a patient with endometritis should be treated as though she has salpingitis. The likelihood that the patient has endometritis–salpingitis can be determined by detecting the presence of plasma cells on histological analysis of the endometrium. Initially, it is likely that the majority of patients with chlamydial and/or gonococcal endometritis may also have a polymicrobial infection involving Gram-positive and Gram-negative facultative and obligate anaerobic bacteria. The risk of polymicrobial infection becomes significant if the patient simultaneously has BV.

Traditionally, PID has been treated with antibiotic regimens that have activity against both *C. trachomatis* and *N. gonorrhoeae* as well as facultative and obligate anaerobic bacteria. Two quinolones have been tested in the treatment of PID: ciprofloxacin and ofloxacin. Trovafloxacin has also been investigated as a possible treatment agent for PID. Several investigators [58–61] found ciprofloxacin to be as effective as clindamycin plus gentamicin in treating PID. In one study [58], ciprofloxacin was not as effective as clindamycin–gentamicin in treating PID, especially in patients with BV. The investigators attributed this to the inferior activity of ciprofloxacin with regard to the anaerobic bacteria that dominate in BV. However, clindamycin plus gentamicin is also synergistic against *C. trachomatis* [62]. Ofloxacin has also received considerable attention regarding its effectiveness in treating PID. Ofloxacin is similar to other quinolones in having reduced efficacy in treating BV, which may be due to its lack of significant activity against obligate anaerobic bacteria [63,64]. However, ofloxacin was found to be as effective as cefoxitin plus doxycycline in the outpatient treatment of PID. Interestingly, *N. gonorrhoeae* was eradicated from all patients in both groups; however, *C. trachomatis* was eradicated from 88% of patients receiving doxycycline and 100% of those receiving ofloxacin [65]. In another study [66], ofloxacin eradicated *C. trachomatis* in 86% of patients, whereas the organism was eradicated in 100% of patients receiving cefoxitin–doxycycline.

The efficacy of quinolones in the treatment of PID was well established in two studies [67,68]. One was a noncomparative study administering ofloxacin, and the other compared pefloxacin–metronidazole to doxycycline–metronidazole. Both studies employed laparoscopy to confirm the diagnosis of PID. In the ofloxacin study, a total of 36 patients were studied, 25 of whom had *N. gonorrhoeae* and 6 *C. trachomatis*. Interestingly, only 1 patient was found to have a polymicrobial infection. Thus, it can be inferred that acute salpingitis is primarily due to *N. gonorrhoeae* or *C. trachomatis*, or both. Preliminary data indicate that trovafloxacin will be as effective as ofloxacin in treating acute salpingitis. In addition, trovafloxacin should be effective in treating complicated PID, because this state of the disease is likely to be polymicrobial and to involve anaerobic bacteria. Trovafloxacin not only has good activity against *N. gonorrhoeae* and *C. trachomatis* but also against facultative and obligate anaerobic bacteria.

PREGNANCY

Quinolones are contraindicated during pregnancy and in the breast-feeding patient. However, in one published study [69] 38 pregnant women received quinolone therapy. Thirty-five of them received norfloxacin or ciprofloxacin for the treatment of a urinary tract infection in the first trimester. No developmental malformations were found in any of the children born to these mothers who received a quinolone during pregnancy. In a rabbit model [70] investigating placental transfer of enrofloxacin and ciprofloxacin, a significant difference in placental clearance of the two quinolones was found. Enrofloxacin had a placental clearance of 0.88 ± 0.13 ml/min and ciprofloxacin 0.06 ± 0.02 ml/min ($p < 0.01$) [28]. This study suggests that enrofloxacin crosses the placenta much more readily than ciprofloxacin, which may explain why when given to pregnant women ciprofloxacin did not seem to have any adverse effect on the fetus. In a large study [71] comparing ciprofloxacin, norfloxacin, ofloxacin, azithromycin, and cefixime in 11,000 patients, 55 pregnant patients received a quinolone, 8 of whom were in the first trimester. None of the newborns had any congenital abnormalities. A new quinolone, prulifloxacin, was administered to pregnant New Zealand white rabbits during the period of organogenesis [72]. Doses of 10, 30, and 100 mg/kg were administered from day 6 to day 18 of gestation. The rabbits were sacrificed on day 29. None of the fetuses exhibited alterations in development of skin, organs, or skeletal structures. Prulifloxacin was also administered to Sprague–Dawley pregnant rats [73] in doses of 30, 300, and 3000 mg of the quinolone from day 8 through day 30 of pregnancy. No developmental abnormalities were noted in any of the fetuses delivered of a mother receiving 30 or 300 mg/kg of prulifloxacin. In animals that received 3000 mg/kg, white spots and a rough surface developed on the kidney, renal tubular nephrosis with crystalline substance was observed, and the weight of the kidney was increased. The fetuses born to these rats had decreased body weight and retarded ossification.

Although these initial studies suggest that the quinolones may be safe to administer to pregnant women, not enough data are available to allow for routine use of these agents in pregnant or breast-feeding women. Therefore, quinolones should not be administered to pregnant or breast-feeding women unless the patient has an infection resistant to all other antimicrobial agents.

CONCLUSION

The use of quinolones for treating patients with surgical and gynecologic diseases will continue. The availability of a broad-spectrum (aerobic and anaerobic) quinolone will increase the opportunities to use a single agent to treat patients with these types of diseases. The convenience of an oral form will be an advantage to patient and surgeon. The final role that this antimicrobial class of drugs assumes in surgery, obstetrics, and gynecology must await further study, which will define not only their efficacy but also their cost-effectiveness.

REFERENCES

1. Von Rosensteil, N., and Adam, D. (1994). Quinolone antibacterials: An update of their pharmacology and therapeutic use. *Drugs* **47**, 872–901.
2. Applebaum, P. C. (1995). Quinolone activity against anaerobes: Microbiological aspects. *Drugs* **49** (Suppl. 2), 76–80.
3. Woodstock, J. M., Andrews, J. M., *et al.* (1997). In vitro activity of BAY 12-8039, a new fluoroquinolone. *Antimicrob. Agents Chemother.* **41**(1), 101–106.
4. Ehrenkranz, N. J., and Meakins, J. L. (1986). Surgical infections. In "Hospital Infections," 3rd ed. (J. V. Bennett and P. S. Brachman, eds.), pp. 685–710. Little, Brown, Boston.
5. Wittmann, D. H., and Schein, M. (1996). Let us shorten antibiotic prophylaxis and therapy in surgery. *Am. J. Surg.* **172** (Suppl. 6A), 26S–32S.
6. Phillips, I., King, A., *et al.* (1988). In vitro properties of the quinolones. In "The Quinolones" (V. T. Andriole, ed.), pp. 83–117. Academic Press, San Diego.

7. Bergan, T. (1988). Pharmacokinetics of fluorinated quinolones. In "The Quinolones" (V. T. Andriole, ed.), pp. 119–154. Academic Press, San Diego.

8. Percival, A. (1996). The appropriate use of quinolones. *Drugs* **52** (Suppl. 2), 34–36.

9. Auger, P., Leclerc, Y., *et al.* (1990). Double blind comparison of pefloxacin and cefazolin as prophylaxis in elective cardiovascular surgery. *J. Antimicrob. Chemother.* **26** (Suppl. B), 75–82.

10. Dellamonica, P., and Bernard, E. (1993). Fluoroquinolones and surgical prophylaxis. *Drugs* **45** (Suppl. 3), 102–133.

11. Girard, A. E., Girard, D., *et al.* (1995). In vivo efficacy of trovafloxacin (cp-99,219), a new quinolone with extended activities against Gram-positive pathogens, streptococcus pneumoniae, and bacteroides fragilis. *Antimocrob. Agents Chemother.* **39**(10), 2210–2216.

12. Data on File, Pfizer Pharmaceuticals.

13. Kernodle, D. S., and Kaiser, A. B. (1994). Comparative prophylactic efficacies of ciprofloxacin, ofloxacin, cefazolin, and vancomycin in experimental model of staphylococcal wound infection. *Antimicrob. Agents Chemother.* **38**(6), 1325–1330.

14. Gold, H. S., and Moellering, R. C. (1996). Antimicrobial drug resistance. *Drug Ther.* **335**(19), 1445–1453.

15. Goldmann, D. A., Weinstein, R. A., *et al.* (1996). Strategies to prevent and control the emergence and spread of antimicrobial-resistant microorganisms in hospitals. *JAMA* **275**(3), 234–240.

16. Galandiuk, S., Polk, H. C., *et al.* (1989). Re-emphasis of priorities in surgical antibiotic prophylaxis. *Surg. Gynecol. Obstet.* **169**, 219–222.

17. Hildebrand III, J. R., Merrill, D. L., *et al.* (1986). Defining appropriate timing of surgical antibiotic prophylaxis. *Infect. Surg.*, pp. 444–457.

18. Amland, P. F., Andenaes, K., *et al.* (1995). A prospective, double-blind, placebo-controlled trial of a single dose of azithromycin on postoperative wound infections in plastic surgery. *Plastic Reconstruc. Surg.* **96**(6), 1378–1383.

19. Vergnaud, M., Morel, C., *et al.* (1989). Pefloxacin plus fosfomycin prophylaxis in cardiac surgery in β-lactam allergic patients. *Pathol. Biol. (Paris)* **37**, 491–495.

20. Karran, S. J., Karran, S. E., *et al.* (1991). Oral prophylaxis: A new approach in elective biliary surgery. *Abstr. 17th Int. Cong. Chemother.*, Berlin. Abstr. #1153.

21. Teng, R., Liston, T. E., *et al.* (1996). Multiple-dose pharmacokinetics and safety of trovafloxacin in healthy volunteers. *J. Antimicrob. Chemother.* **37**(5), 955–963.

22. Andriole, V. T. (1992). Quinolones. In "Infectious Diseases" (S. L. Gorbach, J. G. Bartlett, and N. R. Blacklow, eds.), pp. 244–253. Saunders, Philadelphia.

23. Andriole, V. T. (1988). Clinical overview of the newer 4-quinolone antibacterial agents. In "The Quinolones" (V. T. Andriole, ed.), pp. 155–200. Academic Press, San Diego.

24. Lee, B. Y., McCann, W. J., *et al.* (1989). Optimum management of perforating ulcers of the foot. *Contemp. Surg.* **34**, 25–34.

25. Sales, C. M., and Vieth, F. J. (1995). Management of diabetic foot infection. *Contemp. Surg.* **46**(1), 15–20.

26. Wheat, L. J., Allen, S. D., *et al.* (1986). Diabetic foot infections: Bacteriologic analysis. *Arch. Intern. Med.* **146**, 1935–1940.

27. Scher, K. S., and Steele, F. J. (1988). The septic foot in patients with diabetes. *Surgery* **104**(4), 661–666.

28. Shults, D. W., Hunter, G. C., *et al.* (1989). Value of radiographs and bone scans in determining the need for therapy in diabetic patients with foot ulcers. *Am. J. Surg.* **158**, 525–530.

29. Peterson, L. R., Lissack, L. M., *et al.* (1989). Therapy of lower extremity infections with ciprofloxacin in patients with diabetes mellitus, peripheral vascular disease, or both. *Am. J. Med.* **86**, 801–807.

30. Gentry, L. O., and Rodriguez, G. G. (1990). Oral ciprofloxacin compared with parenteral antibiotics in the treatment of osteomyelitis. *Antimicrob. Agents Chemother.* **34**(1), 40–43.

31. Nichols, R. L., Smith, J. W., *et al.* (1997). Multicenter, randomized study comparing levofloxacin and ciprofloxacin for uncomplicated skin and skin structure infections. *South. Med. J.* **90**(12), 1193–200.

32. Andriole, V. T. (1992). Quinolones. In "Infectious Disease" (S. L. Gorbach, J. G. Bartlett, and N. R. Blacklow, eds.), pp. 244–250. Saunders, Philadelphia.

33. Eckman, M. H., Greenfield, S., *et al.* (1995). Foot infections in diabetic patients: Decision and cost-effectiveness analysis. *JAMA* **273**(9), 712–720.

34. Lipsky, B. A., *et al.* (1999). Safety profile of sparfloxacin, a new fluoroquinolone antibiotic. *Clin. Therap.* **21**(1), 148–159.

35. Bohnen, J. M. A., Solomkin, J. S., *et al.* (1992). Guidelines for clinical care: Anti-infective agents for intra-abdominal infection. *Arch. Surg.* **172**, 83–89.

36. Mosdell, D. M., Morris, D. M., *et al.* (1991). Antibiotic treatment for surgical peritonitis. *Ann. Surg.* **214**(5), 543–549.

37. Christou, N. V., Turgeon, P., *et al.* (1996). Management of intra-abdominal infections: The case for intraoperative cultures and comprehensive broad-spectrum antibiotic coverage. *Arch. Surg.* **131**, 1193–1201.

38. Nichols, R. L. (1996). Surgical infections: Prevention and treatment—1965 to 1995. *Am. J. Surg.* **172**, 68–74.

39. Solomkin, J. S., Reinhart, H. H., *et al.* (1996). Results of a randomized trial comparing sequential intravenous/oral treatment with ciprofloxacin plus metronidazole to imipenem/cilastatin for intra-abdominal infections. *Ann. Surg.* **223**(3), 303–315.

40. Onderdonk, A. B. (1996). Efficacy of trovafloxacin (CP-99,219), a new fluoroquinolone, in an animal model of intra-abdominal sepsis. *Infect. Dis. Clin. Pract.* **5**(3), S117–S119.

41. Nord, C. E. (1998). Use of newer quinolones for the treatment of intraabdominal infections: Focus on clinafloxacin, *Infection* **27**(1), 166–172.

42. Faro, S., Phillips, L. E., and Martens, M. G. (1988). Perspectives on the bacteriology of postoperative obstetric–gynecologic infections. *Am. J. Obstet. Gynecol.* **158**, 694–700.

43. Amsel, R., Totten, C., Spiegel, K. C. S., *et al.* (1983). Nonspecific vaginitis: Diagnostic criteria and microbial and epidemiological association. *Am. J. Med.* **74**, 14–22.

44. Hill, G. B. (1993). The microbiology of bacterial vaginosis. *Am. J. Obstet. Gynecol.* **169**, 450–454.

45. Faro, S., Martens, M. G., Hammill, H. A., *et al.* (1990). Antibiotic prophylaxis: Is there a difference? *Am. J. Obstet. Gynecol.* **162**, 900–907.

46. Benigno, B. B., Evrard, J., Faro, S., *et al.* (1986). A comparison of piperacillin, cephalothin, and cefoxitin in the prevention of postoperative infections in patients undergoing vaginal hysterectomy. *Surg. Gynecol. Obstet.* **163**, 421–427.

47. Brouwer, W. K., Hoogkamp-Korstanje, J. A., and Kuiper, K. M. (1990). Antibiotic prophylaxis in vaginal hysterectomy: Three doses of cefuroxime plus metronidazole versus one dose of ciprofloxacin. *Pharmaceut. Weekbl., Scient. Ed.* **12**, 292–294.

47a. Roy, S., Hemsell, D., Gordon, S., *et al.*, and the Trovafloxacin Surgical Group (1998). Oral trovafloxacin compared with intravenous cefoxitin in the prevention of bacterial infection after elective vaginal or abdominal hysterectomy for nonmalignant disease. *Am. J. Surg.* **176**, 62S–66S.

48. Maccato, M. L., Faro, S., Martens, M. G., and Hammill, H. A. (1991). Ciprofloxacin versus gentamicin/clindamycin for the treatment of postpartum endometritis. *J. Reprod. Med.* **36**, 857–861.

49. Davis, R., and Bryson, H. M. (1994). Levofloxacin: A review of its antibacterial activity, pharmacokinetics, and therapeutic efficacy. *Drugs* **47**, 677–700.

50. Weber, J. T., and Johnson, R. E. (1995). New treatments for *Chlamydia trachomatis* genital infection. *Clin. Infect. Dis.* **20** (Suppl. 1), S66–S71.

51. Faro, S. (1993). Quinolones for the treatment of *Neisseria gonorrhoeae* and *Chlamydia trachomatis. Infect. Dis. Obstet. Gynecol.* **1**, 108–113.

52. Faro, S., Martens, M. G., Maccato, M. L., *et al.* (1991). Effectiveness of ofloxacin in the treatment of *Chlamydia trachomatis* and *Neisseria gonorrhoeae* cervical infection. *Am. J. Obstet. Gynecol.* **164**, 1383–1393.

53. Fedele, L., Caravelli, E., Acaia, B., *et al.* (1990). Enoxacin in the treatment of *Chlamydia trachomatis* genitourinary infection. *Acta. Eur. Fertil.* **21**, 147–149.

54. Jeskanen, L., Karppinen, L., Ingervo, L., Reitamo, S., Happonen, H. P., and Lassus, A. (1989). Ciprofloxacin versus doxycycline in the treatment of uncomplicated urogenital *Chlamydia trachomatis* infection: A double-blind comparative study. *Scand. J. Infect. Dis.* (Suppl.) **60**, 62–65.

55. Schneider, A., Weissenbacher, E. R., Gutschow, K., and Wachter, I. (1987). Ofloxacin versus doxycycline in gynecological infections. *Acta. Eur. Fertil.* **18**, 121–122.

56. MMWR (1993). Sexually transmitted diseases treatment guidelines. *MMWR* **42**, 50–55.

57. Perez, E. J., Aznar, J., Garcia-Iglesias, M. C., and Pascual, A. (1996). Comparative in-vitro activity of sparfloxacin against genital pathogens. *J. Antimicrob. Chemother.* **37** (Suppl. A), 19–25.

58. Apuzzio, J. J., Stankewicz, R., Ganesh, V., *et al.* (1989). Comparison of parenteral ciprofloxacin with clindamycin–gentamicin in the treatment of pelvic infection. *Am. J. Med.* **87**, 148S–151S.

59. Crombleholme, W. R., Schachter, J., Ohm-Smith, M., *et al.* (1989). Efficacy of single agent therapy for the treatment of acute pelvic inflammatory disease with ciprofloxacin. *Am. J. Med.* **87**, 142S–147S.

60. Heinonen, P. K., Teisala, K., Miettinen, A., *et al.* (1989). A comparison of ciprofloxacin with doxycycline plus metronidazole in the treatment of acute pelvic inflammatory disease. *Scand. J. Infect. Dis.* (Suppl.) **60**, 66–73.

61. Hagele, D., and Chysky, V. (1988). Is pelvic inflammatory disease an indication for treatment with ciprofloxacin? *Infection* **16** (Suppl 1), S48–S50.

62. Pearlman, M., Faro, S., Riddle, G. D., and Tortolero, G. (1990). In vitro synergy of clindamycin and aminoglycosides against *Chlamydia trachomatis. Antimicrob. Agents Chemother.* **34**, 1399–1402.

63. Covino, J. M., Black, J. R., Cummings, M., Zwickl, B., and McCormick, W. M. (1993). Comparative evaluation of ofloxacin and metronidazole in the treatment of bacterial vaginosis. *Sex. Transm. Dis.* **20**, 262–264.

64. Nayagam, A. T., Smith, M. D., Ridgway, G. L., *et al.* (1992). Comparison of ofloxacin and metronidazole for the treatment of bacterial vaginosis. *Int. J. STD AIDS* **3**, 204–207.

65. Martens, M. G., Gordon, S., Yarborough, D. R., *et al.* (1993). Multicenter randomized trial of ofloxacin versus cefoxitin and doxycycline in outpatient treatment of pelvic inflammatory disease. *South. Med. J.* **86**, 604–610.

66. Wendel Jr., G. D., Cox, S. M., Bawdon, R. E., *et al.* (1991). A randomized trial of ofloxacin versus cefoxitin and doxycycline in the outpatient treatment of acute salpingitis. *Am. J. Obstet. Gynecol.* **164**, 1390–1396.

67. Soper, D. E., Brockwell, N. J., and Dalton, H. P. (1992). Microbial etiology of urban emergency department acute salpingitis: Treatment with ofloxacin. *Am. J. Obstet. Gynecol.* **167**, 653–660.

68. Witte, E. H., Peters, A. A., Smit, I. B., *et al.* (1993). A comparison of pefloxacin/metronidazole and doxycycline/metronidazole in the treatment of laparoscopically confirmed acute pelvic inflammatory disease. *Eur. J. Obstet. Gynecol. Reprod. Biol.* **50**, 153–158.

69. Berkovitch, M., Pastuszak, A., Gazarian, M., Lewis, M., and Koren, G. (1994). Safety of the new quinolones in pregnancy. *Obstet. Gynecol.* **84**, 535–538.

70. Aramyona, J. J., Garcia, M. A., Fraile, L. J., Abadia, A. R., and Bregante, M. A. (1994). Placental transfer of enrofloxacin and ciprofloxacin in rabbits. *Am. J. Vet. Res.* **55**, 1313–1318.

71. Wilton, L. V., Pearse, G. L., and Mann, R. D. (1996). A comparison of ciprofloxacin, norflox-acin, ofloxacin, azithromycin, and cefixime examined by observational cohort studies. *Br. J. Pharmacol.* **41**, 277–284.

72. Morinaga, T., Fujii, S., Kikumori, M., *et al.* (1996). Reproductive and developmental toxicity studies of prulifloxacin (NM 441), 3: A teratogenicity study in rabbits by oral administration. *J. Toxicol. Sci.* **21**, 207–217.

73. Morinaga, T., Fujii, S., Furukawa, S., *et al.* (1996). Reproductive and developmental toxicity studies of prulifloxacin (NM44), 2: A teratogenicity study in rats by oral administration. *J. Toxicol. Sci.* **21**, 187–208.

CHAPTER 10

Use of the Quinolones for Treatment and Prophylaxis of Bacterial Gastrointestinal Infections

DAVIDSON H. HAMER* and SHERWOOD L. GORBACH[†]

*Division of Geographic Medicine and Infectious Diseases, Department of Medicine, New England Medical Center, Boston, Massachusetts 02111, and [†]Department of Community Health, Tufts University School of Medicine, Boston, Massachusetts 02111

The Quinolones, Third Edition

INTRODUCTION

Gastrointestinal infections cause significant morbidity and mortality in both industrialized and less-developed countries. Foodborne diseases are responsible for approximately 76 million illnesses and 5000 deaths in the United States annually [1]. Medical costs and loss of productivity due to infectious diarrhea amount to $23 billion a year [2]. Given the extensive morbidity and cost of diarrheal disease, prompt, appropriate therapy is vital for the prevention of complications and death due to this common problem. As most episodes of infectious diarrhea are self-limited, the mainstays of treatment are relief of symptoms and rehydration. However, prompt antimicrobial therapy in selected cases may lead to more rapid resolution of symptoms and fewer complications.

If the decision is made to institute antibiotic therapy, identification and sensitivity testing of the enteropathogen should be performed in order to select the most appropriate antimicrobial agent. Fluoroquinolones provide many advantages over other antimicrobial agents used to treat acute gastrointestinal infections, including a broad spectrum of activity against nearly all enteric bacterial pathogens, high fecal concentrations of drug after oral administration, minimal perturbations of the normal intestinal microflora, good patient tolerance, and low levels of resistance. Many of the quinolones have now been used extensively for the treatment and prophylaxis of acute diarrhea.

PHARMACOLOGY

The quinolones are well absorbed after oral administration and are widely distributed in the body. Uptake of the quinolones by macrophages provides an advantage for the treatment of intracellular pathogens such as *Salmonella* spp. Absorption is not diminished by the presence of diarrhea [3]. After oral administration, high intraluminal concentrations are achieved in the bowel lumen and in biliary fluid. In fact, fecal drug concentrations of ciprofloxacin are approximately 10- to 100-fold greater than those attained in serum [3]. Ciprofloxacin levels of 100 to 500 μg/g feces are present during the administration of this drug at a dose of 500 mg b.i.d. during a 5-day period. Therapeutic concentrations of the quinolones are detectable in the feces for up to 5 days after a course of therapy [4,5].

MICROBIOLOGY

The quinolones are highly active *in vitro* against common bacterial enteropathogens, including toxigenic strains of *Escherichia coli*, *Campylobacter jejuni*, *Salmonella* spp., *Shigella* spp., *Vibrio cholerae*, *V. parahaemolyticus*, *Yersinia enterocolitica*, *Aeromonas* spp., and *Plesiomonas shigelloides* [6–8]. The 90%

minimal inhibitory concentrations of all enteropathogens to most quinolones, including newer compounds such as gatifloxacin and moxifloxacin, range from 0.02 to 1.0 µg/ml and are generally less than or equal to 0.025 µg/ml [6–8]. Thus, most bacterial diarrheal pathogens are exquisitely sensitive to the quinolones (see the section on "Antimicrobial Resistance to Quinolones").

EFFECTS ON HUMAN INTESTINAL MICROFLORA

The quinolones exert a strong suppressive effect on aerobic Gram-negative bacteria in the gut, whereas aerobic Gram-positive bacteria are only moderately affected [9]. Ciprofloxacin, ofloxacin, and temafloxacin have been demonstrated to have a stronger suppressive effect on aerobic Gram-positive bacteria in the intestine than other quinolones, such as norfloxacin, lomefloxacin, and pefloxacin. Most quinolones cause little or no suppression of the anaerobic microflora of the gut; however, the new fluoroquinolone gatifloxacin has relatively potent *in-vitro* activity against a number of different Gram-positive and Gram-negative anaerobes [8], and thus is likely to have more potent suppressive effects on the intestinal microflora. When tested in healthy volunteers, oral gatifloxacin led to significant decreases in fecal concentrations of clostridia and fusobacteria, but there was little effect on other anaerobes (10). Within a week after the cessation of quinolone treatment, the intestinal flora return to a state of colonization similar to that of the pretherapy period. Overgrowth by yeasts and the emergence of quinolone-resistant bacteria have not been observed during short-term courses of oral quinolones.

CLINICAL STUDIES

During the last decade, the quinolones have been extensively evaluated for the treatment of acute community-acquired gastroenteritis, traveler's diarrhea, nontyphoidal salmonellosis, typhoid fever, cholera, and shigellosis. Relatively short courses of a quinolone have generally been found to be effective in shortening the duration of diarrhea and associated symptoms. The use of quinolones for prevention of traveler's diarrhea has also been shown to be highly effective. The following sections review many of the studies that have evaluated the efficacy of the quinolones for the treatment and prophylaxis of gastrointestinal infections.

EMPIRICAL THERAPY OF ACUTE DIARRHEA

Placebo-controlled randomized trials of quinolones for the treatment of acute diarrheal disease in adults have generally demonstrated a significant overall effect relative to placebo in terms of clinical cure rate, duration of diarrhea, and microbiologic evidence of eradication of the offending pathogen, when isolated, from the stool (Table I). Differences in study populations, definition of diarrhea, duration of therapy, definitions of cure, the timing of posttherapy microbiological evaluation, and the relative preponderance of different bacterial enteropathogens are reasons for the discrepancies among these studies. None of the studies have found a prolongation of fecal carriage of any bacterial enteropathogen as a result of treatment with a quinolone. One of the two studies that evaluated the efficacy of shorter courses of a quinolone for empiric therapy of acute diarrhea found that both a 3-day course and single-dose therapy with fleroxacin were highly effective [14]. Although Noguerado *et al.* [15] failed to find a significant clinical benefit of single-dose therapy with ofloxacin, this study included a high percentage of patients with *S. enteriditis*.

Although there have been few studies of acute community-acquired gastroenteritis that have compared a quinolone to an alternative antimicrobial agent, one study of adults with acute diarrhea that compared treatment with ciprofloxacin or trimethoprim–sulfamethoxazole (TMP–SMX) vs. placebo found that ciprofloxacin, but not TMP–SMX, shortened the duration of diarrhea and resulted in better microbiological response rates when bacterial pathogens were isolated [12,13]. The single study [15] in Table I that did not show a significant effect of a quinolone for empiric treatment of acute gastroenteritis had a predominance (88% of bacterial isolates) of *S. enteriditis*. Although single-dose ofloxacin did not reduce the intensity or duration of symptoms, the stool cultures of all patients treated became culture-negative for *S. enteriditis* by 48 hours, and there was no relapse after 2 weeks of follow-up. Nevertheless, the results from this and other more recent studies (reviewed below) raise concerns about the efficacy of quinolones for the treatment of nontyphoidal salmonellosis.

Given the clear benefits of quinolones for the treatment of acute community-acquired gastroenteritis as demonstrated by these studies, patients with severe community-acquired diarrhea—defined as diarrhea (more than four fluid stools per day) that had not abated within 3 days in an otherwise healthy person with at least one of the following symptoms: abdominal pain, fever, vomiting, myalgia, and headache—should receive an antimicrobial drug, preferably a quinolone. In this subset of patients with acute diarrhea, there is a high likelihood of isolating a bacterial pathogen (87% in the study by Dryden *et al.* [17]). In this group of patients, quinolone therapy will usually provide prompt relief with a low risk of adverse effects. In addition, because Wistrom *et al.* [13] found that patients who were treated within 48 hours of onset of diarrhea had a much better result from norfloxacin treatment than those treated later in their course, therapy of acute diarrhea with a quinolone should be started at the initial visit to the doctor.

TABLE I Placebo-Controlled Studies of the Efficacy of Quinolones for the Treatment of Acute Bacterial Diarrhea

Reference	Study size (treatment/ placebo)	Treatment drug, dose, and duration of therapy (days)	Clinical response (quinolone/ placebo)	Microbiological cure (quinolone/ placebo)
Pichler et al. [11]	38/38	Ciprofloxacin 500 mg b.i.d. ×5d	97%/66%[a] ($p < 0.001$)	95%/36% ($p < 0.001$)
Goodman et al. [12]	59/58/56 TMP–SMX	Ciprofloxacin 500 mg b.i.d. ×5d or TMP–SMX DS b.i.d. ×5d	95%/77%[b]/87% TMP–SMX ($p < 0.05$)[d]	82%/21%/48% TMP–SMX ($p < 0.001$)
Wiström et al. [13]	301/297	Norfloxacin 400 mg b.i.d. ×5d	63%/51%[b] ($p = 0.003$)	53%/39% ($p = 0.008$)
Butler et al. [14]	110 single dose; 112 3-day course/ 110 placebo	Fleroxacin 400 mg ×1 or qd ×3d	85% single dose; 82% 3-day group/62%[c] ($p < 0.001$)	94% single dose; 93% 3-day group/57% ($p < 0.001$)
Noguerado et al. [15]	57/60	Ofloxacin 400 mg ×1	2.5 ± 2.2/3.4 ± 2.5 days with diarrhea ($p = $ NS) at day 15 ($p = $ NS)	31%/2.9% at 48 hours ($p = 0.0018$); 62%/60%
Ellis-Pegler et al. [16]	40/44	Lomefloxacin 400 mg qd ×5d	85%/73%[b] ($p = 0.1$)	73%/34% ($p = 0.0008$)
Dryden et al. [17]	81/81	Ciprofloxacin 500 mg b.i.d. ×5d	96%/79%[b] ($p < 0.001$)	86%/34% ($p < 0.0001$)

[a]Cure defined as absence of fever and diarrhea within 72 hours.

[b]Cure defined as ≤1 loose stool per 24 hr.

[c]Cure defined as cessation of liquid stools within 2 days of starting treatment.

[d]p value for comparison between ciprofloxacin and placebo. p value for TMP–SMX vs. placebo was not significant.

TRAVELER'S DIARRHEA

The utility of antibiotics including the quinolones for the treatment of traveler's diarrhea has been well established by numerous placebo-controlled clinical trials [18–26]. Ciprofloxacin has been demonstrated to be as effective as TMP–SMX [19]. Three-day courses of ofloxacin, norfloxacin, and ciprofloxacin have all been found to be significantly more effective than placebo for reducing the duration of diarrhea and for microbiologic eradication of bacterial enteropathogens [20–22]. A number of studies [23–25] that have evaluated the efficacy of even shorter courses of quinolones, often as little as a single dose, for the treatment of traveler's diarrhea have shown impressive results. However, the development of ciprofloxacin resistance in travelers with *Campylobacter* enteritis has been associated with clinical relapse after treatment [25]. Quinolones have been well tolerated in all these studies, and their use has not led to prolonged excretion of enteropathogens.

A number of studies [25,27,28] have shown that the most effective relief from symptoms is provided by a combination of an antimicrobial drug and an antimotility drug. In a study [27] of travelers to Mexico, the combined use of loperamide and TMP–SMX curtailed diarrhea within 1 hour, compared to 30 hours with either drug alone and 59 hours with placebo. A study [28] of military personnel in Thailand found that a 3-day course of ciprofloxacin combined with loperamide was more effective than a single dose of ciprofloxacin given either alone or with loperamide. Unfortunately, because this study did not include a reference group treated for 3 days with ciprofloxacin alone, it is not possible to assess how effective the addition of loperamide was relative to the quinolone by itself. However, another study [22] from Egypt failed to show much benefit for a 3-day combination of ciprofloxacin with loperamide relative to ciprofloxacin alone. Although addition of loperamide to a quinolone has not been conclusively demonstrated to improve the efficacy of the antimicrobial in resolving the symptoms of traveler's diarrhea, there have been no adverse effects due to addition of this antimotility agent, even in patients with invasive diarrhea caused by *Shigella* spp.

The use of antibiotics for prevention of traveler's diarrhea is generally not advised because of the risk of side effects incurred during prolonged treatment and the potential for development of antimicrobial resistance. Nevertheless, a single daily dose of a quinolone has been shown to be highly effective for the prevention of diarrhea in travelers. For example, protection rates of 68–94% have been demonstrated with norfloxacin or ciprofloxacin [29–31]. In these studies, the quinolone has generally been well tolerated, with no life-threatening adverse reactions and little development of resistance.

NONTYPHOIDAL SALMONELLOSIS

Although numerous antibiotics have been used to treat nontyphoidal *Salmonella* gastrointestinal infections, most have failed to alter the rate of clinical recovery. In fact, antibiotic therapy often increases the incidence and duration of intestinal carriage of these organisms. Because many *Salmonella* infections are self-limited and the development of strains resistant to one or more antibiotics during treatment frequently occurs, antibiotics should not be employed in most cases of *Salmonella* gastroenteritis.

Despite this general rule, antibiotics should be used when certain disorders are complicated by *Salmonella* gastroenteritis. These include lymphoproliferative disorders; malignant disease; immunosuppressive conditions (AIDS and congenital or acquired forms, including transplantation); known or suspected abnormalities of the cardiovascular system, such as prosthetic heart valves, vascular grafts, aneurysms, and rheumatic or congenital valvular heart disease; the presence of foreign-bodies implanted in the skeletal system; patients with hemolytic anemias; and patients at the extreme ages of life. In addition, treatment should be used in patients with *Salmonella* gastroenteritis when they exhibit signs of severe sepsis—that is, high fever, rigors, hypotension, decreased renal function, and systemic toxicity.

The quinolones, particularly ciprofloxacin and norfloxacin, appeared promising for the treatment of nontyphoidal salmonellosis in early studies [11,32]. However, some more recent studies [13,33–35] have shown that quinolone therapy can cause a high relapse rate and more prolonged fecal excretion of Salmonellae when compared to placebo-treated controls. Many of these studies [33,35] find initial clearance of *Salmonella* spp. during treatment with quinolones and for up to 1 week after treatment, but if longer follow-up is performed, the same species can often be isolated at 2 to 12 weeks after therapy. In addition to potentially leading to an unacceptably high relapse rate and prolonged fecal excretion, treatment with quinolones does not consistently result in a good clinical response in patients with nontyphoidal salmonellosis when compared to placebo controls [14,15,34]. Prolonged fecal excretion of Salmonellae and clinical failure have not been consistently observed in all studies. For example, Dryden *et al.* [17] did show a reduction in symptoms compared to placebo when the case was classified as "severe" (defined as more than four fluid stools per day lasting ≥3 days, with at least one other symptom of infection), and they did not find a prolonged excretion of any pathogen, including nontyphoidal Salmonellae. Consequently, the quinolones should be reserved for more severe cases of salmonellosis or for patients who are at higher risk for complications.

Despite their potential to cause prolonged fecal excretion during the treatment of acute salmonellosis, the quinolones are effective in treating chronic *Salmonella* carriers. Courses of ciprofloxacin or ofloxacin as short as 5–7 days [36,37] to as long as 3–4 weeks have been found to eradicate *Salmonella* carriage [38,39]. However, these studies involved small numbers of patients and variable periods of follow-up. Consequently, before the quinolones can be touted as useful for the treatment of chronic *Salmonella* carriage, larger controlled studies with long-term follow-up are needed. In addition, the minimum duration of treatment and the dosage needed to eradicate *Salmonella* spp. from chronic carriers need to be established.

TYPHOID FEVER

Although chloramphenicol and TMP–SMX have been the treatments of choice for many years, the advent of plasmid-mediated multidrug resistance and newer, potentially more effective antimicrobial agents, such as the quinolones and the third-generation cephalosporins, have led to a reevaluation of the role of these two antibiotics in the treatment of typhoid fever. A number of open-label and randomized comparative studies have demonstrated the efficacy of the quinolones in treating typhoid fever.

A 10- to 14-day course of a quinolone has proved highly effective for the treatment of enteric fever, with cure rates consistently close to 100% [40–57] (Table II). The only exception has been norfloxacin; two studies [40,41] of this agent used for a 14-day period found cure rates of 83 and 90%, respectively. Defervescence generally occurs within 3 to 5 days from the time of initiation of therapy. When treatment of enteric fever (defined as a febrile illness associated with bacteremia with either *S. typhi* or *S. paratyphi*) with a quinolone was compared to chloramphenicol, TMP–SMX, or azithromycin, there was no significant difference in clinical or microbiological efficacy between the two study drugs [31,44,48,51,54,57]. On the other hand, a recent trial [56] that compared a 5-day course of ofloxacin to a 7-day course of cefixime found that the median fever clearance time was significantly longer and there was a higher rate of treatment failure in children treated with cefixime. Three other randomized nonblinded studies [48,51,54] that evaluated duration of fever during therapy found that there was more rapid defervescence in patients treated with the quinolone than in those from the comparator groups. Both ciprofloxacin and ofloxacin have been found to be highly effective therapy for infections due to multidrug-resistant *S. typhi* and *paratyphi* [45–49,56,57]. Long-term fecal carriage of *S. typhi* or relapse of typhoid fever is a very rare event in patients treated with quinolones.

The optimal duration of therapy for typhoid fever with the quinolones has not been fully clarified. Alam *et al.* [46] found that a 10-day course of ciprofloxacin was as effective as a 14-day course, and Uwaydah *et al.* [45] found that a 7- to

TABLE II Treatment of Enteric Fever (*S. typhi* or *S. paratyphi*) with Quinolones

Reference	Type of study	Drug and dosage	Duration of therapy (days)	Cure rate (no. of patients cured/no. treated (%)
Velmonte and Montalban [40]	Open	Norfloxacin 400 mg p.o. b.i.d.	14	10/12 (83.3)
Nalin et al. [41]	Open-label, comparative	Norfloxacin 400 mg p.o. q8h	14	81/90 (90)
Ramirez et al. [42]	Open	Ciprofloxacin 500 mg p.o. b.i.d.	14	36/37 (97.3)
Stanley et al. [43]	Open	Ciprofloxacin 250 mg i.v. q12h or 500 mg p.o. b.i.d.	10–14	26/26 (100)
Limson and Littaua [44]	Open-label, comparative	Ciprofloxacin 500 mg p.o. b.i.d.	10	20/20 (100)
Uwaydah et al. [45]	Open	Ciprofloxacin 500 or 750 mg p.o. b.i.d.	7–13	62/62 (100)
Alam et al. [46]	Open	Ciprofloxacin 500 mg p.o. b.i.d.	10	35/35 (100)
			14	34/34 (100)
Wang et al. [47]	Open	Ofloxacin 10–14		64/64 (100)
Akhtar et al. [48]	Open-label, comparative	Ofloxacin 200 mg p.o. b.i.d.	14	35/35 (100)
Tanphaichitra and Srimuang [49]	Open	Ofloxacin 400 mg p.o. b.i.d.	7–10	35/35 (100)
Zavala-Trujillo et al. [50]	Open	Fleroxacin 400 mg p.o. qd	7	10/10 (100)
			14	10/10 (100)
Arnold et al. [51]	Open-label, comparative	Fleroxacin 400 mg p.o. qd	7	20/24 (83.3)
			14	33/33 (100)
Cristiano et al. [52]	Open	Pefloxacin 400 mg i.v. q8h then p.o. tid	15	30/30 (100)
Ait-Khaled et al. [53]	Open	Pefloxacin 400 mg i.v. or p.o. q12h	7	23/25 (92)
Hajji et al. [54]	Open-label, comparative	Pefloxacin 400 mg p.o. b.i.d.	14	21/21 (100)
Thomsen et al. [55]	Retrospective	Ciprofloxacin 15 mg/kg/d i.v. or 24 mg/kg/d p.o.	7–14	21/21 (100)
Phuong et al. [56]	Open-label, comparative	Ofloxacin 10 mg/kg/d p.o. in 2 divided doses	5	37/38 (97)
Girgis et al. [57]	Open-label, comparative	Ciprofloxacin 500 mg p.o. b.i.d.	7	28/28 (100)

10-day course of ciprofloxacin was adequate therapy for 92% of their cohort. The patients in the latter study who required more than a 10-day course of ciprofloxacin had fever of prolonged duration prior to hospitalization. More recent investigations [49–51,53,56,58,59] have evaluated the effectiveness of shorter courses of therapy with the quinolones. In one study [58], a 6-day course of ciprofloxacin at a dose of 500 mg twice daily led to a cure in 9 of 11 (82%) patients, whereas there was a lower efficacy rate of 67% (8 of 12) in patients treated for only 3 days. A larger study from Algeria [59] found that a 5-day course of ofloxacin at a dose of 200 mg twice a day resulted in a cure rate of 99% (105 of 106 patients). Thus, it appears that courses as short as 5 or 6 days are effective, but shorter courses may lead to an unacceptable failure rate. The duration of fever prior to treatment, the severity of infection at the time of initial presentation, and time to defervescence are factors that must be taken into consideration when determining the duration of quinolone therapy in a patient with enteric fever.

Approximately 1 to 5% of patients with typhoid fever become chronic carriers of *S. typhi*. The quinolone antibiotics, such as ciprofloxacin and norfloxacin, have become the treatment of choice in eradicating the carrier state. In one study [60], a 4-week course of norfloxacin, 400 mg twice per day, resulted in elimination of the typhoid carrier state in 78% (18 of 23) of patients. Ciprofloxacin, administered at a dose of 750 mg twice per day, resulted in elimination of *S. typhi* in 83.3% (10 of 12) of carriers [61]. There was a greater overall incidence of adverse events in the latter study, perhaps as a consequence of the high dose of ciprofloxacin that was used. Reid and Smith [62] found that ciprofloxacin, given at a dose of 500 mg twice per day for 21 to 28 days, eliminated the carrier state in 92% (11 of 12) of patients. Because the lower dose of ciprofloxacin appears to have a similar efficacy, this is recommended pending further research. Reappearance of the carrier state following such treatment is generally associated with gallbladder disease. In persons with gallstones or chronic cholecystitis, cholecystectomy eliminates the carrier state in 85%; however, this procedure is recommended only for those whose profession is not compatible with the typhoid carrier state, such as food handlers and health care providers.

SHIGELLOSIS

Because some cases of invasive diarrhea are mild and self-limited, not all patients require treatment with antibiotics. The major determinant in the decision to employ antibiotics for shigellosis is severity of disease. In practice, moderate and severe cases of dysentery should receive antibiotic therapy. Antibiotics for shigellosis must be absorbed from the bowel in order to reach the population of organisms within the intestinal wall and the lamina propria, and the only effective delivery system is the bloodstream. Treatment options include ampicillin, TMP–

SMX, oral or parenteral third-generation cephalosporins, and fluoroquinolones. The choice of antibiotic is dependent on the *in-vitro* sensitivity pattern of the *Shigella* isolate.

The quinolone antibiotics have been used successfully for the treatment of patients with highly resistant organisms, particularly those acquired in developing countries. A clinical trial of ciprofloxacin vs. ampicillin was conducted in Bangladesh in adult males with shigellosis [63]. Resistance to ampicillin was seen in 60% of isolates, and, not surprisingly, ampicillin treatment failed in two-thirds of these persons. All strains were sensitive to ciprofloxacin, and this antibiotic produced better clinical results (95% clinical cure rate after a 5-day course) than ampicillin even in treating patients with ampicillin-sensitive strains. Two studies [64,65] that compared a 5-day course of a quinolone with nalidixic acid found that the two agents were similar in terms of efficacy, with clinical cures ranging from 72 to 82% at day 5. In both studies, there was more rapid elimination of *Shigella* spp. in patients treated with quinolones than in those receiving nalidixic acid. A study [66] of adult men with shigellosis that compared a 5-day course of ciprofloxacin with azithromycin found that 89% of patients treated with the quinolone were clinically cured at day 5 and that 100% of these patients had microbiological cures. There was no significant difference between the two treatment groups in terms of either clinical or microbiological response. A more recent comparative study of a 3-day course of ciprofloxacin versus single-dose azithromycin also found that both regimens led to complete resolution of symptoms within 1 to 4 days from the time of initiation of therapy [67].

A number of studies have evaluated shorter courses of a quinolone for the treatment of shigellosis. Bennish *et al.* [68] found that single-dose therapy with 1.0 g of ciprofloxacin was as effective as two doses (1.0 g/dose) or a 5-day standard regimen (500 mg b.i.d.) in patients with *Shigella* spp. isolates other than *S. dysenteriae* type 1. However, patients infected with *S. dysenteriae* type 1 responded better to a 5-day course of ciprofloxacin than to single-dose therapy. There was no significant difference between patients treated with a 2-dose regimen when compared to the 10-dose group. Another study [69] that compared a 3-day course of TMP–SMX with either a single dose of 800 mg of norfloxacin or a 3-day course of norfloxacin at a dose of 400 mg twice daily found no difference between the two groups receiving the quinolone, with cure rates at day 5 of 97 and 98% in these patients. There was a trend toward a better clinical outcome in patients treated with norfloxacin than in those receiving TMP–SMX ($p = 0.08$). Single-dose therapy with norfloxacin was also found to be as effective as a 5-day course of TMP–SMX in a Peruvian study of adults with shigellosis [70]. All these studies have been limited to adult patients with dysentery. There have been no serious adverse events in any of these studies, and no development of resistant strains of *Shigella* has been encountered.

The concern about cartilage damage in young children has resulted in few studies of the quinolones for the treatment of shigellosis in pediatric populations. As there is now increasing evidence of the skeletal safety of quinolones in children [71], these drugs are being increasingly studied in pediatric populations. During an outbreak of multiresistant *S. dysenteriae* type 1 in Burundi, infected children were treated with a single dose of pefloxacin [72]. By day 5, 91% of treated children were completely symptom free, and the remainder were substantially improved. None of the children experienced any joint problems during the 4-week period of follow-up. Similarly, a double-blind trial [73] of ciprofloxacin suspension versus pivmecillinam for childhood shigellosis found that ciprofloxacin was clinically successful in 80% of children, and this treatment was not associated with development of arthropathy.

Although early animal and human volunteer studies indicated that the use of antimotility agents in the treatment of invasive diarrhea might lead to prolonged fever and pathogen carriage, a 1993 study [74] challenges this dictum. Treatment of dysenteric patients with a combination of the synthetic antidiarrheal agent, loperamide, and ciprofloxacin resulted in a significantly shortened duration of diarrhea and decreased number of stools when compared to ciprofloxacin alone. The use of loperamide did not lead to prolonged fever or excretion of pathogenic bacilli. Thus, it is evident from this and the studies described above that short a course of a quinolone alone, or in combination with an antimotility drug, is highly effective for the treatment of shigellosis.

CHOLERA AND OTHER VIBRIOS

While oral or parenteral hydration is central to the treatment of cholera, antimicrobial agents are useful as ancillary measures. The quinolones have been found to be highly effective for the treatment of patients with infections due to *V. cholerae*. A double-blind, randomized, placebo-controlled trial [75] of adults with cholera in India found that a 5-day course of norfloxacin was superior to TMP–SMX and placebo in reducing stool output, duration of diarrhea, fluid requirements, and *Vibrio* excretion. A comparative study [76] of 3-day courses of ciprofloxacin, erythromycin, nalidixic acid, pivmecillinam, and tetracycline found that ciprofloxacin with concomitant fluid therapy was the most effective treatment for adults infected with tetracycline-resistant strains of *V. cholerae*. Diarrhea resolved within 72 hours in 93% of patients treated with ciprofloxacin but in only 42% of those receiving tetracycline. As little as 250 mg of ciprofloxacin given daily for 3 days has been shown to be as effective as a standard 3-day course of tetracycline for the treatment of moderate to severe cholera [77].

As observed in studies of shigellosis and traveler's diarrhea, single-dose therapy with a quinolone appears to be highly effective for the treatment of cholera. A single 1-g dose of ciprofloxacin resulted in a successful clinical response in 94% of patients infected with *V. cholerae* O1, whereas only 73% who received single-dose therapy with doxycycline were considered clinical successes [78]. In this study, single-dose treatment with ciprofloxacin also resulted in excellent clinical and bacteriological responses in patients infected with *V. cholerae* O139. Treatment failed in 52% of doxycycline-treated patients who were infected with a tetracycline-resistant strain of *V. cholerae* O1. Resistance to the quinolones has not been observed in any studies that have used these agents for the treatment of cholera.

Although often explosive in onset, disease due to *V. parahaemolyticus* is generally rather short-lived. Patients are usually treated symptomatically. Nevertheless, treatment with a quinolone will lead to a more rapid resolution of diarrhea when compared to control patients receiving placebo [14].

Although clearly effective for the treatment of acute cholera, ciprofloxacin failed to prevent the acquisition of *V. cholerae* O1 infection or the development of diarrhea during a study [79] of prophylaxis of adult household contacts of patients with cholera in Peru. The prophylactic treatment was well tolerated and did not lead to development of resistant isolates. The lack of efficacy of ciprofloxacin may have been partially due to low rates of transmission of cholera during the period of study.

CAMPYLOBACTER

Clinical trials that have included patients with diarrhea caused by *Campylobacter* spp. have generally shown encouraging results with the quinolones [11–13,17]. However, one study [16] that included a large percentage of patients with community-acquired diarrhea due to *Campylobacter* found that lomefloxacin successfully eradicated the pathogen in most patients, but this treatment did not alter clinical outcome. Consequently, although most studies have demonstrated favorable clinical responses to the quinolones in patients with *Campylobacter* diarrhea, the role of these agents for the treatment of this enteropathogen remains unclear. Studies [12,17] of the empiric therapy of community-acquired acute diarrhea where treatment with a quinolone was started at the time of presentation generally showed a favorable clinical response in patients who were subsequently found to have an infection due to *Campylobacter*. Consequently, if treatment with a quinolone is started early in the course of diarrhea, there may be a better response. The development of resistance to the fluoroquinolones during treatment of *Campylobacter* infections has become an increasingly common problem in the United States, Western Europe, and Thailand [80–86].

ANTIMICROBIAL RESISTANCE TO QUINOLONES

A number of the studies [12,13,16,17,81] of quinolones for the acute empiric therapy of community-acquired diarrhea have noted the development of resistant isolates of *Campylobacter* spp., predominantly *C. jejuni*, during treatment. In all of these studies, at the time of the initiation of therapy, the initial isolates of *Campylobacter* were sensitive to the quinolone being investigated. *Campylobacter* spp. resistant to ciprofloxacin have been noted in 4.1% of isolates in England [82], 28.5% of isolates in Spain [83], and 50% of isolates from U.S. military personnel in Thailand [84]. A large study of human *Campylobacter* isolates in Minnesota found a rise in quinolone resistance from 1.3 to 10.2% between 1992 and 1998 [85]. Factors associated with resistance of *Campylobacter* spp. to the quinolones include foreign travel and local patterns of fluoroquinolone use, especially if these agents are used in animal husbandry [85–87].

Although relatively uncommon, resistance to ciprofloxacin has been observed during the treatment of patients with nontyphoidal salmonellosis [88]. The strain of *S. enterica* serotype *typhimurium* known as definitive phage type 104 (DT104) is usually multidrug resistant, but, until the late 1990s, this strain has remained susceptible to the quinolones. A community outbreak of salmonellosis in Denmark during 1998 that appeared to arise from a Danish swine herd was caused by a strain of DT104 that was nalidixic acid resistant and that showed decreased susceptibility to fluoroquinolones *in vitro* [89]. The epidemiological investigation of this outbreak suggested decreased clinical effectiveness of the quinolones in the treatment of these *Salmonella* infections.

Resistance to ciprofloxacin of *S. typhi* appears to be increasing, especially on the Indian subcontinent [90,91], and in Central Asia [92] and Vietnam [93]. While there were no isolates of *S. typhi* or *S. paratyphi* that had an MIC of 0.25 µg/ml or greater in 1991 in a study conducted in India [91], in 1998–99 60% of 50 isolates tested had MICs of 2 µg/ml or greater. In association with the rise in nalidixic acid resistance and decreased susceptibility to ciprofloxacin, clinicians in India and Vietnam have observed a longer time to defervescence and more patients requiring alternative treatments during the late 1990s [91,93].

Resistance of *Shigella* strains to the quinolones remains an uncommon phenomenon, with one study [94] finding quinolone resistance in less than 1% of strains. Strains of *Shigella* acquired during travel outside the United States were more likely to be resistant to the quinolones.

The development of resistance to the quinolones, especially in countries where these drugs are frequently used, will require close surveillance. It is entirely possible that in the foreseeable future these drugs will lose their effectiveness for treating the enteropathogens.

CONCLUSION

The quinolones have been extremely useful for the treatment of acute gastrointestinal infections because of their potent activity against most enteric bacterial pathogens, the high fecal drug concentrations attained after oral administration, good patient tolerance, and low levels of resistance. Placebo-controlled trials of quinolones for the treatment of acute diarrheal disease and traveler's diarrhea in adults have nearly all demonstrated significant effects relative to placebo in terms of clinical cure rate, duration of diarrhea, and microbiologic evidence of eradication of the offending pathogen. In addition, randomized trials that have compared the quinolones to accepted therapies have found that these agents are highly effective for the treatment of shigellosis and cholera.

Although even brief courses of treatment with the quinolones have been found to be effective for many types of diarrheal disease, their utility for the treatment of nontyphoidal salmonellosis remains unclear. Some studies have shown that the quinolones do not consistently result in a good clinical response in patients with nontyphoidal salmonellosis when compared to placebo controls, and that this treatment can result in a high relapse rate and prolonged fecal excretion of Salmonellae. Despite their potential to cause prolonged fecal excretion during the treatment of acute salmonellosis, the quinolones appear to be effective in treating chronic *Salmonella* carriers. The increasing reports of nalidixic acid-resistant strains of *Salmonella* with concomitant reduced susceptibility to the fluoroquinolones suggest that this class of drugs may become less effective in the future.

Courses as brief as 5 to 6 days of either ciprofloxacin or ofloxacin have been found to be highly effective therapy for enteric fever, including infections due to multidrug-resistant *S. typhi* and *paratyphi*. In addition, the quinolones have become the treatment of choice for eradication of *S. typhi* fecal carriage. However, the rising incidence of isolates of *S. typhi* and *S. paratyphi* with decreased susceptibility to the quinolones suggests that the utility of these agents for treatment of enteric fever is declining in some regions of the world.

Although the quinolones have been demonstrated to be potent agents for the treatment of many different types of diarrheal disease, the development of quinolone-resistant strains of *C. jejuni* during treatment is of great concern. The increased use of fluoroquinolones in the poultry and other animal husbandry industries has resulted in a progressive rise in quinolone-resistant strains of both *Campylobacter* and *Salmonella* spp. The rising incidence of quinolone-resistant strains of *S. typhi* emphasizes the importance of the judicious use of the quinolones and effective surveillance for resistant strains.

REFERENCES

1. Mead, P. S., Slutsker, L., Dietz, V., McCaig, L. F., Bresee, J. S., Shapiro, C., Griffin, P. M., and Tauxe, R. V. (1999). Food-related illness and death in the United States. *Emerg. Infect. Dis.* **5**, 607–625.

2. Gorbach, S. L. (1988). Infectious diarrhea. *Infect. Dis. Clin. N. Amer.* **2**, 643–654.

3. Segreti, J., Goodman, L. J., Petrak, R. M., Kaplan, R. L., Parkhurst, G. W., and Trenholme, G. M. (1988). Serum and fecal levels of ciprofloxacin and trimethoprim–sulfamethoxazole in adults with diarrhea. *Rev. Infect. Dis.* **10** (Suppl. 1), S206–S207.

4. Leigh, D. A., Walsh, B., Harris, K., Hancock, P., and Travers, G. (1988). Pharmacokinetics of ofloxacin and the effect on the faecal flora of healthy volunteers. *J. Antimicrob. Chemother.* **22** (Suppl. C), 115–125.

5. Segreti, J., Goodman, L. J., Petrak, R. M., Kaplan, R. L., Levin, S., and Trenholme, G. M. (1985). Serum and stool levels of ciprofloxacin and trimethoprim-sulfamethoxazole in adults with diarrhea. *Abstr. 25th Intersci. Conf. Antimicrob. Agents Chemother.*, Minneapolis. Abstr. #154.

6. Carlson, J. R., Thornton, S. A., DuPont, H. L., West, A. H., and Mathewson, J. J. (1983). Comparative *in vitro* activities of ten antimicrobial agents against bacterial enteropathogens. *Antimicrob. Agents Chemother.* **24**, 509–513.

7. Goodman, L. J., Fliegelman, R. M., Trenholme, G. M., and Kaplan, R. L. (1984). Comparative in vitro activity of ciprofloxacin against *Campylobacter* spp. and other bacterial enteric pathogens. *Antimicrob. Agents Chemother.* **25**, 504–506.

8. Bauerfeind, A. (1997). Comparison of the antibacterial activities of the quinolones Bay 12-8039, gatifloxacin (AM 1155), trovafloxacin, clinafloxacin, levofloxacin and ciprofloxacin. *J. Antimicrob. Chemother.* **40**, 639–651.

9. Nord, C. E. (1995). Effect of the quinolones on the human intestinal microflora. *Drugs* **49** (Suppl. 2), 81–85.

10. Edlund, C., and Nord, C. E. (1999). Ecological effect of gatifloxacin on the normal human intestinal microflora. *J. Chemother.* **11**, 50–53.

11. Pichler, H. E. T., Diridl, G., Stickler, K., and Wolf, D. (1987). Clinical efficacy of ciprofloxacin compared with placebo in bacterial diarrhea. *Am. J. Med.* **82** (Suppl. 4A), 329–332.

12. Goodman, L. J., Trenholme, G. M., Kaplan, R. L., Segreti, J., Hines, D., Petrak, R., Nelson, J. A., Mayer, K. W., Landau, W., Parkhurst, G. W., and Levin, S. (1990). Empiric antimicrobial therapy of domestically acquired acute diarrhea in urban adults. *Arch. Intern. Med.* **150**, 541–546.

13. Wistrom, J., Jertborn, M., Ekwall, E., Norlin, K., Soderquist, B., Stromberg, A., Lundholm, R., Hogevik, H., Lillemor, L., Englund, E., Norrby, S. R., and the Swedish Study Group (1992). Empiric treatment of acute diarrheal disease with norfloxacin: A randomized, placebo-controlled study. *Ann. Intern. Med.* **117**, 202–208.

14. Butler, T., Lolekha, S., Rasidi, C., Kadio, A., Del Rosal, P. L., Iskandar, H., Rubinstein, E., and Pastore, G. (1993). Treatment of acute bacterial diarrhea: A multicenter international trial comparing placebo with fleroxacin given as a single dose or once daily for 3 days. *Am. J. Med.* **94** (Suppl. 3A), 187S–193S.

15. Noguerado, A., Garcia-Polo, I., Isasia, T., Jimenez, M. L., Bermudez, P., Pita, J., and Gabriel, R. (1995). Early single-dose therapy with ofloxacin for empirical treatment of acute gastroenteritis: A randomised, placebo-controlled double-blind clinical trial. *J. Antimicrob. Chemother.* **36**, 665–672.

16. Ellis-Pegler, R. B., Hyman, L. K., Ingram, R. J. H., and McCarthy, M. (1995). A placebo-controlled evaluation of lomefloxacin in the treatment of bacterial diarrhea in the community. *J. Antimicrob. Chemother.* **36**, 259–263.

17. Dryden, M. S., Gabb, R. J. E., and Wright, S. K. (1996). Empirical treatment of severe acute community-acquired gastroenteritis with ciprofloxacin. *Clin. Infect. Dis.* **22**, 1019–1025.

18. Dupont, H. L., and Ericsson, C. D. (1993). Prevention and treatment of traveler's diarrhea. *New Engl. J. Med.* **328**, 1821–1827.

19. Ericsson, C. D., Johnson, P. C., DuPont, H. L., Morgan, D. R., Bitsura, J. A., and de la Cabada, F. J. (1987). Ciprofloxacin or trimethoprim–sulfamethoxazole as initial therapy for traveler's diarrhea. *Ann. Intern. Med.* **106**, 216–220.

20. Dupont, H. L., Ericsson, C. D., Mathewson, J. J., and DuPont, M. W. (1992). Five versus three days of ofloxacin therapy for traveler's diarrhea: A placebo-controlled study. *Antimicrob. Agents Chemother.* **36**, 87–91.

21. Mattila, L., Peltola, H., Siitonen, A., Kyronseppa, H., Simula, I., and Kataja, M. (1993). Short-term treatment of traveler's diarrhea with norfloxacin: A double-blind, placebo-controlled study during two seasons. *Clin. Infect. Dis.* **17**, 779–782.

22. Taylor, D. N., Sanchez, J. L., Candler, W., Thornton, S., McQueen, C., and Echeverria, P. (1991). Treatment of traveler's diarrhea: Ciprofloxacin plus loperamide compared with ciprofloxacin alone. A placebo-controlled, randomized trial. *Ann. Intern. Med.* **114**, 731–734.

23. Steffen, R., Jori, J., DuPont, H. L., Mathewson, J. J., and Sturchler, D. (1993). Treatment of traveler's diarrhea with fleroxacin: A case study. *J. Antimicrob. Chemother.* **31**, 767–776.

24. Salam, I., Katelaris, P., Leigh-Smith, S., and Farthing, M. J. G. (1994). Randomised trial of single-dose ciprofloxacin for travellers' diarrhoea. *Lancet* **344**, 1537–1539.

25. Petruccelli, B. P., Murphy, G. S., Sanchez, J. L., Walz, S., DeFraites, R., Gelnett, J., Haberberger, R. L., Echeverria, P., and Taylor, D. N. (1992). Treatment of traveler's diarrhea with ciprofloxacin and loperamide. *J. Infect. Dis.* **165**, 557–560.

26. Glandt, M., Adachi, J. A., Mathewson, J. J., Jiang, Z. D., DiCesare, D., Ashley, D., Ericsson, C. D., and DuPont, H. L. (1999). Enteroaggregative *Escherichia coli* as a cause of traveler's diarrhea: Clinical response to ciprofloxacin. *Clin. Infect. Dis.* **29**, 335–338.

27. Ericsson, C. D., DuPont, H. L., Mathewson, J. J., West, M. S., Johnson, P. C., and Bitsura, J. M. (1990). Treatment of traveler's diarrhea with sulfamethoxazole and trimethoprim and loperamide. *JAMA* **263**, 257–261.

28. Johnson, P. C., Ericsson, C. D., DuPont, H. L., Morgan, D. R., Bitsura, J. A. M., and Wood, L. V. (1986). Comparison of loperamide with bismuth subsalicylate for the treatment of acute traveler's diarrhea. *JAMA* **255**, 757–760.

29. Johnson, P. C., Ericsson, C. D., Morgan, D. R., DuPont, H. L., and Cabada, F. J. (1986). Lack of emergence of resistant fecal flora during successful prophylaxis of traveler's diarrhea with norfloxacin. *Antimicrob. Agents Chemother.* **30**, 671–674.

30. Wistron, J., Norrby, S. R., Burman, L. G., Lundholm, R., Jellheden, B., and Englund, G. (1987). Norfloxacin versus placebo for prophylaxis against travellers' diarrhoea. *J. Antimicrob. Chemother.* **20**, 563–574.

31. Rademaker, C. M., Hoepelman, I. M., Wolfhagen, M. J., Beumer, H., Rozenberg, Arska, M., and Verhoef, J. (1989). Results of a double-blind placebo-controlled study using ciprofloxacin for prevention of traveler's diarrhea. *Eur. J. Clin. Microbiol. Infect. Dis.* **8**, 690–694.

32. Lopez-Brea, M., Jiminez, M. L., Lopez Lavid, M. C., Padilla, B., and Isasia, T. (1989). Norfloxacin vs. trimethoprim–sulfamethoxazole in the treatment of salmonella gastroenteritis. *Rev. Infect. Dis.* **11** (Suppl. 5), S1153–S1154.

33. Neill, M. A., Opal, S. M., Heelan, J., Giusti, R., Cassidy, J. E., White, R., and Mayer, K. H. (1991). Failure of ciprofloxacin in convalescent fecal excretion after acute salmonellosis: Experience during an outbreak in health care workers. *Ann. Intern. Med.* **114**, 195–199.

34. Sanchez, C., Garcia-Restoy, E., Garau, J., Bella, F., Freixas, N., Simo), M., Lite, J., Sanchez, P., Espejo, E., Cobo, E., and Rodriguez, M. (1993). Ciprofloxacin and trimethoprim–sulfamethoxazole versus placebo in acute uncomplicated *Salmonella* enteritis: A double-blind trial. *J. Infect. Dis* **168**, 1304–1307.

35. Carstedt, G., Dahl, P., Niklasson, P. M., Gullberg, K., Banck, G., and Kahlmeter, G. (1990). Norfloxacin treatment of salmonellosis does not shorten the carrier stage. *Scand. J. Infect. Dis.* **22**, 553–556.

36. Damjanovic, V., Williets, T. H., Glynne-Thomas, D., and van Saene, H. K. F. (1990). Eradication of *Salmonella* by oral ciprofloxacin in food handlers. *Lancet* **335**, 974.

37. Loffler, A., and Graf von Westphalen, H. (1986). Successful treatment of a chronic salmonella excretor with ofloxacin. *Lancet* **I**, 1206.

38. Diridl, G., Pichler, H., and Wolf, D. (1986). Treatment of chronic salmonella carriers with ciprofloxacin. *Eur. J. Clin. Microbiol.* **5**, 260–261.

39. Sammalkorpi, K., Lahdevirta, Makela, T., and Rostila, T. (1987). Treatment of chronic salmonella carriers with ciprofloxacin. *Lancet* **ii**, 164–165.

40. Velmonte, M. A., and Montalban, C. S. (1988). Norfloxacin in the treatment of infections caused by *Salmonella typhi*. *Scand J. Infect. Dis.* **56** (Suppl.) 46–48.

41. Nalin, D. R., Hoagland, V. L., Acuna, G., Bran, J. L., Carillo, C., Gotuzzo, E., Ruiz-Palacios, G., Ramirez, C., and Guerra, J. (1987). Clinical trial of norfloxacin versus chloramphenicol therapy for acute typhoid fever. *Abstr. 15th Int. Cong. Chemother.*, Munksgåard, Copenhagen, pp. 1174–1175.

42. Ramirez, C. A., Bran, J. L., Mejia, C. R., and Garcia, J. F. (1985). Open, prospective study of the clinical efficacy of ciprofloxacin. *Antimicrob. Agents Chemother.* **28**, 128–132.

43. Stanley, P. J., Flegg, P. J., Mandal, B. K., and Beddes, A. M. (1989). Open study of ciprofloxacin in enteric fever. *J. Antimicrob. Chemother.* **23**, 789–791.

44. Limson, B. M., and Littaua, R. T. (1989). Comparative study of ciprofloxacin versus co-trimoxazole in the treatment of salmonella enteric fever. *Infection* **17**, 105–106.

45. Uwaydah, A. K., Al Soub, H., and Matar, I. (1992). Randomized prospective study comparing two dosage regimens of ciprofloxacin for the treatment of typhoid fever. *J. Antimicrob. Chemother.* **30**, 707–711.

46. Alam, M. N., Haq, S. A., Das, K. K., Baral, P. K., Mazid, M. N., Siddique, R. U., Rahman, K. M., Hasan, Z., Khan, M. A. S., and Dutta, P. (1995). Efficacy of ciprofloxacin in enteric fever: Comparison of treatment duration in sensitive and multidrug-resistant *Salmonella*. *Am. J. Trop. Med. Hyg.* **53**, 306–311.

47. Wang, F., Gu, X. Z. M., and Tai, T. (1989). Treatment of typhoid fever with ofloxacin. *J. Antimicrob. Chemother.* **23**, 785–788.

48. Akhtar, M. A., Karamat, K. A., Malik, A. Z., Hashmi, A., Khan, Q. M., and Rasheed, P. (1989). Efficacy of ofloxacin in typhoid fever, particularly in drug-resistant cases. *Rev. Infect. Dis.* **11** (Suppl. 5), S1193.

49. Tanphaichitra, D., and Srimuang, S. (1989). In vitro and clinical evaluation of ofloxacin in urinary tract infection and enteric fever. *Rev. Infect. Dis.* **11** (Suppl. 5), S1190–S1191.

50. Zavala-Trujillo, I., Nava-Zavala, A., Marcano, M. G., and Renteria, M. (1989). Fleroxacin in the treatment of enteric fever and salmanellosis in adults. *Rev. Infect. Dis.* **11** (Suppl. 5), S1188–S1189.

51. Arnold, K., Hong, C.-S., Nelwan, R., Zavala-Trujillo, I., Kadio, A., Oliverira Barros, M. J., and De Garis, S. (1993). Randomized comparative study of fleroxacin and chloramphenicol in typhoid fever. *Am. J. Med.* **94** (Suppl. 3A), 195S–200S.

52. Cristiano, P., Morelli, G., Briante, V., Iovene, M. R., Simioli, F., and Altucci, P. (1989). Clinical experience with pefloxacin in the therapy of typhoid fever. *Infection* **17**, 86–87.

53. Ait-Khaled, A., Zidane, L., Amrane, A., and Aklil, R. (1989). A seven-day pefloxacin course for the treatment of typhoid fever in Algeria. *Rev. Infect. Dis.* **11** (Suppl. 5), S1191.

54. Hajji, M., El Mdaghri, N., Benbachir, M., Marhoum El Filali, K., and Himmich, H. (1988). Prospective randomized comparative trial of pefloxacin versus cotrimoxazole in the treatment of typhoid fever in adults. *Eur. J. Clin. Microbiol. Infect. Dis.* **7**, 361–363.

55. Thomsen, L. L., and Paerregaard, A. (1998). Treatment with ciprofloxacin in children with typhoid fever. *Scand. J. Infect. Dis.* **30**, 355–357.

56. Phuong, C. X. T., Kneen, R., Anh., N. T., Luat., T. D., White, N. J., Parry, C. M., and the Dong Nai Pediatric Center Typhoid Study Group (1999). A comparative study of ofloxacin and cefixime for treatment of typhoid fever. *Pediatr. Infect. Dis. J.* **18**, 245–248.

57. Girgis, N. I., Butler, T., Frenck, R. W., Sultan, Y., Brown, F. M., Tribble, D., and Khakhria, R. (1999). Azithromycin versus ciprofloxacin for treatment of uncomplicated typhoid fever in a randomized trial in Egypt that included patients with multidrug resistance. *Antimicrob. Agents Chemother.* **43**, 1441–1444.

58. Nelwan, R. H. H., Hendarwanto, Zulkarnain, I., *et al.* (1992). Recent results of short-course treatment of typhoid fever with ciprofloxacin. *Abstr. 3rd West. Pac. Cong. Chemother. Infect. Dis.*, Bali. Abstr. #52004.

59. Bryskier, A., Zribi, A., Ould Rouis, B., *et al.* (1992). Typhoid fever: Five day therapy with ofloxacin, preliminary results. *Abstr. 4th Int. Symp. New Quinolones*, Munich. Abstr. #223.

60. Gotuzzo, E., Guerra, J. G., Benavente, L., Palomino, J. C., Carrillo, C., Lopera, J., Delgado, F., Nalin, D. R., and Sabbaj, J. (1988). Use of norfloxacin to treat chronic typhoid carriers. *J. Infect. Dis.* **157**, 1221–1225.

61. Ferreccio, C., Morris, J. G., Valdivieso, C., Prenzel, I., Sotomayor, V., Drusano, G. L., and Levine, M. M. (1988). Efficacy of ciprofloxacin in the treatment of chronic typhoid carriers. *J. Infect. Dis.* **157**, 1235–1239.

62. Reid, T., and Smith, C. (1987). Ciprofloxacin treatment of chronic salmonella excreters. *Chemotherapy* **6** (Suppl. 2), 485–486.

63. Bennish, M. L., Salam, M. A., Haider, R., and Barza, M. (1990). Therapy for shigellosis, II: Randomized, double-blind comparison of ciprofloxacin and ampicillin. *J. Infect. Dis.* **162**, 711–716.

64. Rogerie, F., Ott, D., Vandepitte, J., Verbist, L., Lemmens, P., and Habiyaremye, I. (1986). Comparison of norfloxacin and nalidixic acid for treatment of dysentery caused by *Shigella dysenteriae* type 1 in adults. *Antimicrob. Agents Chemother.* **29**, 883–886.

65. De Mol, P., Mets, T., Lagasse, R., Vandepitte, J., Mutwewingabo, A., and Butzler, J. P. (1987). Treatment of bacillary dysentery: A comparison between enoxacin and nalidixic acid. *J. Antimicrob. Chemother.* **19**, 695–698.

66. Khan, W. A., Seas, C., Dhar, U., Salam, M. A., and Bennish, M. L. (1997). Treatment of shigellosis, V: Comparison of azithromycin and ciprofloxacin. *Ann. Intern. Med.* **126**, 697–703.

67. Shanks, G. D., Smoak, B. L., Aleman, G. M., Oundo, J., Waiyaki, P. G., Dunne, M. W., Petersen, L., and the Acute Dysentery Study Group (1999). Single dose of azithromycin or three-day course of ciprofloxacin as therapy for epidemic dysentery in Kenya. *Clin. Infect. Dis.* **29**, 942–943.

68. Bennish, M. L., Salam, M. A., Khan, W. A., and Khan, A. M. (1992). Treatment of shigellosis, III: Comparison of one- or two-dose ciprofloxacin with standard 5-day therapy: A randomized, blinded trial. *Ann. Intern. Med.* **117**, 727–734.

69. Bassily, S., Hyams, K. C., El-Masry, N. A., Farid, Z., Cross, E., Bourgeois, A. L., Ayad, E., and Hibbs, R. G. (1994). Short-course norfloxacin and trimethoprim-sulfamethoxazole treatment of shigellosis and salmonellosis in Egypt. *Am. J. Trop. Med. Hyg.* **51**, 219–223.

70. Gotuzzo, E., Oberhelman, R. A., Maguiña, C., Berry, S. J., Yi, A., Guzman, M., Ruiz, R., Leon-Barua, R., and Sack, R. B. (1989). Comparison of single-dose treatment with norfloxacin and standard 5-day treatment with trimethoprim-sulfamethoxazole for acute shigellosis in adults. *Antimicrob. Agents Chemother.* **33**, 883–886.

71. Burkhardt, J. E., Walterspiel, J. N., and Schaad, U. B. (1997). Quinolone arthropathy in animals versus children. *Clin. Infect. Dis.* **25**, 1196–1204.

72. Gendrel, D., Moreno, J. L., Nduwimana, M., Baribwira, C., and Raymond, J. (1997). One-dose treatment of pefloxacin for infection due to multidrug-resistant *Shigella dysenteriae* type 1 in Burundi. *Clin. Infect. Dis.* **24**, 83.

73. Salam, M. A., Dhar, U., Khan, A. K., and Bennish, M. L. (1998). Randomised comparison of ciprofloxacin suspension and pivmecillinam for childhood shigellosis. *Lancet* **352**, 522–527.

74. Murphy, G. S., Bodhidatta, L., Echeverria, P., Tansuphaswadikul, S., Hoge, C. W., Imlarp, S., and Tamura, K. (1993). Ciprofloxacin and loperamide in the treatment of bacillary dysentery. *Ann. Intern. Med.* **118**, 582–586.

75. Bhattacharya, S. K., Bhattacharya, M. K., Dutta, P., Dutta, D., De, S. P., Sikdar, S. N., Maitra, A., Dutta, A., and Pal, S. C. (1990). Double-blind, randomized, controlled trial of norfloxacin for cholera. *Antimicrob. Agents Chemother.* **34**, 939–940.

76. Khan, W. A., Begum, M., Salam, M. A., Bardhan, P. K., Islam, M. R., and Mahalanabis, D. (1995). Comparative trial of five antimicrobial compounds in the treatment of cholera in adults. *Trans. R. Soc. Trop. Med. Hyg.* **89**, 103–106.

77. Gotuzzo, E., Seas, C., Echevarría, J., Carrillo, C., Mostorino, R., and Ruiz, R. (1995). Ciprofloxacin for the treatment of cholera: A randomized, double-blind, controlled clinical trial of a single daily dose in Peruvian adults. *Clin. Infect. Dis.* **20**, 1485–1490.

78. Khan, W. A., Bennish, M. L., Seas, C., Khan, E. H., Ronan, A., Dhar, U., Busch, W., and Salam, M. A. (1996). Randomised controlled comparison of single-dose ciprofloxacin and doxycycline for cholera caused by *Vibrio cholerae* O1 or O139. *Lancet* **348**, 296–300.

79. Echevarría, J., Seas, C., Carrillo, C., Mostorino, R., Ruiz, R., and Gotuzzo, E. (1995). Efficacy and tolerability of ciprofloxacin prophylaxis in adult household contacts of patients with cholera. *Clin. Infect. Dis.* **20**, 1480–1484.

80. Segreti, J., Gootz, T. D., Goodman, L. J., Parkhurst, G. W., Quinn, J. P., Martin, B. A., and Trenholme, G. M. (1992). High-level quinolone resistance in clinical isolates of *Campylobacter jejuni*. *J. Infect. Dis.* **165**, 667–670.

81. Wretlind, B., Stromberg, A., Ostlund, L., Sjogren, E., and Kaijser, B. (1992). Rapid emergence of quinolone resistance in *Campylobacter jejuni* in patients treated with norfloxacin. *Scand. J. Infect. Dis.* **24**, 685–686.

82. Gaunt, P. N., and Piddock, L. J. V. (1996). Ciprofloxacin resistant *Campylobacter* spp. in humans: An epidemiological and laboratory study. *J. Antimicrob. Chemother.* **37**, 747–757.

83. Sanchez, R., Fernandez-Baca, V., Diaz, M. D., Muñoz, P., Rodriguez-Creixems, M., and Bouza, E. (1994). Evolution of susceptibilities of *Campylobacter* spp. to quinolones and macrolides. *Antimicrob. Agents Chemother.* **38**, 1879–1882.

84. Kuschner, R. A., Trofa, A. F., Thomas, R. J., Hoge, C. W., Pitarangsi, C., Amato, S., Olafson, R. P., Echeverria, P., Sadoff, J. C., and Taylor, D. N. (1995). Use of azithromycin for the

treatment of *Campylobacter* enteritis in travelers to Thailand, an area where ciprofloxacin resistance is prevalent. *Clin. Infect. Dis.* **21**, 536–541.

85. Smith, K. E., Besser, J. M., Hedberg, C. W., Leano, F. T., Bender, J. B., Wicklund, J. H., Johnson, B. P., Moore, K. A., Osterholm, M. T., and the Investigation Team (1999). Quinolone-resistant *Campylobacter jejuni* infections in Minnesota, 1992–1998. *New Engl. J. Med.* **340**, 1525–1532.

86. Talsma, E., Goettsch, W. G., Nieste, H. L. J., Schrijnemakers, P. M., and Sprenger, M. J. W. (1999). Resistance in *Campylobacter* species: Increased resistance to fluoroquinolones and seasonal variation. Clin. Infect. Dis. **29**, 845–848.

87. Endtz, H. P., Ruijs, G. J., van Klingeren, B., Jansen, W. H., van der Reyden, T., and Mouton, R. P. (1991). Quinolone resistance in campylobacter isolated from man and poultry following the introduction of fluoroquinolones in veterinary medicine. *J. Antimicrob. Chemother.* **27**, 199–208.

88. Piddock, L. J. V., Whale, K., and Wise, R. (1990). Quinolone resistance in salmonella: Clinical experience. *Lancet* **1**, 1459.

89. Molbak, K., Baggesen, D. L., Aarestrup, F. M., Ebbesen, J. M., Engberg, J., Frydendahl, K., Gerner-Smidt, P., Petersen, A. M., and Wegener, H. C. (1999). An outbreak of multidrug-resistant, quinolone-resistant *Salmonella enterica* serotype typhimurium DT104. *New Engl. J. Med.* **341**, 1420–1425.

90. Threlfall, E. J., Ward, L. R., Skinner, J. A., Smith, H. R., and Lacey, S. (1999). Ciprofloxacin-resistant *Salmonella typhi* and treatment failure. *Lancet* **353**, 1590–1591.

91. Chitnis, V., Chitnis, D., Verma, S., and Hemvani, N. (1999). Multidrug-resistant *Salmonella typhi* in India. *Lancet* **354**, 514–515.

92. Tarr, P. E., Kuppens, L., Jones, T. C., Ivanoff, B., Aparin, P. G., and Heymann, D. L. (1999). Considerations regarding mass vaccination against typhoid fever as an adjunct to sanitation and public health measures: Potential use in an epidemic in Tajikistan. *Am. J. Trop. Med. Hyg.* **61**, 163–170.

93. Wain, J., Hoa, N. T. T., Chinh, N. T., Vinh H., Everett, M. J., Diep, T. S., Day, N. P. J., Solomon, T., White, N. J., Piddock, L. J. V., and Parry, C. M. (1997). Quinolone-resistant *Salmonella typhi* in Vietnam: Molecular basis of resistance and clinical response to treatment. *Clin. Infect. Dis.* **25**, 1404–1410.

94. Tauxe, R. V., Puhr, N. D., Wells, J. G., Hargrett-Bean, N., and Blake, P. A. (1990). Antimicrobial resistance of *Shigella* isolates in the USA: The importance of international travelers. *J. Infect. Dis.* **162**, 1107–1111.

CHAPTER 11

Use of the Quinolones in Treatment of Bacterial Meningitis

RODRIGO HASBUN* and VINCENT J. QUAGLIARELLO†

*Tulane University School of Medicine, Section of Infectious Diseases, New Orleans, Louisiana 70118, and Yale University School of Medicine, Section of Infectious Diseases, New Haven, Connecticut 06520-8022

INTRODUCTION

Bacterial meningitis remains a disease with unacceptable morbidity and mortality despite the availability of effective bactericidal antibiotic therapy [1,2]. For example, in a review of 493 episodes of bacterial meningitis in adults from 1962 to 1988 [3], the overall mortality rate was 25% and did not change significantly over the 27-year study. The emergence of antibiotic resistance in *Streptococcus pneumoniae* has further complicated the therapy of bacterial meningitis, and has prompted the development of new antimicrobials.

Some of the new fluorinated quinolones have very important characteristics that make them potentially useful in the therapy of bacterial meningitis: excellent *in-vitro* activity against Gram-negative aerobic microorganisms [4], activity against penicillin and cephalosporin-resistant pneumococci [5–9], and reproducible cerebrospinal fluid penetration [10]. Activity against resistant strains of pneumococci will become more important in the near future as the incidence of β-lactam resistance increases. Despite this, the quinolones have been infrequently used in meningitis because the majority of cases occurred in the pediatric population, where quinolones have been relatively contraindicated. Two major changes have developed more recently: (1) widespread use of the *H. influenzae* conjugate vaccine has shifted the median age of patients with bacterial meningitis from 15 months to 25 years of age, making bacterial meningitis (in countries where vaccination is widespread) more common in adults [11], and (2) more clinical experience has been reported with fluoroquinolones in children, making quinolones a future option in the pediatric population [12].

PHARMACOLOGY

IN-VITRO ACTIVITY OF QUINOLONES AGAINST MENINGEAL PATHOGENS

The quinolones most studied in animal models of meningitis and in humans are ciprofloxacin, ofloxacin, pefloxacin, trovafloxacin, gemifloxacin, gatifloxacin, and moxifloxacin. As shown in Table I, they possess excellent activity against several Gram-negative meningeal pathogens (e.g., *Neisseria meningitidis, Haemophilus influenzae*, and *Escherichia coli*). Although the MBC is more predictive of therapeutic efficacy than the MIC [13], these agents achieve CSF concentrations of from ~4- to ≥50-fold above the MIC_{90} for these Gram-negative meningeal pathogens [14].

The activity of the older quinolones against most Gram-positive meningeal pathogens (staphylococci, streptococci, and *Listeria*) is suboptimal. The CSF concentrations obtained with systemic administration of the quinolones, in most instances, are below the MIC_{90} for these pathogens. The newer quinolones (trovafloxacin, gemifloxacin, moxifloxacin, and gatifloxacin) have much better activity against *S. pneumoniae* (both penicillin-sensitive and penicillin-resistant), *Staphylococcus aureus* (oxacillin-sensitive), *Streptococcus agalactiae*, and *Listeria monocytogenes* (see Table I). The low MIC_{90} (μg/ml) to penicillin-resistant *S. pneumoniae* for the new quinolones (trovafloxacin 0.125, gemifloxacin 0.06,

TABLE I *In-Vitro* Activity of Quinolones against Common Meningeal Pathogens

Organism	Ciprofloxacin	Ofloxacin	Pefloxacin	Trovafloxacin	Gemifloxacin	Moxifloxacin	Gatifloxacin
				MIC$_{90}$ (µg/ml)			
N. meningitidis	<0.001	0.02	0.03	0.005	0.006	0.015[c]	0.008[c]
H. influenzae	0.01	0.03	0.06	0.008–0.03	0.004	0.03–0.06	<0.03
S. pneumoniae[a] (PCN-sensitive)	2.0	2.0	8.0	0.125	0.06	0.06–0.25	0.5
S. pneumoniae[b] (PCN-resistant)	2.0	4.0	NA	0.125	0.06	0.12–0.25	0.5
E. coli	0.02–0.06	0.06	0.13	0.015–4.0	0.015	0.06–1.0	0.06
S. epidermidis	0.25–0.4	0.25	1	0.06	0.015–0.25	2.0	2.0
S. aureus (methicillin-sensitive)	0.5–1.0	0.5	0.5	0.06	0.03	0.12	0.12
S. aureus (methicillin-resistant)	>2.0	1	1	2.0	2.0	2.0	4.0
S. agalactiae	0.5–0.8	1	16	0.25	0.125	0.25	NA
L. monocytogenes	1	2	8	0.25	0.125	0.5	NA

NA = not available. Data from [4–6,8,14,50–55].

[a]MIC < 0.06 µg/ml of PCN.

[b]MIC > 0.1 µg/ml of PCN.

[c]*Neisseria* spp.

moxifloxacin 0.12–0.25, and gatifloxacin 0.5) make these agents attractive
alternatives in the era of drug-resistant pneumococci.

CSF PENETRATION OF THE QUINOLONES *IN VIVO*

Animal Models

Experimental animal models of meningitis have been very important in studying
CSF penetration and the *in-vivo* bactericidal activity of the quinolones [15–17].
Armengaud and colleagues were the first to use experimental models of meningitis to study the quinolones. In their first study [18], pefloxacin achieved
CSF/serum concentrations of ~45% in uninfected dogs and 76% in dogs with
Staphylococcus aureus meningitis. In another study [19], the diffusion of enoxacin
into the CSF in dogs with healthy meninges and with experimental meningitis
was evaluated. After a 1-hour intravenous injection of 12.5 and 25 mg/kg of
enoxacin in three dogs with healthy meninges, the CSF concentration observed
between 90 and 240 minutes averaged 2.6 (1.8–3.3) μg/ml and 6.5 (4.7–8.4) μg/ml
respectively (see Table II). These concentrations greatly exceed the MICs for
Neisseria meningitidis and *Haemophilus influenzae*. The ratio of the CSF/plasma
AUC (area under the curve) was 47% after the 25-mg/kg and 33% after the
12.5-mg/kg dose. Meningitis was then induced with a pathogenic strain of
Staphylococcus aureus, and 18–20 hours later the animals were given 12.5 mg/kg
of enoxacin. The mean CSF concentration in the infected dogs was 4.9 (3.1–6.4)
μg/ml, and the percentage ratio of CSF/plasma AUC was 67.3%. These ratios

TABLE II   CSF Penetration of Quinolones in Animal Models

Antibiotic	CSF/Serum concentration ratio	
	Healthy meninges	Inflamed meninges
Pefloxacin	26–45%	37–76%
Enoxacin	25–37%	50%
Ciprofloxacin	4%	17–39%
Trovafloxacin	NR	17–25%
Moxifloxacin	50%	34–78%
Gatifloxacin	NR	46–56%
Gemifloxacin	NR	9–13%

NR = not reported. Data from [7,9,18–26].

TABLE III Ratios of CSF/Plasma AUCs in Dogs with Inflamed
Meninges: Comparison of Enoxacin with β-Lactam Antibiotics

Antibiotic	CSF/plasma AUCs
Enoxacin	67.3%
Mezlocillin	26.6%
Ceftriaxone	22.4%
Cefuroxime	18.7%
Amoxicillin	18.6%
Cefoxitin	18.5%
Cefamandole	17.4%
Cefotaxime	16.3%

Adapted from Tho *et al.* (1984) [19].

obtained with enoxacin were far superior than those achieved by seven β-lactam antibiotics (see Table III).

Shibl *et al.* [20] evaluated the therapeutic efficacy of pefloxacin in comparison to that of cefotaxime and chloramphenicol in a rabbit model of *E. coli* meningitis. The MIC/MBC of the antibiotics for the *E. coli* strain were as follows: 0.125/0.125 µg/ml for pefloxacin, 0.25/0.5 µg/ml for cefotaxime, and 8/>64 µg/ml for chloramphenicol. In normal uninfected rabbits, pefloxacin had good CSF penetration, ranging from 26 to 33% of simultaneous serum concentration at doses of 5, 15, and 30 mg/kg. The rabbits then received an intracisternal inoculation of 10^5 *E. coli*, and 16 hours later they received one of the three antibiotics. The mean percentage CSF penetration of pefloxacin of infected rabbits was better (51.3%) than with cefotaxime (11.1%) and chloramphenicol (22.3%), and the rate of bacterial killing of pefloxacin was equivalent to that of cefotaxime and superior to chloramphenicol.

Hackbarth *et al.* [21] evaluated ciprofloxacin in a similar rabbit model of *Pseudomonas aeruginosa* meningitis. The geometric mean MIC and MBC (µg/ml) for the test strain were as follows: ciprofloxacin 1/1, ceftazidime 3.5/57, and tobramycin 0.8/2.6.

The CSF percentage penetration of ciprofloxacin in normal rabbits was $4.08 \pm 1.27\%$ (mean ± standard deviation), compared with $18.4 \pm 12.3\%$ in rabbits with meningitis. At 5 mg/kg/hr (a dose that approximates maximum serum levels that are achievable in humans), ciprofloxacin was equally effective in reducing bacterial titers in the CSF as a ceftazidime and tobramycin combination (see Table IV).

Paris *et al.* [7] evaluated trovafloxacin (or CP-99,219) in the therapy of experimental penicillin- and cephalosporin-resistant pneumococcal meningitis in

TABLE IV   Evaluation of Ciprofloxacin in Experimental *P. aeruginosa* Meningitis

Drug dosage (mg/[kg·hr])	Mean concentration (µg/ml)		Mean percentage penetration	Mean $\Delta\log_{10}$ cfu/ml in CSF/hr
	Serum	CSF		
Ciprofloxacin (5)	6.7	0.8	17.3	−0.48
Ceftazidime (25)	109.0	24.8	22.9	−
Ceftazidime plus tobramycin (2.5)	9.9	3.1	32.9	−0.51
Untreated	−	−	−	+0.14

Adapted from Hackbarth *et al.* (1986) [21].

rabbits. The MICs and MBCs of penicillin, ceftriaxone, vancomycin, and CP-99,219 for the two strains used are shown on Table V. The peak and trough concentrations of CP-99,219 in the CSF were 19 and 25% of the serum concentration and were unaffected by concomitant administration of dexamethasone. Using the relatively resistant JM strain of *S. pneumoniae* (MIC = 1 µg/ml), the bacteriologic effects of CP-99,219, vancomycin, and ceftriaxone with or without dexamethasone were evaluated (see Table VI). Vancomycin and CP-99,219 were more effective than ceftriaxone in reducing the bacterial concentrations at 10 but not at 24 hours. Dexamethasone therapy did not significantly reduce the bacteriologic response of any of the three antibiotics.

Kim *et al.* [9] also compared trovafloxacin to standard antimicrobial agents in penicillin-resistant *S. pneumoniae* meningitis in rabbits. The MICs (µg/ml) of the

TABLE V   MICs and MBCs for the *S. pneumoniae* Strains

Antibiotic	JM strain		JG strain	
	MIC[a]	MBC[a]	MIC[a]	MBC[a]
Penicillin	1	1	2	2
Ceftriaxone	1	1	4	4
Vancomycin	0.25	0.5	0.25	0.25
CP-99,219	0.06	0.125	0.06	0.125

Adapted from Paris *et al.* (1995) [7].

[a]Measured in µg/ml.

TABLE VI Comparison of Bacterial Concentrations in CSF of Rabbits Infected with the JM Strain Treated with Vancomycin, Ceftriaxone, or CP-99,219 with or without Dexamethasone

Treatment group	Mean $\Delta \log_{10}$ cfu after 10 and 24 hours of therapy	
Control	+1.0	ND
Vancomycin	−5.5	−6.1
Vancomycin + dexamethasone	−3.9	−3.7
Ceftriaxone	−2.9	−5.6
Ceftriaxone + dexamethasone	−2.2	−2.6
CP-99,219	−4.7	−5.0
CP-99,219 + dexamethasone	−4.8	−3.9

Adapted from Paris et al. (1995) [7].

[a]ND = not done. Death ocurred in most animals at 24 hours.

strain used were: penicillin 4, trovafloxacin 0.25, ceftriaxone 0.25, ampicillin 4, and rifampin 0.5. Trovafloxacin (10 mg/kg) was compared to ceftriaxone (10 mg/kg) and ampicillin (50 mg/kg). All antibiotics, except ampicillin, were given as single intravenous bolus. The results of the investigation are shown in Table VII. Trovafloxacin was very effective in reducing bacterial counts in the CSF, and the addition of ampicillin or rifampin to trovafloxacin did not improve the killing rate.

TABLE VII Comparison of Trovafloxacin, Ceftriaxone, and Ampicillin in Therapy of Experimental Penicillin-Resistant Streptococcus pneumoniae[a] Meningitis

	1 hr concentration (µg/ml)		
	CSF	Serum	$\Delta \log_{10}$ cfu/ml/hr
Trovafloxacin	0.28 ± 0.09	1.66 ± 0.51	−0.50 ± 0.26[b]
Ceftriaxone	0.81 ± 0.66	15.85 ± 7.4	−0.31 ± 0.28[b]
Ampicillin	4.23 ± 2.68	13.11 ± 7.8	−0.23 ± 0.31
Control	−	−	0.00 ± 0.09

Adapted from Kim et al. (1997) [9].

[a]MIC to penicillin = 4.0 µg/ml; MIC to ceftriaxone = 0.25 µg/ml

[b]$p < 0.05$ compared to control.

Lutsar *et al.* [22–23] studied gatifloxacin in experimental pneumococcal and *E. coli* meningitis. In the first study [22], gatifloxacin was used in rabbits infected with a cephalosporin-resistant isolate of *S. pneumoniae* (MICs of 4 μg/ml to ceftriaxone and 0.125 μg/ml to gatifloxacin). The CSF penetration (AUC of CSF divided by AUC of serum) of gatifloxacin ranged from 46 to 56%. The bactericidal activity of gatifloxacin was comparable to a combination of vancomycin and ceftriaxone. In the second study [23], gatifloxacin at 15 mg/kg every 5 hours was compared to meropenem at 75 mg/kg every 5 hours and cefotaxime at 75 mg/kg every 5 hours in experimental meningitis caused by a β-lactamase positive strain of *E. coli*. As shown in Table VIII, gatifloxacin and meropenem had similar bactericidal effect, but both were more rapidly bactericidal than cefotaxime.

Lewandowski *et al.* [24] evaluated gemifloxacin in a rat model with penicillin-sensitive *S. pneumoniae* meningitis and compared it to several other antimicrobials (ciprofloxacin, trovafloxacin, levofloxacin, cefuroxime, cefotaxime, and vancomycin). The *S. pneumoniae* strain was susceptible to all the antimicrobial agents used in the study. The survival rate of the rats at 7 days was 0% in the placebo group and 83% in the gemifloxacin-treated group. This survival rate did not differ significantly between all the antimicrobials (except for trovafloxacin, which had a 60% survival rate).

Schmidt *et al.* [25] compared moxifloxacin with ceftriaxone in rabbits infected by a cephalosporin-sensitive strain of *S. pneumoniae*. The bactericidal activity of 10 mg of moxifloxacin per kg per hour had similar bactericidal efficacy as that of ceftriaxone given at 10 mg/kg/hr. Furthermore, the CSF penetration of moxifloxacin was 37% and was not affected by coadministration of dexamethasone. In another study, Østergaard *et al.* [26] compared moxifloxacin, ceftriaxone,

TABLE VIII   Effect of Bacterial Concentration on the Bactericidal Killing Rate (BKR)

Initial bacterial concentration (cfu/ml)	BKR ($\Delta \log_{10}$ cfu/ml/hr) at 6 hr		
	Gati- floxacin (1 μg/ml)	Meropenem (3 μg/ml)	Cefotaxime (4 μg/ml)
10^5	>0.6	>0.6	0.6
10^6	>0.66	0.58	0.33
10^7	>0.83	0.58	0.25
10^8	>1	0.6	0.16

Adapted from Lutsar *et al.* (1999) [23].

and vancomycin in rabbits infected with penicillin-resistant *S. pneumoniae* (penicillin, ceftriaxone, vancomycin, and moxifloxacin MICs were 1, 0.5, 0.5, and 0.125 µg/ml, respectively). The CSF penetration of moxifloxacin was 50 and 80% in uninfected and infected rabbits, respectively. Moxifloxacin was as effective as ceftriaxone and vancomycin in reducing bacterial counts at all time points tested (3, 5, 10, and 24 hr).

Humans

The CSF penetration of pefloxacin, ofloxacin, ciprofloxacin, and trovafloxacin has been studied. Wolff and colleagues [27] evaluated diffusion of pefloxacin in 15 patients with bacterial meningitis or ventriculitis. All patients were also being treated with other antibiotics, and 14 of them were culture-positive. Three doses of pefloxacin were given at 12-hr intervals to 11 patients intravenously and to 4 patients orally. The CSF concentration of pefloxacin was determined by a high-performance liquid chromatographic (HPLC) assay 2 hours after infusion or 4 hours after ingestion. As shown in Table IX, pefloxacin had very good penetration (52–58%) into both lumbar and ventricular CSF. Dow *et al.* [28] studied the pharmacokinetics of pefloxacin in nine patients with hydrocephalus and noninflamed meninges. A single dose of 400 mg of pefloxacin was administered intravenously, and several CSF samples were obtained through an external ventricular drain. The CSF concentrations of pefloxacin were determined by HPLC at different intervals after the infusion and was found to be ~60% of the plasma concentration (see Table IX). The apparent half-life ($T_{1/2}$) of transfer of pefloxacin from plasma to CSF was 1.26 hr, and the elimination $T_{1/2}$ in CSF was 13.4 hr (i.e., similar to elimination kinetics in serum).

There are two studies evaluating penetration of ofloxacin into human CSF. In the first study [29], ofloxacin was given orally to nine patients with bacterial meningitis, of whom five were culture-proven. All patients were being treated with intravenous amoxicillin. On days 2 and 5, serum and CSF concentrations were determined by HPLC, the results of which are summarized in Table IX. The serum and CSF concentrations were variable, but the CSF ofloxacin trough levels (12 hr after a 200-mg oral dose) still exceeded 0.9 µg/ml and was 52–59% of the serum concentration. Stubner *et al.* [30] evaluated the diffusion of ofloxacin in 17 patients with suspected meningitis, of whom 6 (35%) had a CSF WBC ≥5. Ofloxacin was administered orally at a dosage of 200 mg twice a day, and serum and CSF samples were obtained at 1.5 and 12 hours after dosing. The maximum concentration (at 1.5 hr) varied from 0.5 to 7.75 µg/ml in the serum and between 0.32 and 3.6 µg/ml in the CSF, with a CSF/plasma ratio of 47%. The minimal

TABLE IX   Penetration of the quinolones in human CSF

Quinolone	Dose	Mean concentration (μg/ml)		CSF/ plasma ratio
		Serum	CSF	
Inflamed meninges				
Pefloxacin	7.5 mg/kg	10.3	4.8	58%
	15 mg/kg	20.2	8.3	52%
Ofloxacin	200 mg p.o. b.i.d. × 2 days	3.5	1.8	52%
	200 mg p.o. b.i.d. × 5 days	4	2.4	59%
Ofloxacin	200 mg p.o. b.i.d.	NR	NR	47–87%
Ciprofloxacin	200 mg i.v. q. 12 hr × 3	NR	0.45	26–37%

Quinolone	Dose	T_{max} (hr)		AUC CSF/ serum	CSF/ plasma ratio
		Serum	CSF		
Noninflamed meninges					
Pefloxacin	400 mg i.v.	1	5.5	NR	60%
Ciprofloxacin	500 mg p.o.	3	4	10%	5%
Trovafloxacin	180 mg/m^2 i.v.	0.8	1.1	25%	22–25%

NR = not reported. Data from [17–33].

concentration (at 12 hr) varied from 0.5 to 1.83 μg/ml in the serum and between 0.5 and 1.3 μg/ml in the CSF, with a CSF/plasma ratio of 87% (see Table IX).

The CSF penetration of ciprofloxacin in patients with bacterial meningitis was evaluated by Wolff and colleagues [31]. Three 200-mg doses of ciprofloxacin were administered intravenously at 12-hour intervals during the acute stage of meningitis (between 2 and 4 days after admission). All patients were being treated with other antibiotics. The results are summarized in Table IX. These achievable concentrations were equal or higher than the MICs for most of the Enterobacteriaceae. Another group [32] evaluated ciprofloxacin's CSF penetration in patients with noninflamed meninges in which one dose of 500 mg of ciprofloxacin was given orally to 48 patients undergoing lumbar puncture for diagnostic purposes. The maximum serum and CSF concentrations achieved were 2.7 and 0.14 μg/ml, respectively, and the CSF/plasma ratio was 5% (see Table IX). In a group of 4 patients with meningitis, the mean serum concentrations of ciprofloxacin in serum and CSF were 2.39 and 0.28 μg/ml, respectively, and the CSF/serum ratio was ~12%.

Trovafloxacin is one of the new fluoroquinolones. Arguedas-Mohs and colleagues [33] evaluated its CSF penetration in 21 children undergoing diagnostic lumbar puncture (only one of whom had CSF pleocytosis). CP-116,517, the prodrug of trovafloxacin, was administered at a dose of 180 mg/m^2 intravenously, and serum and CSF samples were obtained at different intervals. The serum and CSF concentrations varied widely (0.5–6.8 and 0.12–1.4 μg/ml, respectively), and the CSF/serum concentration ratio was ~25%. CP-116,517 reached sufficient inflammation-independent peak CSF concentrations that were up to 10 times above the MIC$_{90}$ for *Streptococcus pneumoniae*, regardless of the potential resistance to penicillin or cephalosporins. There are currently no human studies evaluating the CSF penetration of moxifloxacin, gatifloxacin, or gemifloxacin.

MICROBIOLOGY

The more common etiologic agents of bacterial meningitis are shown in Table X. The etiologic organisms differ depending on patient age. For example, *Listeria monocytogenes* and Group B *Streptococci* predominate in the neonatal period; *Streptococcus pneumoniae* and *Neisseria meningitidis* in the 1-month to 4-year age group; *N. meningitidis* in the 5- to 29-year group, and *S. pneumoniae* above 30 years [1]. Because of the introduction of the *Haemophilus influenzae* type b PRP and conjugate vaccine in the mid-1980s, the incidence of *H. influenzae* has dramatically decreased in children and is now an uncommon cause of meningitis [11,34].

TABLE X Etiologic Agents of Bacterial Meningitis in Adults (≥16 years)

Organism	Incidence (%)
Streptococcus pneumoniae	30–50
Neisseria menigitidis	10–35
Staphylococci	5–15
Gram-negative bacilli	1–10
Group B *Streptococcus*	5
Listeria monocytogenes	5
Haemophilus influenzae	1–3

Adapted from Roos *et al.* (1991) [49].

STUDIES OF CLINICAL EFFICACY

CASE REPORTS

The quinolones have been sporadically used in the management of bacterial meningitis. Their major role has been in the therapy of meningitis due to multidrug-resistant Gram-negative agents [10]. For example, a 78-year-old woman developed *Morganella morganii* meningitis after a laminectomy. She was treated with pefloxacin 800 mg intravenously every 12 hours for 7 days with prompt clinical response. She expired 2 days after finishing therapy, but autopsy studies revealed no bacteriological or histological evidence of meningitis [35]. In a second case, a 56-year-old man with *Pseudomonas aeruginosa* meningitis failed to respond to cefotaxime and gentamicin. He was then treated with intravenous ciprofloxacin (200 mg every 12 hr) and tobramycin (120 mg every 8 hr) and recovered fully after 14 days of therapy [36]. In a third case, a premature infant developed ventriculitis due to a multidrug-resistant *Pseudomonas aeruginosa* isolate that failed therapy with netilmicin and colistin. She was then treated with intravenous ciprofloxacin for 28 days and remained without recurrence during a 3-month follow-up period [37]. Furthermore, ciprofloxacin at a dose of 750 mg orally twice a day has been used successfully to prevent relapses in a patient with chronic *Pseudomonas* meningitis [10].

Ciprofloxacin has also been used sporadically to treat cases of neonatal Gram-negative bacillary meningitis [38–40]. Bhutta *et al.* [38] reported a 10-day-old baby with meningitis secondary to a multidrug-resistant *Salmonella paratyphi A*. After failing therapy with cefotaxime and tobramycin, he was treated with intravenous ciprofloxacin with prompt clinical response and had no neurologic sequela at 7-month follow-up. Green *et al.* [39] described two cases of neonatal meningitis, one due to *E. coli* and another caused by *Flavobacterium meningosepticum*. Both patients were treated successfully with intravenous ciprofloxacin and were without sequelae at discharge. Hansen *et al.* [40] described two additional cases of neonatal meningitis caused by *Salmonella* species. In conjunction with other antibiotics, ciprofloxacin was used in the therapy of one of the cases with good clinical response. The patient was free of neurological sequelae at 2-year follow-up.

CHEMOPROPHYLAXIS OF MENINGOCOCCAL MENINGITIS

The risk of meningococcal disease is up to 1000-fold higher among close (i.e., household, day-care, or nursery school) contacts of an index case than in the general population [14]. Rifampin has been most widely used for chemoprophylaxis in the United States but has some clear limitations [41]: failure to eradicate the carrier state in up to 10–25% of patients, development of rifampin resistance, contraindication in pregnancy, and the requirement for 2 days of administration.

There have been several studies evaluating the use of quinolones in eradication of the carrier state of *Neisseria meningitidis*. Pugsley *et al.* [42] enrolled 42 nasopharyngeal carriers of *Neisseria meningitidis* in a double-blind clinical trial, randomly assigning them to receive either 500 mg of ciprofloxacin or placebo every 12 hours for 5 days. All 21 patients in the ciprofloxacin group had negative nasopharyngeal cultures after the third day of therapy, in contrast to the placebo group, in whom 85% of subjects had a positive nasopharyngeal culture for *N. meningitidis* 1 week after finishing therapy. Renkonen *et al.* [43] studied 118 army recruits that were meningococcal carriers and randomly assigned them to receive either 250 mg of ciprofloxacin ($n = 61$) or placebo ($n = 59$) twice a day for 2 days. Meningococcal carriage was eliminated in 96% of subjects given ciprofloxacin and in 13% of those given placebo. After an outbreak of meningococcal meningitis at a naval base, ciprofloxacin was also found to be effective in eradicating meningococcal carriage [44]. Rifampin was initially given for chemoprophylaxis, but it was associated with a 26% failure rate. In the patients that continued to be culture-positive for meningococci, ciprofloxacin in a single oral dose of 500 mg succeeded in eradicating *N. meningitidis* from the pharynx of 97% of the 336 carriers sampled 48–96 hours later, and no persistent carriage was found in the group sampled 11 days later. Pugsley and colleagues [45] gave a single dose of 750 mg of ciprofloxacin to 12 nasopharyngeal carriers of *N. meningitidis*. Two weeks after the administration of ciprofloxacin, eradication of meningococci was documented in 11 subjects (i.e., 92% success rate).

Ofloxacin has also been evaluated in eradicating the nasopharyngeal carriage of *N. meningitidis* [46]. After an outbreak of serogroup B meningococcal disease in a college, 84 of 392 subjects (21%) were found to be carriers of *N. meningitidis*. Three days after receiving a single dose of 400 mg of ofloxacin, all 75 evaluable volunteers were culture-negative for *N. meningitidis*. At 1-month follow-up cultures, 69 of 75 (91.5%) remained culture-negative. No case of meningococcal disease occurred for 6 months.

More recently, ciprofloxacin (single oral dose of 750 mg) was compared to rifampin (600 mg orally twice a day for 2 days) and ceftriaxone (2 g intramuscularly) in a randomized clinical trial in Africa [47]. During an outbreak of meningococcal disease, a total of 1875 contacts were evaluated with nasopharyngeal cultures and randomized to receive either one of the three antibiotics. Those that had a positive nasopharyngeal culture for *Neisseria meningitidis* were evaluated for efficacy. As shown in Table XI, the eradication rates were similar for the three antibiotics, and none of the subjects developed meningococcal disease in the 2 weeks following chemoprophylaxis.

TABLE XI   Efficacy Analysis of Chemoprophylactic Agents Used to Treat Contacts of Persons
with Meningococcal Disease with Positive Nasopharyngeal Culture for *Neisseria meningitidis*

	Ciprofloxacin ($n = 79$)	Rifampicin ($n = 88$)	Ceftriaxone ($n = 41$)
Eradication at day 7 after treatment	88.6%	96.5%	95.1%
Eradication at day 14 after treatment	91.1%	97.7%	97.6%

Adapted from Cuevas *et al.* (1995) [47].

CLINICAL TRIAL OF TROVAFLOXACIN

The first quinolone to be evaluated in a comparative clinical efficacy trial in
patients with meningitis was trovafloxacin. Hopkins and colleagues conducted a
study in Nigeria during an epidemic of meningococcal meningitis [48]. Children
were randomly assigned to receive either trovafloxacin (3 mg/kg i.v. or p.o.) once
a day for 5 days or standard therapy with ceftriaxone (100 mg/kg i.m. or i.v. q.d.
× 5 days). Due to logistic constraints, approximately 80% of the patients assigned
to trovafloxacin received their full course as oral suspension or tablets. The results
are shown in Table XII. Trovafloxacin orally or intravenously was as effective
(90.3%) as ceftriaxone (89.7%) in the therapy of meningococcal meningitis. None
of the patients randomized to trovafloxacin required prolonged or changed
therapy. There were no discontinuations for adverse events and no relapses at 4-
to 6-week follow-up.

TABLE XII   Comparison of Oral or Intravenous Trovafloxacin Versus
Ceftriaxone in the Therapy of Epidemic Meningococcal Meningitis

	Trovafloxacin ($n = 93$)	Ceftriaxone ($n = 97$)
Cure	90.3%	89.7%
Cure with deficit	4.3%	4.1%
Death	5.4%	6.2%

Adapted from Hopkins *et al.* (1996) [48].

CONCLUSION

Bacterial meningitis continues to result in morbidity and mortality despite the availability of effective bactericidal antibiotic therapy. The emergence of antibiotic-resistant *Streptococcus pneumoniae* has further complicated the therapy of bacterial meningitis, prompting the development and use of new antimicrobials. The new fluorinated quinolones have important characteristics that make them potentially useful in the therapy of bacterial meningitis: excellent *in-vitro* activity against Gram-negative aerobic microorganisms, activity against penicillin and cephalosporin-resistant pneumococci, and reproducible cerebrospinal fluid penetration in animal models and in humans. The quinolones have been used in the management of bacterial meningitis due to multidrug-resistant Gram-negative agents, in chemoprophylaxis of contacts of patients with *Neisseria meningitidis* infections, and in the therapy of epidemic meningococcal meningitis in Africa. Despite this, the quinolones have been infrequently used in meningitis because the majority of cases occurred in the pediatric population, where quinolones have been relatively contraindicated. This practice will likely change as more clinical experience is reported with fluoroquinolones in children and adults.

REFERENCES

1. Quagliarello, V. J., and Scheld, W. M. (1997). Treatment of bacterial meningitis. *New Engl. J. Med.* **336**, 708–716.
2. Schech III, W. F., Ward, J. I., Band, J. D., *et al.* (1985). Bacterial meningitis in the United States, 1978 through 1981: The National Bacterial Meningitis Surveillance Study. *JAMA* **253**, 1749–1754.
3. Durand, M. L., Calderwood, S. B., Weber, D. J., *et al.* (1993). Acute bacterial meningitis in adults: A review of 493 episodes. *New Engl. J. Med.* **328**, 21–28.
4. Fitton, A. (1992). The Quinolones: An overview of their pharmacology. *Clin. Pharmacokin.* **22** (Suppl. 1), 1–11.
5. Visalli, M. A., Jacobs, M. R., and Appelbaum, P. C. (1996). Activity of CP 99,219 (trovafloxacin) compared with ciprofloxacin, sparfloxacin, clinafloxacin, lomefloxacin, and cefuroxime against ten penicillin-susceptible and penicillin-resistant pneumococci by time-kill methodology. *J. Antimicrob. Chemother.* **37**, 77–84.
6. Spangler, S. K., Jacobs, M. R., and Appelbaum, P. C. (1992). Susceptibilities of penicillin-susceptible and -resistant strains of *Streptococcus pneumoniae* to RP 59500, vancomycin, erythromycin, PD 131628, sparfloxacin, temafloxacin, Win 57273, ofloxacin, and ciprofloxacin. *Antimicrob. Agents Chemother.* **36**, 856–859.
7. Paris, M. M., Hickey, S. M., Trujilo, M., Shelton, S., and McCracken, G. H. (1995). Evaluation of CP 99,219, a new fluoroquinolone, for treatment of experimental penicillin and cephalosporin-resistant pneumococcal meningitis. *Antimicrob. Agents Chemother.* **39**, 1243–1246.

8. Gootz, T. D., Zaniewski, R., Haskell, S., *et al.* (1996). Activity of the new fluoroquinolone trovafloxacin (CP 99,219) against DNA-gyrase and topoisomerase IV mutants of *Streptococcus pneumoniae* selected *in vitro. Antimicrob. Agents Chemother.* **40**, 2691–2697.

9. Kim, Y. S., Liu, Q. X., Chen, L. L., and Tauber, M. G. (1997). Trovafloxacin in treatment of rabbits with experimental meningitis caused by high-level penicillin-resistant *Streptococcus pneumoniae. Antimicrob. Agents Chemother.* **41**, 1186–1189.

10. Norrby, S. R. (1988). 4-Quinolones in the treatment of infections of the central nervous system. *Rev. Infect. Dis.* **10** (Suppl.), S253–S255.

11. Schuchat, A., Robinson, K., Wenger, J. D., *et al.* (1997). Bacterial meningitis in the United States in 1995. *New Engl. J. Med.* **337**, 970–976.

12. Douibar, S. M., and Snodgrass, W. R. (1989). Potential role of fluoroquinolones in pediatric infection. *Rev. Infect. Dis.* **6**, 878–889.

13. Scheld, W. M., and Sande, M. A. (1983). Bactericidal versus bacteriostatic antibiotic therapy of experimental pneumococcal meningitis in rabbits. *J. Clin. Invest.* **71**, 411–419.

14. Scheld, W. M. (1989). Quinolone therapy for infections of the central nervous system. *Rev. Infect. Dis.* **11** (Suppl.), S1194–S1202.

15. Peterson, L. R. (1986). Animal models: The in-vivo evaluation of ciprofloxacin. *J. Antimicrob. Chemother.* **18** (Suppl. D), 55–64.

16. Gerberding, J. L., Brooks-Fournier, R. A., and Sande, M. A. (1987). Efficacy of ciprofloxacin in animal models of infection: Endocarditis, meningitis, and pneumonia. *Am. J. Med.* **82** (Suppl. 4A), 63–66.

17. Andriole, V. T. (1987). Efficacy of ciprofloxacin in animal models of infection. *Am. J. Med.* **82** (Suppl. 4A), 67–70.

18. Armengaud, M., Tran, V. T., and DiCostanzo, B. (1983). Study of pefloxacin diffusion into serum and CSF in the dog, both with healthy meninges and during experimental meningitis. *Abstr. 13th Int. Cong. Chemother.*, Vol. 5, 110/23-8.

19. Tho, T. V., Armengaud, A., and Davet, B. (1984). Diffusion of enoxacin into the cerebrospinal fluid in dogs with healthy meninges and with experimental meningitis. *J. Antimicrob. Chemother.* **14** (Suppl. Q), 57–62.

20. Shibl, A. M., Hackbarth, C. J., and Sande, M. A. (1986). Evaluation of pefloxacin in experimental *Escherichia coli* meningitis. *Antimicrob. Agents Chemother.* **29**, 409–411.

21. Hackbarth, C. J., Chambers, H. F., Stella, F., Shibl, A. M., and Sande, M. A. (1986). Ciprofloxacin in experimental *Pseudomonas aeruginosa* meningitis in rabbits. *J. Antimicrob. Chemother.* **18** (Suppl. D), 65–69.

22. Lutsar, I., Friedland, I. R., Wubbel, L., *et al.* (1998). Pharmacodynamics of gatifloxacin in cerebrospinal fluid in experimental cephalosporin-resistant pneumococcal meningitis. *Antimicrob. Agents Chemother.* **42**(10), 2650–2655.

23. Lutsar, I., Friedland, I. R., Hasan, S. J., *et al.* (1999). Efficacy of gatifloxacin in experimental *Escherichia coli* meningitis. *Antimicrob. Agents Chemother.* **43**(7), 1805–1807.

24. Lewandowski, T., Berry, V., De Marsch, P., *et al.* (1999). *In vivo* activity of gemifloxacin (SB-265805) in an infant rat meningitis model with *Streptococcus pneumoniae. Abstr. 39th Intersci. Conf. Antimicrob. Agents Chemother.*, San Francisco. Abstr. #1789.

25. Schmidt, H., Dalhoff, A., Stuertz, K., *et al.* (1998). Moxifloxacin in the therapy of experimental pneumococcal meningitis. *Antimicrob. Agents Chemother.* **42**(6), 1397–1401.

26. Østergaard, C., Klitmoller-Sorensen, T., Knudsen, J. D., *et al.* (1998). Evaluation of moxifloxacin, a new 8-methoxyquinolone, for treatment of meningitis caused by a penicillin-resistant pneumococcus in rabbits. *Antimicrob. Agents Chemother.* **42**(7), 1706–1712.

27. Wolff, M., Regnier, B.. Daldoss, C., Nkam, M., and Vachon, F. (1984). Penetration of pefloxacin into cerebrospinal fluid of patients with meningitis. *Antimicrob. Agents Chemother.* **26**, 289–291.

28. Dow, J., Chazal, J., Frydman, A. M., *et al.* (1986). Transfer kinetics of pefloxacin into cerebrospinal fluid after one hour i.v. infusion of 400-mg in man. *J. Antimicrob. Chemother.* **17** (Suppl. B), 81–87.

29. Stahl, J. P., Croize, J., Lefebvre, M. A., *et al.* (1986). Diffusion of ofloxacin into the cerebrospinal fluid in patients with bacterial meningitis. *Infection* (Suppl. 4), pp. S254–S255.

30. Stubner, G., Weinrich, W., and Brands, U. (1986). Study of the cerebrospinal fluid penetrability of ofloxacin. *Infection* (Suppl. 4), pp. S250–S253.

31. Wolff, M., Boutron, L., Singles, E., *et al.* (1987). Penetration of ciprofloxacin into cerebrospinal fluid of patients with bacterial meningitis. *Antimicrob. Agents Chemother.* **31**, 899–902.

32. Kitzes-Cohen, R., Miler, A., Gibboa, A., and Harel, D. (1988). Penetration of ciprofloxacin into the cerebrospinal fluid. *Rev. Infect. Dis.* **10**, S256–S257.

33. Arguedas-Mohs, A., Vargas, S. L., Bradley, J. S., *et al.* (1997). Trovafloxacin CSF penetration and pharmacokinetics in children. *Abstr. 37th Intersci. Conf. Antimicrob. Agents Chemother.*, Toronto. Abstr. #A105.

34. Adams, W. G., Deaver, K. A., Cochi, S. L., *et al.* (1993). Decline of childhood *Haemophilus influenzae* type b (Hib) disease in the Hib vaccine era. *JAMA* **269**, 221–226.

35. Isaacs, R. D., and Ellis-Pegler, R. B. (1987). Successful treatment of *Morganella morganii* meningitis with pefloxacin mesylate [letter]. *J. Antimicrob. Chemother.* **20**, 769–770.

36. Millar, M. R., Bransby-Zachary, M. A., Tompkins, D. S., *et al.* (1986). Ciprofloxacin for *Pseudomonas aeruginosa* meningitis. *Lancet*, p. 1325.

37. Isaacs, D., Slack, M. P. E., Wilkinson, A. R., and Westwood, A. W. (1986). Successful treatment for *Pseudomonas* ventriculitis with ciprofloxacin. *J. Antimicrob. Chemother.* **17**, 535–538.

38. Bhutta, Z., Farooqui, B., and Sturm, W. (1992). Eradication of a multiple drug resistant *Salmonella paratyphi* A causing meningitis with ciprofloxacin. *J. Infect.* **25**, 215–219.

39. Green, S. D. R., Ilunga, F., Cheesbrough, J. S., *et al.* (1993). The treatment of neonatal meningitis due to Gram-negative bacilli with ciprofloxacin: Evidence of satisfactory penetration into the cerebrospinal fluid. *J. Infect.* **26**, 253–256.

40. Hansen, L. N., Eschen, C., and Bruun, B. (1996). Neonatal salmonella meningitis: Two case reports. *Acta Paediatr.* **85**, 629–631.

41. Apicella, M. A. (1995). *Neisseria meningitidis*. In "Principle and Practice of Infectious Diseases," 4th ed. (G. L. Mandell, J. E. Bennett, and R. Dolin, eds.), p. 189.

42. Pugsley, M. P., Dworzack, D. L., Horowitz, E. A., *et al.* (1987). Efficacy of ciprofloxacin in the treatment of nasopharyngeal carriers of *Neisseria meningitidis*. *J. Infect. Dis* **156**, 211–213.

43. Renkonen, O., Sivonen, A., and Visakorpi, R. (1987). Effect of ciprofloxacin on carrier state of *Neisseria meningitidis* in army recruits in Finland. *Antimicrob. Agents Chemother.* **31**, 962–963.

44. Gaunt, P. N., and Lambert, B. E. (1988). Single-dose ciprofloxacin for eradication of pharyngeal carriage of *Neisseria meningitidis*. *J. Antimicrob. Chemother.* **21**, 489–496.

45. Pugsley, M. P., Dworzack, D. L., Roccaforte, J. S., *et al.* (1988). An open study of the efficacy of a single dose of ciprofloxacin in eliminating the chronic nasopharyngeal carriage of *Neisseria meningitidis*. *J. Infect. Dis.* **157**, 852–853.

46. Gilja, O. H., Halstensen, A., Digranes, A., *et al.* (1993). Use of single-dose ofloxacin to eradicate tonsillopharyngeal carriage of *Neisseria meningitidis*. *Antimicrob. Agents Chemother.* **37**, 2024–2026.

47. Cuevas, L. E., Kazembe, P., Mughoho, G. K., *et al.* (1995). Eradication of nasopharyngeal carriage of *Neisseria meningitidis* in children and adults in rural Africa: A comparison of ciprofloxacin and rifampicin. *J. Infect. Dis.* **171**, 728–731.

48. Hopkins, S., Williams, D., Dunne, M., *et al.* (1996). A randomized controlled trial of oral or intravenous trovafloxacin versus ceftriaxone in the treatment of epidemic meningococcal meningitis. *Abstr. 36th Intersci. Conf. Antimicrob. Agents Chemother.*, New Orleans. Abstr. #LB21.

49. Roos, K. L., Tunkel, A. R., and Scheld, W. M. (1991). Acute bacterial meningitis in children and adults. In "Infections of the Central Nervous System" (W. M. Scheld, R. J. Whitley, and D. T. Durack, eds.), pp. 335–409. Raven, New York.

50. Pfaller, M. A., Jones, G. V., Doern, H. S., *et al.* (1999). Survey of blood stream infections attributable to Gram-positive cocci: Frequency of occurrence and antimicrobial susceptibility of isolates collected in 1997 in the United States, Canada, and Latin America from the SENTRY antimicrobial surveillance program. *Diag. Microbiol. Infect. Dis.* **33**, 283–297.

51. Oldland, B. A., Jones, R. N., Verhoef, J., *et al.* (1999). Antimicrobial activity of gatifloxacin 9AM- 1155, CG5501), and four other fluoroquinolones tested against 2,284 recent clinical strains of *Streptococcus pneumoniae* from Europe, Latin America, Canada, and the United States. *Diag. Microbiol. Infect. Dis.* **34**, 315–320.

52. de la Fuente, L., Gimenez, M. J., and Mahadahonda, L. A. (2000). In vitro activity of gemifloxacin and 13 other antimicrobials against 400 Spanish isolates of *Neisseria meningitides* collected between 1998 and 1999. *Abstr. 3rd Eur. Cong. Chemother.*, Madrid.

53. Blondaeau, J. M. (1999). A review of the comparative in-vitro activities of 12 antimicrobial agents, with a focus on five new "respiratory quinolones." *J. Antimicrob. Chemother.* **43** (Suppl. B), 1–11.

54. Barry, A. L., Fuchs, P. C., and Brown, S. D. (1999). Antibacterial activity of moxifloxacin (Bay 12-8039) against aerobic clinical isolates, and provisional criteria for disk susceptibility tests. *Eur. J. Clin. Microbiol. Infect. Dis.* **18**, 305–309.

55. Hoellman, D. B., Lin, G., Jacobs, M. R., and Appelbaum, P. C. (1999). Anti-pneumococcal activity of gatifloxacin compared with other quinolone and non-quinolone agents. *J. Antimicrob. Chemother.* **43**, 645–649.

CHAPTER 12

Use of the Quinolones in Immunocompromised Patients

KENNETH V. I. ROLSTON

Department of Internal Medicine Specialties, Section of Infectious Diseases,
The University of Texas, M. D. Anderson Cancer Center, Houston, Texas 77030

INTRODUCTION

Patients who are unable to resist infection in a normal manner owing to impaired host defenses are referred to as being immunocompromised. With each passing year, the number of patients who are immunocompromised, and consequently at increased risk for infection, continues to rise. The reasons for this increase are varied and include an aging population in whom chronic and/or neoplastic disorders are common; the use of intensive antineoplastic regimens designed to achieve maximal antitumor effect, which also cause substantial and prolonged impairment of host defenses; the ever-expanding role in modern medicine of procedures such as solid organ and bone marrow transplantation, which often require the prolonged use of immunosuppressive therapy; and substantial numbers of patients with acquired immunodeficiency syndrome (AIDS), particularly in developing countries, where treatment options such as highly active antiretroviral therapy (HAART) are limited. Bacterial infections are particularly common in patients with severe (<100 PMN/mm^3) and prolonged (>14 days) neutropenia, in whom they are a major cause of morbidity and mortality [1]. Over the past three decades, substantial progress has been made in the management of these infections, including the development of strategies for infection prevention and the use of empiric antibiotics [2]. The profile of the newer quinolones includes improved antibacterial, pharmacokinetic, and safety features that make them an important part of the armamentarium available to clinicians who treat immuno-compromised patients [3]. This chapter will review the current spectrum of bacterial infections in immunosuppressed patients and discuss the role of the quinolones in infection prevention, empiric antimicrobial therapy, the treatment of specific infections, and the use of sequential (i.v. → p.o.) or oral antimicrobial regimens in moderate-to-low risk febrile neutropenic patients.

RISK FACTORS AND ASSOCIATED INFECTIONS

The risk and spectrum of infection differ considerably in various subsets of immunocompromised patients, and they depend on the specific defect in host defenses that is present in a particular individual [4]. Neutropenia is the factor that most frequently predisposes cancer patients to infection [5]. Although some hematologic malignancies and/or myelodysplastic disorders cause neutropenia, it occurs most often as the result of antineoplastic chemotherapy. The degree and duration of neutropenia are both important factors that influence the frequency and severity of infection. The risk of infection bears an inverse relationship to the neutrophil count and begins to increase only when the neutrophil count falls below 1000/mm^3 [5]. Most serious infections including bacteremias develop in patients with severe and prolonged neutropenia, and virtually every patient with a neutrophil count ≤100/ml for more than 2 weeks will develop an infection. Currently, Gram-positive cocci cause approximately 50–70% of documented bacterial infections in febrile neutropenic patients, with coagulase-negative *Staphylococcus* spp., *Staphylococcus aureus*, viridans streptococci, and the enterococci being the most commonly isolated species (Table I). Enteric bacilli such as *Escherichia coli*, *Klebsiella* spp., and *Pseudomonas aeruginosa* are still the most common Gram-negative isolates, but *Enterobacter* spp., *Citrobacter* spp., *Stenotrophomonas maltophilia*, and *Acinetobacter* spp. have emerged as

TABLE I   The Spectrum of Bacterial Infections in
Immunocompromised Patients

Neutropenia

Common Gram-positive organisms
Coagulase-negative *Staphylococci*
Staphylococcus aureus
α-hemolytic (*viridans*) *Streptococci*
Enterococcus spp. (including VRE)
Corynebacterium jeikeiium
Micrococcus spp.

Uncommon Gram-positive organisms
Bacillus spp.
Streptococcus pneumoniae
β-hemolytic *Streptococci* (Groups A, B, C, G, F)
Stomatococcus mucilaginous
Leuconostoc spp.
Listeria monocytogenes
Rhodococcus equi

Common Gram-negative organisms
Escherichia coli
Pseudomonas aeruginosa
Enterobacter spp.
Citrobacter spp.
Proteus spp.
Stenotrophomonas aeruginosa
Acinetobacter spp.

Uncommon Gram-negative organisms
Pseudomonas spp. (not *aeruginosa*)
Flavobacterium meningosepticum
Flavimonas oryzihabitans
Serratia marcescens
Alcaligenes spp.
Aeromonas spp.

Cellular immune dysfunction

Listeria monocytogenes
Legionella spp.
Mycobacteria (tuberculosis and nontuberculosis)
Nocardia spp.
Salmonella spp.
Rhodococcus equi

Humoral immune dysfunction

Streptococcus pneumoniae
Hemophilus influenzae

---

important pathogens as well [6]. The frequency of certain organisms including *P. aeruginosa* can vary from institution to institution, and it is important to be aware of the specific spectrum of infection in one's own institution when designing empiric antimicrobial regimens [7].

Cell-mediated immunity plays a primary role in protection against intracellular pathogens. T-lymphocytes also have an impact on other aspects of immune function, including regulation of B-lymphocyte function. Patients with defects in cellular immunity (Hodgkin's disease or non-Hodgkin's lymphoma, AIDS, corticosteroid administration, fludarabine therapy) often develop infections caused by mycobacteria, *Salmonella* spp., *Legionella* spp., *Listeria monocytogenes*, *Rhodococcus* spp., and *Nocardia* [4,8,9].

Defects in humoral immunity are present in patients with multiple myeloma, Waldenström's macroglobulinemia, the various "heavy-chain" diseases, and chronic lymphocytic leukemia. These patients are especially susceptible to infections caused by encapsulated organisms such as *Hemophilus influenzae* and *Streptococcus pneumoniae*. The emergence of penicillin resistance among isolates of *S. pneumoniae* (40–60% of isolates in some reports) is of considerable concern and has created the need for alternative agents with reliable activity against such isolates [10,11].

Recipients of solid organ or bone marrow transplantation who are on chronic immunosuppressive therapy and patients with AIDS have many more global immunological deficits and are susceptible to infection with a wide spectrum of microorganisms. Surgically implanted central venous catheters are utilized extensively in patients who require frequent and prolonged vascular access. These catheters greatly facilitate overall patient management but are associated with bacterial and, occasionally, fungal infections. Patients who have undergone splenectomy, such as those with Hodgkin's diseases, are at risk of developing infections caused by *S. pneumoniae*, *H. influenzae*, *Neisseria meningitidis*, *Babesia*, and *Capnocytophaga*. Some of these infections can be extremely severe and rapidly fatal if not recognized and treated promptly. Finally, local factors such as tumor metastases that produce obstruction and operative procedures that result in disruption of normal anatomic barriers play an important role in infections occurring in immunocompromised patients with cancer.

RATIONALE FOR FLUOROQUINOLONE USE

The fluoroquinolones possess several properties that make them attractive agents for use in immunocompromised patients. These include a broad antimicrobial spectrum providing coverage against the Enterobacteriaceae, *P. aeruginosa*, and other *Pseudomonas* species, *Acinetobacter*, *Legionella*, *Flavobacterium menin-*

gosepticium, and even moderate activity against *Stenotrophomonas maltophilia* [12]. The newer-generation quinolones possess greater activity against many Gram-positive pathogens (e.g., the staphylococci, streptococci, *Bacillus* spp., *L. monocytogenes*, and *Corynebacterium jeikeium*) than earlier-generation agents [13–15]. The fluoroquinolones also have activity against *Mycobacterium tuberculosis*, *M. kansasii*, *M. fortuitum*, and *M. avium-intracellulare complex* [16–20]. Most fluoroquinolones have good absorption from the gastrointestinal tract and favorable pharmacokinetics, including good tissue penetration, and accumulation in human macrophages and polymorphonuclear leukocytes, which makes them effective against intracellular pathogens such as *Salmonella*, *Legionella*, and Mycobacteria [21]. The fluoroquinolones have unique mechanisms of action (inhibition of bacterial DNA gyrase and topoisomerase IV) that confer bactericidal activity against many microorganisms and make cross-resistance with other antimicrobial agents less likely [22,23]. They also have a good safety profile and, with few exceptions, are generally well tolerated. Finally, several fluoroquinolones are available for parenteral and oral administration and possess bioequivalence, which makes them more convenient to use than agents available for only parenteral or oral administration, or for whom dosage alterations are necessary when switching from parenteral to oral administration.

EFFECT OF FLUOROQUINOLONES ON ENDOGENOUS MICROFLORA

The effect of the fluoroquinolones on the endogenous microflora of humans has been the subject of extensive study. The quinolones exhibit a selective suppressive effect on the intestinal microflora [24]. The aerobic Gram-negative bacteria are most strongly suppressed by ciprofloxacin, ofloxacin, and norfloxacin, with reduction in colony counts of up to 4–7 log per gram of feces within 3–5 days of starting therapy. On discontinuation of therapy, a return to baseline values occurs within 7–14 days. The aerobic Gram-positive intestinal microflora are influenced less than the aerobic Gram-negative flora, with a moderate decrease in colony counts of enterococcal and staphylococcal isolates. Norfloxacin administration does not have an effect on the anaerobic microflora, and only a slight suppression occurs as a result of administration of ciprofloxacin or ofloxacin. Newer agents such as gemifloxacin also have selective effects on human intestinal microflora and do not cause significant disturbances of the anaerobic flora compared to agents such as clinafloxacin and trovafloxacin, which do [25–27]. The fecal concentrations of most fluoroquinolones are very high and far exceed the minimal inhibitory concentrations for most aerobic and anaerobic bacteria. The discrepancy between the expected effect of these agents based on *in-vitro* activity and high fecal concentrations, and their actual suppressive effect on the fecal flora, can be explained by the mechanisms of inoculum effect and fecal binding of quinolones [24]. The effect of the fluoroquinolones on human oropharyngeal flora is less well studied, and the results have often been contradictory.

INFECTION PREVENTION IN AFEBRILE NEUTROPENIC PATIENTS

Because persistent and profound neutropenia is a consistent marker for the development of serious bacterial infections, one approach for infection prevention has been administration of antimicrobial prophylaxis to such patients. The rationale for this approach is to try and suppress the endogenous intestinal microflora (from which the majority of infections arise) and prevent acquisition of and colonization with potential pathogens from the immediate environment [28]. Some investigators consider elimination of the aerobic flora and preservation of the normal anaerobic intestinal microflora (selective decontamination) to be particularly important because of the ability of anaerobes to prevent colonization with potentially pathogenic aerobes (referred to as "colonization resistance"), probably due to competition for nutrients in the gut [29–31]. Older prophylactic regimens using nonabsorbable drugs (aminoglycosides or polymyxin + vancomycin + nystatin) were shown to suppress the aerobic gastrointestinal flora and reduce the incidence of infection in neutropenic patients in several prospective randomized trials [32–34]. However, compliance with these regimens was poor because of the high frequency of gastrointestinal side effects, and they have largely been replaced by better-tolerated and more effective regimens.

Current choices for antimicrobial prophylaxis include the use of oral absorbable drugs like trimethoprim–sulfamethoxazole (TMP–SMX) and the fluoroquinolones. Trimethoprim–sulfamethazole does significantly lower infection rates compared to placebo-treated control subjects, but does not have a significant impact on overall survival [35–37]. It also provides protection against *Pneumocystis carinii* pneumonia [38]. However, it is inactive against *P. aeruginosa*, is myelosuppressive in some patients, frequently produces cutaneous rashes, and its use can lead to the development of resistant bacterial and fungal overgrowth [2].

The fluoroquinolones norfloxacin, ciprofloxacin, ofloxacin, and pefloxacin have been used extensively for prophylaxis in neutropenic patients. Studies comparing fluoroquinolones to TMP–SMX suggest that the quinolones are equal to or better than TMP–SMX as prophylactic agents [39,40]. Among the quinolones, norfloxacin is less effective than the other agents, probably due to poorer absorption and systemic bioavailability [41,42]. Most studies evaluating quinolone prophylaxis have demonstrated significantly fewer Gram-negative bacillary infections, but no difference, or occasionally an increase, in Gram-positive infections. Combinations of quinolones with penicillin, rifampin, or macrolide antibiotics may significantly reduce the development of Gram-positive bacteremias, particularly those due to streptococci [43–46]. However, they do not appear to reduce overall morbidity in neutropenic patients [47,48].

Chemoprophylaxis with the fluoroquinolones is better tolerated than that with oral nonabsorbable agents or TMP–SMX. Gastrointestinal side effects are infrequent in patients receiving fluoroquinolone prophylaxis, and the frequency of skin rashes and myelosuppression in significantly less than with TMP–SMX [2].

Of concern in patients receiving fluoroquinolone chemoprophylaxis is the development of resistant Gram-negative bacilli such as E. coli, P. aeruginosa, and non-aeruginosa Pseudomonas species [49–54]. Pneumocystis carinii pneumonia may also develop in patients at risk for this infection who are given quinolone chemoprophylaxis. Another potential drawback is that the quinolones have not been licensed for use in infants and children, due to the potential (primarily observed in animals) for producing cartilage erosions in weight-bearing joints [55]. However, growing experience with the compassionate use of these agents in children and their use in patients with cystic fibrosis suggests that their administration in the pediatric population is safe [56,57].

A two-part metaanalysis was conducted to assess the effectiveness of the fluoroquinolones for infection prevention in neutropenic patients [58]. The results of the first part indicate that these agents alone significantly reduce the incidence of Gram-negative infections but not that of Gram-positive infections, and they do not have a significant impact on fever-related morbidity or infection-related mortality. The results of the second part indicate that a combination of fluoroquinolones and agents with Gram-positive activity (penicillin, macrolides) significantly reduces the occurrence of Gram-positive bacteremia, without affecting the incidence of morbidity or mortality due to infection.

Another metaanalysis of quinolone-based chemoprophylaxis in neutropenic patients conducted for the Immunocompromised Host Society examined the role of quinolone prophylaxis versus placebo, and quinolone prophylaxis versus other antimicrobials. In both analyses, there was an overwhelming reduction in aerobic Gram-negative infections. There was no reduction in Gram-positive infections unless the quinolones were used in combination with other antibiotics. Quinolone prophylaxis was associated with a trend toward higher risk for invasive fungal infections (an observation that needs confirmation), and had fewer side effects than other regimens, but no more than placebo (Coleman Rotstein, personal communication, 1999).

The benefits of quinolone prophylaxis must be weighed against the potential disadvantages. Newer fluoroquinolones (e.g., gatifloxacin, moxifloxacin), which

are more potent against many Gram-positive isolates, retain adequate Gram-negative activity, and have longer half-lives, which makes once-daily administration
possible, might be more suitable and convenient than agents such as ofloxacin,
levofloxacin, or ciprofloxacin, and need to be evaluated for this indication in
well-designed comparative clinical trials. The Infectious Diseases Society of
America does not recommend routine use of quinolone prophylaxis, but suggests
that it be used only in high-risk patients with profound and prolonged neutropenia,
for as short a period as possible, in order to derive maximum benefit and limit
the emergence of resistance [2,54].

Infections caused by *S. pneumoniae* are relatively common in patients who
have undergone splenectomy, those with multiple myeloma and acute or chronic
lymphocytic leukemia, and allogeneic bone marrow transplant recipients [4]. The
syndrome of overwhelming pneumococcal sepsis that is frequently associated
with disseminated intravascular coagulation, and often follows a fulminant course
resulting in death, is seen primarily in such patients. Consequently, it was
recommended that these high-risk patients be given a personal supply of an
antibiotic with anti-pneumococcal activity (e.g., amoxicillin/clavulanate), so that
they might initiate preemptive therapy at the first sign of infection, prior to
seeking medical attention. In our experience, this practice has been lifesaving on
many occasions. With current rates of penicillin resistance running around 20%
(higher in some communities), the usefulness of this strategy has been impacted.
The newer-generation quinolones (i.e., levofloxacin, sparfloxacin, gatifloxacin,
gemifloxacin, and moxifloxacin) are the only oral agents with reliable activity
against these organisms [11]. Their use in this setting instead of a penicillin
derivative might be prudent but has not been fully evaluated.

EMPIRIC THERAPY IN FEBRILE
NEUTROPENIC PATIENTS

Standard management of the febrile neutropenic patient consists of prompt
administration of parenteral, broad-spectrum, empiric antibiotic therapy [59]. This
is usually achieved by using combinations (aminoglycoside + β-lactam, vancomycin + β-lactam) or selected broad-spectrum agents (extended-spectrum cephalosporins, carbapenems) as monotherapy [2]. The role of the fluoroquinolones in
empiric therapy has been limited owing to their widespread use as prophylactic
agents. However, susceptibility surveillance studies among Gram-negative bacilli
isolated from cancer patients continue to demonstrate low levels of fluoroquinolone resistance despite extensive clinical use [60]. Several studies have
examined the therapeutic role of the quinolones (primarily ciprofloxacin) used

both as monotherapy and in combination with other antimicrobial agents in febrile neutropenic patients.

Initial experience with parenteral ciprofloxacin (200 mg q 8 hr) monotherapy in 30 neutropenic patients, including several with pneumonia and bacteremia, was associated with a 73% response rate, and demonstrated this quinolone's potential as a therapeutic agent [61]. An early study comparing ceftazidime and ciprofloxacin monotherapy revealed comparable response rates (64% for ceftazidime vs. 71% for ciprofloxacin) and similar times to defervescence for both regimens [62]. Gram-positive bacterial superinfections were more common in patients treated with ciprofloxacin. More recent studies of ciprofloxacin monotherapy have shown both favorable and unfavorable results [63–65]. In the European Organization for Research and Treatment of Cancer (EORTC) prospective randomized trial comparing ciprofloxacin monotherapy and combination therapy with piperacillin plus amikacin in neutropenic patients with lymphoma and solid tumors, the overall success rate with ciprofloxacin (65%) was lower than for the combination regimen (91%, $p = 0.002$), primarily because of poor responses to ciprofloxacin in patients with Gram-positive bacteremia [65]. With Gram-positive organisms now accounting for 50–75% of documented bacterial infections in febrile neutropenic patients, and with many of these organisms being resistant or only moderately susceptible to the quinolones, quinolone monotherapy cannot be recommended as routine initial empiric therapy. However, newer-generation quinolones with adequate Gram-negative activity and enhanced potency against Gram-positive organisms (e.g., gatifloxacin, gemifloxacin, moxifloxacin) might be suitable for monotherapy, particularly in low-risk, febrile, neutropenic patients [15,66,67]. Clinical trials evaluating their therapeutic potential need to be conducted.

Various quinolone-based combination regimens have been evaluated in febrile neutropenic patients with moderate success (Table II). Many of these studies have enrolled relatively few patients, and no firm conclusions can be drawn from them. Ciprofloxacin in combination with vancomycin was administered as initial therapy for febrile neutropenic patients and resulted in an overall response rate of 77% [68]. Ciprofloxacin and pefloxacin have also been used successfully in combination with teicoplanin [69,70]. In another study, ciprofloxacin plus netilmicin was found to be as effective as piperacillin plus netilmicin overall, but the ciprofloxacin regimen was significantly better (86% response rate) than the piperacillin regimen (43% response rate) for Gram-negative bacteremia [71]. In both these studies, it was possible to change from intravenous to orally administered ciprofloxacin after approximately 1 week of therapy. Ciprofloxacin in combination with azlocillin has also been used effectively as initial therapy [72,73]. In another trial, ciprofloxacin combined with benzyl-penicillin was compared to a standard regimen of netilmicillin combined with piperacillin [74]. The overall clinical response rates at the end of therapy were very similar (66 vs.

TABLE II   Efficacy of Fluoroquinolones as Empiric Therapy in Febrile Neutropenic Patients

Reference	Drug(s)	No. of patients[a]	Documented infections		Overall response rate (%)
			Gram+	Gram−	
[61]	Ciprofloxacin	147 (30)	24	18	78
[62]	Ciprofloxacin	21	7	0	71
	vs.				
	Ceftazidime	25	9	8	64
[74]	Ciprofloxacin + benzylpenicillin	50	17	11	66
	vs.				
	Netilmicin + piperacillin	46	16	7	65
[72]	Ciprofloxacin + azlocillin	25	5	4	92[b]
	vs.				
	Ceftazidime + amikacin	54	7	10	92[b]
[65]	Ciprofloxacin	48	8	4	65
	vs.				
	Piperacillin vs. amikacin	53	7	7	91

[a]Number in parentheses represents the numbers of patients that were neutropenic.
[b]Response rates with modification of original regimens.

65%). However, the investigators pointed out that, although streptococci accounted for 18% of isolated pathogens treated with ciprofloxacin plus benzylpenicillin, there were no treatment failures or superinfections with these organisms, indicating a potential advantage for this combination.

On the basis on the aforementioned studies and accumulated clinical experience, combination regimens that include a fluoroquinolone are effective as initial therapy in febrile neutropenic patients. However, they have not been evaluated as thoroughly as other standard regimens and should probably be considered "second-line" regimens. Local quinolone susceptibility patterns should be taken into consideration at individual institutions, and their use as initial therapy should occur primarily in patients who have not been given quinolone chemoprophylaxis.

RISK-BASED THERAPY FOR FEBRILE NEUTROPENIA

Although it has been recognized for some time that the risk for developing infection and complications differs substantially in subsets of febrile neutropenic patients, our ability to predict risk early during the course of a febrile episode has been limited. Only in the 1990s did it become possible to stratify such patients into well-defined risk groups [75,76]. Researchers at the Dana Farber Cancer Institute developed and validated a risk prediction model that accurately identified the medical risk among febrile neutropenic patients using only clinical information available at the onset of the febrile episode. Groups 1–3 were considered high- to moderate-risk patients and were associated with substantial morbidity and mortality. These were primarily hospitalized patients with hematologic malignancies (group 1); outpatients with comorbidity factors such as hypotension, respiratory failure, altered mental status, cord compression, dehydration, and so forth (group 2); and outpatients with unresponsive tumors (group 3). Group 4 consisted of clinically stable outpatients (responsive tumors and no comorbidity) who rarely (3%) developed serious complications and in whom no mortality occurred. These are considered low-risk patients and account for approximately 40% of febrile episodes seen at large cancer centers. The Multinational Association for Supportive Care in Cancer (MASCC) has validated statistically derived risk-prediction rules and has developed the numerical MASCC risk index [77]. Other investigators have used simple clinical criteria in order to select low-risk neutropenic patients, and several clinical trials have now been conducted in evaluating such strategies as

- Hospital-based oral antibiotic therapy

- Initial hospital-based parenteral therapy followed by oral therapy at home (sequential or switch therapy)

- Parenteral, sequential, or oral, outpatient antibiotic therapy

The availability of the newer quinolones has been largely responsible for the success of many of these newer treatment options.

Early clinical experience at the University of Texas M. D. Anderson Cancer Center using oral ciprofloxacin (750 mg every 8 hours) for hospitalized, febrile, nonneutropenic cancer patients was associated with an overall response rate of 85% [78]. In another trial, Malik *et al.* compared oral ofloxacin (400 mg twice daily) to various parenteral combinations (amikacin + carbenicillin, piperacillin, or cloxacillin) for initial therapy of hospitalized febrile neutropenic patients [79]. Response rates with oral ofloxacin were similar to those achieved with combination regimens (53% each). Two published large multicenter trials have provided confirmation that in hospitalized low-risk patients who have fever and neutropenia, oral therapy with quinolone-based regimens (ciprofloxacin plus amoxicillin–clavulanate) is as safe and effective as standard intravenous therapy [80,81]. The equivalence of oral and parenteral therapy has significant implications for the management of febrile neutropenic patients, particularly in countries with limited resources. In the United States, however, hospital-based oral antibiotic therapy will probably not be widely used.

The availability of broad-spectrum oral quinolones has also enabled clinicians to switch febrile neutropenic patients from parenteral to oral regimens after an initial period of stabilization and to discharge them earlier then was previously possible [69,70,82,83]. Patients who are stable enough for early discharge but are unable to tolerate oral therapy because of local factors such as mucositis can be treated with parenteral quinolone-based regimens in an ambulatory setting.

The final step in the evolution of risk-based therapy for febrile neutropenia was evaluation of outpatient therapy in low-risk patients using quinolone monotherapy or quinolone-based combination regimens. Several of these trials are summarized in Table III. Combination oral regimens such as ciprofloxacin or pefloxacin + amoxicillin/clavulanate or ciprofloxacin + clindamycin have been associated with response rates ranging from 87 to 90% [84–86]. Although quinolone monotherapy has also been successfully used in this setting, the current predominance of Gram-positive pathogens in febrile neutropenic patients necessitates the provision of better Gram-positive coverage than currently available quinolones can provide, and combination therapy is the more prudent approach [82,87,88]. Newer quinolones with more potent Gram-positive and Gram-negative activity (e.g., gatifloxacin, moxifloxacin) might be more suitable for monotherapy, and await clinical evaluation.

Despite considerable experience with outpatient therapy for febrile neutropenia, there is some reluctance among clinicians to accept this as a standard of care [89]. The obvious advantages of outpatient therapy include ease of administration, vastly reduced cost of therapy, a reduction in superinfections caused by resistant hospital microflora, improved quality of life, and better utilization of valuable and expensive resources [82,90]. Potential disadvantages include possible noncompliance with oral therapy and development of serious complications (septic shock, hemorrhage) in a relatively unsupervised environment. However, a more recent report issued by the Institute of Medicine indicates that the hospital is not necessarily a safe environment and should provide a strong impetus for outpatient management, particularly in low-risk patients. Careful patient selection and monitoring for lack of response or development of side-effects are key elements for the success of these newer strategies.

TREATMENT OF SPECIFIC INFECTIONS

LEGIONELLOSIS

Infections caused by *Legionella pneumophila* and other *Legionella* species are more common in, but not limited to, immunocompromised patients. Treatment strategies for legionellosis continue to evolve, with older agents such as erythro-

TABLE III Fluoroquinolone Based Empiric Oral Therapy in Cancer Patients with Chemotherapy Induced Neutropenia

Reference	Regimen(s)[a]	No. of patients	Overall response rate (%)[b]	Comments
[78][a]	Ciprofloxacin (750 mg q 8 hr)	46	85%	Nonrandomized inpatient study of oral therapy. Only 8% of patients neutropenic.
[80]	Ciprofloxacin (30 mg/kg, q 8 hr) + amoxicillin/clavulanate (40 mg/kg, q 8 hr) vs. i.v. ceftazidime (90 mg/kg, q 8 hr)	116	71%	Randomized, double-blind, placebo controlled inpatient comparison of oral and parenteral regimens in low-risk patients.
		116	67%	
[81]	Ciprofloxacin (750 mg b.i.d.) + amoxicillin/clavulanate (650 mg t.i.d.) vs. i.v. ceftriaxone (2 g, once daily) + i.v. amikacin (20 mg/kg, once daily)	177	86%	Prospective open-label, multicenter, inpatient comparison of oral and parenteral regimens in low-risk patients.
		176	84%	
[84]	Pefloxacin (400 mg b.i.d.) + amoxicillin/clavulanate (500/125 mg t.i.d.)	68	87%	Nonrandomized, self-administered outpatient therapy. No risk-assessment performed.
[79]	Ofloxacin (400 mg b.i.d.) vs. parenteral antibiotic combinations	60	53%	Inpatient comparative trial of oral vs. parenteral therapy. Not limited to low-risk patients.
		62	53%	
[87]	Ofloxacin (400 mg b.i.d.)	111	83%	Nonrandomized, self-administered outpatient therapy.
[86]	Ciprofloxacin (750 mg q 8 hr) + clindamycin (600 mg q 8 hr) vs. i.v. aztreonam (2 g q 8 hr) + i.v. clindamycin (600 mg q 8 hr)	40	88%	Prospective randomized comparison of outpatient oral and parenteral empiric therapy in low-risk febrile neutropenic patients.
		43	95%	
[88]	Ofloxacin (400 mg b.i.d., inpatients) vs. ofloxacin (400 mg b.i.d., outpatients)	85	78%	Prospective randomized comparison of inpatient and outpatient therapy in low-risk febrile neutropenic patients.
		84	77%	
[85]	Ciprofloxacin (500 mg q 8 hr) + amoxicillin/clavulanate (500 mg q 8 hr) vs. i.v. aztreonam (2 g q 8 hr) + Clindamycin (600 mg q 8 hr)	88	90%	Prospective randomized comparison of oral and parenteral outpatient empiric regimens in low-risk febrile neutropenic patients.
		91	87%	

[a] b.i.d. = twice daily; t.i.d. = three times daily; i.v. = intravenously. [b] Overall response rates shown are without modification of the initial regimen.

mycin being replaced by newer agents such as azithromycin, and the quinolones playing an increasingly important role in the treatment of these infections.

As a class, the fluoroquinolones are very active *in vitro* against *Legionella pneumophila*, with MIC values often ≤0.01 µg/ml for ciprofloxacin, ofloxacin, pefloxacin, and fleroxacin, and such newer agents as sparfloxacin, trovafloxacin, moxifloxacin, gatifloxacin, and gemifloxacin [91–99]. These agents are also often bactericidal against intracellular *L. pneumophila*, and animal studies have shown them to be more effective than erythromycin for infections caused by *L. pneumophila* [100–109]. Although no prospective, controlled, human clinical trials for the treatment of legionellosis exist, ciprofloxacin, ofloxacin, and pefloxacin have all been used successfully for this indication. Parenteral and/or oral therapy with these agents used as monotherapy has been reported to be effective in several patients with documented legionellosis, including patients with severe immunosuppression [110–116]. Occasional failures to these agents have also been described, mostly occurring in patients receiving relatively low doses (400 mg of oral ofloxacin daily or 400 mg of intravenous ciprofloxacin daily) [117–119]. This clinical experience has led to current recommendations for the use of higher doses (800–1000 mg daily) of the quinolones to achieve increased efficacy. Parenteral therapy is preferable in patients who are severely immunocompromised or severely ill. A switch to oral therapy can be made when patients are clinically stable and able to tolerate oral therapy and some initial clinical or radiographic response has been achieved.

The quinolones have also been used in combination with other agents active against *L. pneumophila* (erythromycin, rifampin), but currently there is no clinical evidence to indicate that such combinations are more effective than quinolone monotherapy. The quinolones are considered the agents of choice for the treatment of *L. pneumophila* infection in patients receiving immunosuppressive therapy with cyclosporine and tacrolimus [120]. This is due to the fact that they do not influence cyclosporine or tacrolimus metabolism, in contrast to agents like erythromycin and rifampin.

In summary, although recommendations for the use of the fluoroquinolones for the treatment of legionellosis are based on accumulated clinical experience and not on the basis of controlled clinical trials, these agents have expanded our options for treating this infection. In fact, several experts believe that the quinolones should be considered the agents of choice for the treatment of legionellosis, and have called for a change in the standard of care for these infections [121].

MYCOBACTERIAL INFECTIONS

The quinolones possess *in-vitro* activity against many mycobacterial isolates including *M. tuberculosis*, *M. avium complex*, *M. leprae*, *M. fortuitum*, and *M. kansasii* [20,122–124]. Ofloxacin and ciprofloxacin are second-line oral antituberculous drugs and are not included in standard therapeutic regimens for the treatment of tuberculosis. However, the emergence of multidrug-resistant strains of *M. tuberculosis* has been well documented both in individuals with and without HIV infection [125–134]. Both ofloxacin and ciprofloxacin are proving to be extremely useful in the treatment of patients with multidrug-resistant tuberculosis [135–137]. Both drugs possess excellent *in-vitro* activity against strains of *M. tuberculosis* not previously exposed to them, and ofloxacin has shown substantial activity in animal studies as well [122,138]. Extensive clinical experience from the National Jewish Center for Immunology and Respiratory Medicine and other institutions has led to the development of multiple quinolone-based regimens depending on the pattern of drug resistance [136]. These include the administration of at least three drugs to which the organisms are susceptible for prolonged periods (at least 18–24 months). One report from various hospitals in New York documented the course and outcome of multidrug-resistant tuberculosis in 26 HIV-negative patients [129]. Among these, 16 patients (64%) received a complete course of therapy and had no evidence of relapse. All were treated with at least three drugs that had *in-vitro* activity against their isolates, and all received prolonged treatment (median 568 days) with quinolones. In general, despite long-term high-dose administration (ofloxacin 400 mg twice daily, ciprofloxacin 750 mg twice daily) for the treatment of multidrug-resistant tuberculosis, the quinolones have been well tolerated and are associated with minimal toxicity.

Disseminated infection caused by *Mycobacterium avium complex* is the most common opportunistic bacterial infection in HIV-infected adults [139]. Several reports have indicated that therapy of this infection does result in clinical and microbiological improvement and increased survival [140–142]. However, the most effective treatment for this infection is yet to be determined. Combination regimens that have included ciprofloxacin have been used with moderate success in the treatment of *M. avium complex* infection in HIV-infected individuals. One often recommended four-drug regimen (rifampin, ethambutol, clofazimine, and ciprofloxacin) has been considered standard treatment for *M. avium complex* infection [142–145]. However, this regimen was compared to a three-drug regimen consisting of rifabutin, ethambutol, and clarithromycin [146]. More frequent resolution of bacteremia (69 vs. 29%, $p \leq 0.001$) and better survival (8.6 vs. 5.2 months, $p \geq 0.001$) were found in patients treated with the three-drug regimen. The development of newer quinolones with greater *in-vitro* activity and more favorable pharmacokinetics than those of currently available agents will undoubtedly lead to further investigation into their role in the treatment of *M. avium complex* infection.

M. fortuitum infections of the skin or soft tissues have been successfully treated with ciprofloxacin and ofloxacin. As with other mycobacterial infections, prolonged therapy using a combination of two or three agents with activity against these isolates is recommended because monotherapy is likely to lead to development of resistance.

MISCELLANEOUS INFECTIONS

The quinolones have a high degree of *in-vitro* activity against enteric bacteria, including *Salmonella typhi* and nontyphi *Salmonella* spp. Recurrent infections caused by *Salmonella* spp. are relatively common in HIV-infected individuals [147]. Because of the emergence of resistance among these organisms to conventional antityphoidal agents (ampicillin, TMP–SMX, and chloramphenicol), the quinolones (norfloxacin, ciprofloxacin, ofloxacin, and pefloxacin) have been used extensively for salmonellosis and have been associated with response rates that are superior to conventional therapy [148–150]. The quinolones are also effective in eliminating intestinal excretion of *Salmonella* in chronic carriers, and are now considered the agent of choice for salmonellosis [150]. Some experts recommend the use of secondary quinolone prophylaxis in patients with AIDS to prevent relapsing and recurrent infections [149]. As yet, there is no direct clinical evidence that this approach is of benefit (H. DuPont, personal communication, 2000), and its role must be evaluated in controlled clinical trials, particularly in this new era of HAART, and the subsequent reduction of opportunistic infections in patients with AIDS.

The quinolones have been demonstrated to be of use both for prophylaxis and treatment of traveler's diarrhea. With global travel becoming increasingly more efficient and available, vacationing in areas where traveler's diarrhea is common is quite frequent. Although routine quinolone prophylaxis is not recommended in healthy travelers, it is our practice to suggest such prophylaxis to our immuno-compromised cancer patients when they travel to high-risk areas. This practice is not based on controlled clinical trials but on several years of accumulated clinical experience.

Infections caused by coryneform bacteria (particularly *Corynebacterium jeikeium*), *Bacillus* species, *L. monocytogenes*, and *Rhodococcus* spp. are being recognized more frequently in neutropenic and immunosuppressed patients and may be associated with more severe manifestations in such patients than in immunocompetent individuals [4,6,9,151]. Most fluoroquinolones possess *in-vitro* activity against these organisms and may have a role to play in the treatment of infections caused by them [152,153]. Many quinolones are also active against multidrug-resistant isolates such as *Stenotrophomonas maltophilia* and *Flavobacterium meningosepticum*, which cause infections infrequently, but are associated with substantial morbidity and mortality [66,154,155]. There is *in-vitro* evidence to suggest a role for the quinolones in the treatment of these infections, and they might have an additive or even synergistic effect in combination with other agents [154,156]. However, clinical experience with these agents is limited to anecdotal reports, and they cannot be currently recommended for routine use for these infections.

CONCLUSION

The fluoroquinolones play an important role in overall management of infections in immunosuppressed individuals with several established indications (Table IV). They are effective in reducing infections caused by Gram-negative bacilli in neutropenic patients and, in doing so, are better tolerated and have fewer side effects than alternative prophylactic regimens. Combining them with agents such as rifampin, penicillins, or macrolides significantly reduces the incidence of Gram-positive (particularly streptococcal) infections as well. Some newer-generation agents with broader and more potent Gram-positive activity might be effective when used alone. In neutropenic patients, routine quinolone prophylaxis should be avoided and should only be considered in high-risk patients who are expected to have profound and prolonged neutropenia. With the emergence of penicillin-resistant pneumococci, the newer quinolones will play an important role for prophylaxis/preemptive therapy of such infections in high-risk patients with

TABLE IV   Clinical Indications for Fluoroquinolone Usage in Immunocompromised Patients

Indications	Comments
Chemoprophylaxis in afebrile neutropenic patients.	Reduction in Gram-negative infections. No effect on, or possible increase in Gram-positive infections. Avoid routine use. Emergence of resistant organisms of concern.
Empiric therapy in febrile neutropenic patients.	Monotherapy not recommended. Combine with agents that have better Gram-positive activity. Other regimens preferred in patients receiving fluoroquinolone prophylaxis.
Sequential, oral, and outpatient therapy in moderate- to low-risk febrile neutropenic patients.	Lowered cost of therapy. Greater ease of administration. Fewer nosocomial superinfections.
Therapy of specific infections caused by susceptible organisms.	Based on local susceptibility/resistance patterns (*S. maltophilia, F. meningosepticum, Bacillus* spp. *Rhodococcus* spp. *L. monocytogenes*).
Treatment of legionellosis.	Now considered agents of choice, particularly in patients receiving immunosuppressed therapy.
Treatment of mycobacterial infections.	Useful in combination regimens for multidrug-resistant tuberculosis, *Mycobacterium avium complex*, and other nontuberculosis mycobacteria.
Treatment of salmonellosis.	Agents of choice for acute infection and for chronic carrier stage. Role for prophylaxis not fully determined. Also useful for prophylaxis and treatment of traveler's diarrhea.

defects in humoral immunity. Empiric quinolone monotherapy in febrile neu-tropenic patients should be avoided at least until the newer expanded-spectrum agents have been evaluated. Although quinolone-based combination regimens appear to be effective for the empiric therapy of febrile neutropenia, clinical experience with such regimens is limited, and they should probably only be used as frontline empiric therapy in neutropenic patients not receiving quinolone prophylaxis. Risk-based therapy for febrile neutropenia has become a reality with the availability of the quinolones. The ability to switch from parenteral to oral therapy using the same agent (sequential therapy or switch therapy) has facilitated early discharge of a substantial proportion of moderate-risk neutropenic patients who have been initially stabilized in the hospital. Potent oral quinolones have made it possible to treat low-risk neutropenic patients as outpatients for the entire febrile episode, resulting in a significant reduction in nosocomial superinfections and considerable cost savings. The fluoroquinolones are now considered the drugs of choice for the treatment of *L. pneumophila* infections, particularly in patients receiving immunosuppressive therapy (cyclosporin, tacrolimus). These agents are also useful in the treatment of mycobacterial disease, including multidrug-resis-tant tuberculosis, *M. avium complex* infection, and infection with rapidly growing mycobacteria such as *M. fortuitum*. With the emergence of resistance to conven-tional agents used for treating enteric infections (i.e., *Salmonella*), the quinolones are now the agents of choice for the treatment of these infections, and for eliminating intestinal excretion of *Salmonella* in chronic carriers. With increasing levels of international travel, the quinolones have a significant role to play in the prevention and treatment of traveler's diarrhea. Uncommon infections, such as those caused by *Bacillus* spp., *Corynebacterium jeikeium*, *Rhodococcus* spp., *S. maltophilia*, and *F. meningosepticum* may occasionally respond to quinolone-based regimens. The ever-expanding role of the quinolones and the ease with which they can be used have raised concerns about the emergence of resistance to these agents, and many reports of resistance have already appeared. These valuable agents need to be used judiciously in order to preserve their utility in the years to come.

REFERENCES

1. Pizzo, P. A. (1993). Management of fever in patients with cancer and treatment: Induced neutropenia. *New Engl. J. Med.* **328**, 1323–1332.
2. Hughes, W. T., Armstrong, D., Bodey, G. P., *et al.* (1997). 1997 Guidelines for the use of antimicrobial agents in neutropenic patients and unexplained fever. *Clin. Infect. Dis.* **25**, 551–573.
3. Hooper, D. C. (1998). Expanding uses of fluoroquinolones: Opportunities and challenges. *Ann. Intern. Med.* **129**, 908–910.

4. Rolston, K. V. I., and Bodey, G. P. (1996). Infections in patients with cancer. In "Cancer Medicine," 4th ed. (J. F. Holland, E. Frei III, R. C. Bast Jr., D. W. Kufe, D. L. Morton, and R. R. Weichselbaum, eds.), pp. 3303–3333. Lea & Febiger, Philadelphia.

5. Bodey, G. P., Buckley, M., Sathe, Y. S., and Freireich, E. J. (1966). Quantitative relationships between circulating leukocytes and infection in patients with acute leukemia. *Ann. Intern. Med.* **64**, 328–340.

6. Koll, B. S., and Brown, A. E. (1993). The changing epidemiology of infections at cancer hospitals. *Clin. Infect. Dis.* **17** (Suppl. 2), S322–S328.

7. Rolston, K. V. I., and Tarrand, J. (1999). *Pseudomonas aeruginosa*: Still a frequent pathogen in patients with cancer: 11-year experience from a comprehensive cancer center. *Clin. Infect. Dis.* **13**, 197–257.

8. Berger, B. J., Hussain, F., and Roistacher, K. (1994). Bacterial infections in HIV-Infected patients. In "Infectious Disease Clinics of North America" (A. E. Glatt, ed.), Vol. 89, pp 449–465. Saunders, Philadelphia.

9. Chatzinikolaou, I., Dholokia, N. A., Kontoyiannis, D., Tarrand, J. J., and Rolston, K. V. I. (1999). *Rhodococcus* spp. infection in cancer patients. *Abstr. 37th Ann. Mtg. Infect. Dis. Soc. Amer.*, Philadelphia. Abstr. #128.

10. Teira, R., Tarrand, J., and Rolston, K. (1999). Bacteremia due to penicillin susceptible (PSSP) and penicillin non-susceptible streptococcus pneumoniae (PNSP) in patients with cancer. *Abstr. 4th Int. Symp. Febrile Neutropenia*, Brussels, Abstr. #54.

11. Appelbaum, P., and Klepser, M. E. (1999). Role of the newer fluoroquinolones against penicillin-resistant *Streptococcus pneumoniae*. *Infect. Dis. Clin. Pract.* **8**, 374–382.

12. Rolston, K. V. I., Ho, D. H., LeBlanc, B., Streeter, H., and Dvorak, T. (1997). In-vitro activity of trovafloxacin against clinical bacterial isolates from patients with cancer. *J. Antimicrob. Chemother.* **39** (Suppl. B), 15–22.

13. Rolston, K., Nguyen, H., Messer, M., Ho, D. H., and LeBlanc B. (1991). In vitro activity of sparfloxacin (AT-4140) against bacterial isolates from cancer patients. *Eur. J. Clin. Microbiol. Infect. Dis.* [Special Issue], 546–549.

14. Rolston, K. V. I., LeBlanc, B., and Ho, D. H. (1999). In vitro activity of gatifloxacin against Gram-positive isolates from cancer patients. *Abstr. 39th Intersci. Conf. Antimicrob. Agents Chemother.*, San Francisco. Abstr. #360.

15. Diekema, D. J., Jones, R. N., and Rolston, K. V. I. (1999). Antimicrobial activity of gatifloxacin compared to seven other compounds tested against Gram-positive organisms isolated at 10 cancer-treatment centers. *Diag. Microbiol. Infect. Dis.* **34**, 37–43.

16. Khardori, N., Nguyen, H., Rosenbaum, B., Rolston, K., and Bodey, G. P. (1994). In vitro susceptibilities of rapidly growing mycobacteria to newer antimicrobial agents. *Antimicrob. Agents Chemother.* **38**, 134–137.

17. Yew, W. W., Piddock, L. J., Li, M. S., Lyon, D., Chan, C. Y., and Cheng, A. F. (1994). In-vitro activity of quinolones and macrolides against mycobacteria. *J. Antimicrob. Chemother.* **34**, 343–351.

18. Jacobs, M. R. (1995). Activity of quinolones against mycobacteria. *Drugs* **49** (Suppl. 2), 67–75.

19. Garcia-Rodriguez, J. A., and Gomez-Garcia, A. C. (1993). In-vitro activities of quinolones against mycobacteria. *J. Antimicrob. Chemother.* **32**, 797–808.

20. Ruiz-Serrano, M. J., Alcalá, L., Martinez, M. S., *et al.* (1999). In vitro activity of six quinolones against clinical isolates of *Mycobacterium tuberculosis* susceptible and resistant to first-line antituberculosis drugs. *Abstr. 39th Intersci. Conf. Antimicrob. Agents Chemother.*, San Francisco. Abstr. #1492.

21. Bergan, T. (1988). Pharmacokinetics of fluorinated quinolones. In "The Quinolones" (V. T. Andriole, ed.), pp. 119–154. Academic Press, San Diego.

22. Hooper, D. C. (1993). Quinolone mode of action-new aspects. *Drugs* **45** (Suppl. 3), 8–14.

23. Zhao, X., Xu, C., Domagala, J., and Drlica, K. (1997). DNA topoisomerase targets of the fluoroquinolones: A strategy for avoiding bacterial resistance. *Proc. Natl. Acad. Sci. U.S.A.* **94**, 13991–13996.

24. Nord, C. E. (1995). Effect of quinolones on the human intestinal microflora. *Drugs* **49** (Suppl. 2), 81–85.

25. Appelbaum, P. C. (1995). Quinolone activity against anaerobes: Microbiological aspects. *Drug* **49** (Suppl. 2), 76–80.

26. Goldstein, E. J., and Citron, D. M. (1992). Comparative activity of ciprofloxacin, ofloxacin, sparfloxacin, temafloxacin, CI-960, CI-990, and WIN 57273 against anaerobic bacteria. *Antimicrob. Agents Chemother.* **36**, 1158–1162.

27. Barker, P. J., Sheehan, R., Teillol-Foo, M., Palmgren, A. C., and Nord, C. E. (1999). Effect of gemifloxacin on the normal human intestinal microflora. *Abstr. 39th Intersci. Conf. Antimicrob. Agents Chemother.*, San Francisco. Abstr. #2303.

28. Bodey, G. P. (1984). Current status of prophylaxis of infection with protected environments. *Am. J. Med.* **76**, 678–684.

29. Van der Waaij, D., Berghuis, J. M., and Lekkerkerk, J. E. C. (1971). Colonization resistance of the digestive tract in conventional and antibiotic-treated mice. *J. Hyg.* **69**, 405–411.

30. Verhoef, J. (1993). Prevention of infections in the neutropenic patient. *Clin. Infect. Dis.* **17** (Suppl. 2), S359–S367.

31. Guiot, H. E. L. (1982). Role of competition for substrate in bacterial antagonism in the gut. *Infect. Immun.* **38**, 887–892.

32. Storring, R. A., Jameson, B., McElwain, T. J., Wittshaw, E., Spies, A. S. P., and Gaya, H. (1977). Oral nonabsorbable antibiotics prevent infection in acute nonlymphoblastic leukemia. *Lancet* **ii**, 37–40.

33. Schimpff, S. C. (1980). Infection prevention during profound granulocytopenia: New approaches to alimentary canal microbial suppression. *Ann. Intern. Med.* **93**, 358–361.

34. Schimpff, S. C., Greene, W. H., Young, V. M., Fortner, C. L., Jepsen, L., Cusack, N., Block, J. B., and Wiernik, P. H. (1975). Infection prevention in acute nonlymphocytic leukemia: Laminar air flow room reverse isolation with oral, nonabsorbable antibiotic prophylaxis. *Ann. Intern. Med.* **82**, 351–358.

35. Dekker, A. W., Rozenberg-Arska, M., Sixma, J. J., and Verhoef, J. (1981). Prevention of infection by trimethoprim–sulfamethoxazole plus amphotericin B in patients with acute nonlymphoblastic leukemia. *Ann. Intern. Med.* **95**, 555–559.

36. Gualtier, R. J., Donowitz, G. R., Kaiser, D. L., Hess, C. E., and Sande, M. A. (1983). Double-blind randomized study of prophylactic trimethoprim–sulfamethoxazole in granulocytopenic patients with hematologic malignancies. *Am. J. Med.* **74**, 934–940.

37. Gurwith, M. J., Braunton, J. L., Lank, B. A., Harding, G. K. M., and Ronald, A. R. (1979). A prospective controlled investigation of prophylactic trimethoprim–sulfamethoxazole in hospitalized granulocytopenic patients. *Am. J. Med.* **66**, 248–256.

38. Hughes, W. T., Rivera, G. K., Schell, M. J., Thornton, D., and Lott, L. (1987). Successful intermittent chemoprophylaxis for *Pneumocystis carinii* pneumonitis. *New Engl. J. Med.* **316**, 1627–1632.

39. Kern, W., and Kurrle, E. (1991). Ofloxacin versus trimethoprim–sulfamethoxazole for prevention of infection in patients with acute leukemia and granulocytopenia. *Infection* **19**, 73–80.

40. Liang, R. H., Yung, R. W., Chan, T. K., Chau, P. Y., Lam, W. K., So, S. Y., and Todd, D. (1990). Ofloxacin versus co-trimoxazole for prevention of infection in neutropenic patients following cytotoxic chemotherapy. *Antimicrob. Agents Chemother.* **34**, 215–218.

41. Anonymous (1991). Prevention of bacterial infection in neutropenic patients with hematologic malignancies: A randomized, multicenter trial comparing norfloxacin with ciprofloxacin (The GIMEMA Infection Program, Gruppo Italiano Malattie Ematologiche Maligne dell' Adulto). *Ann. Intern. Med.* **115**, 7–12.

42. D'Antonio, D., Iacone, A., Fioritoni, G., *et al.* (1992). Comparison of norfloxacin and pefloxacin in the prophylaxis of bacterial infection in neutropenic cancer patients. *Drugs Exp. Clin. Res.* **18**, 141–146.

43. Anonymous (1994). Reduction of fever and streptococcal bacteremia in granulocytopenic patients with cancer: A trial of oral penicillin V or placebo combined with pefloxacin (International Antimicrobial Therapy Cooperative Group of the European Organization for Research and Treatment of Cancer). *JAMA* **272**, 1183–1180.

44. Wimperis, J. Z., Baglin, T. P., Marcus, R. E., and Warren, R. E. (1991). An assessment of the efficacy of antimicrobial prophylaxis in bone marrow autografts. *Bone Marrow Transplant.* **8**, 363–367.

45. Fanci, R., Leoni, F., Bosi, A., *et al.* (1993). Chemoprophylaxis of bacterial infections in granulocytopenic patients with ciprofloxacin vs. ciprofloxacin plus amoxicillin. *J. Chemother.* **5**, 119–123.

46. Gilbert, C., Meisenberg, B., Vredenburgh, J., Ross, M., Hussein, A., Perfect, J., *et al.* (1994). Sequential prophylactic oral and empiric once-daily parenteral antibiotics for neutropenia and fever after high-dose chemotherapy and autologous bone marrow support. *J. Clin. Oncol.* **12**, 1005–1011.

47. Bow, E. J., Mandell, L. A., Louie, T. J., Feld, R., Palmer, M., Zee, B., and Pater J. (1996). Quinolone-based antibacterial chemoprophylaxis in neutropenic patients: Effect of augmented gram-positive activity on infectious morbidity. *Ann. Intern. Med.* **125**, 183–190.

48. Hidalgo, M., Hornedo, J., Lumbreras, C., Trigo, J. M., Gomez, C., Perea, S., Ruiz, A., Hitt, R., and Cortes-Funes, H. (1997). Lack of ability of ciprofloxacin–rifampin prophylaxis to decrease infection-related morbidity in neutropenic patients given cytotoxic therapy and peripheral blood stem cell transplants. *Antimicrob. Agents Chemother.* **41**, 1175–1177.

49. Winston, D. J. (1989). Use of quinolone antimicrobial agents in immunocompromised patients. In "Quinolone Antimicrobial Agents" (J. S. Wolfson and D. C. Hooper, eds.), pp. 187–212. American Society for Microbiology, Washington, DC.

50. Carratala, J., Fernandez-Sevilla, A., Tubau, F., Callis, M., and Gudiol, F. (1995). Emergence of quinolone-resistant *Escherichia coli* bacteremia in neutropenic patients with cancer who have received prophylactic norfloxacin. *Clin. Infect. Dis.* **20**, 557–560.

51. Somolinos, N., Arranz, R., Del Rey, M. C., and Himenez, M. L. (1992). Superinfections by *Escherichia coli* resistant to fluoroquinolones in immunocompromised patients [letter]. *J. Antimicrob. Chemother.* **30**, 730–731.

52. Kern, W. V., Androf, E., Oethinger, M., Kern, P., Hacker, J., and Marre, R. (1994). Emergence of fluoroquinolone-resistant *Escherichia coli* at a cancer center. *Antimicrob. Agents Chemother.* **38**, 681–687.

53. Cometta, A., Calandra, T., Bille, J., and Glauser, M. P. (1994). *Escherichia coli* resistant to fluoroquinolones in patients with cancer and neutropenia [letter]. *New Engl. J. Med.* **330**, 1240–1241.

54. Rolston, K. V. I.. (1998). Commentary: Chemoprophylaxis and bacterial resistance in neutropenic patients. *Infect. Dis. Clin. Pract.* **7**, 202–204.

55. Linseman, D. A., Hampton, L. A., and Branstetter, D. G. (1995). Quinolone-induced arthropathy in the neonatal mouse: Morphological analysis of articular lesions produced by pipemidic acid and ciprofloxacin. *Fundam. Appl. Toxicol.* **28**, 59–64.

56. Schaad, U. B. (1994). Use of the new quinolones in pediatrics. *Isr. J. Med. Sci.* **30**, 463–468.

57. Danisovicova, A., Brezina, M., Belan, S., Kayserova, H., Kaiserova, E., Hruskovic, I., Orosova, K., Dluholucky, S., Galova, K., Matheova, E., *et al.* (1994). Magnetic resonance imaging in children receiving quinolones: No evidence of quinolone-induced arthropathy. A multicenter survey. *Chemotherapy* **40**, 209–214.

58. Cruciani, M., Rampazzo, R., Valena, M., Lazzarini, L., Todeschini, G., Messori, A., and Concia, E. (1996). Prophylaxis with fluoroquinolones for bacterial infections in neutropenic patients: A meta-analysis. *Clin. Infect. Dis.* **23**, 795–805.

59. Bodey, G. P. (1984). Antibiotics in patients with neutropenia. *Arch. Intern. Med.* **144**, 1845–1851.

60. Rolston, K. V. I., Elting, L., Waguespack, S., Ho, D. H., LeBlanc, B., and Bodey, G. P. (1996). Survey of antibiotic susceptibility among Gram-negative bacilli at a cancer center. *Chemotherapy* **42**, 348–353.

61. Rolston, K. V. I., Haron, E., Cunningham, C., and Bodey, G. (1989). Intravenous ciprofloxacin for infections in cancer patients. *Am. J. Med.* **87** (Suppl. 5A), 261S–265S.

62. Bayston, K. F., Want, S., and Cohen, J. (1989). A prospective, randomized comparison of ceftazidime and ciprofloxacin as initial empiric therapy in neutropenic patients with fever. *Am. J. Med.* **87** (Suppl. 5A), 269S–273S.

63. Johnson, P. R., Yin, J. A., and Tooth, J. A. (1990). High-dose intravenous ciprofloxacin in febrile neutropenic patients. *J. Antimicrobial. Chemother.* **26** (Suppl. F), 101–107.

64. Johnson, P. R., Liu Yin, J. A., and Tooth, J. A. (1992). A randomized trial of high-dose ciprofloxacin versus azlocillin and netilmicin in the empirical therapy of febrile neutropenic patients. *J. Antimicrob. Chemother.* **30**, 203–214.

65. Meunier, F., Zinner, S. H., Gaya, H., Calandra, T., Viscoli, C., Klastersky, J., and Glauser, M. (1991). Prospective randomized evaluation of ciprofloxacin versus piperacillin plus amikacin for empiric antibiotic therapy of febrile granulocytopenic cancer patients with lymphomas and solid tumors (The European Organization for Research on Treatment of Cancer International Antimicrobial Therapy Cooperative Group). *Antimicrob. Agents Chemother.* **35**, 873–878.

66. Rolston K. V. I., LeBlanc B., and Ho, D. H. (1999). In vitro activity of gatifloxacin against Gram-negative isolates from cancer patients. *Abstr. 39th Intersci. Conf. Antimicrob. Agents Chemother.*, San Francisco. Abstr. #359.

67. Antoniadou, A., Giannakou, P., Bourousi, M., and Giamarellou, H. (1999). In vitro activity of gemifloxacin against 322 Gram-negative nosocomial clinical isolates. *Abstr. 39th Intersci. Conf. Antimicrob. Agents Chemother.*, San Francisco. Abstr. #1496.

68. Smith, G. M., Leyland, M. J., Farrel, I. D., *et al.* (1988). A clinical, microbiological, and pharmacokinetic study of ciprofloxacin plus vancomycin as initial therapy of febrile episodes in neutropenic patients. *J. Antimicrob. Chemother.* **21**, 647–655.

69. Studena, M., Hlavacova, E., Hel'pianska, L., *et al.* (1994). Teicoplanin plus pefloxacin versus teicoplanin plus netilmicin in empiric therapy of febrile patients with cancer and neutropenia: A randomized study of two once-daily regimens in patients with previously inserted catheters. *Chemotherapy* **40**, 431–434.

70. Kelsey, S. M., Collins, P. W., Delord, C., Weinhard, B., and Newland, A. C. (1990). A randomized study of teicoplanin plus ciprofloxacin versus gentamicin plus piperacillin for the empirical treatment of fever in neutropenic patients. *Br. J. Haematol.* **76** (Suppl. 2), 10–13.

71. Chan, C. C., Oppenheim, B. A., Anderson, H., *et al.* (1989). Randomized trial comparing ciprofloxacin plus netilmicin versus piperacillin plus netilmicin for empiric treatment of fever in neutropenic patients. *Antimicrob. Agents Chemother.* **33**, 87–91.

72. Flaherty, J. P., Waitley, D., Elein, B., George, D., Arnow, P., O'Keefe, P., and Weinstein, R. A. (1989). Multicenter, randomized trial of ciprofloxacin plus azlocillin versus ceftazidime plus amikacin for empiric treatment of febrile neutropenic patients. *Am. J. Med.* **87** (Suppl. 5A), 278S–282S.

73. Philpott-Howard, J. N., Barker, K. F., Wade, J. J., Kaczmarski, R. S., Smeldley, J. C., and Mufti, G. J. (1990). Randomized multicentre study of ciprofloxacin and azlocillin versus gentamicin and azlocillin in the treatment of febrile neutropenic patients. *J. Antimicrob. Chemother.* **26** (Suppl. F), 89–99.

74. Kelsey, S. M., Wood, M. E., Shaw, E., and Newland, A. D. (1989). Intravenous ciprofloxacin as empirical treatment of febrile neutropenic patients. *Am. J. Med.* **87** (Suppl. 5A), 274S–277S.

75. Talcott, J. A., Siegel, R. D., Finberg, R., *et al.* (1992). Risk assessment in cancer patients with fever and neutropenia: A prospective, two-center validation of a prediction rule. *J. Clin. Oncol.* **10**, 316–322.

76. Talcott, J. A., Finberg, R., Mayer, R. J., *et al.* (1988). The medical course of cancer patients with fever and neutropenia. *Arch. Intern. Med.* **148**, 2561–2568.

77. Paesmans, M., Rubenstein, E., Boyer, M., Elting, L., Feld, R., Gallagher, J., Herrstedt, J., Rapaport, B., Rolston, K., Talcott J., and Klastersky, J., on behalf of the MASCC Study Section on Infections (1999). The MASCC Risk Index: A multinational scoring system to predict low-risk febrile neutropenic cancer patients. *Abstr. 4th Int. Symp. Febrile Neutropenia*, Brussels, Abstr. #67.

78. Haron, E., Rolston, K. V. I., Cunningham, C., Holmes, F., Umsawasdi, T., and Bodey, G. P. (1989). Oral ciprofloxacin therapy for infections in cancer patients. *J. Antimicrob. Chemother.* **24**, 955–962.

79. Malik, I. A., Abbas Z., and Karim, M. (1992). Randomized comparison of oral ofloxacin alone with combination of parenteral antibiotics in neutropenic febrile patients. *Lancet* **339**, 1092–1096.

80. Freifeld, A., Marchigiani, D., Walsh, T., *et al.* (1999). A double-blind comparison of empirical oral and intravenous antibiotic therapy for low-risk febrile patients with neutropenia during cancer chemotherapy. *New Engl. J. Med.* **341**, 305–311.

81. Kern, W. V., Cometta, A., deBock, R., *et al.* (1999). Oral versus intravenous empirical antimicrobial therapy for fever in patients with granulocytopenia who are receiving cancer chemotherapy. *New Engl. J. Med.* **341**, 312–318.

82. Rolston, K., Rubenstein, E. B., and Freifeld, A. (1996). Early empiric antibiotic therapy for febrile neutropenia patients at low-risk. *Infect. Dis. Clin. N. Amer.* **10** (Suppl. 2), 223–237.

83. Freifeld, A., and Pizzo, P. A. (1996). The outpatient management of febrile neutropenia in cancer patients. *Oncology* **10**(4), 599–612.

84. Gardembas-Pain, M., Desablens, B., Sensebe, L., *et al.* (1991). Home treatment of febrile neutropenia: An empirical oral antibiotic regimen. *Ann. Oncol.* **2**, 485–487.

85. Rolston, K. V. I., Rubenstein, E. B., Elting, L. S., *et al.* (1995). Ambulatory management of febrile episodes in low-risk patients *Abstr. 35th Intersci. Conf. Antimicrob. Agents Chemother.*, San Francisco. Abstr. #2235.

86. Rubenstein, E. B., Rolston, K., Benjamin, R. S., *et al.* (1993). Outpatient treatment of febrile episodes in low-risk neutropenic patients with cancer. *Cancer* **71**, 3640–3646.

87. Malik, I. A., Khan, W. A., Aziz, Z., *et al.* (1994). Self-administered antibiotic therapy for chemotherapy-induced, low-risk febrile neutropenia in patients with nonhematologic neoplasms. *Clin. Infect. Dis.* **19** 522–527.

88. Malik, I. A., Khan, W. A., Karim, M., *et al.* (1995). Feasibility of outpatient management of fever in cancer patients with low-risk neutropenia: Results of a prospective randomized trial. *Am. J. Med.* **98**, 224–231.

89. Finberg, R. W., and Talcott, J. A. (1999). Fever and neutropenia: How to use a treatment strategy [editorial]. *New Engl. J. Med.* **341**, 362–363.

90. Cantor, S. B., Rubenstein, E. B., Elting, L. S., *et al.* (1996)/ Cost-effectiveness analysis of management strategies for low-risk febrile neutropenic cancer patients. *Abst. 8th Int. Symp. Supp. Care Cancer*, Toronto. Abstr. #3.

91. Edelstein, P. H., and Edelstein, M. A. C. (1989). WIN 57273 Is bactericidal for *Legionella pneumophila* grown in alveolar macrophages. *Antimicrob. Agents Chemother.* **33**, 2132–2136.

92. Edelstein, P. H., Edelstein, M. A. C., Weidenfeld, J., and Dorr, M. B. (1990). In vitro activity of sparfloxacin (CI-978; AT-4140) for clinical *Legionella* isolates, pharmacokinetics in guinea pigs, and use to treat guinea pigs with *L. pneumophila* pneumonia. *Antimicrob. Agents Chemother.* **34**, 2122–2127.

93. Chen, S. C., Paul, M. L., and Gilbert, G. L. (1993). Susceptibility of *Legionella* species to antimicrobial agents. *Pathology* **25**, 180–183.

94. Traub, W. H., and Spohr, M. (1984). In vitro antibiotic susceptibility of Legionellaceae: Search for alternative antimicrobial drugs. *Chemotherapy* **30**, 182–187.

95. Gooding, B. B., Erwin, M. E., Barrett, M. S., Johnson, D. M., and Jones, R. N. (1992). Antimicrobial activities of two investigational fluoroquinolones (CI-960 and E4695) against over 100 *Legionella* spp. isolates. *Antimicrob. Agents Chemother.* **36**, 2049–2050.

96. Moffie, B. G., and Mouton, R. P. (1988). Sensitivity and resistance of *Legionella pneumophila* to some antibiotics and combinations of antibiotics. *J. Antimicrob. Chemother.* **22**, 457–462.

97. Gooding, B. B., and Jones, R. N. (1993). In vitro antimicrobial activity of CP-99,219, a novel azabicyclo-naphthyridone. *Antimicrob. Agents Chemother.* **37**, 3449–3453.

98. Edelstein, P. H., Edelstein, M. A. C., and Holzknecht, B. (1992). In vitro activities of fleroxacin against clinical isolates of *Legionella* spp., its pharmacokinetics in guinea pigs, and use to treat guinea pigs with *L. pneumophila* pneumonia. *Antimicrob. Agents Chemother.* **36**, 2387–2391.

99. Dubois, J., and St.-Pierre, C. (1999). In vitro susceptibility and post-antibiotic effect of gemifloxacin against *Legionella* spp. *Abstr. 39th Intersci. Conf. Antimicrob. Agents Chemother.*, San Francisco. Abstr. #2310.

100. Pasculle, A. W., Dowling, J. N., Frola, F. N., McDevitt, D. A., and Levi, M. A. (1985). Antimicrobial therapy of experimental *Legionella micdadei* pneumonia in guinea pigs. *Antimicrob. Agents Chemother.* **28**, 730–734.

101. Dournon, E., Rajagopalan, P., Vilde, J. L., and Pocidalo, J. J. (1986). Efficacy of pefloxacin in comparison with erythromycin in the treatment of experimental guinea pig legionellosis. *J. Antimicrob. Chemother.* **17** (Suppl. B), 41–48.

102. Havlichek, D., Saravolatz, L., and Pohlod, D. (1987). Effect of quinolones and other antimicrobial agents on cell-associated *Legionella pneumophila*. *Antimicrob. Agents Chemother.* **31**, 1529–1534.

103. Kitsukawa, K., Hara, J., and Saito, A. (1991). Inhibition of *Legionella pneumophila* in guinea pig peritoneal macrophages by new quinolone, macrolide and other antimicrobial agents. *J. Antimicrob. Chemother.* **27**, 343–353.

104. Vildé, J. L., Dournon, E., and Rajagopalan, P. (1986). Inhibition of *Legionella pneumophila* multiplication within human macrophages by antimicrobial agents. *Antimicrob. Agents Chemother.* **30**, 743–748.

105. Nowicki, M., Paucod, J. C., Bornstein, N., Meugnier, H., Osoard, P., and Fleurette, J. (1988). Comparative efficacy of five antibiotics on experimental airborne legionellosis in guinea-pigs. *J. Antimicrob. Chemother.* **22**, 513–519.

106. Havlichek, D., Pohlod, D., and Saravolatz, L. (1987). Comparison of ciprofloxacin and rifampicin in experimental *Legionella pneumophila* pneumonia. *J. Antimicrob. Chemother.* **20**, 875–881.

107. Fitzgeorge, R. B., Gibson, D. H., Jepras, R., and Baskerville, A. (1985). Studies on ciprofloxacin therapy of experimental Legionnaires' disease. *J. Infect.* **10**, 194–204.

108. Fitzgeorge, R. B. (1985). The effect of antibiotics on the growth of *Legionella pneumophila* in guinea-pig alveolar phagocytes infected *in vivo* by an aerosol. *J. Infect.* **10**, 189–193.

109. Fitzgeorge, R. B., Baskerville, A., and Featherstone, A. S. R. (1986). Treatment of experimental Legionnaires' disease by aerosol administration of rifampin, ciprofloxacin, and erythromycin [letter]. *Lancet* **1**, 502–503.

110. Edelstein, P. (1995). Antimicrobial chemotherapy for Legionnaires' disease: A review. *Clin. Infect. Dis.* **21** (Suppl. 3), 265–276.

111. Dournon, E., Mayaud, C., Wolff, M., *et al.* (1990). Comparison of the activity of three antibiotic regimens in severe Legionnaires' disease. *J. Antimicrob. Chemother.* **26** (Suppl. B), 129–139.

112. McDonald, K. S., Faoagali, J. L., Tait, G. B., and Moller, P. W. (1980). Legionnaires' disease in a patient with polymyositis. *N.Z. Med. J.* **91**, 451–452.

113. Meyer, R. D. (1991). Role of the quinolones in the treatment of legionellosis. *J. Antimicrob. Chemother.* **28**, 623–625.

114. Peugeot, R. L., Lipsky, B. A., Hooton, T. M., and Pecoraro, R. E. (1991). Treatment of lower respiratory infections in outpatients with ofloxacin compared with erythromycin. *Drugs Exp. Clin. Res.* **17**, 253–257.

115. Singh, N., Muder, R. R., Yu, V. L., and Gayowski, T. (1993). Legionella infection in liver transplant recipients: Implications for management. *Transplantation* **56**, 1549–1551.

116. Winter, J. J., McCartney, C., Bingham, J., Telfer, M., White, L. O., and Fallon, R. J. (1988). Ciprofloxacin in the treatment of severe Legionnaires' disease. *Rev. Infect. Dis.* **10** (Suppl.), S218–S219.

117. Unertl, K. E., Lenhart, F. P., Forst, H., *et al.* (1989). Brief report: Ciprofloxacin in the treatment of legionellosis in critically ill patients including those cases unresponsive to erythromycin. *Am. J. Med.* **87** (Suppl. 5A), 128S–131S.

118. Salord, J.-M., Matsiota-Bernard, P., Staikowsky, F., Kirstetter, M., Frottier, J., and Nauceil, C. (1993). Unsuccessful treatment of *Legionella pneumophila* infection with a fluoroquinolone [letter]. *Clin. Infect. Dis.* **17**, 518–519.

119. Kurz, R. W., Graninger, W., Egger, T. P., Pilcher, H., and Tragl, K. H. (1988). Failure of treatment of *Legionella pneumonia* with ciprofloxacin [letter]. *J. Antimicrob. Chemother.* **22**, 389–391.

120. Hooper, T. L., Gould, F. K., Swinburn, C. R., *et al.* (1988). Ciprofloxacin: A preferred treatment for *Legionella* infections in patients receiving cyclosporin A [letter]. *J. Antimicrob. Chemother.* **22**, 952–953.

121. Edelstein, P. H. (1998). Antimicrobial chemotherapy for legionnaires' disease: Time for a change [editorial]. *Ann. Intern. Med.* **129**, 328–330.

122. Tsukamura, M. (1985). Antituberculosis activity of ofloxacin (DL 8280) on experimental tuberculosis in mice. *Am. Rev. Respir. Dis.* **132**, 915.

123. Tsukamura, M. (1985). In vitro antituberculosis activity of a new antibacterial substance ofloxacin (DL 8280). *Am. Rev. Respir. Dis.* **131**, 348–351.

124. Heifets, L. B., and Lindholm-Levy, P. J. (1987). Bacteriostatic and bactericidal activity of ciprofloxacin and ofloxacin against *Mycobacterium tuberculosis* and *Mycobacterium avium complex. Tuberculosis* **68**, 267–276.

125. MMWR (1991). Nosocomial transmission of multidrug-resistant tuberculosis among HIV-infected persons: Florida and New York, 1988–1991. *Morb. Mortal. Wkly. Rep.* **40**, 585–591.

126. Coronado, V. G., Beck-Sague, C. M., Hutton, M. D., *et al.* (1993). Transmission of multidrug-resistant mycobacterium tuberculosis among persons with human immunodeficiency virus infection in an urban hospital: Epidemiologic and restriction fragment length polymorphism analysis. *J. Infect. Dis.* **168**, 1052–1055.

127. Small, P. M., Shafer, R. W., Hopewell, P. C., *et al.* (1993). Exogenous reinfection with multidrug-resistant *Mycobacterium tuberculosis* in patients with advanced HIV infection. *New Engl. J. Med.* **328**, 1137–1144.

128. Bloch, A. B., Cauthen, G. M., Onorato, I. M., *et al.* (1994). Nationwide survey of drug-resistant tuberculosis in the United States. *JAMA* **271**, 665–671.

129. Telzak, E. E., Sepkowitz, K., Alpert, P., Mannheimer, S., Medard, F., El-Sadr, W., Blum, S., Gagliardi, A., Salomon, N., and Turett, G. (1995). Multidrug-resistant tuberculosis in patients without HIV infection. *New Engl. J. Med.* **333**, 907–911.

130. Frieden, T. R., Sterling, T., Pablos-Mendez, A., Kilburn, J. O., Cauthen, G. M., and Dooley, S. W. (1993). The emergence of drug-resistant tuberculosis in New York City. *N. Engl. J. Med.* **328**, 521–526.

131. Bloch, A. B., Cauthen, G. M., Onorato, I. M., *et al.* (1994). Nationwide survey of drug-resistant tuberculosis in the United States. *JAMA* **271**, 665–671.

132. Edlin, B. R., Tokars, J. I., Grieco, H. M., *et al.* (1992). An outbreak of multidrug-resistant tuberculosis among hospitalized patients with the immunodeficiency syndrome. *New Engl. J. Med.* **326**, 1514–1521.

133. Ben-Dov, I., and Mason, G. R. (1987). Drug-resistant tuberculosis in a southern California hospital: Trends from 1969 to 1984. *Am. Rev. Respir. Dis.* **135**, 1307–1310.

134. Carpenter, J. L., Obnibene, A. J., Gorby, E. W., Neimes, R. E., Koch, J. R., and Perkins, W. L. (1983). Antituberculosis drug resistance in South Texas. *Am. Rev. Respir. Dis.* **128**, 1055–1058.

135. Fischl, M. A., Daikos, G. l., Uttamchandani, R. B., *et al.* (1992). Clinical presentation and outcome of patients with HIV infection and tuberculosis caused by multiple-drug-resistant bacilli. *Ann. Intern. Med.* **117**, 184–190.

136. Iseman, M. D. (1993). Drug therapy: Treatment of multidrug-resistant tuberculosis. *New Engl. J. Med.* **329**, 784–791.

137. Goble, M., Iseman, M. D., Madsen, L. A., Waite, D., Ackerson, L., and Horsburgh Jr., C. R. (1993). Treatment of 171 patients with pulmonary tuberculosis resistant to isoniazid and rifampin. *New Engl. J. Med.* **328**, 527–532.

138. Chen, C.-H., Shih, J.-F., Lindholm-Levy, P. J., and Heifets, L. B. (1989). Minimal inhibitory concentrations of rifabutin, ciprofloxacin, and ofloxacin against *Mycobacterium tuberculosis* isolated before treatment of patients in Taiwan. *Am. Rev. Respir. Dis.* **140**, 987–989.

139. Inderlied, C. B., Kemper, C. A., and Bermudez, L. E. M. (1993). The *Mycobacterium avium complex. Clin. Microbiol. Rev.* **6**, 266–310.

140. Benson, C. A., and Ellner, J. J. (1993). *Mycobacterium avium complex* infection and AIDS: Advances in theory and practice. *Clin. Infect. Dis.* **17**, 7–20.

141. Hoy, J., Mijch, A., Sandland, M., Grayson, L., Lucas, R., and Dwyer, B. (1990). Quadruple drug therapy for *Mycobacterium avium-intracellulare* bacteremia in AIDS patients. *J. Infect. Dis.* **161**, 801–805.

142. Chiu, J., Nussbaum, J., Bozzette, S., *et al.* (1990). Treatment of disseminated *Mycobacterium avium complex* infection in AIDS with amikacin, ethambutol, rifampin, and ciprofloxacin. *Ann. Intern. Med.* **113**, 358–361.

143. Kemper, C. A., Meng, T.-C., Nussbaum, J., *et al.* (1992). Treatment of *Mycobacterium avium complex* bacteremia in AIDS with four-drug oral regimen: Rifampin, ethambutol, clofazidime, and ciprofloxacin. *Ann. Intern. Med.* **116**, 466–472.

144. Horsburgh Jr., C. R. (1991). *Mycobacterium avium complex* infection in the acquired immunodeficiency syndrome. *New Engl. J. Med.* **324**, 1332–1338.

145. Ellner, J. J., Goldberger, M. J., and Parenti, D. M. (1991). *Mycobacterium avium* infection and AIDS: A therapeutic dilemma in rapid evaluation. *J. Infect. Dis.* **163**, 1326–1335.

146. Shafran, S. D., Singer, J., Zarowny, D. P., Phillips, P., Salit, I., Walmsley, S. L., Fong, I. W., Gill, M. J., Rachis, A. R., Lalonde, R. G., Fanning, M. M., and Tsoukas, C. M. (1996). A comparison of two regimens for the treatment of *Mycobacterium avium complex* bacteremia in AIDS: Rifabutin, ethambutol, and clarithromycin versus rifampin, ethambutol, clofazimine, and ciprofloxacin. *New Engl. J. Med.* **335**, 377–383.

147. Celum, C. L., Chaisson, R. E., Rutherford, G. W., *et al.* (1987). Incidence of salmonellosis in patients with AIDS. *J. Infect. Dis.* **156**, 998–1002.

148. Sperber, S. J., and Schleupner, C. J. (1987). Salmonellosis during infection with human immunodeficiency virus. *Rev. Infect. Dis.* **9**, 925–934.

149. Berger, B. J., Hussain, F., and Roistacher, K. (1994). Bacterial infections in HIV-Infected patients. In "Infectious Disease Clinics of North America" (A. E. Glatt, guest ed.), Vol. 8, pp. 449–465. Saunders, Philadelphia.

150. DuPont, H. L. (1993). Quinolones in *Salmonella typhi* infection. *Drugs* **45** (Suppl. 3), 11–124.

151. Martinez-Martinez, L., Joyanes, P., Suárez, A. I., and Perea, E. J. (1999). Activity of Gemifloxacin against clinical isolates of *Listeria monocytogenes* and *Coryneform* bacteria. *Abstr. 39th Intersci. Conf. Antimicrob. Agents Chemother.*, San Francisco. Abstr. #1504).

152. Martinez-Martinez, L., Suarez, A. I., Ortega, M. C., and Perea, E. J. (1994). Comparative in vitro activities of new quinolones against *Coryneform* bacteria. *Antimicrob. Agents Chemother.* **38**, 1439–1441.

153. Cherubin, C. E., and Stratton, C. W. (1994). Assessment of the bactericidal activity of sparfloxacin, ofloxacin, levofloxacin, and other fluoroquinolones compared with selected agents of proven efficacy against *Listeria monocytogenes*. *Diag. Microbiol. Infect. Dis.* **20**, 21–25.

154. Di Pentima, M. C., Mason, E. O., and Kaplan, S. L. (1998). In vitro antibiotic synergy against *Flavobacterium meningosepticum*: Implications for therapeutic options. *Clin. Infect. Dis.* **26**, 1169–1176.

155. Verhagegen, J., and Verbist, L. (1999). In vitro activity of gemifloxacin and other antimicrobials against recent isolates of *Pseudomonas aeruginosa*, *Stenotrophomonas maltophilia*, *Burkholderia cepacia* and *Acinetobacter* spp. *Abstr. 39th Intersci. Conf. Antimicrob. Agents Chemother.*, San Francisco. Abstr. #2306.

156. Vartivarian, S., Anaissie, E., Bodey, G., Sprigg, H., and Rolston, K. (1994). A changing pattern of susceptibility of *Xanthomonas maltophilia* to antimicrobial agents: Implications for therapy. *Antimicrob. Agents Chemother.* **38**, 624–627.

CHAPTER 13

Use of the Quinolones in Skin and Skin Structure (Osteomyelitis) and Other Infections

ADOLF W. KARCHMER

*Chief, Division of Infectious Diseases, Beth Israel Deaconess Medical Center,
Boston, Massachusetts 02215, and Professor of Medicine, Harvard Medical School,
Boston, Massachusetts 02115*

INTRODUCTION

The new fluoroquinolones have a broad spectrum of activity, including activity against many facultative Gram-negative bacteria and aerobic Gram-positive cocci, excellent bioavailability after oral administration, favorable pharmacokinetics, and a good safety profile. Not surprisingly, these compounds have been of great interest for the treatment of patients with skin and associated soft tissue infection and with bone or joint infections. These patients are often not severely ill and hence are candidates for oral therapy initially or following an abbreviated course of intravenous therapy. Increasing experience with ciprofloxacin, ofloxacin, and fleroxacin, and early experience with levofloxacin and trovafloxacin have suggested roles for the quinolones in treatment of skin and skin-structure infection, including osteomyelitis. The recognition of infrequent but severe hepatotoxicity due to trovafloxacin has markedly restricted its use, particularly for the treatment of less severe skin and skin-structure infection. Gatifloxacin, moxifloxacin, and gemifloxacin compounds that have enhanced potency against aerobic and anaerobic Gram-positive cocci and significant, although less predictable, activity against anaerobic Gram-negative bacteria have a potential role in the treatment of skin and skin-structure infections. To date, these compounds have been approved for treatment of respiratory tract infections; however, data defining their role in skin infections is very limited. This chapter will examine the basis for using fluoroquinolones for the treatment of skin and skin-structure infections, the efficacy of the established agents, and the potential of newer agents in this area.

SKIN AND SOFT TISSUE INFECTION

Skin and adjacent soft tissue infections range from cellulitis, erysipelas, lymphangitis, and staphylococcal abscesses to more complex infections, including necrotizing fascitis, synergistic necrotizing gangrene and cellulitis, surgical wound infection, and infections complicating preexisting skin lesions (burns, foot ulcers in patients with diabetes, and decubitus ulcers). In the absence of detected bacteremia or drainable abscesses, recovery of an etiologic agent from patients with cellulitis, erysipelas, or lymphangitis is uncommon. Nevertheless, *Staphylococcus aureus*, *Streptococcus pyogenes*, or occasionally other β-hemolytic streptococci cause most of these infections. The more complex skin and soft tissue infections are associated with preexisting injury to the involved tissue or themselves cause tissue necrosis as a primary process or as a result of local vascular occlusion and infarction. In these patients, facultative Gram-negative and anaerobic bacteria, as well as *S. aureus* and β-hemolytic streptococci, may be causative, and infections are frequently polymicrobial. *Streptococcus agalactiae*, the group B streptococcus, is a frequent cause of significant skin infection in patients with diabetes mellitus. The broad spectrum of the quinolones and their bioavailability by the oral route suggest a potential role for these compounds in the treatment of skin and soft tissue infections.

PHARMACOLOGY

As a class, the quinolones penetrate into skin and adjacent soft tissue well and achieve therapeutically effective concentrations against most susceptible organisms at these sites. Concentrations of ciprofloxacin, ofloxacin, pefloxacin, fleroxacin, levofloxacin, sparfloxacin, trovafloxacin, gatifloxacin, and moxifloxacin in skin approach 100% of those achieved in serum [1–12]. After a brief time lag to allow distribution, these quinolones are found in blister fluid at concentrations equivalent to those found in plasma [6–8,10,11].

MICROBIOLOGY

The majority of skin and associated soft tissue infections occurring in immunocompetent patients without major preexisting skin injury are caused by *S. aureus* or β-hemolytic streptococci, particularly *S. pyogenes*. Nevertheless, infection of these tissues occurring in nosocomial settings (surgical wounds) or at the site of subacute cutaneous ulcers are often caused by other bacteria and are commonly polymicrobial (Table I). The broad range of microorganisms causing these complex infections provides a rationale for quinolone therapy, particularly considering the development of newer agents with enhanced activity against Gram-positive bacteria and retained activity against Gram-negative bacilli (Table II). With the widespread use of quinolones such as ciprofloxacin to treat staphylococcal infection, quinolone-resistant strains of methicillin-susceptible and even more commonly methicillin-resistant *S. aureus* have emerged and disseminated. Although some newer quinolones (e.g., trovafloxacin, moxifloxacin, clinafloxacin, and gemifloxacin) retain significant activity against ciprofloxacin-resistant *S. aureus*, the utility of these agents in the treatment of more serious infections caused by these strains is not established [13,16–19].

Soft tissue infections resulting from human and animal bites are caused not only by *S. aureus* and β-hemolytic streptococci but also by a variety of fastidious or anaerobic bacteria (Table I). While many of the aerobic organisms, particularly *Pasteurella* spp., are highly susceptible to quinolones, some anaerobic species, particularly *Fusobacterium* spp., are less susceptible to ciprofloxacin, ofloxacin, levofloxacin, and sparfloxacin [14,15,20,21]. Trovafloxacin, gemifloxacin, gatifloxacin, and moxifloxacin are active against many of the oral cavity aerobic and anaerobic organisms, especially *Pasteurella* spp., *Peptostreptocuccus* spp., *Prevotella* spp., *Porphyromonas* spp., and some *Fusobacterium* spp. [22–24]. Never-

TABLE I   Microbiology of Complex Skin and Associated Soft Tissue Infection[a]

Surgical wounds (nosocomial)	Decubitus ulcers/ foot ulcers[b]	Animal and human bite wounds
S. aureus	*S. aureus*	*Actinobacillus* spp.
Enterococci	*Streptococcus agalactiae*	*Capnocytophaga* spp.
Coagulase-negative staphylococci	Other streptococci	*Eikenella corrodens*
Escherichia coli	Enterococci	*Moraxella* spp.
Pseudomonas aeruginosa	Coagulase-negative staphylococci	*Pasturella multocida* and other spp.
Other Enterobacteriaceae	Enterobacteriaceae	*S. aureus*
Streptococci	Peptococci	Streptococci
Candida albicans	Peptostreptococci	*Bacteroides tectum[c]*
Bacteroides fragilis group[c]	*Prevotella* species[c]	*Fusobacterium* spp.[c]
	Bacteroides fragilis group[c]	Peptostreptococci
	Other *Bacteroides* species[c]	*Porphyromonas* spp.[c]
	P. aeruginosa	*Prevotella* spp.[c]

Data from [14,42,43,45,46,89].
[a]The pathogenic role some isolates play in these settings is not established.
[b]In patients with diabetes.
[c]Anaerobic Gram-negative bacilli.

theless, the activity of these agents against anaerobes is not entirely predictable, and clinical experience in treating bite infections with these agents is very limited. The susceptibility of the *Bacteroides fragilis* group to earlier quinolones is marginal [15,20,25]. Accordingly, caution is advised when considering use of these agents to treat infections where these anaerobes may play an important role. Trovafloxacin, clinafloxacin, moxifloxacin, and gemifloxacin have significant activity against *B. fragilis* and other anaerobes and hence may have a role in the treatment of the infections caused by these organisms. Nevertheless, many anaerobic species are relatively resistant to these agents—for example, *Bacteroides thetaiotaomicrons*, *Bacteroides distasonis*, and *Bacteroides ovatus*—hence caution is again advised [15,20,21,24,26,27].

CLINICAL STUDIES

As one of the initial fluoroquinolones, ciprofloxacin has been widely studied in the treatment of skin and soft tissue infection. Gentry reviewed the efficacy of

TABLE II   Activity of Quinolones Against the Major Gram-Positive Cocci Causing Skin and Soft Tissue Infection

Quinolone	S. aureus[a] MIC$_{90}^b$	S. pyogenes MIC$_{90}^b$	S. agalactiae MIC$_{90}^b$
Ciprofloxacin	1	1	1
Fleroxacin	1	8	16
Pefloxacin	1	8	32
Ofloxacin	0.5	2	2
Levofloxacin	0.25	1	2
Sparfloxacin	0.125	0.5	0.5
Tosufloxacin	0.06	0.25	0.25
Trovafloxacin	0.06	0.25	0.5
Clinafloxacin	0.03	0.06	0.12
Moxifloxacin	0.12	0.25	0.5
Gatifloxacin	0.25	0.5	0.5
Gemifloxacin	0.06	0.03	0.03

Data from [1,10,16,90-92].

[a]Methicillin-susceptible S. aureus.

[b]Representative minimum inhibitory concentrations in µg/ml for 90% of isolates tested.

ciprofloxacin, generally administered at oral doses of 500 to 750 mg every 12 hours, in open trials treating patients with infected ulcers, wounds, cellulitis, and abscesses, of whom 60% required initial hospitalization [28]. Of 358 patients, 274 (77%) were successfully treated. Of note, infection caused by S. aureus, Enterobacteriaceae, and P. aeruginosa were cured in 73, 100, and 72% of patients. Eradication of methicillin-resistant S. aureus was accomplished in only 48% of infected patients. Ofloxacin at oral doses of 400 mg every 12 hours, as treatment of moderately severe skin and soft tissue infections, has been similarly effective [2].

In comparative studies, fleroxacin and ofloxacin have been as effective as amoxicillin–clavulanate and first- or second-generation oral cephalosporins in the treatment of uncomplicated mild to moderate skin infection [2,29,30]. In studies of over 700 patients, levofloxacin 500 mg daily has been as effective as ciprofloxacin 500 mg every 12 hours, with cure rates of 97 and 94%, respectively [31].

In randomized trials, oral ciprofloxacin and ofloxacin and intravenous fleroxacin have been as effective clinically as cefotaxime or ceftazidime given intravenously for the treatment of complex and serious skin and soft tissue infections caused by Gram-negative bacilli, Gram-positive cocci, and combinations of these two groups of bacteria [32–34] (Table III). The infections treated in these trials have been primarily surgical wound infections, complex cellulitis, soft tissue abscesses, and infected skin ulcers. In addition, randomized trials have demonstrated sequential treatment with intravenous and oral ciprofloxacin to be as effective as intravenous ceftazidime in the treatment of serious skin and skin-structure infections [35–37]. Microbiologic response rates have been high as well. Occasional Gram-negative bacilli, that is, *P. aeruginosa*, *Serratia* spp., and *Enterobacter* spp., have persisted in quinolone and cephalosporin treatment groups [32–34]. Not surprisingly, there was a trend to more persistence of *S. aureus* among ceftazidime-treated patients than those receiving quinolones; however, the differences were not statistically significant. Levofloxacin 500 mg daily intravenously and then orally has been as effective as imipenem/cilastatin 500 mg every 6 hours followed by ciprofloxacin in the treatment of complicated skin and skin-structure infections, with cure rates of 82 and 88%, respectively [31]. *P. aeruginosa* persistence after levofloxacin therapy has been noted.

TABLE III   Comparative Trials of Quinolone Treatment of Moderately Severe or Severe Skin and Soft Tissue Infections

Author [reference]	Antimicrobial therapy/ dose, route (mean days)	Cured/ total evaluable (%)	Antimicrobial therapy/ dose, route (mean days)	Cured/ total evaluable (%)
Gentry [32]	Ciprofloxacin 1.5 g p.o.	164/217 (76)	Cefotaxime 6 g i.v.	162/215 (75)
Fass [35]	Ciprofloxacin 400 mg i.v./ 1–1.5 g p.o.	46/58 (79)	Ceftazidime 2–4 g i.v.	28/39 (72)
Gentry [34]	Ofloxacin 800 mg p.o. (12)	42/43 (98)[a]	Cefotaxime 6 g i.v. (12)	49/50 (98)[a]
Tassler [93]	Fleroxacin 400 mg p.o. (7)	105/114 (92)[a]	Amoxicillin– clavulanate 1.5 g p.o. (7)	55/57 (96)[a]
Parrish [34]	Fleroxacin 400 mg i.v. (7)	74/90 (82)	Ceftazidime 2–6 g i.v. (8)	36/49 (73)
Nicodermo [94][b]	Levofloxacin 500 mg (7)	124/129 (96)[a]	Ciprofloxacin 1 g (10)	116/124 (94)[a]

p.o. = orally, i.v. = intravenously.

[a]Cure plus improved/total evaluable.

[b]Uncomplicated skin and skin structure infection.

More recent studies, available only in abstract form, suggest a high potential in the treatment of skin infections for newer quinolones with enhanced Gram-positive activity. Gatifloxacin 400 mg daily orally achieved a similar clinical outcome and microbiologic eradication rate when compared to levofloxacin 500 mg daily by mouth in treatment (7–10 days) of uncomplicated skin and soft tissue infections in a 400-patient randomized blinded trial [38]. Treatment for 5–10 days with moxifloxacin 400 mg daily by mouth was comparable to cephalexin 500 mg three times daily by mouth (with or without metronidazole) in both clinical response and bacteriologic success in a randomized blinded trial among patients with uncomplicated skin and skin-structure infection [39]. In a randomized investigator-blind trial among patients with severe skin and soft tissue infection, treatment for 7 to 14 days with clinafloxacin 200 mg every 12 hours intravenously was comparable to that with piperacillin–tazobactam 3.375 g every 6 hours in both clinical cure rates (69%, 99/144, vs. 65%, 88/135, respectively) and pathogen eradication (62%, 152/247, vs. 57%, 139/243, respectively) [40].

Polybacterial diabetic foot infections, many of which arise from neuropathic ulcers and are complicated by arterial insufficiency, have been treated effectively with ciprofloxacin and ofloxacin, often using sequential intravenous-to-oral routes of administration [41–43]. Lipsky *et al.* treated diabetic patients with moderately severe foot infections in a randomized nonblinded trial comparing sequential intravenous to oral ofloxacin 400 mg every 12 hours to ampicillin–sulbactam 1.5 to 3.0 g intravenously every 6 hours followed by amoxicillin–clavulanate 625 mg orally every 8 hours. Patients in each arm were treated for an average total course of 20 days [43]. Response rates for soft tissue infections (cured and improved) were 28 of 31 (90%) and 31 of 36 (89%) after treatment with ofloxacin or an aminopenicillin–β-lactamase inhibitor, respectively. Of note, in these studies anaerobic Gram-negative bacteria that are commonly resistant to ciprofloxacin, ofloxacin, levofloxacin, and sparfloxacin were rarely recovered from the infected site. The necessity for treating anaerobic bacteria in diabetic foot infection remains to be elucidated [44,45]. Nevertheless, if a currently available quinolone is used to treat severe limb-threatening infected foot ulcers in diabetics, addition of a second antibiotic effective against anaerobic Gram-negative rods, for example, clindamycin, is prudent [46]. Of interest, non-limb-threatening foot infections in patients with diabetes, that is, those in the absence of full skin thickness ulceration, significant systemic toxicity, and severe arterial insufficiency, are primarily caused by *S. aureus* and streptococci, and are most appropriately treated with anti-staphylococcal targeted antimicrobials rather than quinolones [46,47].

Overall, data from noncomparative and comparative studies indicate that currently available quinolones are highly effective in the treatment of mild uncomplicated and many serious complex skin and soft tissue infections. For those infections where the isolated pathogens are initially susceptible to the quinolone, successful outcomes similar to those achieved with standard β-lactam antibiotic regimens can be anticipated. The earlier quinolones are not optimally potent against β-hemolytic streptococci and should not be used to treat necrotizing (streptococcal) fascitis. Experience with the newer agents with increased potency against streptococci is not available; thus, these are not recommended for treatment of this severe infection. The quinolones are unduly broad-spectrum therapy for treatment of uncomplicated skin infections wherein *S. aureus* and streptococci are the major pathogens. Furthermore, there is increasing quinolone resistance among staphylococci, particularly among methicillin-resistant *S. aureus*, and uncertain clinical utility of the more potent newer compounds. Accordingly, appropriate treatment for these uncomplicated infections utilizes traditional regimens targeting methicillin-susceptible or methicillin-resistant *S. aureus*, as indicated. Alternatively, when complex skin and soft tissue infections caused by Gram-negative bacilli or both Gram-positive cocci and Gram-negative bacilli are encountered, quinolones provide highly effective therapy, if the causative organisms are susceptible. Patients with complex skin and soft tissue infections where anaerobic bacteria play an important pathogenic role—for example, synergistic necrotizing cellulitis, Fournier's gangrene, wound infections caused by fecal flora, some bite wounds, and severe crepitant necrotizing diabetic foot infections—are not ideal candidates for quinolone-only therapy, given the toxicity limitations of trovafloxacin and the very limited experience with moxifloxacin, gemifloxacin, and gatifloxacin [48]. If quinolones are to be used in these settings to treat the facultative Gram-negative bacillus component, an additional agent should be included for treatment of anaerobic organisms.

BONE AND JOINT INFECTION

OSTEOMYELITIS

From the pathogenesis perspective, osteomyelitis can be divided into hematogenous disease and contiguous-focus osteomyelitis, the latter developing as an extension of adjacent soft tissue infection with or without associated vascular insufficiency [49,50]. Hematogenous osteomyelitis occurs more commonly in the long bones of children and may be complicated by subperiosteal abscesses; in adults it may involve long bones but more commonly involves the vertebral bodies. Contiguous-focus osteomyelitis, the most prevalent form of bone infection, occurs as a consequence of the direct introduction of organisms into bone at the time of trauma, at surgery with or without the placement of foreign devices in bone, and as an extension of infection from adjacent soft tissue. A now common form of osteomyelitis is that associated with implanted devices wherein surgery injures bone and the device presents a vulnerable locus for infection [51]. A common and somewhat specific form of contiguous-focus osteomyelitis is that occurring in the feet of patients with diabetes and occasionally in nondiabetic patients with severe peripheral vascular disease [50,52].

The evolution of osteomyelitis from acute to chronic infection has overarching therapeutic significance. Acute osteomyelitis is characterized microscopically by purulence, edema, vascular congestion, and small-vessel occlusion. Osteomyelitis that has persisted untreated for greater than 10 days or that has relapsed after prior treatment is considered chronic and is characterized by microscopic and macroscopic fragments of necrotic bone, the latter called sequestra. While effective therapy of acute osteomyelitis occasionally requires drainage of intramedullary or subperiosteal abscesses, primary treatment relies on antimicrobial agents. Chronic osteomyelitis, however, is infection in an area of impaired host defenses and impaired antibiotic activity. Sequestra act effectively as foreign material to which bacteria adhere and consequently express phenotypic resistance to some antimicrobial agents [53]. Additionally, cultured osteoblasts can internalize *S. aureus*, a common cause of all forms of osteomyelitis, allowing intracellular survival [54]. Quinolones, by virtue of their intracellular penetration and ability to kill metabolically inactive (adherent) organisms may possess inherent therapeutic advantages for the treatment of osteomyelitis [55]. Nevertheless, effective therapy of chronic osteomyelitis requires resection of devitalized bone and necrotic soft tissue, a subject reviewed elsewhere [49,50,56].

PHARMACOLOGY

Measurements of the concentration of quinolones in bone are vulnerable to methodologic problems, including variable extraction techniques and contamination with serum. Furthermore, antibiotic concentrations in bone have not been correlated with efficacy of therapy for osteomyelitis. Nevertheless, the reported concentrations in bone of pefloxacin, ciprofloxacin, ofloxacin, and fleroxacin (Table IV) greatly exceed the MIC_{90}s of most Enterobacteriaceae, equal or exceed the MIC_{90} of methicillin-susceptible *S. aureus*, and often suggest efficacy against *P. aeruginosa*. Maximum bone concentrations generally exceed 1 mg/kg (or 1 mg/liter) and are usually 20 to 50% of peak serum concentration. In one study, the ratio of fleroxacin in bone and serum averaged 1.2 [57]. The pharmacology of the quinolones combined with their broad spectrum of activity make them potentially ideal agents for treating selected forms of osteomyelitis. Specifically, their high degree of bioavailability by the oral route, clearance rates that allow once- or twice-daily dosing, penetration into bone, and the relatively low frequency of associated adverse events, are desirable characteristics for an

TABLE IV   Quinolone Concentrations in Human Bone

Drug [reference]	Patients	Dose (mg)/ route of administration	Maximum concentrations (time after dose)	
			Serum (μg/ml)	Bone
Pefloxacin [95]	23	400 i.v.	3.75 (2hr)	Cortical 0.74 mg/kg (6 hr) Cancellous 1.24 mg/kg (6 hr)
		400/12 h p.o.	7.11 (3 hr)	Cortical 6.26 mg/kg (3 hr) Cancellous 7.72 mg/kg (3 hr)
Pefloxacin [96]	40	800 i.v.	9.26 (1 hr)	7.78 mg/l (1 hr)
Ciprofloxacin [97]	18	500–1000 p.o.	2.9 (2 hr)	0.4–1.6 mg/kg (2 hr)
	10[a]	500–750 p.o.	2.9 (2 hr)	1.4 mg/kg (2 hr)
Ciprofloxacin [98]	20[a]	200 i.v.	2.6	Cortical 1.42 mg/l (1 hr) Cancellous 2.1 mg/l (1 hr)
Ofloxacin [99]	10[a]	400 p.o.	3.45 (1.5 hr)	1.22 mg/l (4.5 hr)
Ofloxacin [100]	23[a]	200 i.v.	7.2	Cortical 0.8 mg/l (4 hr) Cancellous 1.7 mg/l (1.5 hr)
Fleroxacin [57]	4	400 p.o.	4.15 (4 hr)	4.92 mg/kg (4 hr) 0.79–1.86 mg/l (24 hr)
Fleroxacin [85]	40	400 p.o.		1.87–7.13 mg/kg (4 hr) 0.72–5.46 mg/kg (24 hr)[a]

p.o. = orally, i.v. = intravenously.
[a]Infected bone.

antimicrobial agent targeted to osteomyelitis wherein prolonged treatment is required.

MICROBIOLOGY

Optimum antimicrobial treatment of osteomyelitis requires that the causative microorganism and its antibiotic susceptibility be defined. Bone, obtained surgically or by needle biopsy, except when blood culture isolates can be linked to bone infection, is the most reliable source of a microbiologic diagnosis. Cultures obtained from ulcers and fistulae do not correlate sufficiently with the microbiology of underlying infected bone to permit precise decisions regarding antimicrobial therapy. Although *S. aureus* is the most common organism isolated from all clinical forms of osteomyelitis, diverse organisms cause bone infection in various settings (Table V). The microbiology of osteomyelitis associated with

TABLE V   Bacterial Causes of Osteomyelitis Associated with Clinical Predisposition

Hematogenous	Trauma/wound infection	Decubitus ulcers/ foot ulcers[a]	Orthopedic implants
S. aureus	*S. aureus*	*S. aureus*	*S. aureus*
S. agalactiae[b]	Enterobacteriaceae	*S. agalactiae*	Coagulase-negative staphylococci
Escherichia coli[b]	Coagulase-negative staphylococci	Coagulase-negative staphylococci	*Corynebacterium* spp.
Salmonella spp.[c]	Enterococci	Enterococci	Viridans streptococci
P. aeruginosa[d]	*P. aeruginosa*	Enterobacteriaceae	β-hemolytic streptococci
Enterobac- teriaceae[e]		*P. aeruginosa* Peptostreptococci *Bacteroides* spp. *Prevotella* spp.	

[a]In patients with diabetes.
[b]Neonates.
[c]Sickle cell disease.
[d]Injecting narcotic abusers.
[e]Elderly, immunocompromised.

contiguous infection (e.g., penetrating trauma, compound fractures, wound infections, decubitus ulcers, and foot ulcers in diabetics) is not only highly varied but also often polymicrobial. Acute infections of orthopedic devices and adjacent bone are commonly *S. aureus* or other causes of surgical wound infection. In contrast, delayed-onset indolent infections in this setting are often caused by avirulent organisms (e.g., coagulase-negative staphylococci, viridans strepto-cocci, and *Corynebacterium* species). Because of their marked potency against Enterobacteriaceae and their adequate activity against methicillin-susceptible staphylococci, the quinolones are well suited for treatment of the often polymi-crobial contiguous-focus osteomyelitis associated with trauma, wound infections, and cutaneous ulcers.

Animal model studies have provided supportive evidence of the efficacy of quinolones as single agents or as agents in combination therapy of osteomyelitis and septic arthritis. Using negative cultures as endpoints, ciprofloxacin was more effective than tobramycin in a rabbit model of chronic *P. aeruginosa* osteomyelitis and more effective than gentamicin in a model of acute *E. coli* septic arthritis [58,59]. In a rat model of chronic osteomyelitis, ciprofloxacin plus rifampin and pefloxacin plus rifampin reduced the concentration of methicillin-resistant quinolone-susceptible *S. aureus* more effectively than either vancomycin or quinolone alone and were comparable to vancomycin plus rifampin [60,61].

CLINICAL STUDIES

Trials evaluating antimicrobial treatment of osteomyelitis are among the most difficult to perform and, when published, to analyze. With the exception of acute hematogenous osteomyelitis involving long bones and vertebral osteomyelitis, surgical debridement of devitalized bone and soft tissue and removal of foreign material are essential for successful therapy. Unfortunately, surgical intervention cannot be standardized among patients assigned to different regimens and is not comparable between trials. Among patients with chronic contiguous-focus osteomyelitis, the population in whom quinolone treatment trials are usually performed, infection is often polymicrobial and the susceptibility of diverse causative organisms as well as the interaction of organisms may vary among patients. Additionally, the endpoints of treatment, both clinical and microbiological, are difficult to define, and follow-up of patients to detect late relapse, which is typical of chronic osteomyelitis, is generally inadequate. Lastly, the infrequency of osteomyelitis makes trials with significant statistical power to detect different outcomes or reliably establish the comparability of antimicrobials impractical at best.

Open noncomparative trials using ciprofloxacin, pefloxacin, ofloxacin, and fleroxacin have suggested significant efficacy for each agent in the treatment of chronic, primarily contiguous-focus osteomyelitis (Table VI). The major organisms implicated as causing osteomyelitis in these trials have been *S. aureus*, *P. aeruginosa*, and various Enterobacteriaceae. The outcomes reported in these trials must be interpreted cautiously because the duration of follow-up after treatment has either been not stated or less than 12 months. Nevertheless, the studies are encouraging and report combined clinical cure plus improvement rates averaging 83% (range 65–100%) [62–71]. A prolonged course (mean duration 4 months) of ofloxacin or ciprofloxacin for chronic osteomyelitis caused by resistant Gram-negative bacilli was clinically and microbiologically successful in over 66% of patients with 2 to 5 years of follow-up [72]. The organisms most commonly persisting at the conclusion of therapy or at the time of recurrence were *P. aeruginosa* and *S. aureus*, which in some instances had become resistant to the quinolone administered for therapy [62–65,67,70–72]. Additionally, the frequency of adverse events during prolonged treatment was acceptable and discontinuation of the treatment because of adverse events rare. The most commonly reported adverse events were gastrointestinal discomfort, headache, insomnia, rash, abnormal liver function tests, and phototoxicity.

Clinical trials comparing quinolone treatment of osteomyelitis to standard parenteral antibiotic regimens, particularly if patients are randomized to therapy after surgical debridement, provide a more satisfactory appraisal. Comparative trials using ciprofloxacin, ofloxacin, and pefloxacin suggest that the efficacy of these agents is similar to that of β-lactam antibiotics or β-lactams plus aminoglycosides (Table VII) [73–78]. In four trials, the clinical cure rate for the pooled oral ciprofloxacin-treated patients was 82% (77 of 94), while that for patients treated with parenteral regimens was 86% (78 of 91) [73–75,78]. Cure rates in two small studies among patients treated with ofloxacin and pefloxacin were 74 and 85% compared with clinical cure rates of 86 and 85% in patients receiving parenteral regimens, respectively [76,77]. As in the open trials, *P. aeruginosa* and *S. aureus* were the organisms most likely to persist following treatment. Although these data are very encouraging, the limited number of patients studied obviates statistically valid comparisons. Nevertheless, Lew and Waldvogel in reviews of osteomyelitis conclude that for the antimicrobial treatment of osteomyelitis caused by Enterobacteriaceae the efficacy of quinolones is undisputed (microbiologic eradication rates of 92%) and recommend ciprofloxacin 750 mg orally every 12 hr as treatment of choice for these infections [50,79]. Data from open and comparative trials, however, suggest microbiologic failure rates with quinolone treatment of 28, 25, and 23% for osteomyelitis caused by *P. aeruginosa*, *S. aureus*, and *Serratia* spp., respectively; consequently, conventional regimens are preferred to quinolones in these settings [50,79].

The treatment of osteomyelitis involving the bones of the feet in patients with diabetes is challenging. Bone necrosis is often extensive, infection is commonly polymicrobial, achieving soft tissue coverage of overlying ulcers is difficult, and there is often confounding vascular insufficiency. In spite of prolonged courses of ciprofloxacin (mean 120 days) and frequent concomitant use of metronidazole, 7 of 15 patients failed treatment in one study [63]. Peterson *et al.* reported a successful outcome without surgical debridement in 19 of 29 (66%) diabetic patients with pedal osteomyelitis treated with 1.5 or 2.0 g of ciprofloxacin for 3 months [42]. Because the diagnosis of osteomyelitis was based solely on changes in roentgenograms or triple phase bone scans, the diagnosis and consequent favorable response rate may be questioned. Lipsky *et al.* reported 12 of 16 diabetic patients with pedal osteomyelitis cured or improved after treatment with ofloxacin 400 mg every 12 hours for an average of 21 days [43]. Favorable outcomes occurred with similar frequency (75%) in the 12 patients undergoing bone debridement and the 4 who were not treated surgically. Among similar patients randomized to treatment with an aminopenicillin–β-lactamase inhibitor combination for an average of 20 days (initially given intravenously, thereafter orally), these authors reported cure or improvement in 3 of 7. Of note, among patients with foot infection (some without osteomyelitis) treated with ofloxacin, *S. aureus*

TABLE VI Quinolone Treatment of Osteomyelitis[a] in Open Noncomparative Clinical Trials

Drug [reference]	Daily dose/ mean duration	Patients treated surgically/ total	Major causative organisms (no. isolated)	Clinical cure or improved (%)	Bacterio- logic cure/ total (%)
Ciprofloxacin [62]	1.5 g/6–12 wk	15/20	Enterobacteriaceae[b] (7) P. aeruginosa (13)	13 (65)	14 (70)
Ciprofloxacin [63]	1.0–1.5 g/90 d	NA/13	Enterobacteriaceae (7) P. aeruginosa (7) S. aureus (2)	9 (69)	8 (62)
Ciprofloxacin [64]	1.0–3.0 g/139 d	NA/34	Enterobacteriaceae (5) P. aeruginosa (28) S. aureus (3) CNS (3) Enterococci (5)	27 (79)	17 (50)
Ciprofloxacin [65]	1.5 g/12 wk	18/20	P. aeruginosa (10)	19 (95)	18 (90)
Pefloxacin [66]	0.8–1.2 g[c]/45 d	19/20	Enterobacteriaceae (6) P. aeruginosa (3) S. aureus (16	18 (90)	NA
Ofloxacin [67]	600 mg/22 d	105/105	Enterobacteriaceae (23) P. aeruginosa (15) S. aureus (74) CNS (19) Streptococci (10)	98 (93)	NA

Ofloxacin [68]	400 mg[c]/22 d	25/25	*S. aureus*(22) *P. aeruginosa* (1) CNS (1) Streptococci (1) Pasturella (1)	25 (100)	25 (100)
Fleroxacin [69]	400 mg/4.9 d	NA/19	*S. aureus* (15) Enterobacteriaceae (5)	15 (79)	15 (79)
Fleroxacin [70]	400 mg/2–12 wk	NA/26	*S. aureus* (13) Enterobacteriaceae (7) CNS (6) *S. agalactiae* (2)	22 (85)	20 (77)
Fleroxacin [71]	400 mg/30 d	NA/13	*S. aureus* (8) CNS (2) Enterobacteriaceae (3) *Pseudomonas* spp. (1) Streptococci (1)	10 (77)	11 (85)

wk = week, d = day, CNS = coagulase-negative staphylococci, NA = not available.

[a]Osteomyelitis was primarily chronic, related to a contiguous focus of infection but not a foreign device, and often had failed prior treatment.

[b]Enterobacteriaceae include *Escherichia, Citrobacter, Enterobacter, Klebsiella, Morganella, Proteus, Providencia, Salmonella, Serratia,* and *Shigella* spp.

[c]Initial therapy administered intravenously.

TABLE VII Treatment of Osteomyelitis:[a] Oral Quinolones Compared to Standard Parenteral Regimens

Author [reference]	Major organisms isolated (number)	Antimicrobial therapy (mean days)	Cured/total (%)	Antimicrobial therapy[b] (mean days)	Cured/total (%)	Follow-up
Greenberg[c] [73]	Enterobacteriaceae (18) P. aeruginosa (16) S. aureus (4)	Ciprofloxacin 1.5 g/d (>42)	7/14 (50)	Various parenteral agents (>42)	11/16 (69)	≥12 m
Mader [74]	S. aureus (16) CNS (9) P. aeruginosa (8) Enterobacteriaceae (7) Miscellaneous (13)	Ciprofloxacin 1.5 g/d (38)	11/14 (79)	Various parenteral agents (38)[b]	10/12 (83)	>24 m
Gentry[c] [75]	Enterobacteriaceae (33) S. aureus (20) P. aeruginosa (17) Enterococci (4) Miscellaneous (5)	Ciprofloxacin 1.5 g/d (56)	24/31 (77)	Ceftazidime or nafcillin + aminoglycoside (47)	22/28 (79)	≥12 m
Gentry[c] [76]	S. aureus (16) Enterobacteriaceae (15) P. aeruginosa (6) Miscellaneous (2)	Ofloxacin 800 mg/d (56)	14/19 (74)	Cefazolin or ceftazidime (56)	12/14 (26)	≥18 m
Defino[c] [77]	S. aureus (41) Enterobacteriaceae (11) P. aeruginosa (10) Miscellaneous (1)	Pefloxacin 1.2 g/d (28)	23/27 (85)	Cephalothin/cephalexin plus gentamicin (28)	28/33 (85)	≥12 m
Trujillo[c] [78]	Enterobacteriaceae (47) S. aureus (11) P. aeruginosa (7)	Ciprofloxacin 1.0 g/d[d] (75)	35/35 (100)	Ceftriaxone plus amikacin (90)	35/35 (100)	≥12 m

hr = hours; m = months. [a]Patients had contiguous-focus chronic osteomyelitis that had been debrided and all foreign material removed.
[b]Parenteral agents selected based on susceptibility of causative microorganisms.
[c]Randomized nonblinded trials. [d]Initial therapy given intravenously.

and streptococci persisted after therapy in 3 of 10 and 8 of 11 patients, respectively [43]. This again raises the question regarding efficacy of currently available quinolones in treatment of infections caused by Gram-positive cocci. As in other forms of chronic osteomyelitis, debridement or resection of necrotic bone is required for optimal outcome of pedal osteomyelitis in diabetics. Adequately debrided pedal osteomyelitis caused by *S. aureus* or *S. agalactiae* should be treated by appropriately targeted β-lactam antibiotics or vancomycin. When pedal osteomyelitis is caused by Gram-negative bacilli or these plus Gram-positive cocci, a quinolone can be used; however, if anaerobic Gram-negative bacteria are also involved, an agent with antimicrobial activity against the anaerobes should be added [43,44].

Tissue cages implanted subcutaneously in guinea pigs or rats and subsequently infected display many features of foreign device-associated infection and serve as a model for this entity. Treatment with vancomycin or a quinolone has only a modest effect against *Staphylococcus epidermidis* or *S. aureus* in this model [55,80,81]. In contrast, ciprofloxacin plus rifampin sterilized *S. epidermidis*-infected cages, and fleroxacin plus rifampin and fleroxacin plus rifampin and vancomycin markedly reduced the numbers of infecting *S. aureus* and fully sterilized some infected cages [55,80,81]. Furthermore, in this model quinolones were effective in preventing the emergence of rifampin-resistant staphylococci. These and other observations suggest that quinolone–rifampin combinations have promise for treatment of *S. aureus* osteomyelitis [55,60,61,80,81]. In addition, they suggest the potential for treating device-associated staphylococcal infections without removing the foreign material.

Widmer *et al.* reported cure of staphylococcal infection involving orthopedic implants in 10 of 11 patients using prolonged rifampin-containing antimicrobial regimens (8 received ciprofloxacin plus rifampin) [82]. Drancourt *et al.* treated 47 patients who had orthopedic devices (internal fixation, hip, and knee prostheses) infected with *S. aureus* (26 patients) or coagulase-negative staphylococci (21 patients) using very prolonged courses of ofloxacin (600 mg daily) plus rifampin (900 mg daily) [83]. Devices were sterile at the time of removal and replacement in 23 of 26 patients, and infection was eradicated without replacement in 13 of 21 patients. Zimmerli *et al.*, in a randomized prospective trial, treated patients with newly symptomatic (0–21 days) [84] *Staphylococcus aureus* (*n* = 26) or *Staphylococcus epidermidis* (*n* = 7) stable but infected prosthetic hip or knee joints or internal fixation devices with an initial 2 weeks of either intravenous vancomycin or flucloxacillin plus rifampin 450 mg every 12 hours or its placebo orally [84]. After 2 weeks, intravenous therapy was replaced by ciprofloxacin 750 mg every 12 hours, and rifampin or placebo was continued based on initial randomization. Wounds were debrided, but prosthetic material was not removed; antibiotic treatment was continued for 3 to 6 months. Dropouts in the rifampin and placebo arms numbered 6 and 3, respectively. At median follow-up of 35 and 33 months, among those receiving the full course of therapy, all 12 receiving ciprofloxacin plus rifampin and 7 of 12 receiving ciprofloxacin plus placebo were cured and the prosthetic joints were retained. Seven of the dropouts were retreated with ciprofloxacin plus rifampin, and 5 were cured with the device retained. Overall, 16 of 18 randomized to receive rifampin and 9 of 15 receiving placebo were cured. The tissue cage infection studies suggest that rifampin is the ingredient enhancing cure rates in these infections; nevertheless, the quinolones have played a pivotal role in therapy, as well. This approach to the treatment of device infection is promising, but additional experience is required, including comparative trials with either standard antistaphylococcal agents or a quinolone combined with rifampin. Presently, the traditional antimicrobial regimens used for osteomyelitis, including quinolones for episodes caused by Enterobacteriaceae, combined with removal and ultimately replacement of the often loosened and painful orthopedic implants are advocated [51].

Data do not support treatment of *S. aureus* or streptococcal hematogenous osteomyelitis in children (long bones) or adults (vertebrae) with currently available quinolones. As noted previously, the efficacy of current quinolones used alone, compared with conventional antistaphylococcal agents, for treatment of *S. aureus* osteomyelitis is uncertain. For the rare episode of hematogenous osteomyelitis caused by a facultative Gram-negative bacillus, quinolones are likely to provide effective treatment.

SEPTIC ARTHRITIS

Bacterial infections of joints, in the absence of implanted orthopedic devices, are primarily hematogenous in origin. Occasionally, infections arise as a consequence of trauma and direct introduction of organisms or by extension from adjacent infection. The causative organisms of septic arthritis have age-specific distributions: in children less than 5 years of age, *S. aureus*, streptococci (*Streptococcus pneumoniae*, *S. pyogenes*, and *S. agalactiae*), and *Hemophilus influenzae* type B (now markedly reduced by immunization) are major causes; in children above 5 years of age, *S. aureus* and streptococci predominate; in adults *Neisseria gonorrhoeae* are the most common cause of suppurative arthritis; however, nongonococcal arthritis is primarily caused by *S. aureus* and streptococci, and in patients with underlying morbid or immunosuppressive disease by Gram-negative bacilli.

Large trials comparing quinolones and standard parenteral therapy for septic arthritis have not been published. Fleroxacin has been shown to penetrate well into synovial tissue and fluid, with concentrations rapidly approximating those in plasma [57,86]. It is likely that other quinolones also penetrate well into synovial tissue and fluid. Quinolone treatment has been successful in sporadic cases of suppurative arthritis caused by *Salmonella* and *Pasteurella multocida* [86–88]. Among 9 patients with septic arthritis treated with fleroxacin 400 mg daily, episodes caused by *Enterobacter cloacae*, *P. aeruginosa*, *Salmonella* spp., and coagulase-negative staphylococci were cured; in only 1 of the 5 patients with infection caused by fleroxacin-susceptible *S. aureus* was the organism eradicated and clinical cure achieved [70,71]. Quinolones are advocated as alternatives to ceftriaxone treatment of disseminated gonococcal infection and are likely effective therapy for gonococcal arthritis caused by quinolone-susceptible strains.

CONCLUSION

Expanded clinical experience with the quinolones now approved for use in the United States or elsewhere has defined significant roles for these agents in the treatment of skin and soft tissue infection and of bone and joint infection. Quinolones are highly effective and appropriate therapy for complex skin and soft tissue infection caused by facultative Gram-negative bacilli or these organisms in combination with aerobic Gram-positive cocci. Additionally, ciprofloxacin is the recommended agent of choice for the treatment of osteomyelitis caused by Enterobacteriaceae, except *Serratia* spp. Significant failure rates with quinolone therapy of osteomyelitis caused by *S. aureus*, *P. aeruginosa*, and *Serratia* spp., even when these organisms are quinolone susceptible, suggest that other agents be used in these settings. The emergence and dissemination of staphylococci, particularly methicillin-resistant *S. aureus* and *P. aeruginosa* that are resistant to quinolones, may further limit their utility in these infections. The unpredictability of the antibacterial activity of newly available compounds (and the poor activity of earlier ones) against anaerobic Gram-negative bacilli argues for caution in using these agents alone when severe infection due to anaerobes is encountered.

The combination of quinolones plus rifampin may hold great promise for the treatment of *S. aureus* osteomyelitis and for eradication of staphylococcal infections involving prosthetic devices without obligatory device removal. Additional research is warranted in these areas.

In treating these infections, the quinolones provide considerable strategic advantages. Their potency against Gram-negative bacilli and bioavailability with oral administration allow significant simplification of therapy. Oral therapy can replace parenteral therapy, thus reducing hospitalization, avoiding complications of intravenous access, and reducing end-organ toxicities associated with parenteral β-lactam antimicrobials and aminoglycosides. Significant cost savings can be achieved with the judicious use of quinolones in the treatment of skin and soft tissue infections and osteomyelitis. These compounds are an advance in the treatment of these complex and difficult to treat infections.

REFERENCES

1. Davis, R., Markham, A., Balfour, J. A. (1996). Ciprofloxacin: An updated review of its pharmacology, therapeutic efficacy, and tolerability. *Drugs* **51**, 1019–1074.

2. Todd, P. A., and Faulds, D. (1991). Ofloxacin: A reappraisal of its antimicrobial activity, pharmacology and therapeutic use. *Drugs* **42**, 825–876.

3. Andriole, V. T. (1988). Clinical overview of newer quinolone antibacterial agents. In "The Quinolones" (V. T. Andriole ed.), pp. 155–181. Academic Press, San Diego.

4. Panneton, A. C., Bergeron, M. C., and LeBel, M. (1988). Pharmacokinetics and tissue penetration of fleroxacin after single and multiple 400-mg and 800-mg dosage regimens. *Antimicrob. Agents Chemother.* **32**, 1515–1520.

5. Hellum, K. B., Walstad, R. A., Thurman-Neilsen, E., and Dale, L. G. (1989). Fleroxacin pharmacokinetics and penetration into interstitial fluid. *Rev. Infect. Dis.* **11** (Suppl. 5), S1081–S1082.

6. Johnson, J. H., Cooper, M. A., Andrews, J. M., and Wise, R. (1992). Pharmacokinetics and inflammatory fluid penetration of sparfloxacin. *Antimicrob. Agents Chemother.* **36**, 2444–2446.

7. Wise, R., Mortiboy, D., Child, J., and Andrews, J. M. (1996). Pharmacokinetics and penetration into inflammatory fluid of trovafloxacin (CP-99,219). *Antimicrob. Agents Chemother.* **40**, 47–49.

8. Wise, R., Griggs, D., and Andrews, J. M. (1988). Pharmacokinetics of the quinolones in volunteers: A proposed dosing schedule. *Rev. Infect. Dis.* **10** (Suppl. 1), S83–S87.

9. Gerding, D. N., and Hitt, J. A. (1989). Tissue penetration of the new quinolones in humans. *Rev. Infect. Dis.* **11** (Suppl. 5), S1046–S1057.

10. Wise, R., Andrews, J. M., Ashby, J. P., and Marshall, J. (1999). A study to determine the pharmacokinetics and inflammatory fluid penetration of gatifloxacin following, A single oral dose. *J. Antimicrob. Chemother.* **44**, 701–704.

11. Wise, R., Andrews, J. M., Marshall, G., and Hartman, G. (1999). Pharmacokinetics and inflammatory-fluid penetration of moxifloxacin following oral or intravenous administration. *Antimicrob. Agents Chemother.* **43**, 1508–1510.

12. Muller, M., Stab, H., Brunner, M., Moller, J. G., Lackner, E., and Eichler, H. G. (1999). Penetration of moxifloxacin into peripheral compartments in humans. *Antimicrob. Agents Chemother.* **43**, 2345–2349.

13. Endtz, H. P., Mouton, J. W., and den Hollander, J. G. (1997). Comparative *in vitro* activities of trovafloxacin (CP 99,219) agaInst 445 Gram-positive isolates from patients with endocarditis and those with other blood stream infections. *Antimicrob. Agents Chemother.* **41**, 1146–1149.

14. Goldstein, E. J. C., Citron, D. M., Hunt-Gerardo, S., Hudspeth, M., and Merriam, C. V. (1997). Comparative *in vitro* activities of DU-6859a, levofloxacin, ofloxacin, sparfloxacin, and ciprofloxacin against 387 aerobic and anaerobic bite wound isolates. *Antimicrob. Agents Chemother.* **41**, 1193–1195.

15. Nord, C. E. (1996). In vitro activity of quinolones and other antimicrobial agents against anaerobic bacteria. *Clin. Infect. Dis.* **23** (Suppl. 1), S15–S18.

16. Eliopoulos, G. M. (1999). Activity of newer fluoroquinolones *in vitro* against Gram-positive bacteria. *Drugs* **58** (Suppl. 2), 23–28.

17. Jones, M. E., Visser, M. R., Klootwijk, M., Heisig, P., Verhoef, J., and Schmitz, F. J. (1999). Comparative activities of clinafloxacin, grepafloxacin, levofloxacin, moxifloxacin, ofloxacin, sparfloxacin, and trovafloxacin and nonquinolones linozelid, quinupristin-dalfopristin, gentamicin, and vancomycin against clinical isolates of ciprofloxacin-resistant and -susceptible *Staphylococcus aureus* strains. *Antimicrob. Agents Chemother.* **43**, 421–423.

18. Jones, R. N., Beach, M. L., Pfaller, M. A., and Doern, G. V. (1998). Antimicrobial activity of gatifloxacin tested against 1676 strains of ciprofloxacin-resistant Gram-positive cocci isolated from patient infections in North and South America. *Diag. Microbiol. Infect. Dis.* **32**, 247–252.

19. Pong, A., Thomson, K. S., Moland, E. S., Chartrand, S. A., and Sanders, C. C. (1999). Activity of moxifloxacin against pathogens with decreased susceptibility to ciprofloxacin. *J. Antimicrob. Chemother.* **44**, 621–627.

20. Hecht, D. W., and Wexler, H. M. (1996). In vitro susceptibility of anaerobes to quinolones in the United States. *Clin. Infect. Dis.* **23** (Suppl. 1), S2–S8.

21. Aldridge, K. E., Ashcraft, D., and Bowman, K. A. (1997). Comparative *in vitro* activities of trovafloxacin (CP 99,219) and other antimicrobials against clinically significant anaerobes. *Antimicrob. Agents Chemother.* **41**, 484–487.

22. Goldstein, E. J. C., Citron, D. M., Merriam, C. V., Tyrrell, K., and Warren, Y. (1999). Activity of gatifloxacin compared to those of five other quinolones versus aerobic and anaerobic isolates from skin and soft tissue samples of human and animal bite wound infections. *Antimicrob. Agents Chemother.* **43**, 1475–1479.

23. Goldstein, E. J. C., Citron, D. M., Merriam, C. V., Tyrrell, K., and Warren, Y. (1999). Activities of gemifloxacin (SB 265805, LB20304) compared to those of other oral antimicrobial agents against unusual anaerobes. *Antimicrob. Agents Chemother.* **43**, 2726–2730.

24. Goldstein, E. J., Citron, D. M., Warren, Y., Tyrrell, K., and Merriam, C. V. (1999). *In vitro* activity of gemifloxacin (SB265805) against anaerobes. *Antimicrob. Agents Chemother.* **43**, 2231–2235.

25. Felmingham, D., Robbins, M. J., Mathias, I., Ingley, K., Bhogal, H., and Grunenberg, R. N. (1997). European multicenter study of comparative in vitro susceptibility of Gram-negative bacteria to levofloxacin. *Abstr. 8th Eur. Cong. Clin. Microbiol. Infect. Dis.*, Lausanne. Abstr. #P1150.

26. Betriu, C., Gomez, M., Palau, L., Sanchez, A., and Picazo, J. J. (1999). Activities of new antimicrobial agents (trovafloxacin, moxifloxacin, sanfetrinem, and quinupristin–dalfopristin) against *Bacteroides fragilis* group: Comparison with the activities of 14 other agents. *Antimicrob. Agents Chemother.* **43**, 2320–2322.

27. Appelbaum, P. C. (1999). Quinolone activity against anaerobes. *Drugs* **58** (Suppl. 2), 60–64.

28. Gentry, L. O. (1991). Review of quinolones in the treatment of infections of skin and skin structure. *J. Antimicrob. Chemother.* **28** (Suppl. C), 97–110.

29. Smith, J. W., and Nichol, R. L. (1993). Comparison of oral fleroxacin with oral amoxicillin/clavulanate for treatment of skin and soft tissue infections. *Am. J. Med.* **94** (Suppl. 3A), 150S–154S.

30. Powers, R. D. (1993). Open trial of fleroxacin versus amoxicillin/clavulanate in the treatment of infections of skin and soft tissue. *Am. J. Med.* **94** (Suppl. 3A), 155S–158S.

31. Data on File (1966). 300331:2. Raritan, NJ, R.W.J. Pharmaceutical Research Institute. (GENERIC) Ref Type: Report

32. Gentry, L. O., Ramirez-Ronda, C. H., Rodriguez-Noreiga, E., Thadepalli, H., del Rosal, P. L., and Ramirez, C. (1989). Oral ciprofloxacin vs. parenteral cefotaxime in treatment of difficult skin and skin structure infections: A multicenter trial. *Arch. Intern. Med.* **149**, 2579–2583.

33. Gentry, L. O., Rodriguez-Gomez, G., Zeluff, B. J., Koshdel, A., and Price, M. (1989). A comparative evaluation of oral ofloxacin versus intravenous cefotaxime therapy for serious skin and skin structure infections. *Am. J. Med.* **87** (Suppl. 6C), 57S–60S.

34. Parrish, L. C., and Jungkind, D. L. (1993). Systemic antimicrobial therapy for skin and skin structure infections: Comparison of fleroxacin and ceftazidime. *Am. J. Med.* **94** (Suppl. 3A), 166S–173S.

35. Fass, R. L., Plouffe, J. F., and Russell, J. A. (1989). Intravenous/oral ciprofloxacin versus ceftazidime in the treatment of serious infections. *Am. J. Med.* **18** (Suppl. D), 153–157.

36. Gentry, L. O., and Koshdel, A. (1987). Intravenous/oral ciprofloxacin versus intravenous ceftazidime in the treatment of serious Gram-negative infections of skin and skin structure. *Am. J. Med.* **87** (Suppl. 5A), 132S–135S.

37. Dominguez, J., Palma, F., Vega, M. E., *et al.* (1989). Brief report: Prospective controlled randomized non-blind comparison of intravenous/oral ciprofloxacin with intravenous ceftazidime in the treatment of skin or soft tissue infections. *Am. J. Med.* **87** (Suppl. 5A), 136S–137S.

38. Tarshis, G., Miskin, B. M., Jones, T. M., *et al.* (1999). Oral gatifloxacin, 400 mg QD, vs. oral levofloxacin, 500 mg QD, in the treatment of uncomplicated skin and soft tissue infections. *Abstr. 39th Intersci. Conf. Antimicrob. Agents Chemother.*, San Francisco. Abstr. #1075.

39. del Rosal, P. L., Fabian, G., Vickfragoso, R., *et al.* (1999). Efficacy and safety of moxifloxacin vs. cephalexin (with or without metronidazole) in the treatment of mild to moderate uncomplicated skin and skin structure infections. *Abstr. 39th Intersci. Conf. Antimicrob. Agents Chemother.*, San Francisco. Abstr. #1076.

40. Siami, G., Christou, N., Eiseman, I., Carter, C., and Tack, K. (1999). A randomized study of clinafloxacin and piperacillin/tazobactam in severe skin and soft tissue infections. *Abstr. 39th Intersci. Conf. Antimicrob. Agents Chemother.*, San Francisco. Abstr. #1106a.

41. Beam, T. R. Jr., Gutierrez, I., Powell, S., *et al.* (1989). Prospective study of the efficacy and safety of oral and intravenous ciprofloxacin in the treatment of diabetic foot infections. *Rev. Infect. Dis.* **11** (Suppl. 5), S1163–S1163.

42. Peterson, L. R., Lissack, L. M., Canter, K., Fasching, C. E., Clabots, C., and Gerding, D. N. (1989). Therapy of lower extremity infections with ciprofloxacin in patients with diabetes mellitus, peripheral vascular disease, or both. *Am. J. Med.* **86**, 801–808.

43. Lipsky, B. A., Baker, P. D., Landon, G. C., and Fernau, R. (1997). Antibiotic therapy for diabetic foot infections: Comparison of two parenteral-to-oral regimens. *Clin. Infect. Dis.* **24**, 643–648.

44. Gerding, D. N. (1995). Foot infections in diabetic patients: The role of anaerobes. *Clin. Infect. Dis.* **20** (Suppl. C), S283–S288.

45. Johnson, S., Lebahn, F., Peterson, L. P., and Gerding, D. N. (1995). Use of an anaerobic collection and transport swab device to recover anaerobic bacteria from infected foot ulcers in diabetics. *Clin. Infect. Dis.* **20** (Suppl. A), S289–S290.

46. Karchmer, A. W., and Gibbons, G. W. (1994). Foot infections in diabetes: Evaluation and management. In "Current Clinical Topics in Infectious Diseases" (J. S. Remington and M. N. Swartz, eds.), pp. 1–22. Blackwell Scientific, Boston.

47. Lipsky, B. A., Pecoraro, R. E., Larson, S. A., Hanley, M. E., and Ahroni, J. H. (1990). Outpatient management of uncomplicated lower-extremity infections in diabetic patients. *Arch. Intern. Med.* **150**, 790–797.

48. Goldstein, E. J. C. (1996). Possible role for the new fluoroquinolones (levofloxacin, grepafloxacin, trovafloxacin, clinafloxacin, sparfloxacin, and DU-6859a) in the treatment of anaerobic infections: Review of current information on efficacy and safety. *Clin. Infect. Dis.* **23** (Suppl. 1), S25–S30.

49. Waldvogel, F. A., Medoff, G., and Swartz, M. N. (1970). Osteomyelitis: A review of clinical features, therapeutic considerations, and unusual aspects. *New Engl. J. Med.* **282**, 198–322.

50. Lew, D. P., and Waldvogel, F. A. (1997). Osteomyelitis. *New Engl. J. Med.* **336**, 999–1007.

51. Brause, B. D. (1995). Infections with prostheses in bones and joints. In "Principles and Practice of Infectious Diseases" (G. L. Mandell, J. E. Bennett, and R. Dolin, eds.), pp. 1051–1055. Churchill Livingstone, New York.

52. Caputo, G. M., Cavanagh, P. R., Ulbrecht, J. S., Gibbons, G. W., and Karchmer, A. W. (1994). Assessment and management of foot disease in patients with diabetes. *New Engl. J. Med.* **331**, 854–860.

53. Chuard, C., Lucet, J. C., Rohner, P., *et al.* (1991). Resistance of *Staphylococcus aureus* recovered from infected foreign body in vivo to killing by antimicrobials. *J. Infect. Dis.* **163**, 1369–1373.

54. Hudson, M. C., Ramp, W. K., Nicholson, N. C., Williams, A. S., and Nousianen, M. T. (1995). Internalization of *Staphylococcus aureus* by cultured osteoblasts. *Microb. Pathogen.* **19**, 409–419.

55. Widmer, A. F., Frei, R., Rajacic, Z., and Zimmerli, W. (1990). Correlation between *in vivo* and *in vitro* efficacy of antimicrobial agents against foreign body infections. *J. Infect. Dis.* **162**, 96–102.

56. Mader, J. T., and Calhoun, M. (1995). Osteomyelitis. In "Principles and Practice of Infectious Diseases" (G. L. Mandell, J. E. Bennett, and R. Dolin, eds.), pp. 1039–1051. Churchill Livingstone, New York.

57. Weidekamm, E., and Portmann, R. (1993). Penetration of fleroxacin into body tissues and fluids. *Am. J. Med.* **94** (Suppl. 3A), 75S–80S.

58. Norden, C. W., and Shinners, E. (1985). Ciprofloxacin as therapy for experimental osteomyelitis caused by *Pseudomonas aeruginosa*. *J. Infect. Dis.* **151**, 291–294.

59. Bayer, A. S., Norman, D., and Anderson, D. (1985). Efficacy of ciprofloxacin in experimental arthritis caused by *Escherichia coli* in *in vitro–in vivo* correlations. *J. Infect. Dis.* **152**, 811–816.

60. Henry, N. K., Rouse, M. S., Whitesell, A. L., *et al.* (1987). Treatment of methicillin-resistant *Staphylococcus aureus* experimental osteomyelitis with ciprofloxacin or vancomycin alone or in combination with rifampin. *Am. J. Med.* **82**, 73–75.

61. Dworkin, R., Modin, G., Kunz, S., *et al.* (1990). Comparative efficacies of ciprofloxacin, pefloxacin, and vancomycin in combination with rifampin in a rat model of methicillin-resistant *Staphylococcus aureus* chronic osteomyelitis. *Antimicrob. Agents Chemother.* **34**, 1014–1016.

62. Gilbert, D. N., Tice, A. D., Marsh, P. K., *et al.* (1987). Oral ciprofloxacin therapy for chronic contiguous osteomyelitis caused by aerobic Gram-negative bacilli. *Am. J. Med.* **82** (Suppl. 4A), 254–258.

63. Nix, D. E., Cumbo, T. J., Kuritzky, P., Devito, J. M., and Schentag, J. J. (1987). Oral ciprofloxacin in the treatment of serious soft tissue and bone infection. *Am. J. Med.* **82** (Suppl. 4A), 146–153.

64. Swedish Study Group (1988). Therapy of acute and chronic Gram-negative osteomyelitis with ciprofloxacin. *J. Antimicrob. Chemother.* **22**, 221–228.

65. Dan, M., Siegman, I. Y., Pitlik, S., *et al.* (1990). Oral ciprofloxacin treatment of *Pseudomonas aeruginosa* osteomyelitis. *Antimicrob. Agents Chemother.* **34**, 849–852.

66. Gomis, M., Barberan, J., Lopez-Arceo, J., *et al.* (1993). Pefloxacin in the treatment of osteomyelitis. *Drugs* **45** (Suppl. 3), 456–457.

67. Ketteri, R., Beckurtz, T., Stubinger, B., *et al.* (1988). Use of ofloxacin in open fractures and in treatment of post-traumatic osteomyelitis. *J. Antimicrob. Chemother.* **22** (Suppl. C), 159–166.

68. Seibold, R., and Betz, A. (1991). Treatment of post-traumatic osteitis with intravenous ofloxacin. *Clin. Therap.* **13**, 457–459.

69. Stamboulian, D., Barclay, E., Cassetti, I., and Sturba, E. (1990). Treatment of acute osteomyelitis with fleroxacin, a long-acting fluoroquinolone (presented at 3rd Int. Symp. New Quinolones, Vancouver). *Eur. J. Clin. Microbiol. Infect. Dis. Symp. Proc.*, pp. 33–34.

70. Green, S. L. (1993). Efficacy of oral fleroxacin in bone and joint infections. *Am. J. Med.* **44** (Suppl. 3A), 174S–176S.

71. Putz, P. A. (1993). A pilot study of oral fleroxacin given once daily in patients with bone and joint infections. *Am. J. Med.* **94** (Suppl. 3A), 177S–181S.

72. Galanakis, N., Giamarellou, H., and Moussas, T. (1997). Chronic osteomyelitis caused by multiresistant Gram-negative bacteria: Evaluation of treatment with newer quinolones after prolonged follow-up. *J. Antimicrob. Chemother.* **39**, 241–246.

73. Greenberg, R. N., Tice, A. D., Marsh, P. K., *et al.* (1987). Randomized trial of ciprofloxacin compared with other antimicrobial therapy in the treatment of osteomyelitis. *Am. J. Med.* **82** (Suppl. 4A), 266–269.

74. Mader, J. T., Cantrell, J. S., and Calhoun, J. (1990). Oral ciprofloxacin compared with standard parenteral antibiotic therapy for chronic osteomyelitis in adults. *J. Bone Joint Surg.* **72**, 104–110.

75. Gentry, L. O., and Rodriguez-Gomez, G. (1990). Oral ciprofloxacin compared with parenteral antibiotics in the treatment of osteomyelitis. *Antimicrob. Agents Chemother.* **34**, 40–43.

76. Gentry, L. O., and Rodriguez-Gomez, G. (1991). Ofloxacin versus parenteral therapy for chronic osteomyelitis. *Antimicrob. Agents Chemother.* **35**, 538–541.

77. Defino, H. L. A., Moretti, J. E., and Rodrigues-Fuentes, A. E. (1992). Comparative study of the efficacy of pefloxacin versus cephalexin plus gentamicin in the treatment of post-traumatic or post-surgical osteomyelitis. *Rev. Bras. Med.* **49**, 785–790.

78. Trujillo, I. Z., Valladares, G., and Nava, A. (1993). Ciprofloxacin in the treatment of chronic osteomyelitis in adults. *Drugs* **45** (Suppl. 3), 454–455.

79. Lew, D. P., and Waldvogel, F. A. (1995). Quinolones and osteomyelitis: State-of-the-art. *Drugs* **49** (Suppl. 2), 100–111.

80. Lucet, J. C., Herrmann, M., Rohner, P., Auckenthaler, R., Waldvogel, F. A., and Lew, D. P. (1990). Treatment of experimental foreign body infection caused by methicillin-resistant *Staphylococcus, aureus. Antimicrob. Agents Chemother.* **34**, 2312–2317.

81. Chuard, C., Herrmann, M., Vaudaux, P., Waldvogel, F. A., and Lew, D. P. (1991). Successful therapy of experimental chronic foreign-body infection due to methicillin-resistant *Staphylococcus aureus* by antimicrobial combinations. *Antimicrob. Agents Chemother.* **35**, 2611–2616.

82. Widmer, A. F., Gaechter, A., Ochsner, P. E., and Zimmerli, W. (1992). Antimicrobial treatment of orthopedic implant-related infections with rifampin combinations. *Clin. Infect. Dis.* **14**, 1251–1253.

83. Drancourt, M., Stein, A., Argenson, J. N., Zannier, A., Curvale, G., and Raoult, D. (1993). Oral rifampin plus ofloxacin for treatment of *Staphylococcus*-infected orthopedic implants. *Antimicrob. Agents Chemother.* **37**, 1214–1218.

84. Zimmerli, W., Widmer, A. F., Blatter, M., Frei, R., Ochsner, P. E., and the Foreign-Body Infection Study Group (1998). Role of rifampin for treatment of orthopedic implant-related staphylococcal infections: A randomized controlled trial. *JAMA* **279**, 1537–1541.

85. Schmidt, H. G. K., *et al.* (1989). Penetration of fleroxacin into bone and synovial fluid after administration of a single oral dose. *Rev. Infect. Dis.* **2** (Suppl. 5), 1268.

86. Diaz-Tejeiro, R., Diez, J., Maduell, F., Esparza, N., Errasti, P., and Pueroy, A. (1989). Successful treatment with ciprofloxacin of multiresistant *Salmonella* arthritis in a renal transplant recipient. *Nephrol. Dial. Transplant.* **4**, 390–392.

87. Praet, J. P., Peretz, A., Goosens, H., van Laethem, Y., and Famacy, J. P. (1989). Salmonella septic arthritis: Additional 2 cases with quinolone treatment. *J. Rheumatol.* **16**, 1610–1611.

88. Raffi, F., Poirier, P., and Reynaud, A. E. (1989). Arthrite septique a *Pasteurella multocida*: Traitement par une fluoroquinolone. *Presse Med.* **18**, 1482.

89. Centers for Disease Control and Prevention (1996). National Nosocomial Infections Surveillance System. USPHS May.

90. Piddock, L. J. V. (1994). New quinolones and Gram-positive bacteria. *Antimicrob. Agents Chemother.* **38**, 163–169.

91. Eliopoulos, G. M., and Eliopoulos, C. T. (1993). Activity in vitro of the quinolones. In "Quinolone Antimicrobial Agents" (D. C. Hooper and J. S. Wolfson, eds.), pp. 161–193. American Society for Microbiology, Washington, DC.

92. Eliopoulos, G. M., Klimm, K., Eliopoulos, C. T., Ferraro, M. J., and Moellering Jr., R. C. (1993). In vitro activity of CP-99,219, a new fluoroquinolone, against clinical isolates of Gram-positive bacteria. *Antimicrob. Agents Chemother.* **37**, 366–370.

93. Tassler, H. (1993). Comparative efficacy and safety of oral fleroxacin and amoxicillin/clavulanate potassium in skin and soft tissue infection. *Am. J. Med.* **94** (Suppl. 3A), 159S–165S.

94. Nicodermo, A. C., Robledo, J. A., Jasovich, A., and Neto, W. (1998). A multicenter, double-blind, randomised study comparing the efficacy and safety of oral levofloxacin versus ciprofloxacin in the treatment of uncomplicated skin and skin structure infections. *Int. J. Clin. Pract.* **52**, 69–74.

95. Coignard, S., Renard, C., and Lortat-Jacob, A. (1986). Diffusion de la perfloxacine dans le tissue osseux humain. *Med. Mal. Infect.* **7**, 471–474.

96. Davies, A. J., Synot, M., Ashfield, N., *et al.* (1989). Penetration of pefloxacin into bone following a single intravenous dose. *Rev. Infect. Dis.* **11** (Suppl. 5), S1078–S1079.

97. Fong, I. W., Ledbetter, W. H., and Vanderbroucke, A. C. (1986). Ciprofloxacin concentrations in bone and muscle after oral dosing. *Antimicrob. Agents Chemother.* **29**, 405–408.

98. Meissner, A., and Borner, K. (1993). Konzentration von ciprofloxacin im knochengewebe. *Akt. Traumatol.* **23**, 80–84.

99. Wittmann, D. H., and Kotthaus, E. (1986). Further methodological improvement in antibiotic bone concentration measurements: Penetration of ofloxacin into bone and cartilage. *Infection* **14** (Suppl. 4), S270–S273.

100. Meissner, A., Borner, K., and Koeppe, P. (1990). Concentrations of ofloxacin in human bone and in cartilage. *J. Antimicrob. Chemother.* **26** (Suppl. D), 69–74.

CHAPTER 14

Safety Overview

Toxicity, Adverse Effects, and Drug Interactions

RALF STAHLMANN* and HARTMUT LODE†

*Department of Pharmacology and Toxicology, Institute of Clinical Pharmacology and Toxicology, University Hospital Benjamin Franklin, Freie Universität Berlin, 14195 Berlin, Germany, and †Department of Chest and Infectious Diseases, Hospital Zehlendorf, 14109 Berlin, Germany

INTRODUCTION

It is generally more difficult to detect all the side effects of a drug than to prove its effectiveness. Studies on the antimicrobial activity or clinical efficacy of an antibiotic are comparatively easy because investigators know what they are looking for: inhibition of microbes *in vitro* or clinical cure of an infectious disease. It is a planned search for an expected result. However, searching for toxicity is open ended and must be performed without definition of all possible endpoints.

Fluoroquinolones are relatively safe and well-tolerated drugs. Among trials comparing quinolones with other agents, the rate of adverse reactions was very similar in most studies. Under therapeutic conditions, no uniform life-threatening organ toxicity is known that would restrict their clinical use. However, therapy with fluoroquinolones is associated with several hazards and risks that must be considered and weighed against the possible benefits of a quinolone therapy before a compound of this class can be prescribed. Despite routinely performed studies in animals, volunteers, and patients on the safety of drugs before approval, unexpected adverse effects occurred after treatment with fluoroquinolones as observed before with antimicrobials from other classes. Stained teeth in children due to tetracyclines, the effects of certain cephalosporins on blood clotting, or the severe reactions seen with the fluoroquinolone temafloxacin are examples of effects that were noticed only several months or even years after launch of the drug.

The fluoroquinolones temafloxacin, trovafloxacin, and grepafloxacin were taken from the market due to rarely occurring severe adverse reactions. The toxic effects observed with these three drugs differed. The use of *temafloxacin* was associated with a syndrome of hemolysis, renal failure, and thrombocytopenia. The estimated incidence of the syndrome was 1 per 5000 prescriptions—an incidence too low to be detected reliably during clinical studies before marketing. Due to this toxicity, the drug was withdrawn from the market shortly after approval for clinical use in 1992. A similar pattern of adverse effects has not been observed with other fluoroquinolones. The mechanism of this rare side effect is unknown [1,2].

The use of trovafloxacin was associated with severe hepatic reactions in rare cases. A total of 140 patients with severe hepatic reactions became known after the drug had been prescribed worldwide approximately 2.5 million times. In many cases, patients had severe underlying diseases. Details of one of the human cases have been published: a 66-year-old man developed gastrointestinal symptoms and showed increased transaminases after daily treatment with 100 mg trovafloxacin for 4 weeks. A biopsy specimen of the liver showed centrilobular and focal periportal necrosis and eosinophilic infiltration suggesting toxic injury [3,4].

Another quinolone, one that was taken off the market in 1999, was grepafloxacin. Due to an effect of grepafloxacin on cardiac repolarization, manifested as QT interval prolongation on the electrocardiogram, some patients were considered at risk of torsade de pointes when treated with grepafloxacin. Although such events had been reported very rarely, it was withdrawn in all countries. From the toxicological studies performed during preclinical development, it was known that the potential of the drug to induce cardiac arrhythmia was higher than in other quinolones that had been tested as comparators, such as ciprofloxacin [5]. However, since the effect on the QT interval in humans after oral administration was marginal and based on the favorable experience during clinical investigation, it was considered to be without risk to humans.

TOXICITY OF QUINOLONES (STUDIES IN ANIMALS)

GENERAL REMARKS

During routinely performed preclinical studies, fluoroquinolones revealed specific toxicities. The results of these studies, which were mainly conducted by the manufacturers, usually have not been published in peer-reviewed journals, and some of the information given here is taken from material distributed by the drug-producing companies. The relevance of toxicological data from animal experiments certainly diminishes with increasing human information and data from clinical studies. Nevertheless, some preclinical data are described here because they provide a background for evaluation of the tolerability of quinolones in humans. Furthermore, some toxicological data on the quinolones that have not been introduced for therapy might be of interest to the clinically oriented reader.

Although similar studies have been conducted by the companies for all derivatives, the amount of data from these studies published by the manufacturers differs considerably. For this reason, no "balanced" information is given here. A well-founded comparison of toxicity among the fluoroquinolones is not possible for most effects studied because they usually do not derive from comparative studies. Furthermore, important data, such as the pharmacokinetics of a drug in laboratory animals, are not available in most instances. A comprehensive review of the toxicity studies performed with quinolones has been published by Takayama et al. [6].

Effects on Connective Tissue Structures (Cartilage, Tendon)

Effects on Cartilage

Arthropathy in juvenile animals is an extraordinary form of drug toxicity that has been observed with all quinolones tested so far (for a review, see [7–9]). In immature animals, quinolones cause joint cartilage defects, which must be considered irreversible, as shown in juvenile dogs and rats (e.g., [10]). Dogs are especially sensitive to the chondrotoxic action of quinolones, with lesions inducible at rather low-dose levels (10 to 50 mg/kg body weight). This chondrotoxic potential has led to an important restriction on the use of quinolones. They are contraindicated in children and growing adolescents, and during pregnancy and lactation, although the significance of the findings for humans still remains unclear (Table I). There are several published reports of children and adolescents treated with quinolones (mostly norfloxacin and ciprofloxacin), and no definitely drug-related cases of arthropathy have been noted (see, e.g., [11]), but there are several incidences of arthralgia after quinolone therapy (see section on "Musculoskeletal Reactions (Arthralgia, Tendinitis)").

Gait abnormalities in immature dogs were first observed and described in 1977 after oral administration of nalidixic acid, oxolinic acid, and pipemidic acid for 1–15 days at doses of 200–1000 mg/kg. Lesions were confined to the major articulations, such as the hip or shoulder joints. Initially, blisters in the articular cartilage were evident, which then progressed to ulcerative erosions. In most animals, clinical recovery occurred within 2 to 3 weeks; however, the cartilage lesions were present up to 3 months after withdrawal of the drug [12].

Daily oral administration of two times 50-mg pipemidic acid/kg b.w. or more caused lameness in juvenile beagle dogs (2.5–6 months old) that was most pronounced 3–7 days after the start of treatment. At a lower dose (2×15 mg/kg daily), cartilage erosions were still found, but the dogs showed no clinical symptoms. Dogs that were 2.5 to 6 months old were most susceptible to the toxic effect. Mature dogs, aged 12 months or older, showed no clinical signs of arthropathy. Very young animals (1 or 2 weeks old) also seemed to be rather "resistant" to this toxic effect; however, the doses applied were considerably lower. On the assumption that blister formation only takes place with the mechanical pressure of body weight on the cartilage, young dogs were given pipemidic acid and kept hung with their shoulders up so that the joints of the forefeet were free from pressure for a certain period of time. Under these conditions, cartilage alterations after a single oral dose of 500 mg pipemidic

TABLE I   Arthropathy Induced by Quinolones in Juvenile Animals

Compounds	All quinolones tested so far
Animal species	Dog, rat, rabbit, mouse, guinea pig, nonhuman primate, and others (juvenile animals)
Known since	1977 (pipemidic acid, dog)
Dose	For example, 10 mg/kg/d ofloxacin for 1 week (dog) (higher doses in rodents can be explained by differences in pharmacokinetics)
Lesions	Blisters and erosions in articular cartilage of weight-bearing joints (lesions were irreversible)
Mechanism	Probably due to the magnesium-chelating properties of the drugs
Clinical observations	Low risk for acute effects, best experience with ciprofloxacin in cystic fibrosis patients
	Several case reports of arthralgia (mostly with pefloxacin)
Consequence	Quinolones are contraindicated in children and adolescents, in pregnant and breast-feeding women
	for some indications (e.g., cystic fibrosis), treatment with ciprofloxacin seems to be justified.

acid/kg b.w. were observed in the hind legs, but "blister formation was hardly noted in the forefeet." Average plasma levels of the drug 5 and 24 hours after administration were 31.5 and 2.5 mg/liter, respectively [13].

Corresponding results were found with all of the newer fluoroquinolones (e.g., ciprofloxacin, ofloxacin, levofloxacin, fleroxacin, sparfloxacin, moxifloxacin, gatifloxacin, gemifloxacin), but only a few studies have been published in peer-reviewed journals. One exception is difloxacin, which is not available for therapeutic use. The histological and ultrastructural findings with this fluoroquinolone have been described in a series of papers providing detailed information on the pathological alterations [14,15].

Taken together, the available information indicates that all (fluorinated or nonfluorinated) quinolones induce joint cartilage lesions in immature animals from multiple species. The minimal doses are low in dogs (e.g., 10 to 50 mg/kg b.w.), which represent the most sensitive species, but the immature rat is a suitable model for studying the effects more closely [16–20]. Very little is known about the effects of fluoroquinolones during very early postnatal development (e.g., the neonatal period), but at earlier developmental phases the epiphyseal growth plate as well as the articular cartilage layer seem to be susceptible (see section on "Postnatal Studies").

Because the pharmacokinetics of fluoroquinolones differ considerably between rodents and man, data on bioavailability and drug concentrations in plasma or target tissues in animals have to be taken into account if the results from experiments in rats are compared with the clinical situation. For example, due to the poor bioavailability of sparfloxacin in rats after gastric intubation with a high dose of 1800 mg sparfloxacin per kg of body weight, peak concentrations in plasma were less than 20 mg/liter [21]. Oral treatment of juvenile rats with 100 mg ofloxacin per kg b.w. b.i.d. for 5 days corresponds to an exposure that is roughly equivalent to a normal human exposure during therapy with the drug. Concentrations in joint cartilage are approximately three times higher than the corresponding plasma concentrations under these conditions [20].

The exact mechanism of quinolone-induced arthropathy is still unknown. However, some data indicate that the affinity of the drugs for magnesium is probably the crucial initial step. Fluoroquinolones form chelate complexes with divalent and trivalent cations, and their affinity for magnesium is more pronounced than for calcium or other minerals. Immature rats fed a magnesium-deficient diet developed cartilage lesions that could not be distinguished from lesions induced by quinolone treatment [18,22,23]. A possible consequence of depletion of functionally available magnesium in joint cartilage could be production of oxygen-derived reactive species, as observed in chondrocytes from quinolone-treated juvenile rabbits [24]. Some data from experiments performed with other tissues indicate that such radicals can be generated in magnesium deficiency [25]. Finally, chondrocytes and/or cartilage matrix are irreversibly damaged, and the characteristic blisters and clefts are formed. The finding that supplementation with magnesium and tocopherol diminishes quinolone-induced chondrotoxicity in immature rats further emphasizes this hypothesis [26]. Furthermore, it seems noteworthy that a pronounced synergistic toxicity exists between fluoroquinolone treatment and magnesium deficiency. Juvenile rats with a mild magnesium deficiency reacted with joint cartilage lesions when they were treated with low doses of a fluoroquinolone that induced no cartilage toxicity when given to rats with normal magnesium status [20].

Data established in rats at various times during postnatal development showed that magnesium concentration in joint cartilage from 28-day-old rats is significantly lower than in younger or older rats. This might explain the "phase specificity" of quinolone-induced arthropathy, that is, the pronounced sensitivity of immature animals during a certain developmental stage [27].

It is of considerable interest that the similarities between symptoms after quinolone treatment or after a magnesium-deficient diet exist in dogs as well. Lameness and gait alterations closely resembling those associated with quinolone-induced arthropathy have been described in magnesium-deficient beagles. Unfortunately, no joint histology has been performed with cartilage samples from these dogs, and no data are available on the concentration of magnesium in the joint cartilage of this species [28]. More recent comparative studies have shown that ultrastructural changes in canine cartilage are similar after ciprofloxacin treatment and magnesium deficiency [29,30].

Effects on Tendons

The first data on structural changes in tendon and tendon-associated tissues in rats were published by Kato and coworkers [31]. They found that pefloxacin (at 300 and 900 mg/kg) and ofloxacin (900 mg/kg) affected the Achilles tendon in juvenile 4-week-old rats, but not in 12-week-old rats. The quinolone-induced lesions were characterized by edema and mononuclear cell infiltration in the inner sheath of the inner Achilles tendon with infiltration into the adjacent synovial membrane and joint space [31,32]. In a follow-up paper, the authors showed that, out of a series of 10 fluoroquinolones, pefloxacin and fleroxacin were the most toxic derivatives, whereas, for example, sparfloxacin, norfloxacin, and ciprofloxacin were less toxic or produced no lesions even after rather high oral doses [33]. These findings are explainable by major differences in the pharmacokinetics of the compounds: fleroxacin is very well absorbed, while the absorption rates of sparfloxacin or ciprofloxacin are extremely low [21,34].

Interestingly, partial reduction of the incidence of tendonopathies after pefloxacin was obtained by administration of L-NAME (N-nitro-L-arginine methyl ester, a nitric oxide synthase inhibitor). This suggests that nitric oxide partly mediates induction of lesions, which is in agreement with the finding of Hayem and colleagues that radical formation is an important step in the pathogenesis of quinolone-induced arthropathy [24,33]. Simonin and coworkers reported an observation in mice that pefloxacin induces oxidative stress in the Achilles tendon that altered proteoglycan anabolism and oxidized collagen [35].

In an extensive electron microscopic study, tenocytes from rat Achilles tendons showed degenerative alterations, such as multiple vacuoles and vesicles in the cytoplasm, that had developed due to swelling and dilatation of cell organelles. Other indications of cell degradation were the occurrence of cell debris and cell detachment from the extracellular matrix accompanied by a loss of cell–matrix interaction. The tenocytes of Wistar rats that had been treated at day 36 and

sacrificed either 3 or 6 months afterward exhibited similar degenerative alterations. The number of degenerative alterations of tenocytes after ofloxacin
treatment was considerably higher in rats that had received a magnesium-deficient
diet than in rats with normal magnesium status [36].

NEUROTOXICITY

Adverse reactions of the central nervous system are a well-known complication
of therapy with quinolones. The mechanism of CNS toxicity with the quinolones
is unknown. Interestingly, amfonelic acid, which has a chemical structure similar
to that of nalidixic acid, has been developed as a CNS stimulant. In mice, this
compound had effects on locomotor activity similar to those with amphetamine
[37].

Some biochemical work has been done in an attempt to explain the CNS effects
observed under therapeutic conditions. Quinolones inhibit receptor binding of
γ-aminobutyric acid (GABA), an inhibitory neurotransmitter. However, it seems
doubtful that an interaction with GABA receptors could explain the adverse
effects during quinolone therapy. Convulsive seizures can be induced in mice by
concomitant administration of fenbufen and fluoroquinolones. The molecular
target or receptor for the effects of the quinolones on the CNS is unknown. The
GABA antagonistic effects of the quinolones *in vitro* depend on their substituent
at position 7 of the heterocycle. Those derivatives with a free piperazinyl group
show stronger activity in such assays than quinolones with a methylated
piperazine ring. However, the effects of quinolones on binding of ^{3}H-GABA or
^{3}H-muscimol (a GABA receptor agonist) to its receptor are weak and cannot
explain their epileptogenic properties. In the presence of fenbufen or its main
metabolite biphenyl acetic acid, the inhibitory effect of quinolones on GABA
binding is enhanced [38–40].

As receptor-binding studies have so far failed to predict the convulsive potency
of the different fluoroquinolones, the hippocampus slice model was used to study
the neurotoxic effects of a series of fluoroquinolones [41]. Electrophysiological
determination of the field potentials in the CA1 region of the rat hippocampus
slice allowed for assessment of the excitatory potential of the fluoroquinolones.
The drugs were investigated at concentrations comparable to therapeutic concentrations in the brain. All the compounds increased the population spike amplitude
in a concentration-dependent manner. Ofloxacin, ciprofloxacin, and moxifloxacin
were among those that increased the population spike amplitude only moderately,
whereas trovafloxacin, clinafloxacin, and some investigational compounds were

much more excitatory. This *in-vitro* system allows us to investigate the effects of the drugs at varying cation concentrations. Slight changes in magnesium concentrations led to strong amplification of the effects. For example, clinafloxacin (2 μmol/liter) induced an increase of the population spike amplitude of 233% at the physiological Mg^{2+} concentration of 2 mmol/liter. A slight decrease in Mg^{2+} concentration (to 1.75 mmol/liter) very strongly potentiated the clinafloxacin effect [41]. Blocking the ion channel of the NMDA receptor by the antagonist MK-801 counteracts the effects of quinolones in a concentration-dependent manner, pointing to direct involvement of the NMDA-gated ion channel in the excitatory effects of fluoroquinolones. It is of further interest that seizures induced by either quinolones or magnesium deficiency can be antagonized by MK-801 [42,43].

PHOTOTOXICITY, PHOTOMUTAGENICITY, AND PHOTOCARCINOGENICITY

Phototoxicity has been observed with all the known quinolones. It can be estimated by measuring rates of degradation when exposed to UV radiation, by measuring cellular damage *in vitro*, or through *in vivo* models. The *in-vivo* models have the advantage of incorporating such pharmacokinetic aspects as skin penetration. The most phototoxic quinolones are those that induce singlet oxygen and radicals, since these species cause severe tissue damage. Photoreactivity, and thus phototoxicity, is mostly influenced by the substituent in position 8. Drugs that are substituted with an additional chlorine or fluorine atom in this position, such as clinafloxacin, fleroxacin, lomefloxacin, or sparfloxacin, generally exhibit a relatively high phototoxic potential [44].

On the other hand, it has been shown that a methoxy substituent at position 8, as present in the molecules of moxifloxacin or gatifloxacin, significantly increases the stability of quinolones to UV light and that these derivatives exhibit little or no phototoxicity under therapeutic conditions [45]. These structure–phototoxicity relationships have been studied in a mouse model (Table II).

Some quinolones have been shown to be not only phototoxic but photomutagenic and photocarcinogenic as well. As these types of toxicity are obviously related to the physicochemical phenomenon of photoinstability, so we can expect that photostable derivatives such as moxifloxacin are not photomutagenic, and this assumption was corroborated in a series of experiments [46].

In a long-term (up to 78 weeks) phototoxicity study in hairless Skh-1 mice, all of the quinolones tested caused development of skin tumors. The mice were

TABLE II   Phototoxicity of Quinolones in a Mouse Model

Quinolone	Substitution at position 8	Substitution at position 5	Highest dose without phototoxicity (mg/kg b.w.)
Ciprofloxacin	CH	H	>300
Moxifloxacin	COR	H	>300
Ofloxacin	COR	H	>300
Norfloxacin	CH	H	>300
Pefloxacin	CH	H	172
Enoxacin	N	H	100
Fleroxacin	CF	H	18
Sparfloxacin	CF	NH$_2$	18
Desamino-sparfloxacin	CF	H	<10
Lomefloxacin	CF	H	10
CI-934	CF	H	3
Bay 3118	CCl	H	3

Modified after Domagala (1994) [44].

chronically dosed with the test drugs (fleroxacin, ciprofloxacin, lomefloxacin, ofloxacin, nalidixic acid, and 8-methoxypsoralen) and periodically exposed to UV radiation. Differences in latency period and tumor incidence were seen. Except for lomefloxacin, nearly all skin tumors were of benign type. These findings have been confirmed in other laboratories. Their meaning for humans remains unclear, but consequent prevention of exposure to sunlight or artificial UV sources during treatment with quinolones is strongly recommended, and derivatives with a high phototoxic potential should not be used for therapy if less toxic alternatives are available [39,47–50].

NEPHROTOXICITY

Some quinolones, which are only slightly soluble at neutral or alkaline pH conditions (e.g., norfloxacin, ciprofloxacin), induce nephrotoxicity in laboratory animals due to crystallization of the drugs in renal tubules. Crystalluria has also been observed in man with ciprofloxacin and norfloxacin. Extensive studies have been performed on this topic, especially with ciprofloxacin, to clarify the relevance of this laboratory finding and to evaluate a possible risk of nephrotoxicity with therapeutic use of this drug (see section on "Renal Reactions").

In laboratory animals, parenteral application of ciprofloxacin for 4 weeks at daily doses of 80 mg/kg b.w. (rats) or 30 mg/kg b.w. (monkeys) produced nephrotoxic reactions. Acicular crystals were found in the urine sediment and in the distal tubule section of the kidneys. Analysis of this material showed that the crystal-like structure represents a complex of ciprofloxacin and/or its metabolites (magnesium and protein). Inflammatory foreign body reactions of the tubular epithelium and interstitium were observed as a secondary phenomenon. Similar nephropathies have been described after administration of other compounds with poor solubility (e.g., norfloxacin, piromidic acid, cinoxacin). In an attempt to evaluate the phenomenon of crystalluria as a potential hazard during therapy with ciprofloxacin, it should be considered that solubility varies significantly with pH conditions. Ciprofloxacin is only slightly soluble at neutral or alkaline conditions, but its solubility increases considerably as the pH becomes acidic. Alkaline urine conditions are typical for the animal species studied (rat, monkey), whereas human urine is normally slightly acidic [51].

OCULAR TOXICITY

The potential of norfloxacin to produce ophthalmic toxicity has been compared with that of nalidixic acid. Only this older quinolone (100 mg/kg b.w./day), and not norfloxacin (200 mg/kg b.w./day), produced electrical and histopathological changes in the feline retina [52].

Detailed studies on this topic have been conducted with ciprofloxacin in monkeys. No lens densification was found in animals treated for 6 months with doses up to and including 20 mg ciprofloxacin per kg b.w. Biochemical studies (e.g., electrophoretic separation of lens proteins) failed to provide any evidence of lens alteration. Pharmacokinetic studies yielded no evidence of accumulation of ciprofloxacin in lens tissue [51].

A comparative ophthalmotoxicity study with several quinolones was performed in rats. The animals were orally treated daily with 100 mg/kg of levofloxacin, ciprofloxacin, norfloxacin, or nalidixic acid for 2 weeks, and the effects on visual function were examined. Electroretinograms (ERGs) revealed several changes in rats treated with both nalidixic acid and, though less pronounced, norfloxacin. The ERGs from rats treated with levofloxacin or ciprofloxacin were normal [53].

Lens opacities have been detected in beagles during long-term investigation with pefloxacin. A dose of 50 mg/kg b.w. given for 8 months was well tolerated; however, after 100 and 200 mg pefloxacin per kg b.w., lens opacities occurred in a dose-related proportion of animals. Similar toxic effects have been reported for the older quinolone rosoxacin [54].

There was no indication of moxifloxacin-induced changes of the lens in dogs treated orally for 4 weeks with moxifloxacin at doses up to 90 mg/kg and studied by ophthalmoscopy [46].

CARDIOTOXICITY

Preclinical toxicological evaluation of fluoroquinolones showed that they can induce such cardiovascular effects as hypotension or tachycardia after intravenous injection in cats and dogs. Symptoms after infusion of an investigational compound (CP 74,667) at a dose of 5 mg/kg produced a response characterized by cutaneous erythema, facial swelling, occasional tremors, muscular weakness, and a decrease in blood pressure in dogs immediately following dosing [55]. It is unclear if these effects, some of which have been described for other quinolones, are direct responses or if they are induced via histamine release. Few data have been published on electrocardiographic analysis of the quinolone-induced effects on heart function. After chronic oral treatment with 25 mg sparfloxacin, prolongation of the QT interval was observed in dogs [56], while CI-934, another investigational compound, induced multiple, coupled, bigeminal ventricular extrasystoles in dogs at doses of 50 and 100 mg/kg b.w. [57].

The cardiovascular effects of grepafloxacin (1–30 mg/kg i.v.) have been compared with those of ciprofloxacin (1–30 mg/kg i.v.) in anesthetized rabbits. At lower doses, grepafloxacin had little effect on heart rate, but transient and mild increases were observed at 10 and 30 mg/kg. Ciprofloxacin caused a transient dose-related decrease in heart rate. Grepafloxacin caused transient dysrhythmias in one of four (10 mg/kg) and four of four animals (30 mg/kg). At 30 mg/kg one animal developed ventricular tachycardia. Ciprofloxacin did not produce any changes in cardiac rhythm at this dose level, but after a 10-fold higher dose (300 mg/kg) ventricular tachycardia was also observed with ciprofloxacin and lomefloxacin [5].

In a 4-week study, beagles received moxifloxacin at oral doses of 10, 30, or 90 mg/kg once daily. A slightly prolonged QT interval (25 msec longer than pretreatment values) was observed at the highest dose level that leads to peak plasma concentrations of approximately 20 mg/liter (AUC = ~230 mg/liter·hr) and thus represents an exposure that is multifold that of humans during therapy. No other changes (particularly arrhythmias) were observed [46].

REPRODUCTIVE AND DEVELOPMENTAL TOXICITY

Male Fertility

Several quinolones caused fertility disorders that were associated with histopathological changes of the testes. For example, pefloxacin impaired spermatogenesis in rats and dogs after long treatment periods. This quinolone at a dose of 500 mg/kg b.w. induced testicular atrophy after 6 weeks of treatment in rats. Similar effects were obtained with lower doses (100 mg/kg b.w.) in beagles [54]. Testicular atrophy and reduced spermatogenesis were also seen in rats and dogs after treatment with enoxacin. Impaired fertility was noticed in male rats after treatment with 1000 mg enoxacin per kg b.w., an effect that was reversible [58]. In a fertility study with fleroxacin, a reduction in the number of spermatozoa and atrophy of the seminiferous tubules were seen in rats after treatment with 320 mg/kg [59]; in a similarly designed study with moxifloxacin, sperm evaluation revealed treatment-related effects on sperm morphology (head/tail separation) but not on fertility at a dose of 500 mg/kg in rats [46]. Testicular degeneration was observed in dogs after 6 months of treatment with 25 mg trovafloxacin per kg of body weight b.i.d. [60].

Teratogenicity

Prenatal formation of the skeletal system is based on synthesis and differentiation of cartilaginous structures. With respect to the well-known toxic effect of the quinolones on joint cartilage in immature animals, it is remarkable that gross structural defects, such as limb reduction defects, have not been observed with quinolones in the routinely performed teratogenicity tests (segment II studies). Obviously, prenatally formed cartilage reacts much less sensitively to quinolones than joint cartilage.

Routinely performed reproductive toxicity studies with ciprofloxacin revealed no effects on fertility or pre- or postnatal development of offspring. No embryotoxic or teratogenic effects were observed. At the end of the postnatal study, no cartilage changes were histologically detectable in the joints of offspring [61].

Comparatively detailed data on the prenatal toxicity studies have been published for ofloxacin. At a dose of 90 mg/kg b.w., at which the mothers were not affected by treatment, a slight decrease in body weight and a retardation of the degree of ossification were observed in live fetuses. At 810 mg/kg, a dose that induced the same effects on fetuses, the toxic effects in mothers (e.g., weight gain, food intake) were more pronounced. Skeletal variations such as cervical ribs and shortening of the 13th rib, but no gross structural abnormalities, were found. Further investigations revealed that the critical period of occurrence of skeletal variations was days 9 and 10 of gestation. Fetal mortality was significantly increased compared to controls after a dose of 160 mg/kg b.w. in the rabbit and after 810 mg/kg b.w. in the rat [6].

When doses of 300 mg sparfloxacin per kilogram of body weight were given to pregnant rats during organogenesis, fetuses showed an increased incidence of ventricular septal defects. Such defects were not seen in pups after birth, suggesting that this effect was reversible [62,63].

Moxifloxacin was not teratogenic when administered to pregnant rats during organogenesis at oral doses of 500 mg/kg/day (equal to only 0.24 times the maximum recommended human dose based on systemic exposure [AUC]), but decreased fetal body weight and slightly delayed fetal skeletal development were observed [64]. With gatifloxacin, skeletal malformations were observed in fetuses from rats given 200 mg/kg/day orally during organogenesis; no fetotoxicity was seen at oral doses of 50 mg/kg (~0.2 times the maximum human dose based on systemic exposure) [65]. When these data are evaluated, it must be considered that, due to poor bioavailability and/or rapid metabolism of these drugs in pregnant rats, the systemic exposure is rather low though high doses were applied.

A series of nonhuman primate studies have been conducted to further reveal the prenatal toxic potential of norfloxacin, temafloxacin, ciprofloxacin, and fleroxacin. When cynomolgus monkeys were treated during organogenesis with doses from 50 to 300 mg norfloxacin per kilogram per day, there was no evidence of teratogenicity at any dose level, but maternotoxicity and a significant increase in embryolethality occurred at the highest dose level. At the no-observed-effect dose (50 mg/kg), peak plasma concentrations were approximately threefold higher than in humans. Additional studies suggested that the embryotoxic effect may be related to alterations of trophoblast function, namely a reduction in progesterone production [66,67]. Similar to the findings with norfloxacin, prenatal exposure to temafloxacin at 100 mg/kg/day (peak concentration 12 mg/liter) or fleroxacin at 70 mg/kg/day (peak concentration 8 mg/liter) during organogenesis resulted in a significant increase in prenatal loss, whereas ciprofloxacin did not induce embryolethality at doses up to 100 mg/kg/day (peak concentration 4.8 mg/liter) in cynomolgus monkeys [68–70].

With moxifloxacin there was no evidence of teratogenicity when pregnant cynomolgus monkeys were given oral doses of 100 mg/kg (2.5 times the maximum recommended human dose based on systemic exposure), but an increased number of abortions was noticed at these doses that caused frequent vomiting in the monkeys [46].

Postnatal Studies

In so-called segment III studies, which were designed to detect specific toxico-logical hazards during late pregnancy and lactation, no specific toxicity was observed with quinolones. According to a segment III protocol, pregnant and lactating rats usually are treated from day 15 of pregnancy until weaning (postnatal day 21). Although some data indicate that quinolones are excreted with the milk, no quinolone-induced chondrotoxic effects were detected in the offspring under these conditions. One explanation might be the high concentration of magnesium in rat milk (~10 mmol/liter). Possibly, stable chelate complexes are formed with quinolones and divalent cations in milk, reducing the bioavailability of the drugs in the offspring under the conditions of a segment III study. The chondrotoxic effects of quinolones are only detectable with direct treatment of immature rats [71].

A neonatal study was conducted with trovafloxacin mesylate at a dose of 75 mg/kg in immature Sprague–Dawley rats from postnatal day 4 to postnatal day 55. The peak concentration of trovafloxacin was 11.3 mg/liter on study day 1. This treatment induced an apparent interruption of normal growth, which was evident in reduced body size and lower body weights when compared to control animals. The gait alterations observed were the result of morphologic changes in the cartilage of growth plates, which produced changes in the shape and lengths of the long bones in the fore- and hindlimbs of young adult rats [60].

Effects on the epiphyseal growth plate have also been observed with moxifloxacin in immature dogs. When beagle puppies aged 10 to 12 weeks were treated with 90 mg/kg b.w., degeneration of matrix as well as chondrocytes was observed in the epiphyseal plates; however, no effects on the growth plates were reported in 18- to 22-week-old dogs under otherwise identical conditions. Toxic effects on the immature articular cartilage were seen in both studies at 30 and 90 mg/kg, but not at 10 mg/kg b.w. [46].

Corresponding experiments with other quinolones focusing on the effects of the drugs on the epiphyseal growth plate have not been reported so far. Most data in immature rats have been established with single-dose treatment in 4- to 5-week-old rats, and, under these conditions, pathological changes have only been observed in articular cartilage and not in growth plates. Comparative data with chronic exposure to other quinolones in very young animals are needed to clarify the question of whether the effects observed in rats are specific for trovafloxacin or if these irreversible effects on postnatal growth can be induced with other quinolones. The relevance of these results for humans is obscure.

MUTAGENICITY AND CARCINOGENICITY

Since quinolones inhibit gyrase (a topoisomerase II), which is an essential enzyme for the function of the bacterial DNA, it is very important to study the effects of these drugs on mammalian topoisomerases also and to clarify whether quinolones have a mutagenic or carcinogenic potential. In an early study with some of the older quinolones, the prokaryotic topoisomerase II was approximately 100-fold more sensitive to inhibition by quinolones than its eukaryotic counterpart. The order of potency for inhibition of this enzyme was ciprofloxacin > norfloxacin > nalidixic acid > ofloxacin [72].

Although there is no strict correlation between the activity on topoisomerases in bacterial and eukaryotic cells, it has become apparent that derivatives with significantly increased antibacterial activity (especially against Gram-positive bacteria) generally are more toxic to mammalian cells. Furthermore, some fluoroquinolones have been developed that were both potent antibacterial agents and inhibitors of mammalian topoisomerases. Among these are several of the isothiazolo-quinolones, such as A-65281 [73], and also a series of compounds (e.g., CP-115,953) that exhibit only slight structural differences in comparison to those fluoroquinolones that are used clinically as antibacterial agents. CP-115,953 was considered more potent than etoposide against mammalian topoisomerase II and so was the first quinolone reported to have greater activity against eukaryotic topoisomerase II than does an antineoplastic drug in clinical use. A characteristic component of this series of derivatives is the aromatic C-7 substituent. These findings underline the necessity for extensive genotoxicity testing and a careful case-by-case risk–benefit analysis of newly developed antibacterial quinolones [74].

Several reviews have been published on the genotoxicity of quinolones [75–77]. Aside from the routinely performed in-vitro (Ames test) and in-vivo (micronucleus and dominant lethal test in mice) mutagenicity studies, additional tests have been performed to assess the mutagenic potential of fluoroquinolones. Usually, fluoroquinolones were negative in assays for chromosomal aberrations or mutagenicity at the HGPRT⁻ or Na⁺,–K⁺-ATPase loci in mammalian cells. However, the in-vitro unscheduled DNA synthesis test on rat hepatocytes (UDS test) and the mouse lymphoma test yielded positive results for most quinolones tested. Further investigations have been performed (e.g., with ciprofloxacin) to check whether the drug exhibits an effect on DNA repair in rat hepatocytes after in-vivo application (30 and 190 mg ciprofloxacin per kg b.w., given subcutaneously). In contrast to what was observed in vitro, ciprofloxacin did not elicit DNA repair under these conditions [78].

Long-term carcinogenicity studies in animals have been completed with several fluoroquinolones, including norfloxacin, ciprofloxacin, fleroxacin, and levofloxacin. There was no indication of a carcinogenic effect with these drugs after lifelong exposure. For example, levofloxacin was administered with the diet to 50 male and 50 female F344 rats per dosing group for 2 years at 10, 30, or 100 mg/kg. No evidence of drug-related carcinogenicity was found. When ciprofloxacin was given to mice and rats for up to 2 years, no carcinogenic effect was seen in these species. However, under similar conditions, nalidixic acid induced an increased incidence of preputial gland neoplasms in males and clitoral gland neoplasms in female F344/N rats when given a diet containing 2000 and 4000 ppm of the drug [40].

Several studies have indicated that genotoxicity of fluoroquinolones is enhanced under concurrent irradiation with ultraviolet (UV) light (see section on

"Phototoxicity, Photomutagenicity, and Photocarcinogenicity"). Fluoroquinolones, particularly those with an additional fluorine atom in position 8, are unstable when they are exposed to UV radiation. It is probable that the photolysis results in loss of their F-8 atoms as fluoride and highly reactive carbenes are formed [79]. The photomutagenicity of fleroxacin and lomefloxacin, which represent typical drugs with a fluor atom in position 8, has been tested in a variety of assays in comparison to ciprofloxacin. The chromosomal aberration test with V79 cells and the Comet assay with mouse lymphoma cells proved to be exquisitely sensitive toward the photogenotoxic activity of fluoroquinolones (lomefloxacin > fleroxacin > ciprofloxacin). The results underscore the recommendation to avoid excessive light exposure during quinolone therapy [80].

Some quinolones have been shown to be photocarcinogenic (see section on "Phototoxicity, Photomutagenicity, and Photocarcinogenicity"). During treatment with lomefloxacin and other quinolones plus concurrent UV irradiation, skin tumors developed (e.g., [48,81]).

ADVERSE EFFECTS OF FLUOROQUINOLONES IN CLINICAL STUDIES

ADVERSE EFFECTS OF FLUOROQUINOLONES

One of the most difficult tasks in relation to side effects during quinolone therapy is knowing the exact frequency of adverse effects, thus allowing a well-founded comparison with competing drugs. Before the adverse effects observed in clinical situations with quinolones are described here in detail, a few general remarks should be made regarding difficulties in quantification. The number of adverse effects noticed during clinical studies will depend crucially on the technique used for registration. Three methods are customary:

1. Registration of obvious clinical symptoms and laboratory abnormalities
2. The passive interview (i.e., the patient is asked for unusual events during therapy)
3. The active interview (i.e., the patient is asked about specific symptoms suspected or known to be related to the drug investigated).

Of course, all of these techniques have drawbacks. They will either underestimate the frequency of adverse effects or lead to registration of nondrug-related events. This chapter summarizes the adverse reactions as they were noticed primarily during preregistration clinical trials by the manufacturers and, to a lesser extent, after marketing of the drugs. The most reliable comparative data can be expected from randomized double-blind studies, which are discussed separately.

It should be pointed out that the incidences presented in Tables III–XII are only orientational in character and that the data in the tables are not directly comparable.

During clinical trials, the overall frequencies of adverse effects were reported to vary between 4.4 and 20% (Table III). Serious side effects leading to cessation of treatment occurred at frequencies between 0.7 and 4.6% [39,82–84].

Gastrointestinal Reactions

Nausea, diarrhea, vomiting, dyspepsia, and similar symptoms are among the most often-reported side effects during therapy with the quinolones (0.8 to 6.8% of the patients). Cases of antibiotic-associated colitis have only been rarely observed. In comparison to those with other antimicrobials, these frequencies are not extraordinarily high.

Central Nervous System Reactions

Neurotoxicity of quinolones is an important problem that has to be considered when applying these drugs. Qualitatively, a wide spectrum of complications has been observed, and the neurotoxic potential can be regarded as an important

TABLE III   Adverse Reactions of Quinolones

Site	Incidence (%)
Gastrointestinal	0.8–6.8
Central and peripheral nervous system	0.9–4.7
Serious reactions	<0.5
Skin/hypersensitivity	0.4–2.1
Phototoxicity/photoallergy	0.5–2.0
Special senses	Increased ?
Cardiovascular	0.5–2.0
Renal/urogenital/hepatic	0.5–4.5
Blood disorders	0.5–5.3
Musculoskeletal/rheumatological	0.5–2.0
Neuromuscular disorders	Increased ?
Cumulative incidences	4.4–20

Modified after Christ and Esch (1994) [39].

difference from other antibiotics, although after high doses of other antimicrobials (e.g., β-lactam antibiotics) neurotoxic complications are also occasionally observed. With the older nonfluorinated quinolones, such as oxolinic acid or rosoxacin, neurotoxic symptoms such as dizziness were noted in about half of patients.

For a rational evaluation of quinolone neurotoxicity, it is important to distinguish mild reactions of the central nervous system (CNS) from severe reactions that require interruption of therapy. Mild reactions may occur in the form of headache, dizziness, tiredness, or sleeplessness. Furthermore, abnormal vision, restlessness, bad dreams, and so on have been reported in some instances. Severe neurotoxic side effects are rare (<0.5%), but they have been noticed during therapy with most of the quinolones, and this possibility must be considered when a patient is treated with these drugs. This category of side effects includes psychotic reactions, hallucinations, depressions, and grand mal convulsions. These reactions typically start only a few days after the beginning of therapy and stop with cessation of medication [39].

Elderly patients, especially those with pronounced arteriosclerosis, and patients with other impairments of the central nervous system (especially epilepsy) are prone to neurotoxic complications and should be treated with quinolones only under close supervision. There are indications that in elderly patients (over 70 years), mainly with predominantly renally excreted derivatives such as ofloxacin, levofloxacin, or gatifloxacin, slight cumulative effects occur and relatively high plasma levels are achieved with "normal" doses. Therefore, a few pharmacokinetic considerations that might be relevant for neurotoxic reactions to quinolones are given here.

Graber et al. [85] compared the pharmacokinetics of ofloxacin in young (mean 27 years) and elderly (mean 75 years) patients receiving 200 mg twice daily for 1 week. After day 7, there had been drug accumulation in the elderly group, and the half-life was 17.8 hours, compared to 5.7 hours in the younger group. However, from the information available to date, it seems that neurotoxic reactions to quinolones are not strictly correlated with extraordinarily high plasma concentrations. This might be explained by the circumstance that the blood–brain barrier influences the concentrations in brain tissue to a variable extent.

In a large study of 271 patients treated with various quinolones for urinary tract infections, drug concentrations were measured in serum and cerebrospinal fluid (CSF). For example, ratios of CSF/serum concentrations 3 hours after a single 200-mg dose were 0.08 for norfloxacin, 0.13 for ciprofloxacin, and 0.30–0.34 for fleroxacin, ofloxacin, and sparfloxacin [86]. Few data are available for the concentrations of fluoroquinolones in brain tissue. Concentrations of sparfloxacin or ciprofloxacin in brain tissue were measured in a small group of patients undergoing brain surgery. Concentrations showed considerable variability and were approximately 2 to 20 times higher than the corresponding concentrations in cerebrospinal fluid [87].

Skin Reactions (Hypersensitivity, Phototoxicity)

The frequency of hypersensitivity reactions after fluoroquinolones is specified between 0.4 and 2.1%. They include erythema, pruritus, urticaria, rash, and other cutaneous reactions [39,82]. Of special interest are phototoxic reactions that have been described with all the quinolones. Phototoxic risks differ among the various quinolones available for antimicrobial therapy with 8-halogen derivatives (e.g., lomefloxacin, fleroxacin) possessing a high, and methoxy derivatives (e.g., moxifloxacin, gatifloxacin) exhibiting a low potential for phototoxicity. However, it is a general recommendation that patients taking fluoroquinolones avoid sun exposure (see section on "Phototoxicity, Photomutagenicity, and Photocarcino-genicity").

When the phototoxicity of quinolones as a risk of antimicrobial therapy is discussed, it should be remembered that several other groups of antimicrobial agents cause phototoxic reactions. Among these are the often-prescribed sul-fonamides and tetracyclines. During a randomized study with doxycycline and cefuroxime in patients with erythema migrans, phototoxic reactions were noted in 7 of 113 patients (6.2%) taking doxycycline (3 × 100 mg daily) but in none of the patients treated with the cephalosporin [88].

Phototoxic reactions in association with quinolone therapy were first described with nalidixic acid [89]. Erythema developed on all surfaces exposed to the sun, and even several days after stopping the medication bullae began to develop on the dorsal surfaces of the hands and feet.

During a double-blind study comparing three different doses of fleroxacin in patients with urogenital chlamydia infections, phototoxic reactions were observed in 11 and 19% of patients after treatment with 600 and 800 mg fleroxacin, respectively. None of the 26 patients treated with the 400-mg dose showed phototoxicity [90].

A surprisingly high incidence of phototoxic reactions has been observed in cystic fibrosis patients treated with ciprofloxacin. A questionnaire had been sent to 100 patients, and about a third of this group responded. Fifty-two percent of them reported a phototoxic reaction during therapy with the drug [91].

In healthy subjects, an observer-blinded study was performed to investigate the phototoxic potential of ciprofloxacin, lomefloxacin, and trovafloxacin. Minimal erythema doses (MEDs) for a wavelength of 365 nm and other wavelengths were determined prior to dosing and on day 5 of dosing. The ratios of the MEDs at day 5 to baseline MEDs were 0.93 (placebo), 0.56 (trovafloxacin, 200 mg),

0.38 (ciprofloxacin, 500 mg b.i.d.), and 0.24 (lomefloxacin, 400 mg). The values for the three drugs were all significantly different from the values obtained after placebo administration. An overall evaluation showed that ciprofloxacin and lomefloxacin at wavelengths of 335 and 365 nm induced significantly greater reduction in MEDs, and thus showed a greater phototoxic potential than trovafloxacin at these wavelengths [92].

In a comparative study in healthy volunteers, the naphthyridine derivative gemifloxacin (N in position 8 of the molecule) showed a low potential for phototoxicity that was similar to that of ciprofloxacin [93].

As predicted from the preclinical studies, the two 8-methoxy derivatives moxifloxacin and gatifloxacin showed no phototoxicity in volunteers given normal therapeutic doses [94–96].

The relatively high phototoxic potentials of lomefloxacin and sparfloxacin have caused pronounced limitations of their clinical use in some countries. With lomefloxacin, a correlation was found between the concentrations of the drug in skin and the degree of a phototoxic reaction in volunteers. The drug has a long elimination half-life and is taken only once daily. To minimize the risk of phototoxic reactions, it has been recommended to take the drug at night, as concentrations will decline by the next morning [97].

Musculoskeletal Reactions (Arthralgia, Tendinitis)

A clear-cut relationship between quinolones and arthralgia has only been established in animal experiments (see section on "Effects on Cartilage"). If there is a risk of acute chondrotoxicity in humans under therapeutic conditions, it is obviously small. The most extensive experience with quinolone therapy in children comes from patients with cystic fibrosis who were treated with ciprofloxacin (e.g., [11]). Overall, arthralgia occurred in 1.5% of the treatment courses (n = 2030 courses in 1795 children) and resolved without intervention. Interpretation of these data with respect to a causal relationship is complicated by the fact that the disease cystic fibrosis itself is associated with arthropathy [98].

Because the risk of arthropathy may be higher for other fluoroquinolones, and because cartilage lesions are not always associated with clinical symptoms, these studies with ciprofloxacin cannot prove a complete lack of chondrotoxic effects with any quinolone treatment. Furthermore, it cannot be completely excluded that irreversible cartilage alterations arise that may lead to clinical symptoms only after many years.

Several case reports of severe acute arthralgia during therapy with older quinolones as well as during treatment with fluoroquinolones have been published in which the causal relationship remains unclear but which must be considered as important further information. Soon after marketing of the drug, a child with soreness in one wrist during therapy with nalidixic acid was described [99]. Another report described a young woman who developed severe arthralgia with painful joint swelling and limitation of movement during therapy with nalidixic acid. The symptoms started in the small joints of the feet and spread to the knees, hands, wrists, elbows, and shoulders [100]. It should be stressed that these communications were given years before the arthropathogenic potential of the drug was recognized in animal experiments.

The highest incidence of arthropathy in humans reported to date was observed after treatment with pefloxacin. Arthropathies were observed in 8 of 63 (14%) patients with cystic fibrosis during treatment with pefloxacin, but in a similar group of patients treated with ofloxacin no joint complications were observed. These data, while interesting, were not generated from a prospective or direct comparative study. However, all patients were suffering from cystic fibrosis, and two different quinolones were utilized in the same hospital, in some instances even to the same patients. Five patients who did develop arthralgia under treatment with pefloxacin did not show any joint complications during treatment with ofloxacin [101].

Aside from arthralgia, fluoroquinolones can cause tendinitis and rupture of the Achilles tendon even after short-term use. Most cases of tendon disorders have occurred with pefloxacin. Tendinitis with other drugs such as ciprofloxacin, ofloxacin, levofloxacin, norfloxacin, and enoxacin has been reported, but the incidence appears to be lower [39,102,103].

A study from The Netherlands indicated that the incidence of quinolone-induced tendonopathies might be higher than assumed so far. In that retrospective cohort study, patient data as registered by GPs in a source population of approximately 250,000 were analyzed. Achilles tendinitis was identified in 3 of 418 patients treated with ofloxacin, corresponding to a relative risk of 10.1 (95% CI: 2.2 to 46.0) and an excess risk of 15 cases per 100,000 exposure days [104].

In two reports, French colleagues compiled several hundred cases of patients, providing important further information on quinolone-induced tendon disorders [105,106]. Obviously, such effects can occur several weeks or even months after therapy, which is in agreement with data from studies in rats [36]. Some risk factors have been recognized. For example, older patients (>60 years) and those with concomitant use of corticosteroids are at increased risk. However, fluoroquinolone use alone bears the potential to induce tendon lesions.

Some information exists that patients with renal disorders, and in particular those following renal transplantation, are at risk for quinolone-induced tendonopathies [107–109].

Because quinolones are chelating agents with affinity for di- and trivalent cations—such as Ca^{2+}, Mg^{2+}, Zn^{2+} Cu^{2+}, and Al^{3+}—it seems possible that electrolyte disturbances (e.g., magnesium deficiency) might increase the risk of quinolone-induced toxicity [9]. So far, however, the question of whether electrolyte disorders put patients at increased risk of tendon disorders has not been studied systematically.

Cardiovascular Reactions

Hypotension and tachycardia have been seen after treatment with most quinolones, but the cardiotoxic potential of various quinolones differs considerably (see section on "Cardiotoxicity"). Although systematic comparative studies in animals or man have not been published as of yet, available information indicates that sparfloxacin and grepafloxacin possess the highest potential to induce QT prolongation and arrhythmias among those fluoroquinolones that are used or have been used in man.

During preclinical development of sparfloxacin, prolongation of the electrocardiographic QT interval was observed in dogs. Subsequently, the effect of sparfloxacin on the QTc interval in man was studied in phase I trials in healthy volunteers. Results of these studies as well as the results from phase III studies indicate that the increase in QTc interval associated with sparfloxacin is moderate (3% on average). Careful evaluation of clinical data showed that a small number of patients treated with sparfloxacin experienced a QTc interval prolongation to >500 msec, which might be of clinical significance. Few serious adverse cardiovascular events have been reported during postmarketing surveillance of sparfloxacin, and all have occurred in patients with an underlying cardiac condition [110].

After the withdrawal of grepafloxacin from the market due to cardiovascular events, the issue of QT prolongation observed after quinolone use has gained much attention. Because special attention should be paid to the newer quinolones, the databases for the new and old quinolones are not identical. This should be kept in mind when evaluating the situation.

During the clinical development of moxifloxacin, an extensive ECG program was conducted in phase III trials. The "normal" QT interval is 450 msec in males and 470 msec in females, but physiological intraindividual variability is considerable (15 to 70 msec). The CPMP has defined criteria for "significant" QTc prolongations, which include (1) any QT interval >500 msec, (2) any QT interval changes of >60 msec, (3) QT prolongation of >30 msec above the normal value, or (4) changes of >15%. Such "significant" QT prolongations were noticed in 2.8% out of 787 patients, which was less frequent than in the comparator group treated with the macrolide clarithromycin (3.7%, $n = 136$ patients). Therefore, the drug should be avoided in patients with known prolongation of the QT interval, patients with uncorrected hypokalemia, and patients receiving class IA (e.g., quinidine, procainamide) or class III (e.g., amiodarone, sotalol) antiarrhythmic agents due to the lack of clinical experience with moxifloxacin in these patient populations [64].

No QTc phenomena were reported during investigation of levofloxacin. However, a number of cases of torsade de pointes (0.3 per 100,000 treated patients) have emerged during postmarketing surveillance in the United States. The relationship to therapy is uncertain. Generally, the safety of other fluoroquinolones not previously reported to cause effects on the QTc interval or related clinical phenomena should not be assumed, especially if the patient is receiving other agents capable of producing QT prolongation [111].

Renal Reactions

Rarely, cases of acute interstitial nephritis or nephrotoxic reactions as a consequence of crystalluria with elevation of plasma creatinine levels have been noticed during therapy with fluoroquinolones. Crystalluria has been studied most extensively with ciprofloxacin. In healthy volunteers, the influence of urinary pH and hydration was studied after single oral administration of 500 and 1000 mg ciprofloxacin. The urinary pH was varied by giving each person three different diets: aside from one regular diet, either ammonium chloride or sodium bicarbonate was added to acidify or alkalize the urine, respectively. Crystalluria was seen in 3 of 6 (500 mg) and 5 of 6 (1000 mg) subjects with alkalized urine but not in volunteers with acidified urine. Based on the data from clinical investigations, there is no evidence that ciprofloxacin leads to urolithiasis or adversely influences renal function, though it may still be prudent to ascertain urinary acidity when patients are receiving high doses of ciprofloxacin [112].

Other Rarely Registered Adverse Effects

In some cases, hematologic alterations were described such as thrombocytopenia, leukopenia, and anemia. Transient elevations of hepatic enzymes in plasma occurred [39,82]. (See the "Introduction" for a more detailed discussion of the trovafloxacin associated hepatotoxicity.)

ADVERSE EFFECTS OBSERVED IN PREREGISTRATION CLINICAL TRIALS

The tolerability data from clinical trials with the most widely used fluoroquinolones involving several thousand patients are given in Tables IV to XII. It is impossible during a clinical trial to decide with certainty whether an adverse effect is related to the disease treated, to the drug investigated, to other drugs given concomitantly, or to other reasons. The different basis for registration of side effects (definitely, probably, possibly, or remotely related to study drug) must be

considered when interpreting data. Inclusion in the tables herein does not
necessarily mean that the observed effect is induced by a fluoroquinolone.

Norfloxacin

During clinical trials with norfloxacin, an overall frequency of 4.6% of patients
suffered from adverse gastrointestinal events (Table IV). However, since many of
the complaints were made by patients who were receiving chemotherapy for
leukemia, it was the opinion of the investigators that the observed effects were
related to the norfloxacin in only 1.8% of patients. "Neuropsychiatric adverse

TABLE IV   Adverse Events: Norfloxacin (1540 patients)

Effect	Number	Percent
1. Gastrointestinal		**1.8**
Nausea	14	0.9
Abdominal pain	2	0.1
Dyspepsia	4	0.3
Dry mouth	2	0.1
2. Skin and allergic		**0.6**
Rash	3	0.2
Erythema	2	0.1
Pruritus	2	0.1
Urticaria	2	0.1
3. Central nervous system		**1.4**
Headache	5	0.3
Dizziness	7	0.5
Insomnia	2	0.1
Euphoria	2	0.1
4. Special sense		
Taste perversion	3	0.2

Modified after Corrado *et al.* (1987) [52].

Comments:

1. Some patients had more than one adverse experience; therefore, the
number of symptoms exceeds the total number of patients with adverse
experiences, and the total percentages exceed the percentage of patients
with adverse experiences.

2. Only those adverse experiences are presented that were considered
"probably" or "definitely" drug related.

3. Only adverse effects at a frequency >0.1 % are given.

effects" occurred in 4.8% of patients, but only 1.4% were considered probably or definitely related to norfloxacin. The corresponding figures for skin and allergic adverse effects are 1 and 0.6%. Drug-related adverse laboratory experiences were rare (e.g., two cases, or 0.1%, of elevated liver function tests) [52].

Ciprofloxacin

In 168 (9.9%) of 1690 patients receiving ciprofloxacin during clinical trials, 263 adverse reactions were reported (Table V). One hundred and fifty-two systemic reactions were considered probably or possibly drug related. Of these, 135 (89%) were judged to be of mild or moderate severity and 17 were considered severe.

TABLE V   Adverse Events: Ciprofloxacin (1690 patients)

Effect	Number	Percent
1. Gastrointestinal		**5.0**
Nausea	27	1.6
Diarrhea	25	1.5
Vomiting	12	0.7
Dyspepsia	6	0.4
Abdominal pain	5	0.3
Anorexia	4	0.2
Flatulence	3	0.2
2. Skin and allergic		**1.4**
Rash	14	0.8
Pruritus	8	0.5
3. Central nervous system		**1.6**
Dizziness	9	0.5
Asthenia/tiredness	6	0.4
Headache	5	0.3
Eye disorder	4	0.2

Modified after Bayer (1986, 1987) [113,61].

Comments:

1. Some patients had more than one adverse experience; therefore, the number of symptoms exceeds the total number of patients with adverse experiences, and the total percentages exceed the percentage of patients with adverse experiences.

2. Only those adverse experiences are presented that were considered "highly probably," "probably," or "possibly" drug related.

3. Only adverse effects at a frequency >0.1% are given.

Twenty-three local adverse reactions (15%) were reported in 151 parenterally treated patients. In all patients, therapy commenced with a bolus injection; better tolerance was achieved if the drug was administered as a short infusion of 30 minutes duration. No further local reactions were observed after preparation of the drug solution was changed (excess lactate reduced from 1.3 to 0.1%). Measurements of clinical laboratory parameters showed basically mild to moderate changes in liver function tests (e.g., elevation of SGOT and SGPT) in 77 patients (4.6%). Therapy was discontinued in three patients because of increased levels of liver enzymes. There was no evidence of nephrotoxicity, and no crystalluria was detected during phase II and III clinical trials [61,113].

An analysis of data from more than 1000 patients treated with ciprofloxacin in controlled clinical trials for >30 days showed that most adverse effects occurred early during therapy with little increase in frequency over time. No previously unknown adverse effects were noted [114].

Ofloxacin (Levofloxacin)

In 1985, the overall incidence of side effects during clinical studies with ofloxacin was reported as 4.1% [115]. These early clinical trials were conducted in Japan, and the data reflected experience with 4785 patients (Table VIa). Meanwhile, these data have been confirmed using an even greater number of patients. Among nearly 16,000 patients treated with ofloxacin in phase II to IV clinical trials worldwide, adverse drug events occurred with an overall incidence of 4.3 per 100 patients. The patients were requested to report to their physician all symptoms occurring during a clinical study with ofloxacin. The data presented here, however, represent only those adverse effects that were attributed to the study drug by the physician. Side effects related to the gastrointestinal tract (e.g., nausea, vomiting, diarrhea) were reported most frequently (2.6%). CNS effects (e.g., headache, dizziness) were registered in 0.9% of the patients, and the incidence of hypersensitivity reactions was reported as 0.5% [116].

A different pattern of side effects was noticed from postmarketing surveillance in Germany. The most frequent adverse effects were related to the nervous system, followed by hypersensitivity reactions and gastrointestinal symptoms (Table VIb). Probably, physicians expected gastrointestinal symptoms to occur during antiinfective treatment, so that these effects were less frequently reported than the more striking CNS symptoms [116].

Levofloxacin is the optical S-(−) isomer of ofloxacin, which is significantly more active than the R-(+) isomer; *in vitro* it is generally twice as potent as the racemate ofloxacin. In comparative trials with ofloxacin, at half the daily dosage of ofloxacin, it showed reduced incidence of adverse effects [117].

TABLE VIa   Adverse Events: Ofloxacin (4785 patients)

Effect	Number	Percent
1. Gastrointestinal		**3.2**
Nausea/vomiting	32	0.7
Diarrhea/soft stool	31	0.7
Gastrointestinal pain	18	0.4
Gastrointestinal discomfort	31	0.7
Anorexia	21	0.4
2. Skin and allergic		**0.7**
Rash	20	0.4
Pruritus	7	0.2
3. Central nervous system		**0.9**
Dizziness	13	0.3
Headache	10	0.2
Insomnia	15	0.3

Modified after Anonymous (1985) [115].

Comments:

1. Some patients had more than one adverse experience; therefore, the number of symptoms exceeds the total number of patients with adverse experiences, and the total percentages exceed the percentage of patients with adverse experiences.

2. Only those events are reported as a side effect if the physician attributed it to ofloxacin.

3. Only adverse effects at a frequency >0.1% are given.

Enoxacin

During phase II studies with enoxacin in Japan, 2530 patients were treated and 156 side effects (6.2%) in 117 patients (4.6%) were recorded (Table VII). Transient alterations of laboratory indices were noticed in 35 patients (e.g., 12 patients with pathological liver function tests and 18 patients with hematological alterations) [58,118].

Pefloxacin

The data in Table VIII represent the side effects experience after pefloxacin treatment in 781 patients. In 10 of the 33 cases of gastrointestinal reactions, the side effects led to withdrawal of treatment. In seven instances, the gastrointestinal disturbances were due to taking 800 mg in a single dose [54].

TABLE VIb   Adverse Drug Events First Reported after the Launch of Ofloxacin

Classification	Events as reported	Number of events
Nervous system	Hallucination	20
	Psychotic reaction	12
	Impairment of vision	7
	Impairment of taste	5
	Impairment of smell	4
Symptoms of	Quincke's oedema	15
hypersensitivity	Dyspnoea	15
(isolated or	Anaphylactic reaction	12
combined)	Urticaria	10
	Shock reactions	6
	Glottal oedema	6
Blood dyscrasia	Leukocytopenia	6
	Thrombopenia	6
	Bone marrow depression	6
Myalgia, arthralgia		15

Modified after Jüngst and Mohr (1987) [116].

Fleroxacin

More than 4000 patients treated orally with fleroxacin in preregistration clinical trials were evaluable for safety (Table IX). The overall rate of adverse reactions was 10% for those given 200 mg daily (n = 623) and 20% for those given 400 mg daily (n = 3611). The most frequent adverse reactions involved the GI tract (11%) and the CNS (9%). Insomnia was the most commonly reported adverse effect. With doses greater than 400 mg the adverse effect rates were higher, for example, 44% (385 of 878) in patients receiving the 600-mg dose. Photosensitization was rare with the 200- and 400-mg dose regimens but rose to 5% with a 600-mg dose [119].

In an early double-blind evaluation of oral fleroxacin, using 400, 600, or 800 mg once daily for 7 days to treat uncomplicated genital infections, high rates of adverse reactions were observed. Severe insomnia was seen in 2 of 26 (8%) patients treated with 400 mg daily, but in 16 of 26 patients (62%) treated with the highest dose, which is not licensed or recommended for therapy [90].

TABLE VII   Adverse Events: Enoxacin (2530 patients)

Effect	Number	Percent
1. Gastrointestinal		**3.8**
Nausea	32	1.3
Stomach discomfort	11	0.4
Abdominal pain	11	0.4
Anorexia	11	0.4
Diarrhea	10	0.4
Vomiting	5	0.2
Other	16	0.6
2. Skin and allergic		**0.7**
Rash	14	0.6
3. Central nervous system		**1.2**
Dizziness	10	0.4
Sleepiness	5	0.2
Headache	6	0.2
Insomnia	3	0.1

Modified after Young (1985) [118] and Parke-Davis & Company (1986) [58].

Comments:

1. Some patients had more than one adverse experience; therefore, the number of symptoms exceeds the total number of patients with adverse experiences, and the total percentages exceed the percentage of patients with adverse experiences.

2. Only adverse effects at a frequency >0.1% are given.

Sparfloxacin

A total of 1040 patients with lower respiratory tract infections were evaluated (Table X). A similar number of patients received a comparator regimen (amoxicillin 1000 mg t.i.d., plus ofloxacin 200 mg b.i.d. in one study, or amoxicillin/clavulanic acid 500/125 mg t.i.d., or erythromycin 1000 mg b.i.d.). The incidence and severity of drug-related adverse effects and the incidence of drug discontinuation due to adverse effects were not different among patients treated with sparfloxacin compared to those who received a comparator antibacterial agent. Gastrointestinal reactions were the most common adverse effects (sparfloxacin 11.4%, comparators 20.8%). Photosensitivity was observed in 8 of 370 (2.2%)

TABLE VIII   Adverse Events: Pefloxacin (781 patients)

Effect	Number	Percent
1. Gastrointestinal	33	**4.2%**
Nausea	*	
Vomiting	*	
Epigastric pain	*	
2. Skin and allergic	19	**2.4%**
Photosensitivity reactions	10	
Ichthyerythematous reactions	9	
3. Central nervous system	9	**1.1%**
Insomnia	2	0.3
Headache	2	0.3
Dizziness	1	0.13
Faintness	1	0.13
Agitation	1	0.13
Listlessness	1	0.13
Fits	1	0.13
4. Muscle pain/arthralgia	7	**0.9%**

Modified after Laboratoire Roger Bellon (1985) [54].

* = no frequencies of individual adverse experiences are given.

Comments:

1. Some patients had more than one adverse experience; therefore, the number of symptoms exceeds the total number of patients with adverse experiences, and the total percentages exceed the percentage of patients with adverse experiences.

2. Only adverse effects at a frequency >0.1% are given.

patients with an acute exacerbation of chronic obstructive pulmonary disease (AE–COPD) and in 13 of 670 (1.9%) patients with community-acquired pneumonia treated with sparfloxacin (comparator groups 0.1 and 0%, respectively). In both the sparfloxacin and comparator antibacterial treatment groups, the incidence of any adverse effect was twice as high in patients with pneumonia as in patients with AE–COPD, suggesting that the disease itself was responsible for a number of the reported adverse effects. Overall, sparfloxacin appeared to be as well tolerated as other antibacterial regimens commonly used to treat lower respiratory tract infections [120].

TABLE IX   Adverse Events: Fleroxacin (4234 patients; dose 200 or 400 mg daily)

Effect	Number	Percent
1. Gastrointestinal	**467**	**11**
Nausea	318	8
Diarrhea	40	0.9
Vomiting	67	2
Constipation	30	0.7
2. Skin	**111**	**3**
Photosensitivity	24	0.6
3. Central nervous system	**374**	**9**
Insomnia	157	4
Headache	105	2
Dizziness	96	2
4. Miscellaneous		
Fatigue	47	1

Modified after Geddes (1993) [119].

Comments:

1. Some patients had more than one adverse experience; therefore, the number of symptoms exceeds the total number of patients with adverse experiences, and the total percentages exceed the percentage of patients with adverse experiences.

Moxifloxacin

Metaanalysis of data from 20 phase II and phase III studies involving almost 5000 patients treated with moxifloxacin (400 mg/day in most patients) indicated that adverse effects were primarily mild and transient. Therapy was discontinued in 3.8% of patients. The most frequent events were nausea (7.2%) and diarrhea (5.7%). Dizziness occurred in 2.8% of patients [95]. Detailed data on the tolerability of moxifloxacin in clinical trials that were presented as a poster are shown in Table XI [121].

Gatifloxacin

Analysis of pooled data from clinical trials of oral gatifloxacin at 400 mg/day (n = 3021) and comparator antibacterial agents (including ciprofloxacin, levoflox-

TABLE X   Adverse Events: Sparfloxacin (1040 patients)

Effect	Number	Percent
1. Gastrointestinal		**11.4**
Nausea	15	1.4
Diarrhea	27	2.6
Vomiting	23	2.2
Dyspepsia	7	0.7
Flatulence	1	0.1
Miscellaneous	35	3.4
2. Skin		**5.1**
Rash, urticaria	23	2.2
Pruritus	5	0.5
Angioedema	1	0.1
Phototoxicity	21	2.0
Miscellaneous	24	2.3
3. Central nervous system		**4.2**
Insomnia, sleep disorder	13	1.3
Somnolence	1	0.1
Confusion	3	0.3
Agitation, anxiety, delirium	10	1.0
Convulsion	1	0.1

Modified after Rubinstein (1996) [120].

Comments:

1. Some patients had more than one adverse experience; therefore, the number of symptoms exceeds the total number of patients with adverse experiences, and the total percentages exceed the percentage of patients with adverse experiences.

acin, cephalosporins, and macrolides, $n = 2111$) showed that the most common adverse effects in patients treated with gatifloxacin were nausea (8%), diarrhea (4%), headache (4%), and dizziness (3%); there was no evidence of phototoxicity, crystalluria, or tendinitis. Of 3629 subjects treated with 200 to 400 mg gatifloxacin in clinical trials, adverse effects prompted discontinuation in 107 patients (2.9%). The data are shown in Table XII [96,122].

ADVERSE EFFECTS OBSERVED IN COMPARATIVE DOUBLE-BLIND STUDIES

Since the information from double-blinded studies is of special interest, not only regarding the efficacy of a drug but also in considering the objectivity of

TABLE XI   Adverse Events: Moxifloxacin (4370 patients, 400 mg/d)

Effect	Number	Percent
1. Gastrointestinal		
Nausea	339	7.8
Diarrhea	258	5.9
Vomiting	76	1.7
Abdominal pain	86	2
Dyspepsia	59	1.4
2. Central nervous system		
Dizziness	127	2.9
Headache	87	2
3. Miscellaneous		
Taste perversion	46	2
Abnormal liver function test	52	1.2

Modified after Springsklee *et al.* (2000) [121].

TABLE XII   Adverse Events: Gatifloxacin (3021 patients, 400 mg/d)

Effect	Number	Percent
1. Gastrointestinal		
Nausea	252	8
Diarrhea	117	4
Vomiting	55	2
Dyspepsia	46	2
Abdominal pain	56	2
Dry mouth	43	1
2. Central nervous system		
Headache	107	4
Dizziness	86	3
Insomnia	33	1
3. Miscellaneous		
Vaginitis	106	6
Taste perversion	46	2

Modified after Breen *et al.* (1999) [122].

tolerability reports, the results of some major double-blind studies with fluoroquinolones are shown in Table XIII. Of course, such a study design does not
guarantee a better estimation of the causal relationship of an observed adverse
effect than do open studies, but it does offer a chance for rational comparison of
drugs in this respect.

In one large double-blind study, overall tolerability with norfloxacin was
significantly better than that with cotrimoxazole [123]. In several double-blind
studies, ciprofloxacin has been compared to other antibiotics or placebo. Tolerability of ciprofloxacin was significantly better than with cotrimoxazole in
patients treated for urinary tract infections [124]. However, the tolerability of
doxycycline was superior to ciprofloxacin when both drugs were compared in
patients with nongonococcal urethritis [125].

Pichler *et al.* [126] reported on 85 adult patients with acute diarrhea who
received either 500 mg ciprofloxacin twice daily or placebo for 5 days. Side
effects occurred in both treatment groups at the same rate. Transient elevation of
serum transaminase levels was detected in three patients in the ciprofloxacin
group and in two patients in the placebo group. Epigastric pain and leukopenia
was registered in two patients of the ciprofloxacin group. Two patients in the
placebo group suffered from nausea and epigastric pain, and rash was found in
one patient in the placebo group.

In double-blind studies, the incidence of side effects with ofloxacin was similar
to that with pipemidic acid (5.5 vs. 5.5% [127], 8.5 vs. 7.8% [128]) and
amoxicillin (4.8 vs. 4.0% [129], 5.7 vs. 5.7% [130]), and less than or equal to that
with cefaclor (2.3 vs. 5.4% [131], 8.1 vs. 8.4% [132]). These data from Japanese
studies are given unchanged as published by Monk and Campoli-Richards [133].

Fleroxacin was less well tolerated than amoxicillin or norfloxacin in patients
treated for chronic bronchitis or urinary tract infection [134–136]. At least one
adverse effect was experienced by 31% of the patients treated over 7 days with
fleroxacin (200 mg once daily) for urinary tract infection compared to 26% of
those treated with ciprofloxacin (250 mg twice daily). Adverse effects were
comparable among the treatment groups, but insomnia was more frequent in
patients who received fleroxacin [137].

The efficacy and tolerability of fleroxacin (400-mg single dose or once daily
for 3 days) was compared to placebo in patients with acute bacterial diarrhea.
Adverse effects judged by the investigators to be related to the trial medication
were reported in 7% of patients treated with placebo and in 6% of patients treated
with fleroxacin (same incidence for both fleroxacin-treated groups, not significantly different from the placebo group) [138].

No significant differences in tolerability were seen when sparfloxacin was
compared to various antibacterial regimens for respiratory tract infections or with
ciprofloxacin for urinary tract infections (e.g., [139–142]).

TABLE XIII Adverse Reactions with Fluoroquinolones Observed in Double-Blind Clinical Trials

Fluoro-quinolone	No. of patients	% ADR	Compara-tive drug	No. of patients	% ADR	Signi-ficantly different	Indication	Reference
Norfloxacin	658	34	TMP–SMX	216	49	*	UTI	UTI Study Group (1987) [123]
	148	16	TMP–SMX	148	10		Bacterial diarrhea	Loleka et al. (1988) [188]
Ciprofloxacin	103	17	TMP–SMX	100	32	*	UTI	Grubbs et al. (1992) [124]
	282	14	Cefotaxime	288	12		Skin infections	Gentry et al. (1989) [189]
	110	36	Doxycycline	52	19	#	Nongonococcal urethritis	Hooton et al. (1990) [125]
Fleroxacin	102	41	Amoxicillin	92	15	#	ABECB	Chodosh (1993) [134]
	313	19	Amoxicillin	310	9	#	ABECB	Ulmer (1993) [136]
	321	31	Ciprofloxacin	324	26		UTI	Iravani (1993) [137]
	287	26	Norfloxacin	292	14	#	UTI	Pummer (1993) [135]
	160	6	Placebo	170	7		Bacterial diarrhea	Butler et al. (1993b) [138]
	172	6	(Placebo	170	7)			
Sparfloxacin	110	44	Amoxicillin plus Ofloxacin	101	56		CAP	Portier et al. (1996) [140]
	370	22	Coamoxiclav	363	26		AE-COPD	Allegra et al. 1996 [139]
	193	10	Cefuroximaxetil	184	8.1		Purulent sinusitis	Gehanno et al. (1996) [141]
	344	27	Ciprofloxacin	340	24		Complicated UTI	Naber et al. (1996) [142]
Levofloxacin	177	29	Coamoxiclav	168	29		CAP	Carbon et al. (1999) [190]
	561	20	Cefuroximaxetil	271	18		AECB	Shah et al. (1999) [191]
Moxifloxacin	288	33	Trovafloxacin	302	37		Sinusitis	Baz et al. (1999) [192]
	194	35	Clarithromycin	188	34		CAP	Fogarty et al. (1999) [193]
	322	21	Clarithromycin	327	22		AECB	Wilson et al. (1999) [194]
	302	30	Clarithromycin	312	33		AECB	Chodosh et al. (2000) [195]
	223	37	Cefuroximaxetil	234	26	#	Sinusitis	Burke et al. (1999) [143]
Gatifloxacin	209	28	Levofloxacin	208	32		CAP	Sullivan et al. (1999) [145]

*Tolerability of fluoroquinolone was significantly better than tolerability of comparative drug. #Tolerability of comparative drug was significantly better than the tolerability of fluoroquinolone. ABECB = acute bacterial exacerbation of chronic bronchitis; CAP = community-acquired pneumonia; UTI = urinary tract infection.

Moxifloxacin has been compared with several other antimicrobial agents in a series of large comparative double-blind trials reviewed more recently [95]. A selection of data from such trials is given in Table XIII. In patients with lower respiratory tract infections, moxifloxacin was associated with adverse reactions at similar incidences as the macrolide clarithromycin. Gastrointestinal events (e.g., nausea, diarrhea) were the most commonly reported events with both agents. Dizziness seemed to be more common with moxifloxacin (3 to 5 vs. 1%), and taste perversion occurred more often with clarithromycin (0 to 2 vs. 3.5 to 8%). Compared to amoxicillin, moxifloxacin was associated with a similar overall incidence of drug-related adverse effects. However, a higher rate of adverse effects was noticed with moxifloxacin compared to cefuroxime axetil (31 vs. 23% and 37 vs. 26%). Nausea was significantly more common with moxifloxacin than with cefuroxime axctil in one trial (11 vs. 4%), but not in another (4 vs. 2%) [143,144]. Compared with trovafloxacin, moxifloxacin was associated with a similar overall incidence of adverse effects (33 vs. 37%), a slightly higher incidence of gastrointestinal reactions (22 vs. 16%), but a lower incidence of CNS events (8 vs. 24%).

More than 400 patients with community-acquired pneumonia were evaluated in a double-blind study comparing the efficacy and safety of levofloxacin and gatifloxacin. Incidences of total adverse effects were similar in both groups (28 vs. 32%). Nausea and diarrhea occurred more often in the levofloxacin-treated patients (9 vs. 6% and 6 vs. 3%). In both groups, 4% of the patients reported insomnia. Drug-related adverse effects led to cessation of therapy in five (gatifloxacin) and three (levofloxacin) patients [145].

In a similarly designed study, gatifloxacin (n = 207) was compared with clarithromycin (n = 205) in patients with pneumonia. Among the gastrointestinal adverse effects, taste perversion (6 vs. 11%), abdominal pain (1 vs. 5%), and diarrhea (6 vs. 13%) were less common in gatifloxacin-treated patients than in clarithromycin-treated patients. Nausea was reported by a similar percentage of patients in both groups (9 vs. 8%). Four percent of gatifloxacin patients and 3% of clarithromycin patients reported dizziness. Adverse effects or laboratory abnormalities led to discontinuation of the study medication in 14 (gatifloxacin) and 11 (clarithromycin) patients [146].

DRUG INTERACTIONS

Several types of interactions between quinolones and other xenobiotics have been described: *in-vitro* interactions during testing of antimicrobial activity, interactions with antacids during the absorption phase, interactions affecting the renal excretion of some derivatives, and, last but not least, inhibition of the hepatic metabolism of concomitantly administered drugs [147–150].

INFLUENCE OF pH AND MAGNESIUM ON ANTIBACTERIAL ACTIVITY OF QUINOLONES *IN VITRO*

Detailed studies have been published on the influence on the antibacterial activity of quinolones of lowering the pH of the test medium [151,152]. The activity of 10 different quinolones against *E. coli* KL16 was investigated at four pH values between 5.6 and 8.3, which covers the pH range of urine. It was found that the nature of the substituent at the C7 position determines the kind of alteration of antibacterial activity with changing pH values. For derivatives with a piperazine ring at C7, activity became progressively less as the pH fell. Compounds without a piperazine substituent exhibited a progressive increase in activity as the pH was reduced. In addition, it was found that, except for cinoxacin, a high urinary concentration of magnesium generally caused further antagonism of the antimicrobial activity of quinolones at all pH values tested.

In 22 urine isolates, an increase of mean ciprofloxacin MIC from 0.22 mg/liter in an Mg-free medium (pH 6.0) to 0.71 mg/liter in a medium with 11.2 mg/dl magnesium was determined [152]. Similar results have been published with other quinolones, such as fleroxacin [153].

INTERACTIONS BETWEEN QUINOLONES AND ANTACIDS

Antacids have been described as inhibitors of absorption for ciprofloxacin, ofloxacin, and fleroxacin [150,154]. In these studies, 10 doses of Maalox™ gel, each containing 600 mg $Mg(OH)_2$ and 900 mg $Al(OH)_3$, were administered within 24 hours before administration of the quinolone. Contemporary administration of 500 mg ciprofloxacin and Maalox resulted in a drastic decrease in plasma peak concentrations and the area under the curve (AUC mean from 7.4 to 0.7 mg/liter·hr). The Maalox-induced reduction in gastrointestinal absorption was less pronounced for ofloxacin or fleroxacin (Table XIV).

The degree of interaction between quinolones and mineral antacids strongly depends on the time between the intake of drugs. It is most pronounced when antacids are taken shortly before the quinolone (up to 2 hr) but is less pronounced and probably without clinical relevance if the antacid is taken 2 hours or more after intake of the quinolone (see, e.g., [155,156]).

Significant reductions in the bioavailability of fluoroquinolones (e.g., ciprofloxacin) have been described when the antibacterial was taken together with other drugs that contain metal ions, for example, didanosin-containing tablets that contain magnesium cations [157], or multivitamin preparations with zinc or drugs that contain iron [158]. Significant reductions in absorption of various quinolones also occurred after concomitant intake with sucralfate, an aluminum-containing drug [159–162].

TABLE XIV   Bioavailability of Ciprofloxacin, Ofloxacin, and Fleroxacin

Medication**	C_{max} (mg/l)	T_{max} (min)	AUC_{tot} (h x mg/l)
A. Ofloxacin			
200 mg ofloxacin (O)	2.2 ± 0.4	77 ± 39	14.6 ± 2.7
O plus breakfast	$1.7 \pm 0.4*$	$102 \pm 49*$	13.6 ± 2.1
O plus ranitidine	2.2 ± 0.4	65 ± 34	14.3 ± 1.5
O plus Maalox®	$0.5 \pm 0.1*$	90 ± 30	$4.5 \pm 1.2*$
B. Ciprofloxacin			
250 mg ciprofloxacin (C)	1.6 ± 0.3	57 ± 13	5.6 ± 1.0
C plus breakfast	$0.9 \pm 0.5*$	41 ± 16	5.4 ± 0.7
500 mg ciprofloxacin (C)	1.8 ± 0.4	72 ± 16	7.4 ± 1.2
C plus ranitidine	1.7 ± 0.4	84 ± 34	8.2 ± 1.9
C plus Maalox®	$0.13 \pm 0.1*$	80 ± 16	$0.7 \pm 0.3*$
C. Fleroxacin			
400 mg fleroxacin (F)	5.2 ± 1.9	78 ± 66	56.2 ± 12.9
F plus breakfast	4.3 ± 1.3	144 ± 108	54.9 ± 11.6
F plus ranitidine	5.2 ± 2.1	72 ± 42	60.1 ± 15.3
F plus Maalox®	3.6 ± 1.0	108 ± 90	41.6 ± 12.2

Modified after Höffken et al. 1988 [163] and Deppermann and Lode (1993) [150].

Influence of breakfast and concomitant administered drugs in two groups of healthy volunteers (5 males/5 females in each group). C_{max} = maximum plasma concentration; T_{max} = time at which peak concentration is calculated; AUC = area under the concentration–time curve

*$p < 0.05$ compared to values after administration of drug alone.

**Dosage of concomitant administered drugs (24 hr prior to dosing of quinolone): (1) Maalox® 10 times 1 portion of gel (0.6 g $Mg(OH)_2$ and 0.9 g $Al(OH)_3$]; (2) three times 150 mg ranitidine orally.

However, histamine (H2) receptor blockers that reduce gastric acidity (ranitid-ine, cimetidine) but do not contain metal cations did not significantly alter the bioavailability of fluoroquinolones [150,163,164].

The influence of several drugs that alter gastric mobility on the pharmacokinetics of ciprofloxacin and ofloxacin has also been studied. Pirenzipine and *N*-butyl-scopolamine, antimuscarinic drugs that delay gastric emptying, prolonged the time until maximum serum concentration was achieved but did not alter the AUC or urine recovery of the drugs. However, absorption of ciprofloxacin was accelerated when metoclopramide, a drug that accelerates gastric emptying, was administered immediately prior to administration of ciprofloxacin [165].

Table XV gives an overview on interactions of the newer fluoroquinolones moxifloxacin, gatifloxacin, and gemifloxacin in comparison with ciprofloxacin and levofloxacin.

In summary, all fluoroquinolones show dose-dependent, clinically relevant interactions with mineral antacids and other drugs that contain divalent or trivalent cations (for a review, see [166]). Simultaneous oral administration must be avoided. Absorption of the drugs on the antacid gel or altered solubility of the quinolones at different pH values leading to altered absorption characteristics of the drugs have been discussed as possible explanations for the effects observed. However, the most significant reason for these effects is probably formation of chelate complexes between the antibacterials and the metal ions. Some data on the mode of antibacterial action of quinolones suggest that the drugs bind to a DNA–gyrase complex via a magnesium ion [167]. This means that probably all quinolones with antibacterial activity will exhibit an affinity to magnesium and other di- or trivalent cations.

INFLUENCE OF BREAKFAST OR DAIRY PRODUCTS ON THE BIOAVAILABILITY OF QUINOLONES

A standard breakfast had a significant effect on the absorption of ciprofloxacin (Table XIV). A concomitant breakfast decreased the peak concentrations and delayed absorption of ciprofloxacin, ofloxacin, or fleroxacin but without altering the bioavailability (AUC) of the drugs [150,163].

The effects of calcium-rich dairy products on the absorption of fluoroquinolones have been studied. Pronounced alterations have been observed when milk or yoghurt were taken together with ciprofloxacin, and similar interactions have

TABLE XV Fluoroquinolones and Interaction with Other Drugs and Foods[a]

	Ciprofloxacin	Levofloxacin	Moxifloxacin	Gatifloxacin	Gemifloxacin
Quinolones may interfere with the metabolism of the following: Increased level of:					
Theophylline	↑↑	–	–	–	–
Caffeine	↑↑	–	?	?	?
Warfarin	slight to ↑[b]	–	–	–	–
Absorption of the quinolones is affected when administered concomitantly with the following:					
Aluminium- or magnesium-containing antacids	↓↓↓	↓↓↓	↓↓↓	↓↓↓	↓↓↓↓
Calcium-containing antacids	↓↓	→	↓[d]	→	?
Ferrous sulfate	↓↓↓	↓↓	↓↓↓	↓↓↓	↓↓
Sucralfate	↓↓↓↓	↓↓↓[c]	↓↓↓[c]	?	↓↓↓
Dairy products	↓↓	↓[c]	→	?	?
Food	↓[d]	–	↓[d]	?	→

Modified after Dembry et al. (1999) [83].

[a]Four arrows indicate >75% change; three arrows indicate 50–75% change; two arrows indicate 25–49% change, and one arrow indicates <25% change. Dashes indicate that no significant effect was documented.

[b]The effect of warfarin metabolism is variable.

[c]A decrease in absorption of the fluoroquinolone is documented; however, the actual percentage decrease is not clear.

[d]Absorption delayed with no effect on total bioavailability.

been described with norfloxacin. The bioavailability of ofloxacin was not significantly altered [168,169].

INTERACTIONS IN RENAL ELIMINATION

More than 50% of total ciprofloxacin clearance is due to renal elimination [170]. The renal clearance of ciprofloxacin is about nine times higher than the creatinine clearance, indicating renal tubular secretion. The influence of 1 g probenecid on elimination of ciprofloxacin was studied in healthy volunteers in a double-blind study. Probenecid was shown to have no effect on peak concentrations and elimination half-life but reduced the extent of urinary excretion and increased the AUC significantly [165].

Pretreatment with probenecid (500 mg) twice daily for 2 days had no significant effect on the kinetics of moxifloxacin [171]. Under similar conditions, the half-life of gatifloxacin, which is mainly excreted via the kidney, was prolonged by 44% [65].

INTERACTIONS BETWEEN QUINOLONES AND THEOPHYLLINE

During treatment of lower respiratory tract infections with 2×600 mg enoxacin daily, interactions with theophylline metabolism were first noticed. Eight of 10 patients who received enoxacin plus the bronchodilator experienced serious nausea and vomiting, and two persons also complained of tachycardia and headaches. In all patients, high theophylline plasma levels were measured (17–41 mg/liter); on discontinuation of theophylline therapy, the complaints disappeared after 2 days [172].

In a systematically performed study, Wijnands et al. [173] determined the pharmacokinetic variables of theophylline in eight patients with COLD (chronic obstructive lung disease) undergoing maintenance theophylline treatment (300–600 mg twice daily) alone and after comedication with five different quinolone derivatives. The daily dosage of chemotherapeutic agents was two times 400 mg for 6 days, except for ciprofloxacin and nalidixic acid, which were given 500 mg b.i.d. Significant increases in theophylline plasma concentrations were seen with enoxacin (111%) and, to a lesser degree, also during coadministration of pefloxacin (20%) and ciprofloxacin (23%). The pharmacokinetic variables were not changed during concomitant administration of ofloxacin and nalidixic acid.

However, other data indicate that there might be a slight but statistically significant interaction between theophylline and ofloxacin [174].

No significant influences on theophylline metabolism were found with fleroxacin [175], sparfloxacin [176], or the newer quinolones levofloxacin, moxifloxacin, gatifloxacin, and gemifloxacin (Tables XV and XVI).

Fuhr *et al.* [177,178] have conducted *in-vitro* studies with human liver microsome preparations and showed that the cause of interaction between some quinolones and methylxanthines is competitive inhibition of metabolism. Data indicate that quinolones specifically inhibit the cytochrome P450 isoform CYP1A2. A nitrogen atom in the 7-piperazinyl group is essential for this interaction. The nitrogen atom is possibly the site that binds to the trivalent iron ion (Fe^{3+}) in the catalytic center of cytochrome P450 and inhibits methylxanthine metabolism [179].

TABLE XVI   Effects of Fluoroquinolones on Pharmacokinetics of Theophylline

		Increase in serum theophylline (%)	
Quinolone	Daily dose (mg)	C_{max} (mg/l)	AUC (mg/l × hr)
Enoxacin	600	+74	+84
Pefloxacin	400	+17	+19
Ciprofloxacin	600	+17	+22
Ofloxacin	600	+ 9	+11
Levofloxacin	300	−	−
Norfloxacin	600	−	
Lomefloxacin	600	−	−
Fleroxacin	400	−	−
Sparfloxacin	300	−	−
Moxifloxacin	400	−	−
Gatifloxacin	400	−	−
Gemifloxacin	320	−	−

Modified after Niki *et al.* (1992) [196].

C_{max} = maximum theophylline plasma concentration; AUC = area under the concentration–time curve of theophylline; − = less than 4% increase or decrease.

Five healthy male volunteers. Theophylline: 200 mg b.i.d, 4 days, followed by quinolones for 5 to 7 days. Values for theophylline were obtained on day 5 or day 7 of concomitant treatment (or similar study design).

Pharmacokinetic parameters were statistically significantly different, except for ofloxacin.

In summary, concomitant treatment of patients with theophylline and enoxacin, pefloxacin, and ciprofloxacin should be avoided. If simultaneous therapy with theophylline and these drugs is necessary, theophylline plasma concentrations should be carefully monitored and dosage adjusted. A significant interaction of other fluoroquinolones (e.g., levofloxacin, sparfloxacin, moxifloxacin, gatifloxacin, or gemifloxacin) with the metabolism of methylxanthines is not likely.

INTERACTIONS BETWEEN QUINOLONES AND CAFFEINE

Interactions between quinolones have also been demonstrated with caffeine, which is closely related to theophylline. The metabolism pathways of both methylxanthines are similar. Corresponding results after simultaneous treatment with theophylline were found with the impact of ofloxacin (200 mg b.i.d.), ciprofloxacin (250 mg b.i.d.), and enoxacin (400 mg b.i.d.) on the pharmacokinetic behavior of caffeine in 12 healthy male volunteers using a crossover study design. After coadministration of a single oral caffeine dose (200–230 mg, equal to 3–4 cups of coffee) with ofloxacin (5-day treatment), the pharmacokinetics of caffeine (measured by elimination half-life, total body clearance, and volume of distribution) was not changed at all or was only minimally altered; however, moderate interference was noticed with ciprofloxacin (15% prolongation of elimination half-life) and a pronounced effect occurred during coadministration of enoxacin. Elimination half-life was prolonged from 3.3 to 11.8 hours (mean values), the maximum plasma concentration was increased by 41% (3.9–5.5 mg/liter), and total body clearance was reduced by 78% [180,181].

A rather pronounced influence of ciprofloxacin on the caffeine metabolism was seen in another study in healthy volunteers. The elimination half-life of caffeine increased from 5.2 to 8.2 hours, and clearance was reduced by 38% [182].

Most of the other quinolones have not been studied extensively for a possible interaction with caffeine, or they have only little or no influence on caffeine metabolism. The likelihood for an interaction with caffeine is probably similar to that for an interaction with theophylline.

INTERACTIONS WITH DIGOXIN

Interactions of drugs with digoxin deserve special attention, since digoxin possesses such a small therapeutic index. A general lack of interaction between digoxin and other drugs should not be claimed on the basis of a statistical analysis with a limited number of subjects. If the effect of a concomitantly given drug on the kinetic behavior of digoxin is of considerable variability, statistical tests will fail to detect a significant difference under these conditions, but some individuals may nevertheless be at risk of severe adverse effects. In such situations, a statement that no interaction occurs would be misleading.

Highly variable interactions between digoxin and fluoroquinolones have been described with at least two drugs: gatifloxacin and moxifloxacin [7,65]. Gemifloxacin seems to be free of such risks, as indicated by one study in 14 subjects [93]. As not all studies have been published in detail and direct comparative studies are missing, it is hardly possible to evaluate the risks of such interactions with other quinolones. As long as the mechanism of such interaction remains unclear, considerable uncertainties exist. So far it can only be speculated that increased digoxin levels might be due to increased bioavailability caused by eradication of digoxin-metabolizing gut flora by the drugs.

The findings with gatifloxacin are described in detail on the U.S. package insert for Tequin [65]. Overall, only a modest increase in peak concentration and AUC value (12 and 19%) was noted in 8 of 11 healthy volunteers who received gatifloxacin and digoxin. In 3 of 11 subjects, however, a significant increase in digoxin concentrations was observed. In these three subjects, digoxin AUC increased by 66 to 104%! Therefore, patients taking digoxin plus gatifloxacin (and possibly moxifloxacin and other quinolones!) should be monitored for signs and/or symptoms of toxicity. If signs and symptoms are observed, serum digoxin concentrations should be determined and digoxin dosage adjusted as appropriate [65].

INTERACTIONS BETWEEN QUINOLONES AND OTHER DRUGS

The most important cytochrome P450 isoform for drug metabolism is CYP3A4, which metabolizes macrolides, nifedipine, midazolam, cyclosporine, and many other agents. As mentioned previously, some quinolones obviously inhibit the CYP1A2 isoform. Because this inhibition seems to be rather specific, significant interactions between fluoroquinolones and other drugs that are metabolized by hepatic cytochrome P450 are not very likely. Nevertheless, in several studies, the possible interactions between fluoroquinolones, mostly enoxacin or ciprofloxacin, have been investigated.

When the possibility of interactions between fluoroquinolones and other drugs is considered, two important aspects should be kept in mind that complicate the situation. First, the amount of some cytochrome P450 enzymes expressed in human liver exhibits considerable variability. Thus, an individual risk for an interaction might exist, though no major effects are recognizable if average data are compared. Second, some drugs that inhibit cytochrome P450 enzymes may also cause induction of these enzymes. An induction of CYP1A2 has been described in rat liver CYP450 after multiple-dose treatment with enoxacin [183].

Several publications indicate that ciprofloxacin may have significant effects on phenytoin metabolism. For example, a significant decrease in phenytoin concentrations to subtherapeutic levels and seizures have been described in a 61-year-old man soon after the start of concomitant ciprofloxacin treatment (750 mg b.i.d.). As a consequence, the phenytoin doses were doubled, once again yielding therapeutic plasma levels. However, phenytoin intoxication ensued after discharge from the hospital when the ciprofloxacin was discontinued. This case underscores the need for clinical suspicion of drug interactions in any patient requiring a substantial change in drug dosage [184].

The effects of coadministration of enoxacin and warfarin were investigated in six healthy male volunteers. Enoxacin caused a significant prolongation of the elimination half-life of (R)-warfarin (from 36.8 ± 14.2 to 52.2 ± 14.7 hr; mean $\pm$ SD), but it had no effect on the pharmacokinetics of the pharmacologically more active (S)-enantiomer. No statistically significant change in the anticoagulant response to warfarin was found [185]. Similarly, the newer fluoroquinolones levofloxacin, moxifloxacin, gatifloxacin, and gemifloxacin had no effect on the pharmacokinetics/pharmacodynamics of warfarin in healthy volunteers (Table XV).

No significant interaction was detected between ciprofloxacin and diazepam [186] or the immunosuppressive cyclosporine [187]. No other evidence of clinically relevant interactions between the fluoroquinolones and other drugs exist at this point in time.

REFERENCES

1. Norrby, S. R., and Lietman, P. S. (1993). Safety and tolerability of fluoroquinolones. *Drugs* **45** (Suppl. 3), 59–64.
2. Blum, M. D., Graham, D. J., and McCloskey C. A. (1994). Temafloxacin syndrome: review of 95 cases. *Clin. Infect. Dis.* **18**, 9046–9050.
3. Trovan™, U.S. Package Insert, 1999.
4. Chen, H. J. L., Bloch, K. J., and Maclean, J. A. (2000). Acute eosinophilic hepatitis from trovafloxacin. *New Engl. J. Med.* **342**, 359–360.
5. Stahlmann, R., and Schwabe, R. (1997). Safety profile of grepafloxacin as compared with other fluoroquinolones. *J. Antimicrob. Chemother.* **40** (Suppl. A), 83–92.
6. Takayama, S., Watanabe, T., Akiyama, Y., Ohura, K., Harada, S., Matsuhashi, K., Mochida, K., and Yamashita, N. (1986). Reproductive toxicity of ofloxacin. *Arzneim.–Forsch./Drug Res.* **36**, 1244–1248.

7. Gough, A. W., Kasali, O. B., Sigler, R. E., and Baragi, V. (1992). Quinolone arthropathy: Acute toxicity to immature cartilage. *Toxicol. Pathol.* **20**, 436–450.

8. Stahlmann, R., Förster, C., and van Sickle, D. (1993). Quinolones in children: Are concerns over arthropathy justified? *Drug Saf.* **9**. 397–403.

9. Stahlmann, R., and Lode, H. (1999). Toxicity of quinolones. *Drugs* **58** (Suppl. 2), 37–42.

10. Förster, C., Kociok, K., Shakibaei, M., Merker, H.-J., and Stahlmann, R. (1996a). Quinolone-induced cartilage lesions are not reversible in rats. *Arch. Toxicol.* **70**, 474–481.

11. Schaad, U., Wedgwood, J., Ruedeberg, A., Kraemer R., and Hampel, B. (1997). Ciprofloxacin as antipseudomonal treatment in patients with cystic fibrosis. *Pediatr. Infect. Dis. J.* **16**, 106–111.

12. Ingham, B., Brentnall, D. W., Dale, E. A., and McFadzean, J. A. (1977). Arthropathy induced by antibacterial fused *N*-alkyl-4-pyridone-3-carboxylic acids. *Toxicol. Lett.* **1**, 21–26.

13. Tatsumi, H., Senda, H., Yatera, S., Takemoto, Y., Yamayoshi, M., and Ohnishi, K. (1978). Toxicological studies on pipemidic acid, V: Effect on diarthrodial joints of experimental animals. *J. Toxicol. Sci.* **3**, 357–367.

14. Burkhardt, J. E., Hill, M. A., Carlton, W. W., and Kesterson, J. W. (1990). Histologic and histochemical changes in articular cartilages of immature Beagle dogs dosed with difloxacin, a fluoroquinolone. *Vet. Pathol.* **27**. 162–170.

15. Burkhardt, J. E., Hill, M. A., Turek, J. J., and Carlton, W. W. (1992). Ultrastructural changes in articular cartilage of immature beagle dogs dosed with difloxacin, a fluoroquinolone. *Vet. Pathol.* **29**. 230–238.

16. Kato, M., and Onodera, T. (1988). Morphological investigation of cavity formation in articular cartilage induced by ofloxacin in rats. *Fundam. Appl. Toxicol.* **11**. 110–119.

17. Stahlmann, R., Merker, H.-J., Hinz, N., Webb, J., Heger, W., and Neubert, D. (1990). Ofloxacin in juvenile non-human primates and rats: Arthropathia and drug plasma concentrations. *Arch. Toxicol.* **64**. 193–204.

18. Förster, C., Kociok, K., Shakibaei, M., Merker, H.-J., Vormann, J., Günther, T., and Stahlmann, R. (1996b). Integrins on joint cartilage chondrocytes and alterations by magnesium deficiency in immature rats. *Arch. Toxicol.* **70**, 261–270.

19. Stahlmann, R., Vormann, J., Günther, T., Förster, C., Zippel, U., Lozo, E., Schwabe, R., Kociok, K., Shakibaei, M., and Merker, H.-J. (1997a). Effects of quinolones, magnesium deficiency or zinc deficiency on joint cartilage in rats. *Mg. Bull.* **19**. 7–22.

20. Schwabe, R., Lozo, E., Baumann-Wilschke, I., and Stahlmann, R. (1999). Chondrotoxicity and target tissue kinetics of ofloxacin in immature rats after multiple doses. *Drugs* **58** (Suppl. 2), 385–387.

21. Stahlmann, R., Zippel, U., Förster, C., Shakibaei, M., Merker, H.-J., and Borner, K. (1998). Chondrotoxicity and toxicokinetics of sparfloxacin in juvenile rats. *Antimicrob. Agents Chemother.* **42**, 1470–1475.

22. Stahlmann, R., Förster, C., Shakibaei, M., Vormann, J., Günther, T., and Merker, H.-J. (1995). Magnesium deficiency induces joint cartilage lesions in juvenile rats which are identical with quinolone-induced arthropathy. *Antimicrob. Agents Chemother.* **39**. 2013–2018.

23. Shakibaei, M., Kociok, K., Förster, C., Vormann, J., Günther, T., Stahlmann, R., and Merker, H.-J. (1996). Comparative evaluation of ultrastructural changes in articular cartilage of juvenile rats after treatment with ofloxacin and in magnesium-deficient rats. *Toxicol. Pathol.* **24**. 580–587.

24. Hayem, G., Petit, P. X., Levacher, M., Gaudin, C., Kahn, M. F., and Pocidalo, J. J. (1994). Cytofluorometric analysis of chondrotoxicity of fluoroquinolone antimicrobial agents. *Antimicrob. Agents Chemother.* **38**, 243–247.

25. Merker, H.-J., Günther, T., Höllriegl, V., Vormann, J., and Schümann, K. (1996). Lipid peroxidation and morphology of rat testis in magnesium deficiency. *Andrologia* **28**, 43–51.

26. Stahlmann, R., Schwabe, R., Pfister, K., Lozo, E., Shakibaei, M., and Vormann, J. (1999). Supplementation with magnesium and tocopherol diminishes quinolone-induced chondrotoxicity in immature rats. *Drugs* **58** (Suppl. 2), 393–394.

27. Vormann, J., Förster, C., Zippel, U., Lozo, E., Günther, T., Merker, H.-J., and Stahlmann, R. (1997). Effects of magnesium deficiency on magnesium and calcium content in bone and cartilage in developing rats in correlation to chondrotoxicity. *Calc. Tiss. Intern.* **61**, 230–238.

28. Syllm-Rapoport, I., Strassburger, I., Grüneberg, D., and Zirbel, C. (1958). Über den experimentellen Magnesium-Mangel beim Hund. *Acta Biol. Med. Germ.* **1**, 141–163.

29. Stahlmann, R., Kühner, S., Shakibaei, M., Schwabe, R., Flores, J., Evander, S. A., and van Sickle, D. C. (2000a). Chondrotoxicity of ciprofloxacin in immature Beagle dogs; immunohistochemistry, electron microscopy and drug plasma concentrations. *Arch. Toxicol.* **73**, 564–572.

30. Stahlmann, R., Kühner, S., Shakibaei, M., Flores, J., Vormann, J., and van Sickle, D. C. (2000b). Effects of magnesium deficiency on joint cartilage in immature Beagle dogs: Immunohistochemistry, electron microscopy and mineral concentrations. *Arch. Toxicol.* **73**, 573–780.

31. Kato, M., Takada, S., Kashida, Y., and Nomura, M. (1995). Histological examination on Achilles tendon lesions induced by quinolone antibacterial agents in juvenile rats. *Toxicol. Pathol.* **23**, 385–392.

32. Kashida, Y., and Kato, M. (1997b). Characterization of fluoroquinolone-induced Achilles tendon toxicity in rats: Comparison of toxicities of 10 fluoroquinolones and effects of antiinflammatory compounds. *Antimicrob. Agents Chemother.* **41**, 2389–2393.

33. Kashida, Y., and Kato, M. (1997a). Toxic effects of quinolone antibacterial agents on the musculoskeletal system in juvenile rats. *Toxicol. Pathol.* **25**, 635–643.

34. Schwabe, R., Zippel, U., Förster, C., Baumann-Wilschke, I., and Stahlmann, R. (1996). Plasma concentrations and chondrotoxicity of three fluoroquinolones in juvenile rats. *Naunyn-Schmiedeberg's Arch. Pharmacol.* **354** (Suppl. 1), R28 [Abstr. #10].

35. Simonin, M. A., Gegout-Pottie, P., Minn, A., Gillet, P., Netter, P., and Terlain, B. (2000). Pefloxacin-induced achilles tendon toxicity in rodents: Biochemical changes in proteoglycan synthesis and oxidative damage to collagen. *Antimicrob. Agents Chemother.* **44/4**, 867–872.

36. Shakibaei, M., Pfister, K., Schwabe, R., Vormann, J., and Stahlmann, R. (2000). Ultrastructure of Achilles tendons of rats treated with ofloxacin and fed a normal or magnesium-deficient diet. *Antimicrob. Agents Chemother.* **44**(2), 261–266.

37. Aceto, M. D., Harris, L. S., Lesher, G. Y., Pearl, J., and Brown, T. G. (1967). Pharmacologic studies with 7-benzyl-1-ethyl-1,4-dihydro-4-oxo-1,8-naphthyridine-3-carboxylic acid. *J. Pharmacol. Exp. Ther.* **158**, 286–293.

38. Akahane, K., Sekiguchi, M., Une, T., and Osada, Y. (1989). Structure-epileptogenicity relationship of quinolones with special reference to their interaction with gamma-aminobutyric acid receptor sites. *Antimicrob. Agents Chemother.* **33**, 1704–1708.

39. Christ, W., and Esch, B. (1994). Adverse reactions to fluoroquinolones in adults and children. *Infect. Dis. Clin. Pract.* **3** (Suppl. 3). S168–S176.

40. Takayama, S., Hirohashi, M., Kato, M., and Shimada, H. (1995). Toxicity of quinolone antimicrobial agents. *J. Toxicol. Env. Health* **45**. 1–45.

41. Schmuck, G., Schürmann, A., and Schlüter, G. (1998). Determination of the excitatory potencies of fluoroquinolones in the central nervous system by an *in vitro* model. *Antimicrob. Agents Chemother.* **42**, 1831–1836.

42. de Sarro, G., Nava, F., Calapai, G., and de Sarro, A. (1997). Effects of some excitatory amino acid antagonists and drugs enhancing γ-aminobutyric acid neurotransmission on pefloxacin-induced seizures in DBA/2 mice. *Antimicrob. Agents Chemother.* **41**, 427–434.

43. Nakamura, M., Abe, S., Goto, Y., Chishaki, A., Akazawa, K., and Kato, M. (1994). In vivo assessment of prevention of white-noise-induced seizure in magnesium-deficient rats by *N*-methyl-D-aspartate receptor blockers. *Epilepsy Res.* **17**. 249–256.

44. Domagala, J. M. (1994). Structure–activity and structure–side effect relationship for the quinolone antibacterials. *J. Antimicrob. Chemother.* **33**, 685–706.

45. Marutani, K., Matsumoto, M., Otabe, Y., Nagamuta, M., Tanaka, K., Miyoshi, A., Hasegawa, T., Nagano, H., Masubara, S., Kamide, R., *et al.* (1993). Reduced phototoxicity of a fluoroquinolone antibacterial agent with a methoxy group at the 8 position in mice irradiated with long-wavelength UV light. *Antimicrob. Agents Chemother.* **37/10**. 2217–2223.

46. von Keutz, E., and Schlüter, G. (1999). Preclinical safety evaluation of moxifloxacin, a novel fluoroquinolone. *J. Antimicrob. Chemother.* **43** (Suppl. B), 91–100.

47. Johnson, B. E., Gibbs, N. K., and Ferguson, J. (1997). Quinolone antibiotic with potential to photosensitize skin tumorigenesis. *J. Photochem. Photobiol. Biol.* **37**, 171–173.

48. Klecak, G., Urbach, F., and Urwyler, H. (1997). Fluoroquinolone antibacterials enhance UVA-induced skin tumors. *J. Photochem. Photobiol. Biol.* **37**, 174–181.

49. Mäkinen, M., Forbes, P. D., and Stenbäck, F. (1997). Quinolone antibacterials: A new class of photochemical carcinogens. *J. Photochem. Photobiol. Biol.* **37**, 182–187.

50. Bulera, S. J., Theiss, J. C., Festerling, T. A., and de la Iglesia, F. A. (1999). In vitro photogenotoxic activity of clinafloxacin: A paradigm predicting photocarcinogenicity. *Toxicol. Appl. Pharmacol.* **156**. 222–230.

51. Schlüter, G. (1986). Toxicology of ciprofloxacin. In "Proceedings of the First International Ciprofloxacin Workshop" (H. C. Neu and H. Weuta, eds.), pp. 61–70. Excerpta Medica, Amsterdam.

52. Corrado, M. L., Struble, W. E., Peter, C., Hoagland, V., and Sabbaj, J. (1987). Norfloxacin: Review of safety studies. *Am. J. Med.* **82** (Suppl. 6B), 22–26.

53. Nomura, M., Yamada, M., Yamamura, H., Kajimura, T., and Takayama, S. (1992). Ophthalmotoxicity and ototoxicity of the new quinolone antibacterial agent levofloxacin in Long Evans rats. *Arzneim.-Forsch./Drug Res.* **42**, 398–403.

54. Laboratoire Roger Bellon (1985). Peflacine (pefloxacin) product monograph.

55. Butler, L. D., Biehl, M. L., Beierschmitt, W. P., Beutler, N. J., Parzych, B. M., and Coleman, G. L. (1993a). Preclinical systemic toxicity studies of CP 74,667, a quinolone antimicrobial agent [Abstr. #1471]. *Toxicologist* **13**, 376.

56. Rhone Poulenc Rorer (1994). Sparfloxacin monograph. ADIS Press, Wellington.

57. Macallum, E., Houston, B., and Smith, G. (1993). Subchronic toxicity of a quinolone antibacterial agent in Beagle dogs [Abstr. #1473]. *Toxicologist* **13**, 377.

58. Parke-Davis & Company (1986). Enoxacin. Zusammenfassung der Forschungsergebnisse, Stand Juni 1986.

59. Suzuki, H., Takahashi, T., Sato, Y., and Abe, Y. (1990). Fertility study of fleroxacin in rats. *Chemotherapy* **38** (Suppl. 2), 261–271.

60. Pfizer (1996). Trovafloxacin Investigator's Brochure.

61. Bayer, A. G. (1987). Ciprobay®. Ciprofloxacin Standard Information, Bayer Leverkusen.

62. Funabashi, H., Mukumoto, K., Shigematsu, K., Nishimura, K., and Ohnishi, K. (1991a). Reproductive and developmental toxicity studies of sparfloxacin: Teratogenicity study in rats. *Yakuri Chiryou* **19**, 1257–1274.

63. Funabashi, H., Mukumoto, K., Imura, Y., Nishimura, K., and Ohnishi, K. (1991b). Reproductive and developmental toxicity studies of sparfloxacin: Perinatal and postnatal study in rats. *Yakuri Chiryou* **19**, 1275–1289.

64. Avelox™ (moxifloxacin hydrochloride) Tablets, U.S. Package Insert, 1999.

65. Tequin™ (gatifloxacin). U.S. Package Insert, 1999.

66. Cukierski, M. A., Prahalada, S., Zacchei, A. G., Peter, C. P, Rodgers, J. D., Hess, D. L., Cukierski, M. J., Tarantal, A. F., Nyland, T., Robertson, R. T., and Hendrickx, A. G. (1989). Embryotoxicity studies of norfloxacin in cynomolgus monkeys, I: Teratology studies and norfloxacin plasma concentration in pregnant and non-pregnant monkeys. *Teratology* **39**, 39–52.

67. Cukierski, M. A., Hendrickx, A. G., Prahalada, S., Tarantal, A. F., Hess, D. L. Lasley, B. L., Peter, C. P, Tarara, R., and Robertson, R. T. (1992). Embryotoxicity studies of norfloxacin in cynomolgus monkeys, II: Role of progesterone. *Teratology* **46**, 429–438.

68. Schlüter, G. (1989). Ciprofloxacin: Toxicologic evaluation of additional safety data. *Am. J. Med.* **87** (Suppl. 5A), 37–39.

69. Tarantal, A. F., Lehrer, S. B., Lasley, B. L., and Hendrickx, A. G. (1990). Developmental toxicity of temafloxacin hydrochloride in the long-tailed macaque (*Macaca fascicularis*). *Teratology* **42**, 233–242.

70. Hummler, H., Richter, W. F., and Hendrickx, A. G. (1993). Developmental toxicity of fleroxacin and comparative pharmacokinetics of four fluoroquinolones in the cynomolgus macaque (*Macaca fascicularis*). *Toxicol. Appl. Pharmacol.* **122**, 34–45.

71. Stahlmann, R., Chahoud, I., Thiel, R., Klug, S., and Förster, C. (1997b). Developmental toxicity of three antimicrobial agents observed in non-routine studies only. *Reproduct. Toxicol.* **11**. 1–7.

72. Hussy, P., Maass, G., Tümmler, B., Grosse, F., and Schomburg, U. (1986). Effect of 4-quinolones and novobiocin on calf thymus DNA polymerase alpha primase complex, topoisomerases I and II, and growth of mammalian lymphoblasts. *Antimicrob. Agents Chemother.* **29**, 1073–1078.

73. Kohlbrenner, W. E., Wideburg, N., Weigl, D., Saldivar, A., and Chu, D. T. W. (1992). Induction of calf thymus topoisomerase II-mediated DNA breakage by the antibacterial isothiazolo-quinolones A-65281 and A-65282. *Antimicrob. Agents Chemother.* **36**, 81–86.

74. Gootz T. D., and Osheroff, N. (1993). Quinolones and eukaryotic topoisomerases. In "Quinolone Antimicrobial Agents" (D. C. Hooper and J. S. Wolfson, eds.), pp. 139–160. American Society for Microbiology, Washington, DC.

75. Gootz, T. D., Barrett, J. F., and Sutcliffe, J. A. (1990). Inhibitory effects of quinolone antibacterial agents on eucaryotic topoisomerases and related test systems. *Antimicrob. Agents Chemother.* **34**, 8–12.

76. Fort, F. L. (1992). Mutagenicity of quinolone antibacterials. *Drug Saf.* **7**, 214–222.

77. Albertini, S., Chételat, A. A. Miller, B., Muster, W., Pujadas, E., Strobel, R., and Gocke, E. (1995). Genotoxicity of 17 gyrase and four mammalian topoisomerase II poisons in prokaryotic and eukaryotic test systems. *Mutagenesis* **110**, 343–351.

78. McQueen, C. A., and Williams, G. M. (1987). Effects of quinolone antibiotics in tests for genotoxicity. *Am. J. Med.* **82** (Suppl. 4A), 94–96.

79. Martinez, L. J., Li, G., and Chignell, C. F. (1997). Photogeneration of fluoride by the fluoroquinolone antimicrobial agents lomefloxacin and fleroxacin. *Photochem. Photobiol.* **65**, 599–602.

80. Chételat, A. A., Albertini, S., and Gocke, E. (1996). The photomutagenicity of fluoroquinolones in tests for gene mutation, chromosomal aberration, gene conversion, and DNA breakage (Comet assay). *Mutagenesis* **11**, 497–504.

81. Loveday, K. S. (1996). Interrelationship of photocarcinogenicity, photomutagenicity and phototoxicity. *J. Photochem. Photobiol. Biol.* **63**, 369–372.

82. Adam, D., Andrassy, K., Christ, W., Heinrich, D., Höffler, D., Knothe, H., Lode, H., Matthias, F. R., Müller-Oerlinghausen, B., Neubert, D., Pichler, H., Rüther, E., Schmidt, L., Stahlmann, R., Stille, W., and Weber, E. [Arbeitsgemeinschaft "Arzneimittelsicherheit" der Paul-Ehrlich-Gesellschaft für Chemotherapie] (1987). Verträglichkeit der Gyrase-Hemmer. *Münch. Med. Wochenschr.* **129**, 45–46.

83. Dembry, L. M., Farrington, J. M., and Andriole, V. T. (1999). Fluoroquinolone antibiotics: Adverse effects and safety profiles. *Infect. Dis. Clin. Pract.* **8**. 421–428.

84. Lipsky, B. A., and Baker, C. A. (1999). Fluoroquinolone toxicity profiles: A review focusing on newer agents. *Clin. Infect. Dis.* **28**, 352–364.

85. Graber, H., Ludwig, E., Arr, M., and Lányi, P. (1986). Difference in multiple-dose pharmacokinetics of ofloxacin in young and aged patients *Abstr. 1st Int. Symp. New Quinolones*, Geneva. Abstr. #94.

86. Kawahara K., Kawahara, M., Goto, T., and Ohi, Y. (1991). Penetration of sparfloxacin into the human spinal fluid: A comparative study with 5 other fluoroquinolones. *Chemotherapy* **39**, 149–157.

87. Davey, P. G., Charter, M., Kelly, S., Varma, T. R. K., Jacobson, I., Freeman, A., Precious, E., and Lambert, J. (1994). Ciprofloxacin and sparfloxacin penetration into human brain tissue and their activity as antagonists of $GABA_A$ receptor of rat vagus nerve. *Antimicrob. Agents Chemother.* **38**, 1356–1362.

88. Luger S. W., Paparone, P., Wormser, G. P., Nadelman, R. B., Grunwaldt, E., Gomez, G., Wisniewski, M., and Collins, J. J. (1995). Comparison of cefuroxime axetil and doxycycline in treatment of patients with early Lyme disease associated with erythema migrans. *Antimicrob. Agents Chemother.* **39**, 661–667.

89. Brauner, G. J. (1975). Bullous photoreaction to nalidixic acid. *Am. J. Med.* **58**, 576–580.

90. Bowie, W. R., Willetts, V., and Jewesson, P. J. (1989). Adverse reactions in a dose-ranging study with a new long-acting fluoroquinolone, fleroxacin. *Antimicrob. Agents Chemother.* **33**, 1778–1782.

91. Burdge, D. R., Nakielna, E. M., and Rabin, H. R. (1995). Photosensitivity associated with ciprofloxacin use in adult patients with cystic fibrosis. *Antimicrob. Agents Chemother.* **39**, 793.

92. Ferguson, J., McEwen, J., Patterson, B. E., Purkins, L., Colman, P. J., and Willavize, S. A. (1996). An open, observer-blinded, placebo-controlled, randomized, parallel-group study to investigate the phototoxic potential of trovafloxacin, ciprofloxacin and lomefloxacin. *Abstr. 36th Intersci. Conf. Antimicrob. Agents Chemother.*, New Orleans. Abstr. #A15.

93. Vousden, M., Ferguson, J., Richards, J, Bird, N., and Allen, A. (1999). Evaluation of phototoxic potentials of gemifloxacin in healthy volunteers compared with ciprofloxacin. *Chemotherapy* **45**. 512–520.

94. Man, I., Murphy, J., and Ferguson, J. (1999). Fluoroquinolone phototoxicity: A comparison of moxifloxacin and lomefloxacin in normal volunteers. *J. Antimicrob. Chemother.* **43** (Suppl. B). 77–82.

95. Barman Balfour, J. A., and Lamb, H. M. (2000). Moxifloxacin: A review of its clinical potential in the management of community-acquired respiratory tract infections. *Drugs* **59**(1), 115–139.

96. Perry, C. M., Barman Balfour, J. A., and Lamb, H. M. (1999). Gatifloxacin. *Drugs* **58**(4), 683–696.

97. Lowe, N. J. Fakouhi, T. D., Stern, R. S., Bourget, T., Roniker, B., and Swabb, E. A. (1994). Photoreactions with a fluoroquinolone antimicrobial: Evening versus morning dosing. *Clin. Pharmacol. Ther.* **56**, 587–591.

98. Hampel, B., Hullmann, R., and Schmidt, H. (1997). Ciprofloxacin in pediatrics: Worldwide clinical experience based on compassionate use—safety report. *Pediatr. Infect. Dis. J.* **16**, 127–129.

99. McDonald, D. F., and Short, H. B. (1964). Usefulness of nalidixic acid in treatment of urinary infection. *Antimicrob. Agents Chemother.* **4**, 628–631.

100. Bailey, R. R., Natale, R., and Linton, A. L. (1972). Nalidixic acid arthralgia. *Can. Med. Assoc. J.* **107**, 604–607.

101. Pertuiset, E., Lenoir, G., Jehanne, M., Douchan F., Guillot, M., and Menkes, C. J. (1989). Tolerance articulaire de la pefloxacine et de l'ofloxacine chez les enfants et adolescents atteints de mucoviscidose. *Rev. Rheumatol.* **56**, 735–740.

102. Carrasco, J. M., Gacia, B., Andujar, C., Garrote, F., de Juana, P., and Bermejo, T. (1997). Tendinitis associated with ciprofloxacin [letter]. *Ann. Pharmacother.* **31**, 120.

103. Lewis, J. R., Gums, J. G., and Dickensheets, D. L. (1999). Levofloxacin-induced bilateral Achilles tendonitis. *Ann. Pharmacother.* **33**, 792–795.

104. Van der Linden, P. D., van de Lei, J., Nab, H. W., Knol, A., and Stricker, B. H. Ch. (1999). Achilles tendinitis associated with fluoroquinolones. *Br. J. Clin. Pharmacol.* **48**, 433–437.

105. Royer, R. J., Pierfitte, C., and Netter, P. (1994). Features of tendon disorders with fluoroquinolones. *Therapie* **49**, 75–76.

106. Pierfitte, C., and Royer, R. J. (1996). Tendon disorders with fluoroquinolones. *Therapie* **51**, 419–420.

107. Bailey, R. R., Kirk, J. A., and Peddie, B. A. (1983). Norfloxacin-induced rheumatic disease. *N.Z. Med. J.* **96**, 590.

108. Borderie, P., Marcelli, C., Leray, H., Mourad, G., Hérisson, C., Mion, C., and Simon, L. (1992). Ruptures spontanees du tendon d'Achille aprés transplantation rénale: Role favorisant des fluoroquinolones [abstract]. *Rev. Rhum.* **59**, E22.

109. Marti, H. P., Stoller, R., and Frey, F. J. (1998). Fluoroquinolones as a cause of tendon disorders in patients with renal failure/renal transplants. *Br. J. Rheumatol.* **37**(3), 343–344.

110. Jaillon, P., Morganroth, J., Brumpt, I., Talbot, G., and the Sparfloxacin Safety Group (1996). Overview of electrocardiographic and cardiovascular safety data for sparfloxacin. *J. Antimicrob. Chemother.* **37**, Suppl. A, 161–167.

111. Ball, P., Mandell, L., Niki, Y., and Tillotson, G. (1999). Comparative tolerability of the newer fluoroquinolone antibacterials. *Drug Saf.* **21** (5), 407–421.

112. Thorsteinsson, S. B., Bergan, T., Oddsdottir, S., Rohwedder, R., and Holm, R. (1986). Crystalluria and ciprofloxacin: Influence of urinary pH and hydration. *Chemotherapy* **32**, 408–417.

113. Bayer, A. G. (1986). Ciprofloxacin Product Monograph. ADIS Press, Wellington.

114. Segev, S., Yaniv, I., Haverstock, D., and Reinhart, H. (1999). Safety of long-term therapy with ciprofloxacin: Data analysis of controlled clinical trials and review. *Clin. Infect. Dis.* **28**, 299–308.

115. Anonymous (1985). Ofloxacin profile. In "Ofloxacin: A New Quinolone Antibacterial Agent. Proceedings of a Workshop Held at the 14th International Congress of Chemotherapy, Kyoto" (S. Mitsuhashi and G. K. Daikos, eds.), pp. 3–13, University of Tokyo Press.

116. Jüngst, G., and Mohr, R. (1987). Side effects of ofloxacin in clinical trials and in postmarketing surveillance. *Drugs* **34** (Suppl. 1), 144–149.

117. Davis, R., and Bryson, H. M. (1994). Levofloxacin: A review of its antibacterial activity, pharmacokinetics and therapeutic efficacy. *Drugs* **47**, 677–700.

118. Young, L. S. (1985). Clinical experience with the newer quinolones. In "DNA-gyrase Inhibitors: The Present and the Future" (J. G. Collee, ed). *Res. Clin. Forum* **7**, 97–114.

119. Geddes, A. M. (1993). Safety of fleroxacin in clinical trials. *Am. J. Med.* **94** (Suppl. 3A), 201S–203S.

120. Rubinstein, E. (1996). Safety profile of sparfloxacin in the treatment of respiratory tract infection. *J. Antimicrob. Chemother.* **37** (Suppl. A), 145–160.

121. Springsklee, M., Reiter, C., and Meyer, J. M. (2000). Safety and tolerability of moxifloxacin (MXF) [abstr. #260]. *Antiinfect. Drugs Chemother.* **17**(1), 90.

122. Breen, J., Skuba, K., and Grasela, D. (1999). Safety and tolerability of gatifloxacin, an advanced-generation, 8-methoxy fluoroquinolone. *J. Respir. Dis.* **20**(11) (Suppl.), S70–S76.

123. Urinary Tract Infection Study Group (1987). Coordinated multicenter study of norfloxacin versus trimethoprim–sulfamethoxazole treatment of symptomatic urinary tract infections. *J. Infect. Dis.* **155**, 170–177.

124. Grubbs, N. C., Schultz, H. J., Henry, N. K., Ilstrup, D. M., Muller, S. M., and Wilson, W. R. (1992). Ciprofloxacin versus trimethoprim-sulfamethoxazole: Treatment of community-acquired urinary tract infections in a prospective, controlled, double-blind comparison. *Mayo Clin. Proc.* **67**, 1163–1168.

125. Hooton, T. M., Rogers, E., Medina, T. G., Kuwamura, L. E., Ewers, C., Roberts, P. L., and Stamm, W. E. (1990). Ciprofloxacin compared with doxycycline for nongonococcal urethritis: Ineffectiveness against *Chlamydia trachomatis* due to relapsing infection. *JAMA* **264**, 1418–1421.

126. Pichler, H. E. T., Diridl, G., Stickler, K., and Wolf, D. (1987). Clinical efficacy of ciprofloxacin compared with placebo in bacterial diarrhea. *Am. J. Med.* **82** (Suppl. 4A), 329–332.

127. Kawamura, S., Fujimaki, Y., Iwasawa, T., Sasaki, T., Yanai, O., *et al.* (1984). A comparative double blind study of DL-8280 and pipemidic acid in suppurative otitis media. *Otologia Fukuoka* **30**, 642–670.

128. Kishi, H., Nito, H., Saito, I., Nishimura, Y., Niijima, T., *et al.* (1984). Comparative studies of DL-8280 and pipemidic acid in complicated urinary tract infections by double-blind method. *Acta Urologica Japonica* **30**, 1307–1355.

129. Sasaki, T., Unno, T., Tomiyama, T., Yamai, O., Iwasawa, T., *et al.* (1984). Evaluation of clinical effectiveness and safety of DL-8280 in acute lacunar tonsillitis–in comparison with amoxicillin by double-blind method. *Otologia Fukuoka,* **30**, 484–513.

130. Takase, Z., Komoto, K., Katayama, M., Matsuda, S., Kashiwagura, T., *et al.* (1986). Comparative clinical study of ofloxacin (OFLX) and amoxicillin (AMPC) on the infectious disease in the field of obstetrics and gynecology. *Chemotherapy (Tokyo)* **34**. 33–63.

131. Fujita, K., Nakano, M., Nonami, E., Shishiba, T., Katsumata, M., *et al.* (1984). Comparative clinical study of DL-8280 and cefaclor for suppurative skin and soft tissue infections by a double-blind method. *Kansenshogaku-Zasshi* **58**, 793–819.

132. Fujimori, I., Kobayashi, Y., Obana, M., Saito, A., Tomizawa, M., *et al.* (1984). Comparative clinical study of ofloxacin and cefaclor in bacterial bronchitis, *Kansenshogaku-Zasshi* **58**, 832–861.

133. Monk, J. P., and Campoli-Richards, D. M. (1987). Ofloxacin. A review of its antibacterial activity, pharmacokinetic properties and therapeutic use. *Drugs* **33**, 346–391.

134. Chodosh, S. (1993). Efficacy of fleroxacin versus amoxicillin in acute exacerbations of chronic bronchitis. *Am. J. Med.* **94** (Suppl. 3A), 131S–135S.

135. Pummer, K. (1993). Fleroxacin versus norfloxacin in the treatment of urinary tract infections: A multicenter, double-blind, prospective, randomized, comparative study. *Am. J. Med.* **94** (Suppl. 3A), 108S–113S.

136. Ulmer, W. (1993). Fleroxacin versus amoxicillin in the treatment of acute exacerbations of chronic bronchitis. *Am. J. Med.* **94** (Suppl. 3A), 136S–141S.

137. Iravani, A. (1993). Multicenter study of single-dose and multiple-dose fleroxacin versus ciprofloxacin in the treatment of uncomplicated urinary tract infections. *Am. J. Med.* **94** (Suppl. 3A), 89S–96S.

138. Butler, T., Loleka, S., Rasidi, C., Kadio, A., del Rosal, P. L., Iskandar, H., Rubinstein, E., and Pastore, G. (1993b). Treatment of acute bacterial diarrhea: A multicenter international trial comparing placebo with fleroxacin given as a single dose or once daily for 3 days. *Am. J. Med.* **94** (Suppl. 3A), 187S–194S.

139. Allegra, L., Konietzko, N., Leophonte, P., Hosie, J., Pauwels, R., Guyen, J. N., and Petitpretz, P. (1996). Comparative safety and efficacy of sparfloxacin in the treatment of acute exacerbations of chronic obstructive pulmonary disease: A double-blind, randomised, parallel, multicentre study. *J. Antimicrob. Chemother.* **37** (Suppl. A), 93–104.

140. Portier, H., May, Th., Proust, A., and the French Study Group (1996). Comparative efficacy of sparfloxacin in comparison with amoxycillin plus ofloxacin in the treatment of community-acquired pneumonia. *J. Antimicrob. Chemother.* **37** (Suppl. A), 83–91.

141. Gehanno, P., Berche, P., and the Sinusitis Study Group (1996). Sparfloxacin versus cefuroxime axetil in the treatment of acute purulent sinusitis. *J. Antimicrob. Chemother.* **37** (Suppl. A), 105–114.

142. Naber, K. G., di Silverio, F., Geddes, A., and Guibert, J. (1996). Comparative efficacy of sparfloxacin versus ciprofloxacin in the treatment of complicated urinary tract infection. *J. Antimicrob. Chemother.* **37** (Suppl. A), 135–144.

143. Burke, T., Villanueva, C., Mariano Jr., H., Huck, W., Orchard, D., Haverstock, D., Heyd, A., Church, D., and the Sinusitis Infection Study Group (1999). Comparison of moxifloxacin and cefuroxime axetil in the treatment of acute maxillary sinusitis. *Clin. Ther.* **21**(10), 1664–1677.

144. Siegert, R., Gehanno, P., Nikolaidas, P., and the Moxifloxacin Study Group (2000). A comparison of the safety and efficacy of moxifloxacin (BAY 12-8039) and cefuroxime axetil in the treatment of acute bacterial sinusitis in adults. *Respir. Med.*. In press.

145. Sullivan, J. G., McElroy, A. D., Honsinger, R. W., McAdoo, M., Harrison, B. J., Plouffe, J. F., Gotfried, M., and Mayer, H. (1999). Treating community-acquired pneumonia with once-daily gatifloxacin vs. once-daily levofloxacin. *J. Respir. Dis.* **20**(11) (Suppl.), S49–S59.

146. Ramirez, J. A., Nguyen, T.-H., Tellier, G., Coppola, G., Bettis, R. B., Dolmann, A., St.-Pierre, C., and Mayer, H. (1999). Treating community-acquired pneumonia with once-daily gatifloxacin vs. twice-daily clarithromycin. *J. Respir. Dis.* **20**(11) (Suppl.), S40–S48.

147. Lode, H. (1988). Drug interactions with quinolones. *Rev. Infect. Dis.* **10** (Suppl. 1), S132–S136.

148. Davies, B. I., and Maesen, F. P. V. (1989). Drug interactions with quinolones. *Rev. Infect. Dis.* **11** (Suppl. 5), S1083–S1090.

149. Janknegt, R. (1990). Drug interactions with quinolones. *J. Antimicrob. Chemother.* **26** (Suppl. D), 7–29.

150. Deppermann, K. M., and Lode, H. (1993). Fluoroquinolones. Interaction-profile of enteral absorption. *Drugs* **45** (Suppl. 3). 65–72.

151. Smith, J. T., and Ratcliff, N. T. (1986). Effect of pH and magnesium on the *in vitro* activity of ciprofloxacin. In "Proceedings of the First International Ciprofloxacin Workshop" (H. C. Neu and H. Weuta, eds.), pp. 12–16. Excerpta Medica, Amsterdam.

152. Machka, K., and Braveny, I. (1984). Inhibitorische Wirkung verschiedener Faktoren auf die Aktivität von Norfloxacin. In "Gyrase—Hemmer I" (W. Stille, D. Adam, H.-U. Eickenberg, H. Knothe, G. Ruckdeschel, and C. Simon, eds.), *Fortschr. Antimikrob. Antineoplast. Chemother.* **3/5**, 557–561.

153. Chapman, J. S., and Georgopapadakou, N. H. (1990). Routes of quinolone permeation in *Escherichia coli. Antimicrob. Agents Chemother.* **32**, 438–442.

154. Höffken, G., Borner, K., Glatzel, P. D., Koeppe, P., and Lode, H. (1985a). Reduced enteral absorption of ciprofloxacin in the presence of antacids (letter). *Europ. J. Clin. Microbiol.* **4**, 345.

155. Flor, S., Guay, D. R. P., Opsahl, J. A., Tack, K., and Matzke, G. R. (1990). Effects of magnesium–aluminium hydroxide and calcium carbonate antacids on bioavailability of ofloxacin. *Antimicrob. Agents Chemother.* **34**, 2436–2438.

156. Nix, D. E., Wilton, J. H., Ronald, B., Distlerath, L., Williams, V. C., and Norman, A. (1990). Inhibition of norfloxacin absorption by antacids. *Antimicrob. Agents Chemother.* **34**. 432–435.

157. Sahai, J., Gallicano, K., Oliveras, L., Khaliq, S., Hawley-Foss, N., and Garber, G. (1993). Cations in the didanosine tablet reduce ciprofloxacin bioavailability. *Clin. Pharmacol. Ther.* **53**, 292–297.

158. Polk, R. E., Healy, D. P., Sahai, J., Drwal, L., and Racht, E. (1989). Effect of ferrous sulfate and multivitamins with zinc on absorption of ciprofloxacin in normal volunteers. *Antimicrob. Agents Chemother.* **33**, 1841–1844.

159. Parpia, S. H., Nix, D. E., Hejmanowski, L. G., Goldstein, H. R., Wilton, J. H., and Schentag, J. J. (1989). Sucralfate reduces the gastrointestinal absorption of norfloxacin. *Antimicrob. Agents Chemother.* **33**, 99–102.

160. Garrelts, J. C., Godley, P. J., Peterie, J. D., Gerlach, E. H., and Yakshe, C. C. (1990). Sucralfate significantly reduces ciprofloxacin concentrations in serum. *Antimicrob. Agents Chemother.* **34**, 931–933.

161. Lehto, P., and Kivistö, K. T. (1994). Effect of sucralfate on absorption of norfloxacin and ofloxacin. *Antimicrob. Agents Chemother.* **38**, 248–251.

162. Teng, R., Dogolo, L. C., Willavize, S., Friedman, H. L., and Vincent, J. (1996). Effect of sucralfate, calcium carbonate, and ferrous sulfate on the bioavailability of trovafloxacin. *Abstr. 20th Int. Cong. Chemother.*, Sydney. Abstr. #186.

163. Höffken, G., Lode, H., Wiley, R., Glatzel, T. D., Sievers, D., Olschewski, T., Borner, K., and Koeppe, P. (1988). Pharmacokinetics and bioavailability of ciprofloxacin and ofloxacin, effect of food and antacid intake. *Rev. Infect. Dis.* **10** (Suppl. 1), 138–139.

164. Patterson, B. E., Purkins, L., Oliver, S. D., and Willavize, S. A. (1996). An open, placebo-controlled, two-way crossover study to investigate the effects of cimetidine on the steady-state pharmacokinetics of trovafloxacin. *Abstr. 7th Int. Cong. Chemother.*, Hong Kong. Abstr. #71.019.

165. Wingender, W., Beermann, D., Förster, D., Graefe, K.-H., and Kuhlmann, J. (1986). Interactions of ciprofloxacin with food intake and drugs. In "Proceedings of the First International Ciprofloxacin Workshop" (H. C. Neu and H. Weuta, eds.), pp. 136–140. Excerpta Medica, Amsterdam.

166. Lomaestro, B. M., and Bailie, G. R. (1995). Absorption interactions with fluoroquinolones: 1995 update. *Drug Saf.* **12**(5), 314–333.

167. Palù, G., Valisena, S., Ciarrocchi, G., Gatto, B., and Palumbo, M. (1992). Quinolone binding to DNA is mediated by magnesium ions. *Proc. Natl. Acad. Sci. U.S.A.* **89**, 9671–9675.

168. Neuvonen, P. J., Kivistö, K. T., and Lehto, P. (1991). Interference of dairy products with the absorption of ciprofloxacin. *Clin. Pharmacol. Ther.* **50**, 498–502.

169. Neuvonen, P. J., and Kivistö, K. T. (1992). Milk and yoghurt do not impair the absorption of ofloxacin. *Br. J. Clin. Pharmacol.* **33**, 346–348.

170. Höffken, G., Lode, H., Prinzing, C., Borner, K., and Koeppe, P. (1985b). Pharmacokinetics of ciprofloxacin after oral and parenteral administration. *Antimicrob. Agents Chemother.* **27**, 375–379.

171. Stass, H., and Kubitzka, D. (1999). Interaction profile of moxifloxacin. *Drugs* **58** (Suppl. 2). 235–236.

172. Wijnands, W. J. A., van Herwaarden, C. L. A., and Vree, T. B. (1984). Enoxacin raises plasma theophylline concentrations [letter]. *Lancet* **II**, 108–109.

173. Wijnands, W. J. A., Vree, T. B., and van Herwaarden, C. L. A. (1986). The influence of quinolone derivatives on theophylline clearance. *Br. J. Clin. Pharmacol.* **22**, 677–683.

174. Gregoire, S. L., Grasela Jr, Th. H., Freer, J. P., Tack, K. J., and Schentag, J. J. (1987). Inhibitiion of theophylline clearance by coadministered ofloxacin without alteration of theophylline effects. *Antimicrob. Agents Chemother.* **31**, 375–378.

175. Parent, M., St-Laurent, M., and LeBel, M. (1990). Safety of fleroxacin coadministered with theophylline to young and elderly volunteers. *Antimicrob. Agents Chemother.* **34**, 1249–1253.

176. Okimoto, N., Niki, Y., Sumi, M., Nakagawa, Y., and Soejima, R. (1991). Effect of sparfloxacin on serum concentration of theophylline. *Chemotherapy* **39** (Suppl. 4), 158–160.

177. Fuhr, U., Anders, E. M., Mahr, G., Sörgel, F., and Staib, A. H. (1992). Inhibitory potency of quinolone antibacterial agents against cytochrome P4501A2 activity in vivo and in vitro. *Antimicrob. Agents Chemother.* **36**. 942–948.

178. Fuhr, U., Strobl, G., Manaut, F., Anders, E. M., Sörgel, F., Lopez-De-Brinas, E., Chu, D. T. W., Pernet, A. B., Mahr, G., Sanz, F., and Staib, A. H. (1993). Quinolone antibacterial agents: Relationship between structure and *in vitro* inhibition of the human cytochrome P450 isoform CYP1A2. *Mol. Pharmacol.* **43**. 191–199.

179. Mizuki, Y., Fujiwara, I., and Yamaguchi, T. (1996). Pharmacokinetic interactions related to the chemical structures of fluoroquinolones. *J. Antimicrob. Chemother.* **37** (Suppl. A), 41–55.

180. Staib, A. H., Harder, S., Mieke, S., Beer, C., Stille, W., and Shah, P. (1987). Gyrase-inhibitors impair caffeine elimination in man. *Meth. Find. Exp. Clin. Pharmacol.* **9**(3), 193–198.

181. Stille, W., Harder, S., Mieke, S., Beer, C., Shah, P. M., Frech, K., and Staib, A. H. (1987). Decrease of caffeine elimination in man during co-administration of 4-quinolones. *J. Antimicrob. Chemother.* **20**, 729–734.

182. Healy, D. P., Polk, R. E., Kanawati, L., Rock, D. T., and Mooney, M. L. (1989). Interaction between oral ciprofloxacin and caffeine in normal volunteers. *Antimicrob. Agents Chemother.* **33**, 474–478.

183. Schulz, T. G., Stahlmann, R., Edwards, R. J., Debris, K., Davies, D. S., and Neubert, D. (1995). Enoxacin is an inducer of CYP1A2 in rat liver. *Biochem. Pharmacol.* **50**. 1517–1520.

184. Pollak, P. T., and Slayter, K. L. (1997). Hazards of doubling phenytoin dose in the face of an unrecognized interaction with ciprofloxacin. *Ann. Pharmacother.* **31**, 61–64.

185. Toon, S., Hopkins, K. J., Garstang, F. M., Aarons, L., Sedman, A., and Rowland, M. (1987). Enoxacin–warfarin interaction: Pharmacokinetic and stereochemical aspects. *Clin. Pharmacol. Ther.* **42**, 33–41.

186. Wijnands, W. J. A., Trooster, J. F. G., Teunissen, P. C., Cats, H. A., and Vree, T. B. (1990). Ciprofloxacin does not impair the elimination of diazepam in humans. *Drug Metab. Dispos.* **18**, 954–957.

187. Tan, K. K. C., Trull, A. K., and Shawket, S. (1989). Co-administration of ciprofloxacin and cyclosporine: Lack of evidence for pharmacokinetic interaction. *Br. J. Clin. Pharmacol.* **28**, 185–187.

188. Loleka, S., Patanachareon, S., Thanangkul, B., and Vibulbandhitkit, B. (1988). Norfloxacin versus co-trimoxazole in the treatment of acute bacterial diarrhoea: A placebo controlled study. *Scand. J. Infect. Dis.* **56** (Suppl.), 35–45.

189. Gentry, L. O., Ramirez-Ronda, C. H., Thadepalli, H., del Rosal, P. L., and Ramirez, C. (1989). Oral ciprofloxacin vs. parenteral cefotaxime in the treatment of difficult skin and skin structure infections: A multicenter trial. *Arch. Intern. Med.* **149**, 2579–2583.

190. Carbon, C., Ariza, H., Rabie, W. J., Salvarezza, C. R., Elkharrat, D., Rangaraj, M., and Decosta, P. (1999). Comparative study of levofloxacin and amoxycillin/clavulanic acid in adults with mild-to-moderate community-acquired pneumonia. *Clin. Microbiol. Infect.* **5**. 724–732.

191. Shah, P. M., Maesen, F. P., Dolmann, A., Vetter, N., Fiss, E., and Wesch, R. (1999). Levofloxacin versus cefuroxime axetil in the treatment of acute exacerbations of chronic bronchitis: Results of a randomized, double-blind study. *J. Antimicrob. Chemother.* **43/4**. 529–539.

192. Baz, M. N., Jannetti, W., Villanueva, C., Burke, T., Pause, C., Wang, L., Church, D., Heyd, A., and the Sinusitis Infection Study Group (1999). The efficacy and tolerability of moxifloxacin compared to trovafloxacin in the treatment of acute sinusitis. *Today's Therap. Trends* **17**(4). 303–319.

193. Fogarty, C., Grossman, C., Williams, J., Haverstock, D., and Church, D., for the Community-Acquired Pneumonia Study Group (1999). Efficacy and safety of moxifloxacin vs. clarithromycin for community-acquired pneumonia. *Infect. Med.* **16**(11), 748–763.

194. Wilson, R., Kubin, R., Ballin, I., Deppermann, K.-M., Bassaris, H. P., Leophonte, P., Schreurs, Ad, J. M., Torres, A., and Sommerauer, B. (1999). Five-day moxifloxacin therapy compared with 7-day clarithromycin therapy for the treatment of acute exacerbations of chronic bronchitis. *J. Antimicrob. Chemother.* **44**. 501–513.

195. Chodosh, S., DeAbate, C. A., Haverstock, D., Aneiro, L., Church, D., and the Bronchitis Study Group (2000). Short-course moxifloxacin therapy for treatment of acute bacterial exacerbations of chronic bronchitis. *Respir. Med.* **94**. 18–27.

196. Niki, Y., Hashiguchi, K., Okimoto, N., and Soejima, R. (1992). Quinolone antimicrobial agents and theophylline. *Chest* **101**, 881.

CHAPTER 15

Use of the Quinolones in Pediatrics

URS B. SCHAAD

Department of Pediatrics, University of Basel, CH-4005 Basel, Switzerland

INTRODUCTION

Since the mid-1980s, there has been dramatic progress in the development of the derivatives of nalidixic acid, the fluoroquinolones, which are now an established class of antimicrobials. They are rapidly bactericidal and have an extended antimicrobial spectrum that includes *Pseudomonas*, Gram-positive cocci, and intracellular pathogens. They have advantageous pharmacokinetic properties such as absorption from the gastrointestinal tract, excellent penetration into many tissues, and good intracellular diffusion.

The fluoroquinolones have been effective in the treatment or prevention of a variety of bacterial infections in adults, including infections of the respiratory and urinary tracts, skin and soft tissue, bone and joint, and eye and ear. Overall, they are generally well tolerated; the most frequent adverse events during treatment are gastrointestinal disturbances, reactions of the central nervous system (CNS), and skin reactions [1,2].

The use of fluoroquinolones in children has been limited because of their potential to induce arthropathy in juvenile animals [3–5]. This extraordinary form of age-related drug toxicity has been demonstrated with all the fluoroquinolones tested thus far and has led to important restrictions: their use has been considered to be contraindicated in children, in growing adolescents, and during pregnancy and lactation. However, since the mid-1980s, many children have received treatment with fluoroquinolones, mainly ciprofloxacin [6], because they are the only oral antimicrobials with potential activity against such multiply resistant and difficult-to-treat infections as *Pseudomonas aeruginosa* infections in children with cystic fibrosis, complicated urinary tract infections, and enteric infections in developing countries. Many investigators have reported their experience in the use of ciprofloxacin and other fluoroquinolones on "compassionate use"-based protocols. Results indicate that prolonged therapy with the fluoroquinolones is effective and well tolerated in pediatric patients, with no significant evidence of arthropathy, bone abnormalities, or other serious adverse events [6].

ANIMAL DATA

QUINOLONE ARTHROPATHY

Quinolones, both the older compounds and the newer derivatives, have induced changes in the immature cartilage of the weight-bearing joints in all laboratory animals tested (Table I). These animals include mice [7], rats [8], dogs [3,9], marmosets [10], guinea pigs [11], rabbits [12], and ferrets [13]. The occurrence of quinolone arthropathy is limited to juvenile animals with the exception of pefloxacin, which produced characteristic lesions in both skeletally immature and mature dogs [14]. Juvenile dogs are generally more sensitive to the arthropathic effects of quinolones than are other species [15].

TABLE I   Quinolone Arthropathy

Juvenile animals
All quinolones tested
All laboratory animals tested
Especially weight-bearing joints
"Typical" histopathology: blisters, fissures, erosions, and destruction
Mechanisms: ↓ DNA synthesis
↓ Magnesium ions
Monitoring
Histopathologic studies
Magnetic resonance imaging
Ultrasound
Patients
No documentation of unequivocal quinolone-induced arthropathy.

HISTOPATHOLOGY

Typical histopathological lesions (Table I) after quinolone treatment of juvenile animals include fluid-filled blisters, fissures, erosions, and clustering of chondrocytes, usually accompanied by noninflammatory joint effusion. Under the electron microscope, necrosis of the chondrocytes and swelling of the mitochondria are observed initially, followed by disruption of extracellular matrix and formations of fissures [10]. Loss of collagen and glycosaminoglycan is an early sequela to degeneration of chondrocytes [9,10,16]. When clinically manifested, the quinolone-induced joint lesions present as acute arthritis, including limping and swelling.

Although the clinical manifestations of lameness in dogs resolve in spite of continued dosing [15], complete resolution of structural changes in affected cartilage has not been reported. Magnetic resonance imaging (MRI) of joints in affected immature rabbits identified thickened articular cartilage, surface irregularities consistent with ruptured vesicles, and separation of opposing articular surfaces consistent with synovial effusion [17]. After various recovery periods up to 17 weeks, healing of quinolone arthropathy is incomplete in rats [18]. In dogs, the lesions also fail to achieve complete microscopic resolution after withdrawal periods of 14 [19] or 30 days [20]. Results of multiple experimental studies have corroborated the importance of weight-bearing forces in the development of quinolone arthropathy [9,20].

Animal experiments have shown dose dependency that varies according to the species of animal and according to the drug being studied. This could be explained by either true heterogeneity of arthropathogenicity or differences in pharmacokinetics [3–5,7–10]. There are few good comparative data because many animal studies have compared only two products. Moreover, little is known about the critical intraarticular cartilage concentrations of fluoroquinolones required for induction of lesions in this tissue [21,22].

POSSIBLE MECHANISMS

The histopathologic changes described in the previous section were formerly believed to be pathognomonic for quinolone arthropathy [21]; however, selective nutritional deprivation of magnesium [23,24] and injection of various other agents into joint spaces [25] have produced similar lesions in rats.

The specific mechanism(s) responsible for initiation of quinolone arthropathy has not been determined. *In-vitro* studies of cartilage from various species have implicated inhibitions of synthesis of either collagen or glycosaminoglycans [26–32]. Quinolone-induced oxidative injury to chondrocytes has been described [33,34], as well as inhibition of chondrocytes, DNA synthesis [27,32,35], and compromised mitochondrial integrity [31,32,35]. It is unclear whether any of these disorders are primary or secondary events.

The most recent, and perhaps most plausible, postulate for the mechanism of induction of quinolone arthropathy involves chelation of magnesium ions by quinolones, resulting in changed function of chondrocyte surface integrin receptors. Signal transduction via integrins seems to play a role in the maintenance of cartilage matrix integrity [36,37]. Chondrocytes adjacent to fissures in the articular cartilage of rats dosed with ofloxacin had reduced integrin expression [18], and this observation was confirmed in mice [38]. Further support for this hypothesis is that nutritional magnesium deficiency in juvenile rats induced articular cartilage lesions that were histologically and ultrastructurally identical to those of quinolone arthropathy [23,24]. Combination of ofloxacin administration and magnesium deficiency produced greater cartilage damage than either did alone. In addition, the normal magnesium concentrations in the joint cartilage of rats fall to a nadir at the time of early postnatal growth, coinciding with the period of vulnerability for the seemingly similar magnesium deficiency and quinolone-induced cartilage lesions [39].

Age is the single most critical factor in the sensitivity of animals to development of quinolone arthropathy. Dogs develop quinolone arthropathy when exposed at older than 2 weeks or younger than 8 months [20], whereas rats are susceptible shortly after birth to the age of 8 weeks [8]. Pefloxacin is the reported exception, as histologically confirmed arthropathy was produced in both juvenile and adult dogs after prolonged exposure [4]. Because the period of increased sensitivity to development of quinolone arthropathy in dogs corresponds with the period of maximal growth, a high rate of growth could be a contributing factor [15].

Whether differences in growth can be incorporated into animal-versus-human risk assessments is unclear. Dogs initially outgrow children by a wide margin. A beagle pup gains 8 kg during the period between 1 and 6 months of age. In contrast, a child of similar age gains only 4 kg over the same period. Such differences become even more pronounced when comparing the periods of growth from birth to adulthood in animals and humans. Assuming a growth span from birth to adulthood of 1 year for a dog and 18 years for a human, a day of growth (and quinolone treatment) in a juvenile dog would correspond to 18 days of growth in a young child [40]. It is possible that the extremely rapid extrauterine growth rates of the skeletons of laboratory animals is an explanation for their relative sensitivity to the chondrotoxic effects of quinolones.

TENDOPATHY

Other musculoskeletal adverse effects of quinolones are tendinitis and tendon rupture. Usually the Achilles tendon is involved. Clinical information on quinolone-induced tendopathy is relatively scarce. The first cases of tendinitis in association with norfloxacin therapy were published as early as 1983 [41]. The majority of patients with quinolone-associated tendopathy are older than 60 years, and most cases have occurred with pefloxacin [42]. Clinical experience indicates that patients undergoing corticosteroid treatment are prone to quinolone-induced tendon disorders.

A 1999 analysis of a retrospective epidemiological cohort survey on 1841 fluoroquinolone-treated adult patients in The Netherlands reported an incidence of Achilles tendinitis compared to controls (9406 patients that were treated with amoxicillin, trimethoprim, cotrimoxazole, or nitrofurantoin) of 0 for norfloxacin, 2.8× for ciprofloxacin, and 10.1× for ofloxacin [43].

Earlier animal experiments in juvenile rats described edema and mononuclear cell infiltration in the inner sheath of the Achilles tendon, with infiltration into the adjacent synovial membrane and joint space [44,45]. Only young subjects were sensitive. More recent electron microscopic studies with Achilles tendon specimens from ofloxacin-treated rats reported similar pathological features as described by the same research group in cartilage [46]. The typical degenerative alterations included cytoplasmatic vacuoles and vesicles, cell degradation, and loss of cell–matrix interaction. Toxicity was higher when multiple ofloxacin doses were given and when juvenile rats were used. As observed before for quinolone-induced cartilage lesions [23], magnesium deficiency also enhanced the toxic effects on tenocytes. It was concluded that experimental quinolone-associated arthropathy and quinolone-associated tendopathy probably represent the same toxic effect on cellular components (e.g., chondrocyte, tenocyte) of connective tissue.

PHARMACOKINETICS

The pharmacokinetic data on fluoroquinolones (Table II) in pediatric patients are still limited, and for neonatal patients anecdotal only [47–55]. The results of available studies, most of which were conducted in cystic fibrosis patients, indicate that systemic clearance is increased in young children. This has led to recommendations for higher doses of ciprofloxacin in the 14-to-28-kg weight group [53–55]. In general, fluoroquinolones are rapidly absorbed from the gastrointestinal tract. However, the range for bioavailability is vast, with norfloxacin being as low as 10–29% and ofloxacin as high as 80–90%. All of the newer compounds except norfloxacin have excellent tissue and intracellular penetration at the recommended therapeutic doses. Quinolones are generally excreted either predominantly in the urine (often as parent compound) or through the bile, in which some undergo enterohepatic recirculation.

CLINICAL EXPERIENCES

TOLERABILITY

Clinical adverse effects associated with fluoroquinolone use occur in 5 to 15% of adult and pediatric patients and necessitate discontinuation of treatment in 1 to 2% [56–61]. The most frequent adverse effects are gastrointestinal reactions (nausea, abdominal discomfort, vomiting, and diarrhea), followed by minor CNS

TABLE II   Current Dosage Recommendations

Drug	Route[c]	Dose (mg/kg)	No. of doses/day	Max. daily dose (mg)
Ciprofloxacin	p.o.	15–20	2	1500
	i.v.	10–15	2	800
Ofloxacin[a]	p.o.	7.5	2	800
	i.v.	5	2	600
Norfloxacin[b]	p.o.	10–15	2	800

[a]Majority of pediatric experience in cystic fibrosis patients.

[b]Majority of pediatric experience in urinary tract infection.

[c]p.o. = by mouth, i.v. = intravenously.

disorders (headache, dizziness, agitation, insomnia, and, rarely, seizures), and skin rashes (allergic and, rarely, photosensitive). Discrete laboratory test changes are found in 1 to 4% of patients and include elevated enzymes, leukopenia, and eosinophilia. Both clinical and laboratory adverse effects are always reversible.

More severe adverse effects include nephrotoxicity (crystalluria, interstitial nephritis) [62], anaphylaxis [63], hemolysis, cardiotoxicity (prolongation of the QT interval, dysrhythmia) [64], and hepatotoxicity (eosinophilic hepatitis, liver failure) [65]. Based on *in-vitro* and animal experiments, it has been suggested that damage to eukaryotic DNA, the ocular lens, and cartilage may also occur in patients [56,57]. No unequivocal evidence of such reactions in relation to quinolone therapy has yet been documented. Prospective outcome evaluation of 200 pregnancies exposed to fluoroquinolones did not detect any teratogenic potential of this drug class [66].

It must be remembered that several of the new fluoroquinolone compounds had to be withdrawn after clinical introduction due to either poor tolerability (e.g., phototoxicity, central nervous system effects) or severe adverse events (e.g., hemolysis, hypoglycemia, cardiotoxicity, hepatotoxicity).

DEVELOPMENT OF RESISTANCE

As we enter the new millennium, our position for treating infectious diseases is precarious, to say the least. The emergence of pathogens with resistance to available antibiotics is an increasing threat worldwide. The answer is no longer new drugs, but decreasing emergence of resistance. Bacterial resistance is usually selected by overuse or inappropriate use (misuse) of antibiotics. Overuse (e.g., for viral infection, as prophylaxis, many veterinarian indications) reflects inadequate knowledge and unavailable diagnostic methods. Appropriate use includes not only classical selection of an optimum antibiotic but also individual optimization of both dosage and duration of therapy [67,68].

Bacteria can become resistant to quinolones by mutations in the target molecules (gyrase protein, topoisomerase) or by active drug efflux. With regard to quinolone resistance, great variations exist between bacterial species, clinical settings, and local epidemiology. Nevertheless, resistance is always more commonly encountered in hospital practice than in community-acquired infections. Horizontal spread of resistant strains among hospitalized patients or carriers in close contact (e.g., family, day care) plays a significant role in diffusion of resistance.

Well-defined antibiotic policies, good hygiene measures, and strong infection control programs represent key points for limiting the spread of antibiotic resistance.

QUINOLONE-ASSOCIATED ARTHRALGIA

So far, there is no documentation of unequivocal quinolone-induced arthropathy in humans (Table I). Joint swelling or pain concurrent with quinolone therapy were described in both case reports and various multipatient studies. These data have been reviewed and analyzed [40].

The case reports of quinolone-associated effusion and arthralgia in children and adolescents [69–76] draw attention to the possibility for the occurrence of chondrotoxicity. Reports implicating pefloxacin are clearly overrepresented. There were no long-term sequelae in any of the cases, with the exception of the one described by Chevalier *et al.* [76], in which other etiologies cannot be ruled out. Because the areas of articular cartilage (the site for initiation of quinolone arthropathy of animals) were not evaluated for the presence of primary changes, the comparability of these cases to that of quinolone arthropathy of animals remains uncertain. Adequate evaluation of articular cartilage for the presence of primary changes appears warranted for credible publication of any future cases. Magnetic resonance imaging, which is able to identify quinolone-induced alterations in rabbit articular cartilage [17] and which is capable of detecting articular cartilage defects in humans as small as those caused in dogs by quinolones [3,17,77], seems to be the appropriate method. Nevertheless, adequate histopathologic studies would be the most appropriate technique for detecting cartilage lesions comparable to quinolone arthropathy in animals [78]. Ultrasound examination of knee and hip joints allow detection of articular effusion and measurement of the thickness of the synovia, and sometimes also the cartilage. Ultrasound, therefore, is useful for screening purposes before and after quinolone therapy.

To date, various multipatient studies have described use of ciprofloxacin, nalidixic acid, norfloxacin, or ofloxacin in more than 10,000 skeletally immature patients [78–101]. Occurrence of arthralgia was never beyond the level expected as a result of the underlying disease, especially cystic fibrosis. Any association between quinolone administration and occurrence of musculoskeletal events must be considered in light of the estimated 4% prevalence of arthralgia among children with cystic fibrosis, which rises to 7 or 8% in adolescents [102]. In most cases, concurrent joint disease is explained by hyperimmune mechanisms, so-called cystic fibrosis arthropathy, or hypertrophic pulmonary osteoarthropathy. In addition to clinical monitoring, more rigorous evaluations for detection of any subtle joint changes collectively included MRI in 116, ultrasound in 55, and histopathology in 2 patients. Long-term follow-up was conducted up to several years after quinolone treatment. Moreover, as measured in various multipatient studies, none of the evaluated quinolones (ciprofloxacin, ofloxacin, and nalidixic acid) had negative effects on the linear growth of children. The exception of these studies without unusually high incidence of articular symptoms and signs is a review of 63 pediatric patients with cystic fibrosis treated with pefloxacin [103]. The authors describe nine (14%) predominately adolescent patients with joint manifestations in conjunction with treatment. Two of these cases should probably be excluded because the manifestations were present at the onset of treatment in one and began 6 days after completion of treatment in another. The patients followed a pattern of swelling of the large joints, predominately the knees, with complete resolution and no long-term sequelae. Most notable in this report is that five of the patients with joint manifestations later tolerated therapeutic courses of ofloxacin without any problems.

By end of 1994, there were 1795 case report forms on file with data on individual juvenile patients treated with ciprofloxacin [59,60]. Arthralgia with and without clinical signs of arthritis occurred in 31 treatment courses out of 2030 (1.5%), and 26 of the patients were between 12 and 17 years of age and 28 of them had cystic fibrosis. The outcome was good, and there was no unequivocal documentation of ciprofloxacin-induced arthropathy in any case. The most recent experience is a prospective randomized comparative study of oral ciprofloxacin (15 mg of kg b.i.d.) with conventional ceftazidime–tobramycin for treatment of acute bronchopulmonary exacerbations associated with *P. aeruginosa* in 108 pediatric and adolescent cystic fibrosis patients [101]. Before and after the 2-week treatments, ultrasound examinations were performed in 96 patients (48 patients in both treatment groups) and nuclear magnetic resonance imaging scans in 29 patients (14 patients treated with ciprofloxacin and 15 patients treated with ceftazidime–tobramycin). No evidence of any cartilage toxicity was found.

STUDIED INDICATIONS

Table III provides the potential indications for therapeutic use of the new quinolones in pediatric patients.

Cystic Fibrosis

Chronic relapsing bronchopulmonary infection is the principal cause of morbidity and mortality in patients with cystic fibrosis [104]. *Pseudomonas aeruginosa* becomes the predominant pathogen in the sputum of these patients, occurring in up to 90% of patients. Antipseudomonal chemotherapy has been repeatedly shown to be beneficial in the treatment of bronchopulmonary exacerbations in cystic fibrosis patients; also, there is usually no clear correlation between clinical and bacteriologic outcomes [105,106]. Numerous controlled studies have shown that

TABLE III Present Potential Indications for Therapeutic Use of the New Quinolones in Pediatric Patients

Pathologic or special conditions	Infectious disease	Pathogens	Duration of therapy	Comments	References
Cystic fibrosis	Bronchopulmonary exacerbation	*P. aeruginosa* (*S. aureus*)	2–3 wk	p.o. or i.v./p.o.	[6,78,79,81,85,87,96,97,101,103]
Disturbed urinary outflow	Urinary tract infection (complicated)	*P. aeruginosa* (Gram-negative enteric bacteria)	2–3 wk	p.o. According to *in-vitro* susceptibility	[6,88]
Multidrug resistance	Enteric infection (invasive)	*Shigella, Salmonella, Vibrio cholerae, E. coli*	5–7–14 days	p.o. Cave: misuse/overuse	[6,82,86,92–94,111,112]
Chronic suppuration (>6 wk)	Otitis media perforata	*P. aeruginosa* (*S. aureus*)	2–4 wk	p.o. Plus regular aural toilet	[6,113]
Neutropenia in cancer patients[a]	Bacterial infection	Gram-negative and Gram-positive bacteria	1–2 wk	p.o. Preliminary experience only	[6,83,99,100,114]
Nasopharyngeal carrier state[a]	Prevention of meningitis	*N. meningitidis*	Single dose	p.o. Preliminary experience only	[6,111,115]
Multidrug resistance[a]	Bacterial meningitis	*N. meningitidis S. pneumoniae H. influenzae*	1–2 wk	i.v./p.o. Preliminary experience only	[6,40,116]

[a]NOT recommended outside of adequately controlled studies.

combination therapy with β-lactams and aminoglycosides gives the best results [107–109]. However, increased resistance has been noted with these agents [110], and the intravenous route of administration usually necessitates hospitalization. Thus, the fluoroquinolones, particularly ciprofloxacin, with high activity against *P. aeruginosa*, made oral therapy possible for the first time in these patients.

Since its introduction in 1987, ciprofloxacin has been widely used in pediatric cystic fibrosis patients [6,78,81,85,87,96,97,101]. Compared to ciprofloxacin, experience with ofloxacin [6,79] or pefloxacin [103] is much less. All these studies demonstrated that clinical improvements to fluoroquinolone therapy—in the majority of trials with oral ciprofloxacin—were equivalent to conventional parenteral antipseudomonal combination therapy despite differences in bacteriologic suppression rates. Importantly, ciprofloxacin and ofloxacin therapies were well tolerated and, as outlined previously, not associated with a higher rate of musculoskeletal adverse events. Oral fluoroquinolone therapy in cystic fibrosis patients offers the advantage of reduced hospital stay and no requirement of serum-level monitoring. So far, development of ciprofloxacin resistance of *P. aeruginosa* in cystic fibrosis patients was found to be rare and usually transient, without any clinical correlation [96,97,101].

Complicated Urinary Tract Infection

Complicated urinary tract infections result from inadequate drainage of urine. More than 90% of the causative pathogens are Gram-negative enteric bacteria and *P. aeruginosa*. Current treatment options are less than optimal because of the emergence of multiresistant organisms and nonresponding infections, and the need for hospitalization as a result of parenteral drug administration. Fluoroquinolones allow oral administration, and norfloxacin has been shown to be safe and effective for the treatment of pediatric patients with complicated urinary tract infections [6,88].

Enteric Infections

Gastrointestinal infections cause severe morbidity and significant mortality among infants and young children worldwide, especially in developing countries, and multidrug resistance is increasing in strains of *Shigella*, *Salmonella*, *Virbrio cholerae*, and *Escherichia coli* [6,111]. The only antimicrobial class that at this stage appears to have predictable activity against all of these gastrointestinal pathogens is the fluoroquinolone. In addition, the fluoroquinolones have several advantageous pharmacodynamic features relevant to treatment of gastrointestinal infections: high activity in both feces and bile, and wide distribution after absorption into body fluids, with uptake into phagocytes.

Several studies have shown that oral ciprofloxacin is efficacious and safe therapy of invasive diarrheal disease in children in the developing world [6,82,86,92–94,111,112]. The most urgently needed efforts include avoidance of misuse (e.g., suboptimal dosing because of relatively expensive cost) and overuse (e.g., inadequate indication) promoting the development of antibiotic resistance [111,112].

Chronic Ear Infections

Chronic suppurative otitis media can be defined as otorrhea through a perforated tympanic membrane or tympanotomy tube for a duration of 6 weeks or longer and may predispose patients to serious intratemporal and intracranial complications. *Pseudomonas aeruginosa* is almost always isolated from such cases. Treatment with systemic antimicrobials and aural lavage are efficacious when cholesteatoma is absent. Fluoroquinolones are the only available oral agents with adequate antipseudomonal activity, thus reducing the inconveniences associated with parenteral administration and hospitalization.

Limited experience indicates that oral ciprofloxacin combined with regular oral cleansing is effective and safe for this rare chronic ear infection [113].

Neutropenia in Cancer Patients

Neutropenia represents a predictable consequence of many cancer chemotherapy regimens, rendering the patient at increased risk for invasive bacterial pathogens. The risk from the endogenous bacterial flora, including the Gram-negative bacteria residing in the gastrointestinal tract, is well documented. Therefore, the use of fluoroquinolones to selectively decontaminate the gastrointestinal tract could help to prevent infection in neutropenic patients. However, such experience is currently very preliminary [83,114].

Numerous clinical trials since the mid-1960s have demonstrated that not only antibiotic combinations but also antibiotic monotherapies may help to cure patients with fever and neutropenia. Ongoing studies indicate that oral ciprofloxacin is an effective therapeutic option for managing the febrile neutropenic pediatric cancer patient identified to be at low risk according to depth and duration of neutropenia [6,99,100].

Central Nervous System Infections

Eradication of nasopharyngeal carriage of *Neisseria meningitidis* is an important tool for the control of meningococcal disease in both developed and developing countries. Limited experience suggests that in children a single oral dose of ciprofloxacin achieves more than 90% eradication rates that favorably compare to 2-day rifampin or intramuscular ceftriaxone (single-dose) regimens [111,115].

Fluoroquinolones have good penetration into the cerebrospinal fluid (CSF) and have been used successfully for treatment of CNS infections in adults. There are various published case reports of successful treatment of infants and children with Gram-negative bacterial meningitis and ventriculitis [6,116].

NEWEST COMPOUNDS

Ongoing research on chemical modifications of the quinolones is aimed at: (1) more potent derivatives, (2) less frequent resistance, (3) better penetration into CSF and CNS, and (4) improved patient tolerability. Some of the newer compounds have achieved many of these goals. Of major interest for pediatricians are effective CSF penetration and improved activity against Gram-positive pathogens, while maintaining excellent Gram-negative coverage. The newer quinolones have increased activity against staphylococci, including methicillin-resistant strains, against streptococci, including multiple-drug resistant pneumococci, and against *Mycoplasma* and *Chlamydia* [117–120].

Pneumococci moderately or highly resistant to penicillin G, other β-lactams, and also to other antibiotic classes are a worldwide challenge. Clinical failures in the treatment of meningitis and otitis media caused by penicillin-resistant isolates of *Streptococcus pneumoniae* have been observed [121,122].

Newer quinolones such as the fluoroquinolones gatifloxacin, moxifloxacin, gemifloxacin, and des-F(6)-quinolone (T-3811ME, BMS-284756) are potential options for the treatment of bacterial meningitis and respiratory tract infections (e.g., pneumonia, otitis media) in pediatric patients. The *in-vitro* activity of these agents covers all bacteria that commonly cause these infections, including strains of *S. pneumoniae* resistant to β-lactams and to other antibiotics [118–120]. Their pharmacodynamic properties in animals and adult patients are favorable, and include good penetration at various sites of infection such as the cerebrospinal and middle ear fluids, and are suitable for a once-daily dosing regimen. Several experimental meningitis studies documented bacterial killing rates comparable or superior to currently recommended β-lactam and carbapenem regimens [123–126].

It is concluded that well-designed clinical studies should be conducted to assess the efficacy and safety of some of the newest quinolone compounds, such as gatifloxacin, gemifloxacin, moxifloxacin, and des-F(6)-quinolone, in pediatric bacterial meningitis and respiratory tract infections.

RECOMMENDATIONS

Based on the available experimental and clinical data (Table III) on both the safety and efficacy of the fluoroquinolones, pediatric patients suffering from specific infections complicated by pathologic or special conditions should not be deprived of the therapeutic advantages that these agents have to offer. However, the quinolone antibiotics should never be used in pediatrics for routine treatment when alternative safe and effective antimicrobials are known.

To date, potential pediatric indications for the available fluoroquinolones (especially ciprofloxacin; for some indications, also ofloxacin and norfloxacin) include bronchopulmonary exacerbation in cystic fibrosis, complicated urinary tract infection, and invasive gastrointestinal infection. Based on preliminary experience, further potential pediatric indications that clearly require additional controlled studies are chronic suppurative otitis media, neutropenia in cancer patients, eradication of nasopharyngeal carriage, and CNS infections.

CONCLUSION

Quinolone arthropathy, as described in juvenile animals, has not yet presented in children and adolescents. The clinical observations described in temporal relationship to quinolone use are reversible episodes of arthralgia with and without effusions that do not lead to long-term sequelae when discontinued. Overall, the fluoroquinolones have been safe and effective in the treatment of selected bacterial infections in pediatric patients. There are clearly defined indications for these compounds in children who are ill.

The excellent antibacterial and pharmacodynamic properties of some of the newest quinolones (e.g., gatifloxacin, gemifloxacin, moxifloxacin, and des-F(6)-quinolone) indicate that these agents might become needed alternatives for treatment of childhood bacterial CNS and respiratory tract infections.

REFERENCES

1. Stahlmann, R. (1990). Safety profile of the quinolones. *J. Antimicrob. Chemother.* **26** (Suppl. D), 31–44.

2. Stahlmann, R., and Lode, H. (1988). The quinolones—Safety overview: Toxicity, adverse events, and drug interactions. In "The Quinolones" (V. T. Andriole, ed.), pp. 201–233. Academic Press, London.

3. Gough, A., Barsoum, N. J., Mitchell, L., McGuire, E. J., and de la Iglesia, F. A. (1979). Juvenile canine drug-induced arthropathy: Clinicopathological studies on articular lesions caused by oxolinic and pipemidic acids. *Toxicol. Appl. Pharmacol.* **51**, 177–187.

4. Christ, W., Lehnert, T., and Ulbrich, B. (1988). Specific toxicologic aspects of the quinolones. *Rev. Infect. Dis.* **10** (Suppl. 1), 141–146.

5. Schluter, G. (1989). Ciprofloxacin: Toxicologic evaluation of additional safety data. *Am. J. Med.* **87** (Suppl. 5A), 37–39.

6. Schaad, U. B., Salam, M. A., Aujard, Y., Dagan, R., Green, S. D. R., Peltola, H., Rubio, T. T., Smith, A. L., and Adam, D. (1995). Use of fluoroquinolones in pediatrics: Consensus report of an International Society of Chemotherapy commission. *Pediatr. Infect. Dis. J.* **14**, 1–9.

7. Linseman, D. A., Hamptom, L. A., and Branstetter, D. G. (1995). Quinolone-induced arthropathy in the neonatal mouse: Morphological analysis of articular lesions produced by pipemidic acid and ciprofloxacin. *Fundam. Appl. Toxicol.* **28**, 59–64.

8. Kato, M., and Onodera, T. (1988). Morphological investigation of cavity formation in articular cartilage induced by ofloxacin in rats. *Fundam. Appl. Toxicol.* **11**, 110–119.

9. Burkhardt, J. E., Hill, M. A., Cartlon, W. W., and Kesterson, J. W. (1990). Histologic and histochemical changes in articular cartilages of immature beagle dogs dosed with difloxacin, a fluoroquinolone. *Vet. Pathol.* **27**, 162–170.

10. Stahlmann, R., Merker, H. J., Hinz, N., Chahoud, I., Webb, J., Heger, W., and Neubert, D. (1990). Ofloxacin in juvenile non-human primates and rats: Arthropathia and drug plasma concentrations. *Arch. Toxicol.* **64**, 193–204.

11. Bendele, A. M., Hulman, J. F., Harvey, A. K., Hrubey, P. S., and Chandrasekhar, S. (1990). Passive role of articular chondrocytes in quinolone-induced arthropathy in guinea pigs. *Toxicol. Pathol.* **18**, 304–312.

12. Sharpnack, D. D., Mastin, J. P., Childress, C. P., and Henningsen, G. M. (1994). Quinolone arthropathy in juvenile New Zealand white rabbits. *Lab. Anim. Sci.* **44**, 436–442.

13. Ewing, P. J., and Ness, D. K. (1995). Quinolone arthropathy in juvenile ferrets. *Vet. Pathol.* **32**, 599.

14. Christ, W., and Lehnert, T. (1990). Toxicity of the quinolones. In "The New Generation of Quinolones" (C. Siporin, C. L. Heifetz, and J. M. Domagala, eds.). Marcel Dekker, New York.

15. Burkhardt, J. E. (1996). Review of quinolone arthropathy in the dog. *Chemother. J.* **5** (Suppl. 13), 14–18.

16. Burkhardt, J. E., Hill, M. A., and Carlton, W. W. (1992). Morphologic and biochemical changes in articular cartilages of immature beagle dogs dosed with difloxacin. *Toxicol. Pathol.* **20**, 246–252.

17. Gough, A., Johnson, R., Campbell, E., Hall, L., Tylor, J., Carpenter, A., Black, W., Basrur, P. K., Baragi, V. M., Sigler, R., and Metz, A. (1996). Quinolone arthropathy in immature rabbits treated with the fluoroquinolone PD 117596. *Exp. Toxicol. Pathol.* **48**, 225–232.

18. Forster, C., Kociok, K., Shakibaei, M., Merker, H. J., Vormann, J., Gunther, T., and Stahlmann, R. (1996). Integrins on joint cartilage chondrocytes and alterations by ofloxacin or magnesium deficiency in immature rats. *Arch. Toxicol.* **70**, 261–270.

19. Gough, A. W., Barsoum, N. J., Renlund, R. C., Sturgess, J. M., and de la Iglesia, F. A. (1985). Fine structural changes during reparative phase of canine drug-induced arthropathy. *Vet. Pathol.* **22**, 82–84.

20. Tatsumi, H., Senda, H., Yatera, S., Takemoto, Y., Yamayoshi, M., and Ohnishi, K. (1978). Toxicological studies on pipemidic acid, V: Effect on diarthrodial joints of experimental animals. *J. Toxicol. Sci.* **3**, 357–367.

21. Gough, A. W., Kasali, O. B., Sigler, R. E., and Baragi, V. (1992). Quinolone arthropathy: Acute toxicity to immature cartilage toxicity. *Toxicol. Pathol.* **20**, 436–439.

22. Stahlmann, R., Forster, C., and Vansickle, D. (1993). Quinolones in children: Are concerns over arthropathy justified? *Drug Saf.* **9**, 397–403.

23. Stahlmann, R., Forster, C., Shakibaei, M., Vormann, J., Gunther, T., and Merker, H. J. (1995). Magnesium deficiency induces joint cartilage lesions in juvenile rats which are identical to quinolone-induced arthropathy. *Antimicrob. Agents Chemother.* **39**, 2013–2018.

24. Shakibaei, M., Kociok, K., Forster, C., Vormann, J., Gunther, T., and Merker, H. J. (1996). Comparative evaluation of ultrastructural changes in articular cartilage of ofloxacin-treated and magnesium-deficient immature rats. *Toxicol. Pathol.* **24**, 580–587.

25. Takada, S., Kato, M., and Takayama, S. (1994). Comparison of lesions induced by intraarticular injections of quinolones and compounds damaging cartilage components in rat femoral condyles. *J. Toxicol. Environ. Health* **42**, 73–88.

26. Amacher, D. E., Schomaker, S. J., Gootz, T. D., and McGuirk, P. R. (1989). In "In Vitro Toxicology: New Directions" (M. A. Goldberg, ed.), pp. 307–312. Mary Ann Liebert, New York.

27. Brand, H. S., van Kampen, G. P. J., and van der Korst, J. K. (1990). Effect of nalidixic acid, pipemidic acid, and cinoxacin on chondrocyte metabolism in explants of articular cartilage. *Clin. Exp. Rheumatol.* **8**, 393–395.

28. Burkhardt, J. E., Hill, M., Carlton, W., and Lamar, C. (1991). Difloxacin reduces gylcosamino-glycan synthesis in organ cultures of articular cartilage. In "In Vitro Toxicology: Mechanisms and New Technology" (M. A. Goldberg, ed.), pp. 371–377. Mary Ann Liebert, New York.

29. Schroter-Kermani, C., Hinz, N., Risse, P., Stahlmann, R., and Merker, H. J. (1992). Effects of ofloxacin on chondrogenesis in murine cartilage organoid culture. *Toxicol. In Vitro* **6**, 465–474.

30. Burkhardt, J. E., Hill, M. A., Lamar, C. H., Smith, G. N., and Carlton, W. W. (1993). Effects of difloxacin on the metabolism of glycosaminoglycans and collagen in organ cultures of articular cartilage. *Fundam. Appl. Toxicol.* **20**, 257–263.

31. Hildebrand, H., Kempka, G., Schluter, G., and Schmidt, M. (1993). Chondrotoxicity of quinolones *in vivo* and *in vitro*. *Arch. Toxicol.* **67**, 411–415.

32. Kato, M., Takada, S., Ogawara, S., and Takayama, S. (1995). Effect of levofloxacin on glycosaminoglycan and DNA synthesis of cultured rabbit chondrocytes at concentrations inducing cartilage lesions *in vivo*. *Antimicrob. Agents Chemother.* **39**, 1979–1983.

33. Hayem, G., Petit, P. X., Levacher, M., Gaudin, C., Kahn, M. F., and Pocidalo, J. J. (1994). Cytofluorometric analysis of chondrotoxicity of fluoroquinolone antimicrobial agents. *Antimicrob. Agents Chemother.* **38**, 243–247.

34. Thuong-Guyot, M., Domarle, O., Pocidalo, J. J., and Hayem, G. (1994). Effects of fluoroquinolones on cultured articular chondrocytes: Flow cytometric analysis of free radical production. *J. Pharmacol. Exp. Ther.* **271**, 1544–1549.

35. Mont, M. A., Mathur, S. K., Frondoza, C. G., and Hungerford, D. S. (1996). The effects of ciprofloxacin on human chondrocytes in cell culture. *Infection* **24**, 151–155.

36. Ruoslahti, E. (1991). Integrins. *J. Clin. Invest.* **87**, 1–5.

37. Hynes, R. O. (1992). Integrins: Versatility, modulation, and signaling in cell adhesion. *Cell* **69**, 11–25.

38. Shakibaei, M., Forster, C., Merker, H. J., and Stahlmann, R. (1995). Effects of ofloxacin in integrin expression on epiphyseal mouse chondrocytes *in vitro*. *Toxicol. In Vitro* **9**, 107–116.

39. Vormann, J., Forster, C., Zippel, U., Lozo, E., Gunther, T., Merker, H. J., and Stahlmann, R. (1997). Effects of magnesium deficiency on magnesium calcium content in bone and cartilage in developing rats in correlation to chondrotoxicity. *Calcif. Tissue Int.* **61**, 230–238.

40. Burkhardt, J. E., Walterspiel, J. N., and Schaad, U. B. (1997). Quinolone arthropathy in animals compared to observations in children. *Clin. Infect. Dis.* **25**, 1196–1204.

41. Bailey, R. R., Kirk, J. A., and Peddie, B. A. (1983). Norfloxacin-induced rheumatic disease. *N.Z. Med. J.* **96**, 590.

42. Royer, R. J., Pierfitte, C., Netter, P. (1994). Features of tendon disorders with fluoroquinolones. *Therapie* **49**, 75–76.

43. Van der Linden, P. D., van de Lei, J., Nab, H. W., Knol, A., and Stricker, B. H. Ch. (1999). Achilles tendinitis associated with fluoroquinolones. *Br. J. Clin. Pharmacol.* **48**, 433–437.

44. Kato, M., Takada, S., Kashida, Y., and Nomura, M. (1995). Histological examination on Achilles tendon lesions induced by quinolone antibacterial agents in juvenile rats. *Toxicol. Pathol.* **23**, 385–392.

45. Kashida, Y., and Kato, M. (1997). Characterization of fluoroquinolone-induced Achilles tendon toxicity in rats: Comparison of toxicities of 10 fluoroquinolones and effects of anti-inflammatory compounds. *Antimicrob. Agents Chemother.* **41**, 2389–2393.

46. Shakibael, M., Pfister, K., Schwabe, R., Vormann, J., and Stahlmann, R. (2000). Ultrastructure of Achilles tendons of rats treated with ofloxacin and fed a normal or magnesium-deficient diet. *Antimicrob. Agents Chemother.* **44**, 261–266.

47. Bannon, M. J., Stutchfield, P. R., Weindling, A. M., and Damanovic, V. (1989). Ciprofloxacin in neonatal *Enterobacter cloacae* septicaemia. *Arch. Dis. Child.* **64**, 1388–1389.

48. Cohen, R., Bompard, Y., Danan, C., Auffrant, C., and Aujard, Y. (1990). Indication des quinolones chez le nouveau-né. In "Pharmacol périnatale" (Y. Aujard, E. Autret, and E. Jacqa-Aigrain, eds.), pp. 517–529. Paquiseaued, Angers.

49. LeBel, M., Bergeron, M. G., Vallée, F., Fiset, C., Chassé, G., Bigonesse, P., and Rivard, G. (1986). Pharmacokinetics and pharmacodynamics of ciprofloxacin in cystic fibrosis patients. *Antimicrob. Agents Chemother.* **30**, 260–266.

50. Goldfarb, J., Wormser, G. P., Inchiosa, M. A., Guiden, G., Diaz, M., and Mascia, A. V. (1986). Single-dose pharmacokinetics of oral ciprofloxacin in patients with cystic fibrosis. *J. Clin. Pharmacol.* **26**, 222–226.

51. Blumer, J. L., Stern, R. C., Myers, C. M., *et al.* (1985). Pharmacokinetics and pharmacodynamics of ciprofloxacin in cystic fibrosis. *Abstr. 14th Int. Cong. Chemother.*, Kyoto.

52. Stutman, H. R., Shalit, I., Marks, M. I., Greenwood, R., Chartrand, S. A., and Hillman, B. C. (1987). Pharmacokinetics of two dosage regimens of ciprofloxacin during a two-week therapeutic trial in patients with cystic fibrosis. *Am. J. Med.* **82** (Suppl. 4A), 142–145.

53. Peltola, H., Vaarala, M., Renkonen, O., and Neuvonen, P. J. (1992). Pharmacokinetics of single dose of oral ciprofloxacin in infants and small children. *Antimicrob. Agents Chemother.* **36**, 1086–1090.

54. Schaeffer, H. G., Stass, H., Wedgwood, J., Hampel, B., Fischer, C., Kuhlmann, J., and Schaad, U. B. (1996). Pharmacokinetics of ciprofloxacin in pediatric cystic fibrosis patients. *Antimicrob. Agents Chemother.* **40**, 29–34.

55. Rubio, T. T., Miles, M. V., Lettieri, J. T., Kuhn, R. J., Echols, R. M., and Church, D. A. (1997). Pharmacokinetic disposition of sequential intravenous/oral ciprofloxacin in pediatric cystic fibrosis patients with acute pulmonary exacerbation. *Pediatr. Infect. Dis. J.* **16**, 112–117.

56. Wolfson, J. S. (1989). Quinolone antimicrobial agents: Adverse effects and bacterial resistance. *Eur. J. Clin. Microbiol. Infect. Dis.* **8**, 1080–1092.

57. Norrby, S. R. (1991). Side-effects of quinolones: Comparison between quinolones and other antibiotics. *Eur. J. Clin. Microbiol. Infect. Dis.* **10**, 378–383.

58. Schaad, U. B. (1991). Use of quinolones in pediatrics. *Eur. J. Clin. Microbiol. Infect. Dis.* **10**, 355–360.

59. Chysky, V., Kapila, K., Hullmann, R., Arcieri, G., Schacht, P., and Echols, R. (1991). Safety of ciprofloxacin in children: Worldwide clinical experience based on compassionate use—emphasis on joint evaluation. *Infection* **19**, 289–296.

60. Hampel, B., Hullmann, R., and Schmidt, K. (1997). Ciprofloxacin in pediatrics: Worldwide clinical experience based on compassionate use safety report. *Pediatr. Infect. Dis. J.* **16**, 127–129.

61. Lipsky, B. A., and Baker, C. A. (1999). Fluoroquinolone toxicity profiles: A review focusing on newer agents. *Clin. Infect. Dis.* **28**, 352–364.

62. Simpson, J., Watson, A. R., Mellersh, A., Nelson, C. S., and Dodd, K. (1991). Typhoid fever, ciprofloxacin, and renal failure. *Arch. Dis. Child.* **60**, 1083–1084.

63. Miller, M. S., Gaido, F., Rourk Jr., M. H., and Spock, A. (1991). Anaphylactoid reactions in ciprofloxacin in cystic fibrosis patients. *Pediatr. Infect. Dis. J.* **10**, 164–165.

64. Adamantidis, M. M., Dumotier, B. M., Caron, J. F., and Bordet, R. (1998). Sparfloxacin but not levofloxacin or ofloxacin prolongs cardiac repolarization in rabbit Purkinje fibers. *Fundam. Clin. Pharmacol.* **12**, 70–76.

65. Chen, H. J. L., Bloch, K. J., and Maclean, J. A. (2000). Acute eosinophilic hepatitis from trovafloxacin. *New Engl. J. Med.* **342**, 359–360.

66. Loebstein, R., Addis, A., Ho, E., Andreou, R., Sage, S., Donnenfeld, A. E., Schick, B., Bonati, M., Moretti, M., Lalkin, A., Pastuszak, A., and Koren, G. (1998). Pregnancy outcome following gestational exposure to fluoroquinolones: A multicenter prospective controlled study. *Antimicrob. Agents Chemother.* **42**, 1336–1339.

67. Moellering, R. C. (1995). Past, present, and future of antimicrobial agents. *Am. J. Med.* **99** (Suppl. 6A), 11–18.

68. Polk, R. (1999). Optimal use of modern antibiotics: Emerging trends. *Clin. Infect. Dis.* **29**, 264–274.

69. Kesseler, A., LaCassie, A., Hugot, J. P., Talon, P., Thomas, D., and Astier, L. (1989). Arthropathies consécutives a l'administration de péfloxacine chez un adolescent atteint de mucoviscidose. *Ann. Peadiatr.* (*Paris*) **36**, 275–278.

70. McDonald, D. F., and Short, H. B. (1964). Usefulness of nalidixic acid in treatment of urinary infection. *Antimicrob. Agents Chemother.* **4**, 628–631.

71. Alfaham, M., Holt, M. E., and Goodchild, M. C. (1987). Arthropathy in a patient with cystic fibrosis taking ciprofloxacin. *Br. Med. J.* **295**, 699.

72. Ollier, S., Laroche, M., Arlet, P., Montane, P., Durroux, R., and LeTallec, Y. (1990). Arthropathie a la péfloxacine. *Rev. Rhum. Mal. Osteoartic.* **5** (Suppl. 9), 671.

73. Jawad, A. S. M. (1989). Cystic fibrosis and drug-induced arthropathy. *Br. J. Rheumatol.* **28**, 179–180.

74. Seigneuric, C., Plantavid, M., Bouygues, D., Cassou, M., Amar, J., and Cascarigny, F. (1990). Manifestations articulaires sous péfloxacine chez l'adolescent. *La Presse Méd.* **19**, 428.

75. LeLoet, X., Fessard, C., Noblet, C., Sait, L., and Moore, N. (1991). Severe polyarthropathy in an adolescent treated with pefloxacin. *J. Rheumatol.* **18**, 1941–1942.

76. Chevalier, X., Albengres, E., Voisin, M. C., Tillement, J. P., and Larget-Piet, B. (1992). A case of destructive polyarthropathy in a 17-year-old youth following pefloxacin treatment. *Drug Saf.* **7**, 310–314.

77. Gylys-Morin, V. M., Hajek, P. C., Sartoris, D. J., and Resnick, D. (1987). Articular cartilage defects: Dectectability in cadaver knees with MR. *Am. J. Radiol.* **148**, 1153–1157.

78. Schaad, U. B., Sander, E., Wedgwood, J., and Schaffner, T. (1992). Morphologic studies for skeletal toxicity after prolonged ciprofloxacin therapy in two juvenile cystic fibrosis patients. *Pediatr. Infect. Dis. J.* **11**, 1047–1049.

79. Meyer, H. (1987). Ofloxacin in cystic fibrosis. *Drugs* **34** (Suppl. 1), 177–179.

80. Schaad, U. B., and Wedgwood-Krucko, J. (1987). Nalidixic acid in children: Retrospective matched controlled study for cartilage toxicity. *Infection* **15**, 165–168.

81. Scully, B. E., Nakatomi, M., Ores, C., Davidson, S., and Neu, H. C. (1987). Ciprofloxacin therapy in cystic fibrosis. *Am. J. Med.* **82** (Suppl. 4A), 196–201.

82. Salam, M. A., and Bennish, M. L. (1988). Therapy for shigellosis, I: Randomized, double-blind trials of nalidixic acid in childhood shigellosis. *J. Pediatr.* **113**, 901–907.

83. Cruciani, M., Concia, E., Navarra, A., Perversi, L., Bonetti, F., Arico, M., and Nespoli, L. (1989). Prophylactic co-trimoxazole versus norfloxacin in neutropenic children: Prospective randomized study. *Infection* **17**, 65–69.

84. Black, A., Redmond, A. O. B., Steen, H. J., and Oborska, I. T. (1990). Tolerance and safety of ciprofloxacin in pediatric patients. *J. Antimicrob. Chemother.* **26** (Suppl. F), 25–29.

85. Rubio, T. T. (1990). Ciprofloxacin in the treatment of *Pseudomonas* infection in children with cystic fibrosis. *Diag. Microbiol. Infect. Dis.* **13**, 153–155.

86. Cheesbrough, J. S., Illunga Mwema, F., Green, S. D. R., and Rillotson, G. S. (1991). Quinolones in children with invasive salmonellosis. *Lancet* **338**, 127.

87. Schaad, U. B., Stoupis, C., Wedgwood, J., Tschaeppeler, H., and Vock, P. (1991). Clinical radiologic and magnetic resonance monitoring for skeletal toxicity in pediatric patients with cystic fibrosis receiving a three-month course of ciprofloxacin. *Pediatr. Infect. Dis. J.* **10**, 723–729.

88. Fujii, R. (1992). The use of norfloxacin in children in Japan. *Adv. Antineopl. Chemother.* **11**, 219–232.

89. Karande, S. C., and Kshirasager, N. A. (1993). Adverse drug reaction monitoring of ciprofloxacin in pediatric practice. *Indian Pediatr.* **20**, 181–187.

90. Danisovicova, A., Brezina, M., Belan, S., Kayserova, H., Kaiserova, E., Hruskovic, I., Orosova, K., Dluholucky, S., Gallova, K., Matheova, E., Marinova, I., and Krcmery, V. (1994). Magnetic resonance imaging in children receiving quinolones: No evidence of quinolone-induced arthropathy. *Chemotherapy* **40**, 209–214.

91. Arico, M., Bossi, G., Caselli, D., Cosi, G., Villa, A., Beluffi, G., and Genovese, E. (1995). Long-term magnetic resonance survey of cartilage damage in leukemic children treated with fluoroquinolones. *Pediatr. Infect. Dis.* **14**, 713–714.

92. Pradham, K. M., Arora, N. K., Jena, A., Susheela, A. K., and Bhan, M. K. (1995). Safety of ciprofloxacin therapy in children: Magnetic resonance images, body fluid levels of fluoride and linear growth. *Acta Pediatr.* **84** (Suppl. 5), 555–560.

93. Hien, T. T., Bethell, D. B., Hoa, N. T. T., Wain, J., Diep, T. S., Phi, L. T., Cuong, B. M., Thanh, P. T., Walsh, A. L., Day, N. P. J., and White, N. J. (1995). Short course of ofloxacin for treatment of multidrug-resistant typhoid. *Clin. Infect. Dis.* **20**, 917–923.

94. Rathore, M. H., Bux, D., and Hasan, M. (1996). Multidrug-resistant *Salmonella typhi* in Pakistani children: Clinical features and treatment. *South. Med. J.* **89**, 235–237.

95. Bethell, D. B., Hien, T. T., Phi, L. T., Day, N. P. S., Vinh, H., Duong, N. M., Len, N. V., Chuong, L. V., and White, N. J. (1996). Effects on growth of single short courses of fluoroquinolones. *Arch. Dis. Child.* **74**, 44–46.

96. Church, D. A., Kanga, J. F., Kuhn, R. J., Rubio, T. T., Spohn, W. A., Stevens, J. C., Painter, B. G., Thurberg, B. E., Haverstock, D. C., Perroncel, R. Y., Echols, R. M., and the Cystic Fibrosis Study Group (1997). Sequential ciprofloxacin therapy in pediatric cystic fibrosis: Comparative study vs. ceftazidime/tobramycin in the treatment of acute pulmonary exacerbations. *Pediatr. Infect. Dis. J.* **16**, 97–105.

97. Schaad, U. B., Wedgwood, J., Ruedeberg, A., Kraemer, R., and Hampel, B. (1997). Ciprofloxacin as antipseudomonal treatment in patients with cystic fibrosis. *Pediatr. Infect. Dis. J.* **16**, 106–111.

98. Jick, S. (1997). Ciprofloxacin safety in a pediatric population. *Pediatr. Infect. Dis. J.* **16**, 130–134.

99. Freifeld, A., and Pizzo, P. (1997). Use of fluoroquinolones for empirical management of febrile neutropenia in pediatric cancer patients. *Pediatr. Infect. Dis. J.* **16**, 140–146.

100. Redmond, A. O. (1997). Risk–benefit experience of ciprofloxacin use in pediatric patients in the United Kingdom. *Pediatr. Infect. Dis. J.* **16**, 147–149.

101. Richard, D. A., Nousia-Arvanitakis, S., Sollich, V., Hampel, B. J., Sommerauer, B., Schaad, U. B., and the Cystic Fibrosis Study Group (1997). Oral ciprofloxacin versus intravenous ceftazidime plus tobramycin in pediatric cystic fibrosis patients: Comparison of antipseudomonas efficacy and assessment of safety using ultrasonography and magnetic resonance imaging. *Pediatr. Infect. Dis. J.* **16**, 572–578.

102. Phillips, B. M., and David, T. J. (1986). Pathogenesis and management of arthropathy in cystic fibrosis. *J. Roy. Soc. Med.* **79** (Suppl. 12), 44–50.

103. Pertuiset, E., Lenoir, G., Jehanne, M., Douchain, F., Guillot, M., and Menkes, C. J. (1989). Tolérance articulaire de la péfloxacine et de l'ofloxacine chez les enfants et adolescents atteints de mucoviscidose. *Rev. Rhum. Mal. Osteoartic.* **56**, 735–740.

104. Marks, M. I. (1981). The pathogenesis and treatment of pulmonary infections in patients with cystic fibrosis. *J. Pediatr.* **98**, 173–179.

105. Hoiby, N., Friis, B., Jense, K., *et al.* (1982). Antimicrobial chemotherapy in CF patients. *Acta Pediatr. Scand.* **71** (Suppl. 310), 75–100.

106. Smith, A. L. (1986). Antibiotic therapy in cystic fibrosis: Evaluation of clinical trials. *J. Pediatr.* **108**, 866–870.

107. Schaad, U. B., Desgrandchamps, D., and Kraemer, R. (1986). Antimicrobial therapy of *Pseudomonas* pulmonary exacerbations in cystic fibrosis: A prospective evaluation of netilmicin plus azlocillin versus netilmicin plus ticarcillin. *Acta Pediatr. Scand.* **75**, 128–138.

108. Schaad, U. B., Wedgwood-Krucko, J., Guenin, U., Buehlmann, R., and Kraemer, R. (1989). Antipseudomonal therapy in cystic fibrosis: Aztreonam and amikacin versus oral ceftazidime and amikacin administered intravenously followed by oral ciprofloxacin. *Eur. J. Clin. Microbiol. Infect. Dis.* **8**, 858–865.

109. Schaad, U. B., Wedgwood-Krucko, J., Suter, S., and Kraemer, R. (1987). Efficacy of inhaled amikacin as adjunct to intravenous combination therapy (ceftazidime and amikacin) in cystic fibrosis. *J. Pediatr.* **111**, 599–605.

110. Prince, A. S., and Neu, H. C. (1981). Activities of new β-lactam antibiotics against isolates of *Pseudomonas aeruginosa* from patients with cystic fibrosis. *Antimicrob. Agents Chemother.* **20**, 545–546.

111. Green, S., and Tillotson, G. (1997). Use of ciprofloxacin in developing countries. *Pediatr. Infect. Dis. J.* **16**, 150–159.

112. Salam, M. A., Dhar, U., Khan, W. A., and Bennish, M. L. (1998). Randomised comparison of ciprofloxacin suspension and pivmecillinam for childhood shigellosis. Lancet 352, 522-527.

113. Lang, R., Goshen, S., and Raas-Rothschild, A. (1992). Oral ciprofloxacin in the management of chronic suppurative otitis media without cholesteatoma in children. *Pediatr. Infect. Dis. J.* **11**, 925–929.

114. Patrick, C. C. (1997). Use of fluoroquinolones as prophylaxis agents in patients with neutropenia. *Pediatr. Infect. Dis. J.* **16**, 135–139.

115. Cuevas, L. E., Kazembe, P., Mughogho, G. K., Tilloston, G. S., and Hart, C. A. (1995). Eradication of nasopharyngeal carriage of *Neisseria meningitidis* in children and adult in rural Africa: A comparison of ciprofloxacin and rifampicin. *J. Inf. Dis.* **171**, 728–731.

116. Krcmery, V., Filka, J., Uher, J., Kurak, H., Sagat, T., Tuharsky, J., Novak, I., Urbanova, T., Kralinsky, K., Mateicka, F., Krcmeryova, T., Jurga, L., Sulcova, M., Stencl, J., and Krupova, I. (1999). Ciprofloxacin in treatment of nosocomial meningitis in neonates and in infants: Report of 12 cases and review. *Diag. Microbiol. Infect. Dis.* **35**, 75–80.

117. Barry, A. L., Fuchs, P. C., and Brown, S. D. (1996). In vitro activities of five fluoroquinolone compounds against strains of *Streptococcus pneumoniae* with resistance to other antimicrobial agents. *Antimicrob. Agents Chemother.* **40**, 2431–2433.

118. Schmitz, F.-J., Verhoef, J., Fluit, A. C., and the SENTRY Participants Group (1999). Comparative activities of six different fluoroquinolones against 9,682 clinical bacterial isolates from 20 European university hospitals participating in the European SENTRY surveillance programme. *Int. J. Antimicrob. Agents* **12**, 311–317.

119. Takahata, M., Mitsuyama, J., Yamashiro, Y., Yonezawa, M., Araki, H., Todo, Y., Minami, S., Watanabe, Y., and Narita, H. (1999). *In vitro* and *in vivo* antimicrobial activities of T-3811ME, a novel des-F(6)-quinolone. *Antimicrob. Agents Chemother.* **43**, 1077–1084.

120. Hardy, D., Amsterdam, D., Mandell, L. A., and Rotstein, C. (2000). Comparative *in vitro* activities of ciprofloxacin, gemifloxacin, grepafloxacin, moxifloxacin, ofloxacin, sparfloxacin, trovafloxacin, and other antimicrobial agents against bloodstream isolates of Gram-positive cocci. *Antimicrob. Agents Chemother.* **44**, 802–805.

121. John, C. C. (1994). Treatment failure with use of a third-generation cephalosporin for penicillin-resistant pneumococcal meningitis: Case report and review. *Clin. Infect. Dis.* **18**, 188–193.

122. Gehanno, P., N'Guyen, L., Derriennic, M., Pichon, F., Goehrs, J.-M., and Berche, P. (1998). Pathogens isolated during treatment failures in otitis. *Pediatr. Infect. Dis. J.* **17**, 885–890.

123. Nau, R., Schmidt, T., Kaye, K., Froula, J. L., and Taeuber, M. G. (1995). Quinolone antibiotics in the therapy of experimental pneumococcal meningitis in rabbits. *Antimicrob. Agents Chemother.* **39**, 593–597.

124. Lutsar, I., Friedland, I. R., Wubbel, L., McCoig, C. C., Jafri, H. S., Ng, W., Ghaffar, F., and McCracken Jr., G. H. (1998). Pharmacodynamics of gatifloxacin in cerebrospinal fluid in experimental cephalosporin-resistant pneumococcal meningitis. *Antimicrob. Agents Chemother.* **42**, 2650–2655.

125. Lutsar, I., Friedland, I. R., Jafri, H. S., Wubbel, L, Ng, W., Ghaffar, F., and McCracken Jr., G. H. (1999). Efficacy of gatifloxacin in experimental *Escherichia coli* meningitis. *Antimicrob. Agents Chemother.* **43**, 1805–1807.

126. Smirnov, A., Wellmer, A., Gerber, J., Maier, K., Henne, S., and Nau, R. (2000). Gemifloxacin is effective in experimental pneumococcal meningitis. *Antimicrob. Agents Chemother.* **44**, 767–770.

CHAPTER 16

The Quinolones

Prospects

VINCENT T. ANDRIOLE

Yale University School of Medicine, New Haven, Connecticut 06520-8022

INTRODUCTION

The future prospects of the quinolones were first reviewed more than a decade ago [1], and subsequent updates on these prospects were published more recently [2–4]. Although continued progress has occurred in our understanding of the chemistry and molecular mechanism of quinolone action on pathogenic bacteria, as well as factors that induce the development of quinolone resistance, concomitant toxicity caused by some of the more recently approved compounds is almost impossible to predict until new agents are introduced into clinical use. Additionally, the successful future for a specific class of therapeutic drugs may be determined by a number of major factors, including improved clinical efficacy, minimal toxicity and greater safety, better patient compliance, reduced but equally effective duration of therapy, unique binding to target sites that leads to delayed or preventable induction of resistance, especially for antimicrobial agents, and optimal cost–benefit ratios [4].

Clearly, the quinolones have captured the interest of many investigators from numerous scientific disciplines, and this interest has contributed greatly to the scientific advancements that have occurred during 1998 and 1999. These observations suggest that the prospects are excellent for future advances in quinolone research.

MOLECULAR MECHANISMS OF THE QUINOLONES: KEY DISCOVERIES

The quinolone antibacterial agents were not isolated from growing organisms but were synthesized by chemists. Thus, the history of the newer quinolone agents began with the discovery of nalidixic acid in 1962 as an accidental byproduct during the synthesis of the antimalarial compound chloroquine, which led to the development of the newer quinolones [5]. Other important discoveries followed and contributed to the rapid expansion of the newer quinolones. In particular, the knowledge that bacteria are faced with a major topological problem since each organism contains a chromosome that is composed of double-stranded DNA 1300 μm long and yet the average bacterium is only 2 μm long and 1 μm wide led to the studies by Worcel [6], who observed how the chromosome was packed in *Escherichia coli* and found that it is subdivided into about 65 regions, which he termed *domains*. Each domain, on average about 20 μm long, is attached to an RNA core, and the size of each domain is reduced by supertwisting of each domain. Supertwisting occurs in most bacteria against the normal direction of the helical state of DNA in its linear form and is termed *negative supertwisting* [7,8]. Crumplin and Smith [9] discovered that nalidixic acid acted on chromosome replication in *E. coli* and caused abnormal accumulation of single-stranded DNA precursors of molecular weight 18.8×10^6 daltons, and that there would be about 66 of these per chromosome, which agreed with the number of domains of supercoiling [10]. They also concluded that, when each chromosomal domain was supercoiled, it was also transiently nicked, and that when supercoiling was completed, the single-stranded DNA state was abolished by the sealing action of an enzyme that was specifically inhibited by the quinolone nalidixic acid [8,9].

Gellert *et al.* [11] identified the enzyme that nicks double-stranded chromosomal DNA, introduces negative supercoils, and then seals the nicked DNA, and termed it DNA gyrase or *E. coli* topoisomerase II [12,13]. Thus, the enzymic activity proposed earlier that year by Crumplin and Smith [9] was established. This discovery led to a better understanding of the molecular basis for the potent antibacterial effects of the newer quinolones. We now know that there are four DNA topoisomerases in bacteria. Specifically, topoisomerases I and III are not very sensitive to inhibition by the quinolones. Instead, topoisomerase II (DNA gyrase) and IV are the two major targets of the fluoroquinolones. Topoisomerase II has four subunits, of which two A monomers and two B monomers have been identified [14,15]. Topoisomerase IV, the second target of the quinolones, shares several properties with topoisomerase II (DNA gyrase), and also has a tetrameric structure with A and B subunits that are encoded by the *parC* and *parE* genes. Topoisomerase IV is involved with decatenation of the linked DNA molecules and appears to be the principal enzyme for separating replicated DNA molecules in the bacterial cell [16].

The topoisomerases have been found in every organism examined [7,17], perform specialized functions in the bacterial cell, and are essential for cell growth. For these reasons, topoisomerases II and IV represent lethal targets for the quinolones [16]. Even so, the bactericidal activity of the quinolones may be reduced significantly if RNA or protein synthesis is inhibited since these drugs have a concentration that is most bactericidal, so that higher or lower concentrations demonstrate reduced bactericidal activity [10]. This paradoxical effect of decreased killing at greater concentrations is most probably caused by dose-dependent inhibition of RNA synthesis [18]. The key point is that identification of DNA gyrase has provided the opportunity to develop new quinolone compounds that may have increased activity against DNA gyrase [19].

Another major advance that contributed to the rapid expansion of the newer quinolones was the ability to manipulate the nucleus of the 4-quinolones. The basic molecule has been modified at the N-1 position, with different groups added to the C-6, C-7, and C-8 positions [4,20]. These modifications result in major changes in the antimicrobial activity, pharmacokinetics, and metabolic properties of the quinolones. Specific changes include the addition of a fluorine atom at position C-6, which enhances DNA gyrase inhibitory activity and provides activity against staphylococci; addition of a second fluorine group at position C-8, which results in increased absorption and a longer half-life and may possibly increase phototoxicity; addition of a piperazine group at position C-7, which provides the best activity against aerobic Gram-negative organisms and results in increased activity against staphylococci and adds activity against *Pseudomonas*; ring alkylation, which improves Gram-positive activity and half-life [21]; substitution of a methyl group for the piperazine group, which results in increased absorption and a longer half-life; and addition of a cyclopropyl group at position N-1, an amino group at position C-5, and a fluorine group at C-8, which results in increased activity against *Mycoplasma* and *Chlamydia* [4]. Similarly, adding a fluorine or a chlorine at C-8 in combination with an N-1 cyclopropyl further enhances antibacterial activity [22]. Also, addition of a methoxy group at C-8 instead of a halide targets both DNA gyrase and topoisomerase IV, and probably decreases the possibility of development of fluoroquinolone resistance [21,23]. An excellent review by Gootz and Brighty of the significance of current structural alterations in the quinolone nucleus and the impact of these alterations on antimicrobial activity, pharmacokinetics, and adverse events appears in Chapter 2 of this edition.

MICROBIOLOGY

The early *in-vitro* studies of the very first group of newer quinolones demonstrated that these compounds were highly active against enteric Gram-negative aerobic bacteria and other aerobic Gram-negative organisms, particularly *Haemophilus* species [2,24]. However, they were only moderately active against *Pseudomonas aeruginosa*, and were active against staphylococci, but with the potential for development of resistance by these organisms. In fact, ciprofloxacin was the most active against *Pseudomonas aeruginosa* and presently continues to be the most potent antipseudomonal quinolone. These early compounds were only moderately active against streptococci, especially *Streptococcus pneumoniae* [2,24], and had poor activity against anaerobes [25]. The newer fluoroquinolones have greatly enhanced activity against *Streptococcus pneumoniae*, including penicillin-resistant strains, and against anaerobes, including *Bacteroides fragilis*, other *Bacteroides* species, *Clostridium* spp., *Fusobacterium* spp., *Peptostreptococcus* spp., *Veillonella* spp., and most *Prevotella* species [4,22,24–31]. The newer fluoroquinolones can be grouped according to their relative antipneumococcal and antianaerobic activity such as sparfloxacin, tosufloxacin, gatifloxacin, pazufloxacin, and grepafloxacin, which are much more active than earlier quinolones; and trovafloxacin, clinafloxacin, sitafloxacin, moxifloxacin, and gemifloxacin, which are the most active [4,24–32]. These newer compounds represent clear advances in potency, though some have unacceptable toxicity.

The potential for the development of resistance has been and still is a major concern and was observed during our early clinical experience with some infecting organisms even though spontaneous single-step mutation frequency for the newer quinolones was 1000-fold less than that for nalidixic acid, and mutant strains might still be susceptible to clinically achievable drug concentrations. Plasmid-mediated resistance to the newer quinolones had not yet been documented among clinical isolates, except for one report in a methicillin-resistant strain of *Staphylococcus aureus* [33]. Early studies of resistance indicated that mutations in the *gyrA* gene of topoisomerase II in clinical isolates of *Staphylococcus aureus* conferred resistance to the quinolones. Similar results were found for *P. aeruginosa*, *Escherichia coli*, *Neisseria gonorrhoeae*, *Klebsiella*, and *Citrobacter freundii* [4,20,34]. Also, earlier work suggested that the newer 4-quinolones might act slightly differently and affect both the A and B subunits of the DNA gyrase, since mutations that affect the B subunit were observed to alter bacterial sensitivity to the 4-quinolones [10,35,36].

Quinolone resistance may also result from changes in quinolone permeation. Genes (*nfx*B and *cfx*B) that decrease the expression of OmpF at the posttranscriptional level decrease accumulation of norfloxacin in cells, and porin-deficient bacterial mutants become more resistant to quinolones [34,37]. More recent advances in the development of the newest quinolones indicate that some of these compounds have activity against quinolone-resistant bacteria [16,22]. Potent activity against quinolone-resistant strains (particularly quinolone-resistant *S. aureus* and *P. aeruginosa*) is exhibited by the quinolones clinafloxacin and sitafloxacin, which have a C-8 chlorine atom [16,22,38]. Also, the newest quinolones with a C-8 methoxy group (e.g., moxifloxacin and gatifloxacin) have improved activity against quinolone–resistant *S. aureus* [39-42].

Current intense investigations into the mechanisms responsible for the development of resistance, particularly pneumococcal and staphylococcal resistance that occurs with induction of amino-acid changes in the *parC* and *parE* genes of topoisomerase IV (in pneumococci) and in *gyrA* genes (in staphylococci) are likely to lead to improved compounds for the treatment of infections caused by these bacteria in the near future. The results of these studies are likely to produce compounds that are more resistant to rapid development of resistance [43–49]. Furthermore, as we learn more about quinolone resistance mechanisms, as well as the effects of structure–activity relationships on mechanisms of resistance, we may be able to select particular quinolones to adapt to specific clinical situations [50]. For example, more recent studies have advanced our understanding of the more important amino-acid mutations in *parC* and *gyrA* and their impact on the level of resistance to *Streptococcus pneumoniae* for each of the newer fluoroquinolones, and demonstrate that the level of resistance is different and varies among these quinolones [51,52]. These observations, as they relate to *Streptococcus pneumoniae*, are especially cogent since decreased susceptibility to fluoroquinolones has been observed in some clinical isolates of *Streptococcus pneumoniae*, probably as a consequence of selective pressures from increased fluoroquinolone use [53]. Similarly, the importance of the presence of efflux pumps in quinolone resistance in *Escherichia coli* has been more clearly characterized [54].

Continued investigation into the mechanisms of bacterial resistance to fluoroquinolones will hopefully lead to better methods of prevention or at least lead to delayed development of quinolone resistance.

PHARMACOKINETICS

Important and practical pharmacologic aspects of the newer quinolones include excellent oral absorption, good tissue distribution with excellent interstitial fluid levels, significant entry into phagocytic cells, and excellent urinary concentrations after oral administration [55]. Advances in our understanding of structure–activity relationships has improved the pharmacokinetics (i.e., longer half-life and tissue penetration appropriate for once-daily dosing) of some of the newest quinolones, including grepafloxacin, sparfloxacin, trovafloxacin, moxifloxacin, gatifloxacin, gemifloxacin, and sitafloxacin (DU-6859a) [21,22,56,57].

Key observations that led to the development of newer compounds with improved pharmacokinetics included [4,16,22]:

- alkylation of the quinolone, which improves half-life and tissue penetration, possibly by increasing the lipophilicity of the quinolone

- adding two methyl groups to the C-7 piperazine ring, which increases oral efficacy

- an amino group at C-5, which increases lipophilicity

- a naphthyridone nucleus, i.e., a nitrogen in the 1 and 8 positions of the nucleus, improves pharmacokinetics when an azabicyclo-hexane sidechain is present at the C-7 position

- a halogen in the C-8 position improves *in-vivo* activity but may also contribute to phototoxicity

- chemical manipulations of the C-7 sidechain to improve structure–activity relationships, which may also affect specific antimicrobial activity, alter the incidence of adverse events and serious toxicity, as well as improve pharmacokinetics and pharmacodynamics.

CLINICAL USES

Many infectious diseases can be treated successfully with oral quinolone therapy. Specifically, respiratory infections such as acute bacterial exacerbations of chronic bronchitis, community-acquired pneumonia and sinusitis, both uncomplicated and some complicated urinary tract infections, as well as bacterial prostatitis, skin and soft tissue infections, and bone and joint infections respond well to oral quinolone therapy [4,58–62]. Also, gastrointestinal infections, particularly infectious diarrhea caused by toxigenic *E. coli*, *Salmonella* (including typhoid and paratyphoid fevers, and the chronic *Salmonella* carrier state), *Shigella*, *Campylobacter*, *Aeromonas*, and *Vibrio* species, as well as *Plesiomonas shigelloides*, are highly responsive to oral quinolone therapy [4,58,63]. In addition, some sexually transmitted diseases (i.e., gonococcal, chlamydial, and chancroid infections) and pelvic infections can be cured with oral quinolone therapy [4,58,64]. Extensive clinical studies have provided substantial evidence of efficacy with some of the newer quinolones in these infectious diseases. However, it is important to emphasize that not all fluoroquinolones have been approved for use in all of the infections mentioned above. Unfortunately, physicians who use fluoroquinolones interchangeably (i.e., for unapproved indications) should realize there is no scientific evidence of efficacy unless the drug has been approved for use in a specific indication.

As an example, levofloxacin has not been approved for gastrointestinal infections; moxifloxacin and gatifloxacin have only been approved for respiratory infections such as acute bacterial exacerbations of chronic bronchitis, community-acquired pneumonia, and sinusitis. In contrast, clinical studies with trovafloxacin demonstrated excellent efficacy in intraabdominal infections, in some postoperative surgical abdominal infections, as well as certain obstetrical/gynecological infections, because of the antianaerobic (including *B. fragilis*) spectrum of this quinolone [65]. Also, trovafloxacin has been shown to be highly efficacious in the treatment of meningococcal meningitis. Thus, this is the first of the newest quinolones to demonstrate excellent penetration through the blood–brain barrier and clinical efficacy in a most serious infectious disease [66,67]. Unfortunately, the clinical use of trovafloxacin has been severely restricted in the United States and withdrawn from use in other countries because of rare but severe hepatotoxicity [68]. In addition, during the past decade we have accumulated much more clinical experience in the utility of the newer quinolones in the treatment and prevention of infections in immunocompromised patients [69].

Currently, respiratory infections (acute bacterial exacerbations of chronic bronchitis, community-acquired pneumonia, and sinusitis) appear to be the primary targets for clinical use of the most recently approved quinolones, moxifloxacin and gatifloxacin.

ADVERSE EVENTS

Toxicity with the early quinolones was low, usually appearing within the first 7 to 10 days of therapy and frequently noted within the first several days. In general, adverse reactions occur with similar frequencies in young and elderly patients [68,70]. However, CNS side effects may occur more commonly in elderly patients, except with trovafloxacin, which has a lower incidence of CNS side effects in patients aged 65 and older than in younger patients [68,70,71]. Also, adverse events for both oral and intravenous preparations of fluoroquinolones appear to increase with increasing dose and duration of therapy [68,70]. Compared with other commonly used antimicrobial agents, the fluoroquinolones can be considered relatively safe [4,21,68,70]. Gastrointestinal disturbances (anorexia, nausea, diarrhea, vomiting, dyspepsia, and abdominal discomfort) are the adverse reactions reported most frequently (2–11%). However, grepafloxacin had the highest rate (15.8%) of nausea [68]. Central nervous system (CNS) reactions (1–7%) may occur in the form of headache, dizziness, tiredness, vertigo, syncope, restlessness, insomnia, tinnitus, and sensory changes [4,21,68,70]. Severe neurotoxic reactions are rare (<0.5%) and include psychotic reactions, hallucinations, depression, and grand mal seizures, which are reversible with cessation of therapy. These direct CNS effects correlate roughly with quinolone binding at the $GABA_A$ receptors in the brain, blocking γ-aminobutyric acid (GABA), leading to CNS stimulation [4,21,68,70]. CNS side effects were the most common adverse events observed with ofloxacin and were higher than those reported with levofloxacin. Similarly, CNS side effects with grepafloxacin were higher with the 600-mg dose, and were also higher with sparfloxacin than with ciprofloxacin. CNS side effects were also the most common adverse event reported with trovafloxacin [68]. Hypersensitivity reactions are rare (0.4–2%) and include erythema, pruritus, urticaria, and rash. Equally rare are episodes of hypotension, tachycardia, nephrotoxic reactions (crystalluria) with elevated serum creatinine levels, thrombocytopenia, leukopenia, and anemia.

Moderate to severe phototoxicity, manifested by an exaggerated sunburn reaction, has been observed in patients exposed to direct sunlight while receiving some members of the quinolone class. Quinolones that accumulate in high concentrations in skin have a higher risk of producing phototoxicity, and are associated with fluorination at the C-8 position; it is predictably more common and potentially more severe with lomefloxacin, fleroxacin, and sparfloxacin [21,68,70]. Phototoxicity, in descending order, is much lower with grepafloxacin, ofloxacin, ciprofloxacin, and levofloxacin, and is lowest with trovafloxacin [68]. It has not been reported with moxifloxacin and gatifloxacin.

Quinolone-associated arthropathy is a potential adverse reaction in humans. Substantial experience with the use of quinolones in children indicates little evidence of quinolone-induced arthropathy in man [68,70,72,73]. Quinolones should be avoided during pregnancy and in nursing mothers because some quinolones are excreted into breast milk [74], and their safety has not been established.

Some fluoroquinolones show dose-dependent interactions with aluminum/ magnesium-containing antacids, so that simultaneous oral administration should be avoided. Interactions between some of the early fluoroquinolones and theophylline or caffeine have also been observed [68,70].

Hepatotoxicity. Transient elevations in liver enzymes have been observed rarely with the fluoroquinolones [4,68,70]. The most important hepatotoxicity data occurred in postmarketing surveillance of trovafloxacin. From February 1998 through May 1999, 2.6 million prescriptions were written for trovafloxacin, and 152 patients were reported to have a serious hepatic adverse event: a rare incidence rate of 0.00585. Of these 152 patients, 65 developed jaundice and 87 did not, which represents an incidence of 0.0025 in jaundiced patients. Also, 73 of these 152 patients had or were receiving other hepatotoxic drugs, and 61 of the 152 were known to have liver disease prior to receiving trovafloxacin. Furthermore, of the 65 patients who developed jaundice and/or liver failure, this finding was unrelated to trovafloxacin in 25 and possibly drug related in 40 (25 of these latter 40 patients had an uneventful recovery).

Hepatotoxicity was manifested in two different clinical patterns. Thirty-eight patients developed eosinophilia with eosinophilic infiltration of the liver, suggesting a hypersensitivity hepatitis that resolved in 29 (76%) patients with discontinuation of trovafloxacin. The second pattern was more of a direct hepatotoxic effect similar to isoniazid hepatotoxicity with centrolobular infiltration, sometimes with hepatic necrosis. Although the hepatic reactions occurred between 1 and 60 days after the start of therapy, the risk of serious hepatic injury appeared to increase with treatments of 14 days or longer. Overall, there were four patients who received a liver transplant (one of whom died from Gram-negative sepsis posttransplant) and five other deaths.

On careful review of these patients, only one patient had an unequivocal cause-and-effect relationship between trovafloxacin therapy and hepatic toxicity. This patient received a liver transplant and has had an uneventful recovery. As a result, trovafloxacin use in the United States has been limited to use in serious infections in hospitalized patients with careful monitoring of liver function tests. Trovafloxacin in other countries has been withdrawn from clinical use.

Minimal elevations in liver function tests have occurred in less than 1% of patients treated with moxifloxacin and gatifloxacin.

Cardiovascular Effects. Normal intraindividual variation in QTc intervals ranges from 15 to 70 msec. Because of this variation and differences in formulations and doses of agents used in clinical trials, large numbers of patients may need to be treated with a drug to definitively evaluate any QTc-prolonging effect. However, dose-related prolongation of the QTc interval was a new potential side effect of fluoroquinolones noted during clinical trials of sparfloxacin when a mean prolongation of 10 msec (less than 3% greater than normal) was observed in 1.3% of patients taking sparfloxacin and was related to the maximum peak concentration of sparfloxacin [68].

Prolongation of the QTc interval without significant arrhythmias was noted with grepafloxacin during premarketing clinical trials. Later, however, rare cases of significant arrhythmias including torsade de pointes were reported among the 2.65 million patients treated with grepafloxacin in the United States. This risk to patient safety led to voluntary withdrawal of grepafloxacin from clinical use in November 1999. The cardiovascular effects of moxifloxacin have been studied intensively because early clinical trials (400 mg per day) in patients with paired valid ECGs demonstrated a QTc prolongation of 6 ± 26 msec. Of note, QTc prolongations were also noted in comparator groups (clarithromycin, cephalexin, cefuroxime, and amoxicillin). Three moxifloxacin-treated patients (0.38%) and one patient on a comparator (0.13%) had a prolonged final QTc interval reading (i.e., >500 msec). No ventricular arrhythmias or cardiovascular events related to QTc interval prolongation were noted in any group during these trials. Postmarketing surveillance for moxifloxacin has revealed no episodes of torsade de pointes or clinically significant arrhythmias to date in over 1,000,000 treated patients.

Other drugs associated with prolongation of the QTc interval (e.g. erythromycin, clarithromycin, cisapride, and terfenadine) are metabolized by the cytochrome P450 enzyme system. Moxifloxacin is not primarily metabolized by the cytochrome P450 enzyme system and does not require dose adjustment for renal or liver impairment. Thus, the risk of QTc prolongation with moxifloxacin when administered concomitantly with medications hepatically eliminated should be low.

The potential for gatifloxacin-induced QTc prolongation has been studied in a small number (55) of human volunteers who had 76 paired valid ECGs. Abnormal QTc intervals (defined as greater than 450 msec) were observed in none of the patients, and the mean change in QTc interval was 2.9 ± 16.5 msec. Nevertheless, the Food and Drug Administration in the United States has added package insert warnings with levofloxacin, moxifloxacin, and gatifloxacin regarding potential QTc interval prolongation as a potential class effect of fluoroquinolones. Fluoroquinolones should not be administered concomitantly with class IA drugs that have class III properties (e.g., quinidine, procainamide) or class III (e.g., amiodarone, sotalol) antiarrhythmic agents.

The quinolones may interact to varying degrees with other drugs, including warfarin, H2 receptor antagonists, cyclosporine, rifampin, and nonsteroidal antiinflammatory drugs (NSAIDs). Concomitant administration of an NSAID with a quinolone may increase the risk of CNS stimulation and convulsive seizures.

Disturbances of blood glucose, including symptomatic hyper- and hypoglycemia, have been reported, usually in diabetic patients receiving concomitant treatment with an oral hypoglycemia agent or insulin. In these patients, careful monitoring of blood glucose is recommended, and the quinolone should be discontinued if a hypoglycemic reaction occurs [4,68,70].

QUINOLONES: FUTURE DEVELOPMENTS

Earlier reviews on the future of the quinolones described the potential for chemical modifications that might lead to improved quinolones, including (1) more potent derivatives, (2) less frequent selection of resistance, (3) better CNS/cerebrospinal fluid penetration, and (4) better patient tolerability [2–4]. These earlier reviews also suggested that future developments might provide compounds with greater activity against staphylococci, streptococci (particularly enterococci and S. pneumoniae), corynebacteria, Listeria, Chlamydia, Mycoplasma, Legionella, and anaerobes.

Future developments may also provide us with compounds that have greater activity against those organisms that are currently difficult to treat, such as mycobacteria, Pseudomonas, Stenotrophomonas, and Alcaligenes [2–4].

Some of the newest chemical modifications have accomplished many of the goals described earlier [2–4]. Currently available newer quinolones and some under development (1) are more potent, (2) are less susceptible to development of resistance, and (3) penetrate effectively into the CNS/cerebrospinal fluid. Also, current studies indicate that some of the newer fluoroquinolones (trovafloxacin, moxifloxacin, gatifloxacin, and gemifloxacin) have increased activity against staphylococci, including methicillin-resistant strains, as well as strains resistant to earlier quinolones, and against streptococci, particularly *S. pneumoniae* [4,29, 38,75–78], including strains of pneumococci that are penicillin resistant. Also, some of the newest quinolones are active against enterococci but unfortunately are not optimally active. Furthermore, during the past few years we have learned that many of the newer fluoroquinolones are not only active *in vitro*, but are also clinically effective against infections caused by *Mycoplasma pneumoniae, Chlamydia pneumoniae,* and *Legionella.* Of signal importance is the newest development that has resulted in excellent antianaerobic activity manifested *in vitro* and clinically by trovafloxacin, clinafloxacin, and moxifloxacin. Some of these newest agents also have activity against *Stenotrophomonas maltophilia* and other recalcitrant aerobic Gram-negative bacteria. This subject, that is, the *in-vitro* activity of the newer quinolones, is reviewed in detail by Phillips, King, and Shannon in this edition (Chapter 3).

Further developments may also provide newer quinolones with greater activity against new targets, such as the causative agents for malaria, Lyme disease, nocardiosis, toxoplasmosis, pneumocystosis [79], and leishmaniasis [80], DNA viruses, fungi, and quinolone-resistant bacteria. In addition, new compounds used alone or in combination with other agents may provide more effective killing or may lower the risk of developing bacterial resistance.

Another key potential for the quinolones would be to develop new compounds with higher specific affinity for the DNA of human malignant cells. Earlier studies evaluated the activity of some quinolone congeners against eukaryotic topoisomerase II [81–85]. Success in this area may require the development of effective agents that can be used either alone or in combination with other chemotherapeutic agents. However, the limiting factor may well be the toxicity of these compounds. Even so, the potential of developing quinolones to kill or interfere with the growth of human malignant cells, even if used in combination with other cancer chemotherapeutic agents, would provide sufficient economic and humane rewards to justify investment in their development.

CURRENT QUINOLONE STATUS AND CLASSIFICATION (see Tables I and II)

Many new fluoroquinolones have been synthesized during the past decade. Some offer important advantages over compounds developed earlier. Others will never

TABLE I   Current Quinolone Status

U.S. approved

Norfloxacin	1986
Ciprofloxacin	1987
Ofloxacin	1991
Temafloxacin[a]	1992
Enoxacin	1992
Lomefloxacin	1992
Sparfloxacin	1996
Levofloxacin	1996
Grepafloxacin[b]	1997
Trovafloxacin[c]	1997
Gatifloxacin	1999
Moxifloxacin	1999

Available outside the United States

Pefloxacin
Fleroxacin
Tosufloxacin

Under development

Gemifloxacin
Rufloxacin
Pazufloxacin
Clinafloxacin
Sitafloxacin
Prulifloxacin
Premafloxacin
Nadifloxacin
Balofloxacin
CFC-222
CS-940
HSR-903
CG-5501
DW-116
BMS-284756

[a]Withdrawn 1992.
[b]Withdrawn 1999.
[c]Restricted use in United States, 1999.

be available for clinical use. The currently available newer quinolones in clinical use within the United States and their dates of approval include norfloxacin (1986), ciprofloxacin (1987), ofloxacin (1991), enoxacin (1992), lomefloxacin (1992), sparfloxacin (1996), levofloxacin (1996), trovafloxacin (1997), gatiflox-acin (1999), and moxifloxacin (1999). Temafloxacin, approved in 1992, was withdrawn from clinical use in 1992 because of a hemolytic anemia–uremic

TABLE II   A Practical Microbiologic
Classification of Quinolones

Designed for ease of clinical selection

First generation
 Nalidixic acid
 Oxolinic acid
 Cinoxacin
 Piromidic acid
 Pipemidic acid
 Flumequine

Second generation
 Norfloxacin
 Ciprofloxacin[a]
 Enoxacin
 Fleroxacin
 Lomefloxacin
 Ofloxacin
 Levofloxacin
 Rufloxacin

Third generation[b]
 Sparfloxacin
 Tosufloxacin
 Gatifloxacin
 Pazufloxacin
 Grepafloxacin

Fourth generation[c]
 Trovafloxacin
 Clinafloxacin
 Sitafloxacin
 Moxifloxacin
 Gemifloxacin

[a]Most potent against *Pseudomonas*.
[b]More potent against *Pneumococcus* and anaerobes than earlier compounds were.
[c]Most potent against *Pneumococcus* and anaerobes.

syndrome in treated patients; and grepafloxacin, approved in 1997, was withdrawn in 1999 because of cardiac toxicity, that is, arrhythmias and torsade de pointes. The quinolones available outside the United States include pefloxacin, fleroxacin, and tosufloxacin. In addition, a number of newer quinolones are in various phases of clinical investigation. These include gemifloxacin, rufloxacin, pazufloxacin, clinafloxacin, and sitafloxacin (DU-6859a) [4,22,86]. Other quinolones in various stages of early development include prulifloxacin (PD-140288), premafloxacin, nadifloxacin, balofloxacin, CFC-222, CS-940, HSR-903, CG-5501, and DW-116 [4,22,87–89]. Of these, it is anticipated that gemifloxacin will soon be approved for clinical use in the United States.

A new subclass of quinolones is also under early investigation. Compounds in this subclass, which includes BMS-284756 (T-3811) [90], are desfluorinated, so that the fundamental C-6 fluorine is replaced, most often by an amino radical, which produces an aminoquinolone group of compounds [90]. Clearly, any list of new compounds is likely to be incomplete.

A practical microbiologic classification of the quinolones was first presented six years ago, at which time the quinolones were separated into generations (Table II) in a manner similar to the prior classification of cephalosporins by generation. There are a number of ways to categorize quinolones, for example, by their chemical structure, by their structure–activity relationships, by their specific *in-vitro* spectrum of antimicrobial activity, or by their clinical efficacy. Such classifications are clearly arbitrary. Thus, the classification that appears in Table II represents an update of the initial one presented six years ago. It is based on potency and the newest spectrum of antibacterial activity against "problem" bacterial organisms. This definition was selected because it is in keeping with the classification of cephalosporins into generations and is the most practical classification for clinical use. Different classifications based on chemical structure have been proffered by others [16,91]. Unfortunately, a uniform classification of the quinolones has not yet been agreed upon. Hopefully, one will be specifically defined in the near future.

CONCLUSION

This review has attempted to emphasize the importance of the fluoroquinolones in clinical medicine, and the advances already accomplished during the past decade. These advances have led to the introduction of new compounds that are innovative and have improved clinical applications. The molecular mechanism of action of these compounds may provide potential uses in clinical medicine in areas other than their role as antibacterial agents.

The newer fluoroquinolones that are currently available and those that are under development are categorized and classified by their current stage of development as well as their enhanced and broadened spectrum of antibacterial activity. The classification described herein categorizes the quinolones into *generations*, similar to the prior classification of cephalosporins by generations.

The data presented indicate that the quinolones have captured the interest of investigators and clinicians and that they may have the potential for use in clinical medicine other than their proven efficacy as antibacterial agents. However, even if the quinolones continue to be used only as antibacterial agents, their future role in clinical medicine is likely to be considerable.

REFERENCES

1. Neu, H. C. (1988). The quinolones: Prospects. In "The Quinolones" (V. T. Andriole, ed.), pp. 235–254. Academic Press, London.
2. Andriole, V. T. (1993). The future of the quinolones. *Drugs* **45** (Suppl. 3), 1–7.
3. Andriole, V. T. (1994). Future role and uses of the quinolones. In "Quinolones: The Present and the Future" (H. C. Neu, ed.), *Infect. Dis. Clin. Pract.* **3**, S211.
4. Andriole, V. T. (1999). The future of the quinolones. *Drugs* **58** (Suppl. 2), 1–5.
5. Lesher, G. Y., Froelich, E. J., Gruett, M. D., *et al.* (1962). Naphthyridine derivatives. A new class of chemotherapeutic agents. *J. Med. Pharmacol. Chem.* **5**, 1063.
6. Worcel, A. (1974). Studies on the folded chromosome of *E. coli*. In "Mechanism and Regulation of DNA Replication" (A. R. Kolber and M. Kohiyama, eds.), pp. 201–224, Plenum, New York and London.
7. Wang, J. C. (1974). Interactions between DNAs and enzymes: The effect of superhelical turns. *J. Mol. Biol.* **87**, 797.
8. Smith, J. T., and Lewin, C. S. (1988). Chemistry and mechanisms of action of the quinolone antibacterials. In "The Quinolones" (V. T. Andriole, ed.), pp. 23–81. Academic Press, London.
9. Crumplin, G. C., and Smith, J. T. (1976). Nalidixic acid and bacterial chromosome replication. *Nature* **260**, 643–645.
10. Smith, J. T. (1984). Awakening the slumbering potential of the 4-quinolone antibacterials. *Pharm. J.* **233**, 299.
11. Gellert, M., Mizuuchi, K., O'Dea, M. H., *et al.* (1976). DNA gyrase. *Proc. Natl. Acad. Sci. U.S.A.* **73**, 3872.
12. Gellert, M., Mizuuchi, K., O'Dea, M. H., *et al.* (1977). Nalidixic acid resistance: A second genetic character involved in DNA gyrase activity. *Proc. Natl. Acad. Sci. U.S.A.* **74**, 3872.
13. Sugino, A., Peebles, C. L., Krenzer, K. N., *et al.* (1977). Mechanism of action of nalidixic acid: Purification of *E. coli* Nal A gene production and its relationship to DNA gyrase and a novel nicking–closing enzyme. *Proc. Natl. Acad. Sci. U.S.A.* **74**, 4767.
14. Higgins, N. P., Peebles, C. L., Sugino, A., *et al.* (1978). Purification of subunits of *Escherichia coli*, DNA gyrase and reconstitution of enzymic activity. *Proc. Natl. Acad. Sci. U.S.A.* **75**, 1773.
15. Pedrini, A. (1979). Nalidixic acid. In "Antibiotics" (F. E. Hahn, ed.), Vol. 5. Springer-Verlag, Berlin.
16. Gootz, T. D., and Brighty, K. E. (1998). Chemistry and mechanism of action of the quinolone antibacterials. In "The Quinolones," 2nd ed. (V.T. Andriole, ed.), pp. 29–80. Academic Press, San Diego.
17. Wang, J. C. (1985). DNA topoisomerases. *Annu. Rev. Biochem.* **54**, 665.
18. Crumplin, G. C., and Smith, J. T. (1975). Nalidixic acid: An anti-bacterial paradox. *Antimicrob. Agents Chemother.* **8**, 251.

19. Andriole, V. T. (1992). Quinolones. In "Infectious Diseases" (S. Gorbach, ed.), pp. 244–253. Saunders, Philadelphia.

20. Neu, H. C. (1992). Quinolone antimicrobial agents. *Annu. Rev. Med.* **43**, 465–486.

21. Domagala, J. M. (1994). Structure–activity and structure–side-effect relationships for the quinolone antibacterials. *J. Antimicrob. Chemother.* **33**, 685–706.

22. Gootz, T. D., and Brighty, K. E. (1996). Fluoroquinolone antibacterials: SAR, mechanism of action, resistance, and clinical aspects. *Med. Res. Rev.* **16**, 433–486.

23. Zhao, X., Xu, C., Domaglia, J., *et al.* (1997). DNA topoisomerase targets of the fluoroquinolones: A strategy for avoiding bacterial resistance. *Proc. Natl. Acad. Sci. U.S.A.* **94**, 13991–13996.

24. Phillips, I., King, A., and Shannon, K. (1988). *In vitro* properties of the quinolones. In "The Quinolones" (V. T. Andriole, ed.), pp. 83–118. Academic Press, London.

25. Phillips, I., King, A., and Shannon, K. (1998). *In vitro* properties of the quinolones. In "The Quinolones" (V. T. Andriole, ed.), pp. 81–116. Academic Press, San Diego.

26. Aldridge, K. E., and Ashcraft, D. S. (1997). Comparison of the *in vitro* activities of BAY 12-8039, a new quinolone, and other antimicrobials against clinically important anaerobes. *Antimicrob. Agents Chemother.* **41**, 709–711.

27. Applebaum, P. C. (1995). Quinolone activity against anaerobes: Microbiological aspects. *Drugs* **49** (Suppl. 2), 76–80.

28. Aldridge, K. E., Ashcraft, D., and Bowman, K. A. (1997). Comparative *in vitro* activities of trovafloxacin (CP-99,219) and other antimicrobials against clinically significant anaerobes. *Antimicrob. Agents Chemother.* **41**, 484–487.

29. Hecht, D. W., and Wexler, H. M. (1996). *In vitro* susceptibility of anaerobes to quinolones in the United States. *Clin. Infect. Dis.* **23** (Suppl. 1), S2–S8.

30. Goldstein, E. J. C. (2000). Review of the *in vitro* activity of gemifloxacin against Gram-positive and Gram-negative anaerobic pathogens. *J. Antimicrob. Chemother.* **45** (Suppl. S1), 55–65.

31. Ackermann, G., Schaumann, R., Pless, B., *et al.* (2000). Comparative activity of moxifloxacin *in vitro* against obligately anaerobic bacteria. *Eur. J. Clin. Microbiol. Infect. Dis.* **19**, 228–232.

32. Andriole, V. T. (1998). The quinolones: Prospects. In "The Quinolones" (V. T. Andriole, ed.), pp. 417–429. Academic Press, San Diego.

33. Tanaka, M., Ishii, H., Sato, K., Osada, Y., and Nishino, T. (1991). Characterization of high-level quinolone resistance in methicillin-resistant *Staphylococcus aureus*. *Abstr. 31st Intersci. Conf. Antimicrob. Agents Chemother.*, Chicago. p. 233.

34. Aoyama, H., Fujimaki, K., Sato, K., Tadashi, F., Inoue, M., *et al.* (1988). Clinical isolate of *Citrobacter freundii* highly resistant to new quinolones. *Antimicrob. Agents Chemother.* **32**, 922–924.

35. Inoue, S., Ohue, T., and Yamagishi, J. (1978). Mode of incomplete cross-resistance among pipemidic, piromidic, and nalidixic acid. *Antimicrob. Agents Chemother.* **14**, 240.

36. Yamagishi, J., Yoshida, H., and Yamayoshi, M. (1986). Nalidixic acid resistant mutations of the *gyrB* gene of *Escherichia coli*. *Mol. Gen. Genet.* **204**, 367.

37. Nikaido, H., and Thanassi, D. G. (1993). Penetration of lipophilic agents with multiple protonation sites into bacterial cells: Tetracyclines and fluoroquinolones as examples. *Antimicrob. Agents Chemother.* **37**, 1393–1399.

38. Kitamura, A., Hoshino, K., Kimura, Y., Jayakawa, I., and Sato, K. (1995). Contribution of the C-8 substituent of DU-6859a, a new potent fluoroquinolone, to its activity against DNA gyrase mutants of *Pseudomonas aeruginosa*. *Antimicrob. Agents Chemother.* **39**, 1467–1471.

39. Hosaka, M., Kinoshita, S., Toyama, A., Otsuki, M., and Nishino, T. (1995). Antibacterial properties of AM-1155, a new 8-methoxy quinolone. *J. Antimicrob. Chemother.* **36**, 293–301.

40. Ito, T., Matsumoto, M., and Nishino, T. (1995). Improved bactericidal activity of Q-35 against quinolone-resistant staphylococci. *Antimicrob. Agents Chemother.* **39**, 1522–1525.

41. Kitani, H., Kuroda, T., Moriguchi, A., Ao, H., Hirayama, F., Ikeda, Y., and Kawakita, T. (1997). Synthesis and structural optimization of 7-3(3,3-disubstituted-1-pyrrolidinyl)-1-cyclopropyl-6-fluoro-1,4-dihydro-8-methoxy-4-oxo-3-quinoline carboxylic acids as antibacterial agents. *Bioorg. Med. Chem. Lett.* **7**, 515–520.

42. Maejima, T., Senda, H., Iwatani, W., Tatsumi, Y., Arika, T., Fukui, H., Shibata, T., Nakano, J., and Naito, T. (1995). Potent antibacterial activity of S-32730, a new fluoroquinolone against gram-positive bacteria including quinolone-resistant MRSA. *Abstr. 35th Intersci. Conf. Antimicrob. Agents Chemother.*, San Francisco. Abstr. #F189.

43. Taba, H., and Kusano, N. (1998). Sparfloxacin resistance in clinical isolates of *Streptococcus pneumoniae*: Involvement of multiple mutations in *gyrA* and *parC* genes. *Antimicrob. Agents Chemother.* **42**, 2193–2196.

44. Bebear, C. M., Renaudin, H., Charron, A., *et al.* (1998). Alterations in topoisomerase IV and DNA gyrase in quinolone-resistant mutants of *Mycoplasma hominis* obtained *in vitro. Antimicrob. Agents Chemother.* **42**, 2304–2311.

45. Gonzalez, I., Georgious, M., Alcaide, F., *et al.* (1998). Fluoroquinolone resistance mutations in the *parC, parE* and *gyrA* genes of clinical isolates of viridans group streptococci. *Antimicrob. Agents Chemother.* **41**, 2792–2798.

46. Pan, X. S., and Fisher, L. M. (1998). DNA gyrase and topoisomerase IV are dual targets of clinafloxacin action in *Streptococcus pneumoniae. Antimicrob. Agents Chemother.* **42**, 2810–2816.

47. Piddock, L. J. V., Johnson, M., Ricci, V., *et al.* (1998). Activities of new fluoroquinolones against fluoroquinolone-resistant pathogens of the lower respiratory tract. *Antimicrob. Agents Chemother.* **42**, 2956–2960.

48. Dong, Y., Xu, C., Zhao, X., *et al.* (1998). Fluoroquinolone action against mycobacteria: Effects of C08 substituents on growth, survival and resistance. *Antimicrob. Agents Chemother.* **42**, 2978–2984.

49. Tanaka, M., Onodera, Y., Uchida, Y., *et al.* (1998). Quinolone resistance mutations in the GrlB protein of *Staphylococcus aureus. Antimicrob. Agents* **Chemother. 42**, 3044–3046.

50. Alovero, F. L., Pan, X. S., Morris, J. E., *et al.* (2000). Engineering the specificity of antibacterial fluoroquinolones: Benzenesulfonamide modifications at C-7 of ciprofloxacin change its primary target in *Streptococcus pneumoniae* from topoisomerase IV to gyrase. *Antimicrob. Agents Chemother.* **44**, 320–325.

51. Jones, M. E., Sahm, D. F., Martin, N., *et al.* (2000). Prevalence of *gyrA, gyrB, parC,* and *parE* mutations in clinical isolates of *Streptococcus pneumoniae* with decreased susceptibilities to different fluoroquinolones and originating from worldwide surveillance studies during the 1997–1998 respiratory season. *Antimicrob. Agents Chemother.* **44**, 462–466.

52. Morrissey, I., and George, J. T. (2000). Purification of pneumococcal type II topoisomerase and inhibition by gemifloxacin and other quinolones. *J. Antimicrob. Chemother.* **45** (Suppl. A), 101–106.

53. Chen, D. K., McGeer, A., De Azavedo, J. C., *et al.* (1999). Decreased susceptibility of *Streptococcus pneumoniae* to fluoroquinolones in Canada. *New Engl. J. Med.* **341**, 233–239.

54. Oethinger, M., Kern, W., Jellen-Ritter, A. S., *et al.* (2000). Ineffectiveness of topoisomerase mutations in mediating clinically significant fluoroquinolone resistance in *E. coli* in the absence of the AcrAB efflux pump. *Antimicrob. Agents Chemother.* **44**, 10–13.

55. Bergan, T. (1998). Pharmacokinetics of the fluoroquinolones. In "The Quinolones" (V. T. Andriole, ed.), pp. 144–182. Academic Press, San Diego.

56. Imada, T., Miyazaki, S., Nishida, M., Yamaguchi, K., and Goto, S. (1992). *In vitro* and *in vivo* antibacterial activities of a new quinolone, OPC-17116. *Antimicrob. Agents Chemother.* **36**, 573–579.

57. Kimura, Y., Atarashi, S., Kawakami, K., Sato, K., and Hayakawa, I. (1994). (Fluorocyclopropyl) quinolones, 2: Synthesis and stereochemical structure–activity relationships of chiral 7-(7-amino-5-azaspiro[2.4]heptan-5-yl)-1-(2-fluorocyclopropyl) quinolone antibacterial agents. *J. Med. Chem.* **37**, 3344–3352.

58. Andriole, V. T. (1988). Clinical overview of the newer 4-quinolone antibacterial agents. In "The Quinolones" (V. T. Andriole, ed.), pp. 155–200. Academic Press, London.

59. Andriole, V. T. (1996). Quinolones. In "Current Infectious Disease Drugs" (V. T. Andriole, ed.), pp. 148–163. Current Medicine, Philadelphia.

60. Niederman, M. (1998). Treatment of respiratory infections with quinolones. In "The Quinolones" (V. T. Andriole, ed.), pp. 229–250. Academic Press, San Diego.

61. Nicolle, L. E. (1998). Use of quinolones in urinary tract infection and prostatitis. In "The Quinolones" (V. T. Andriole, ed.), pp. 183–202. Academic Press, San Diego.

62. Karchmer, A. W. (1998). Use of the quinolones in skin and skin structure (osteomyelitis) and other infections. In "The Quinolones" (V. T. Andriole, ed.), pp. 327–349. Academic Press, San Diego.

63. Hamer, D. H., and Gorbach, S. L. (1998). Use of the quinolones for the treatment and prophylaxis of bacterial gastrointestinal infections. In "The Quinolones" (V. T. Andriole, ed.), pp. 267–285. Academic Press, San Diego.

64. DiCarlo, R. P. and Martin, D. H. (1998). Use of the quinolones in sexually transmitted diseases. In "The Quinolones" (V. T. Andriole, ed.), pp. 203–227. Academic Press, San Diego.

65. Faro, S. and Weigelt, J. (1998). Use of quinolones in surgery and obstetrics and gynecology. In "The Quinolones" (V. T. Andriole, ed.), pp. 251–266. Academic Press, San Diego.

66. Hopkins, S., Williams, D., Dunne, M., *et al.* (1996). A randomized controlled trial of oral or intravenous trovafloxacin vs. ceftriaxone in the treatment of epidemic meningococcal meningitis. *Abstr. 36th Intersci. Conf. Antimicrob. Agents Chemother.*, New Orleans. *Late Breaker* **21**, 5.

67. Hasbun, R. and Quagliarello, V. J. (1998). Use of the quinolones in treatment of bacterial meningitis. In "The Quinolones" (V. T. Andriole, ed.), pp. 287–301. Academic Press, San Diego.

68. Dembry, L. M., Farrington, J. M. and Andriole, V. T. (1999). Fluoroquinolone antibiotics: Adverse effects and safety profiles. *Infect. Dis. Clin. Pract.* **8**, 9–16.

69. Rolston, K. V. I. (1998). Use of the quinolones in immunocompromised patients. In "The Quinolones" (V. T. Andriole, ed.), pp. 303–326. Academic Press, San Diego.

70. Stahlmann, R., and Lode, H. (1988). Safety overview: Toxicity, adverse effects and drug interactions. In "The Quinolones" (V. T. Andriole, ed.), pp. 201–233. Academic Press, London.

71. Williams, D. J., and Hopkins, S. (1998). Safety and tolerability of intravenous to oral treatment and single-dose intravenous or oral prophylaxis with trovafloxacin. *Am. J. Surg.* **176** (Suppl. 6A), S74–S79.

72. Adam, D. (1989). Use of quinolones in pediatric patients. *Rev. Infect. Dis.* **11** (Suppl. 5), 1113–1116.

73. Church, D. A., and Echols, R. M. (1997). Ciprofloxacin use in pediatric and cystic fibrosis patients: Proceedings of a symposium. *Pediatr. Infect. Dis. J.* **16**, 89–162.

74. Giamarellou, H., Kilokythas, E., Petrikkos, G., *et al.* (1989). Pharmacokinetics of three newer quinolones in pregnant and lactating women. *Am. J. Med.* **87** (Suppl. 5A), 49–51.

75. Cunha, B. A., Hussain Qadri, S. M., Ueno, Y., Walters, E. A., and Domenico, P. (1997). Antibacterial activity of trovafloxacin against nosocomial Gram-positive and Gram-negative isolates. *J. Antimicrob. Chemother.* **39** (Suppl. B), 29–34.

76. Felmingham, D., Robbins, M. J., Ingley, K., Mathias, I., *et al.* (1997). *In vitro* activity of trovafloxacin, a new fluoroquinolone, against recent clinical isolates. *J. Antimicrob. Chemother.* **39** (Suppl. B), 43–50.

77. Klugman, K. P., and Gootz, T. D. (1997). *In vitro* and *in vivo* activity of trovafloxacin against *Streptococcus pneumoniae.* *J. Antimicrob. Chemother.* **39** (Suppl. B), 51–56.

78. Sefton, A. M., Maskeell, J. P., Rafay, A. M., Whiley, A., and Williams, J. D. (1997). The *in vitro* activity of trovafloxacin, a new fluoroquinolone, against Gram-positive bacteria. *J. Antimicrob. Chemother.* **39** (Suppl. B), 57–62.

79. Bartlett, M. S., Queener, S. F., Tidwell, R. R., *et al.* (1991). 8-aminoquinolines from Walter Reed Army Institute for research for treatment and prophylaxis of *Pneumocystis* pneumonia in rat models. *Antimicrob. Agents Chemother.* **35**, 277–282.

80. Fornet, A., Barriios, A. A., Munoz, V., *et al.* (1993). 2-substituted quinoline alkaloids as potential antileishmanial drugs. *Antimicrob. Agents Chemother.* **37**, 859–863.

81. Kohlbrenner, W. E., Wideburg, N., Weigl, D., Saldivar, A., and Chu, D. T. W. (1992). Induction of calf thymus topoisomerase II-mediated DNA breakage by the antibacterial isothiazoloquinolones A-65281 and A-65282. *Antimicrob. Agents Chemother.* **36**, 81–86.

82. Robinson, M. J., Martin, B. A., Gootz, T. D., *et al.* (1991). Effects of quinolone derivatives on eukaryotic topoisomerase II: A novel mechanism for enhancement of enzyme-mediated DNA cleavage. *J. Biol. Chem.* **266**, 14585–14592.

83. Robinson, M. J., Martin, B. A., Gootz, T. D., McGuirk, P. R., and Osheroff, N. (1992). Effects of novel fluoroquinolones on the catalytic activities of eukaryotic topoisomerase II: Influence of the C-8 fluorine group. *Antimicrob. Agents Chemother.* **36**, 751–756.

84. Yamashita, Y., Ashizawa, T., Morimoto, M., Hosomi, J., and Nakano, H. (1992). Antitumor quinolones with mammalian topoisomerase II mediated DNA cleavage activity. *Cancer Res.* **52**, 2818–2822.

85. Froelich-Ammon, S. J., McGuirk, P. R., Gootz, T. D., Jefson, M., and Osheroff, N. (1993). Novel 1–8 bridged chiral quinolones with activity against topoisomerase II: Stereospecificity of the eukaryotic enzyme. *Antimicrob. Agents Chemother.* **37**, 646–651.

86. Appelbaum, P., Ball, A. P., Logan, M. N., and Wood, M. J. (Eds.) (2000). Gemifloxacin: Potency and performance. *J. Antimicrob. Chemother.* **45** (Suppl. S1), 1–110.

87. Kim, J. H., Kang, J. A., Kim, Y. G., *et al.* (1997). *In vitro* and *in vivo* antibacterial efficacies of CFC-222, a new fluoroquinolone. *Antimicrob. Agents Chemother.* **41**, 2209–2213.

88. Miyazaki, S., Domon, H., Tateda, K, *et al.* (1997). *In vitro* and *in vivo* anitbacterial activities of CS-940, a new fluoroquinolone, against isolates from patients with respiratory infections. *Antimicrob. Agents Chemother.* **41**, 2582–2585.

89. Meyerhoff, C., Dilger, C., Yoon, S. J., *et al.* (1998). Safety, tolerability and pharmacokinetics of the new long-acting quinolone DW-116 after single and multiple dosing in healthy subjects. *Antimicrob. Agents Chemother.* **42**, 349–361.

90. Carbone, M., Fera, M. T., Cecchetti, V., *et al.* (1997). *In vitro* activities of new quinolones against *Helicobacter pylori.* *Antimicrob. Agents Chemother.* **41**, 2790–2792.

91. Ball, P. (1998). The quinolones: History and overview. In "The Quinolones" (V. T. Andriole, ed.), pp. 1–28. Academic Press, San Diego.

Index